Comprehensive Psychiatric Nursing

Comprehensive Psychiatric Nursing

Judith Haber,
R.N., M.A.

Instructor of Psychiatric Mental Health Nursing
Norwalk Community College

Anita M. Leach,
R.N., M.A.

Psychiatric Nurse Co-ordinator
Danbury Hospital

Sylvia M. Schudy,
R.N., M.A.

Director of Nursing Education
Norwalk Community College

Barbara Flynn
Sideleau,
R.N., M.S.N.

Assistant Professor of Nursing
Fairfield University

McGraw-Hill Book Company A Blakiston Publication

New York / St. Louis / San Francisco / Auckland
Bogotá / Düsseldorf / Johannesburg / London / Madrid
Mexico / Montreal / New Delhi / Panama / Paris
São Paulo / Singapore / Sydney / Tokyo / Toronto

Notice

Medicine is an ever-changing science. As new research and clinical experience broaden our knowledge, changes in treatment and drug therapy are required. The editors and the publisher of this work have made every effort to ensure that the drug dosage schedules herein are accurate and in accord with the standards accepted at the time of publication. Readers are advised, however, to check the product information sheet included in the package of each drug they plan to administer to be certain that changes have not been made in the recommended dose or in the contraindications for administration. This recommendation is of particular importance in regard to new or infrequently used drugs.

Comprehensive Psychiatric Nursing

4567890DODO7832109

This book was set in Helvetica Light by Black Dot, Inc. The editors were Mary Ann Richter and Henry C. De Leo; the designer was J. Paul Kirouac, A Good Thing, Inc.; the production supervisor was Angela Kardovich. The part-opening drawings were done by Henry C. De Leo, and all other drawings were done by J & R Services, Inc.
R. R. Donnelley & Sons Company was printer and binder.

Library of Congress Cataloging in Publication Data
Main entry under title:

Comprehensive psychiatric nursing.

    "A Blakiston publication."
    Bibliography: p.
    Includes Index.
    1. Psychiatric nursing. I. Haber, Judith. [DNLM: 1. Community mental health services.
2. Psychiatric nursing. WY160 C737]
RC440.C58   610.73'68   77-23375
ISBN 0-07-025384-6

To Our Significant Others

Contents

Lists of Contributors

Judith Ackerhalt, R.N., B.S., M.S.

Assistant Professor, Graduate Mental
Health-Psychiatric Nursing Program
Adelphi University School of Nursing
Garden City, Long Island, New York

Ann Bello, R.N., B.S., M.A.

Instructor, Nursing
Norwalk Community College
Norwalk, Connecticut

Mary Ann Bohner, R.N., B.S.

Clinical Staff Nurse
Memorial Sloan Kettering Cancer Center
New York, New York

June N. Brodie, R.N., B.S., M.S., Ph.D.

Director, Graduate Program
Department of Nursing
Herbert H. Lehman College of the
City University of New York

Katharine J. Burns, R.N., B.S., M.A.

Herbert H. Lehman College
Bronx, New York
Private Practice, New York City

Margaret A. Colliton, R.N., B.S.N., M.S.N., D.Sc.N.

Private Practice and Consultation
New Haven, Connecticut

Judith Gregorie D'Afflitti, R.N., B.S., M.S.

Clinical Instructor, Department of Psychiatry,
Yale University Lecturer,
Department of Psychology
Quinnipiac College
Hamden, Connecticut

Donna Kaye Diers, R.N., B.N.S., M.S.N.

Dean and Associate Professor
Yale School of Nursing
New Haven, Connecticut

Hope Fox, R.N., B.S., M.A.

Assistant Professor of Nursing
Molloy College
Rockville Centre, New York
Psychotherapist, Private Practice

Karen Davis Frank, R.N., B.S., M.A.

Clinical Specialist, Pediatric Service
Psychiatric–Mental Health Nursing
Elizabeth General Hospital and Dispensary
Elizabeth, New Jersey

Jane N. Gorman, R.N., B.A., B.S.N., M.S., D.N.S.

Assistant Clinical Professor
Department of Mental Health and Community
Nursing, School of Nursing
University of California
San Francisco, California

M. Leah Gorman, R.N., B.S., M.A., Ed.D.

Acting Chief, Psychiatric Nursing Education
Branch, Division Manpower Training Programs
National Institute of Mental Health
Rockville, Maryland

Loretta Kawalec Guise, R.N., B.S., M.S.

Psychiatric Nurse-Clinician
Alcoholism Rehabilitation Unit
Veterans Administration Hospital
West Haven, Connecticut

Judith Haber, R.N., B.S., M.A.

Instructor, Psychiatric–Mental Health Nursing
Norwalk Community College
Norwalk, Connecticut
Clinical Specialist in Psychiatric-
Mental Health Nursing

Eugenia McAuliffe Kelly, R.N., B.S., M.A.

Assistant Director of Psychiatric Nursing
Psychiatric Nursing Consultant
Consultation/Liaison Service
Coney Island Hospital/Affiliate Maimonides
Medical Center, Department of Psychiatry
Brooklyn, New York

Mary Jane Kennedy, R.N., B.S.N.E., M.A., M.S.N.

Director of Nursing
Yale University Health Services
New Haven, Connecticut

Judith Belliveau Krauss, R.N., B.S.N., M.S.N.

Assistant Dean
Yale School of Nursing
New Haven, Connecticut

Anita M. Leach, R.N., B.S., M.A.

Psychiatric Nurse Co-ordinator
Danbury Hospital
Danbury, Connecticut

Suzanne Lego, R.N., B.S.N., M.S., Ph.D.

Psychotherapist and Psychoanalyst,
Private Practice
New York City and Demarest, New Jersey

Nada Light, R.N., B.S., M.A.

Associate Professor
Graduate Program in Child Psychiatric Nursing
Columbia University School of Nursing
New York, New York

Elizabeth M. Maloney, R.N., B.S., M.A., Ed.D.

Associate Professor
Department of Nursing Education
Teachers' College, Columbia University
New York, New York

Roberta Mattheis, R.N., B.S.N., M.S.N.

Chairman, Parent Education
Mercer Island Preschool Association
Mercer Island, Washington

Lenora J. McClean, R.N., B.S.N., M.A., Ed.D.

Assistant Dean
Educational Programs and Development
School of Nursing
Health Sciences Center
State University of New York at Stony Brook
Stony Brook, New York

Judith Meyer, R.N., B.S.N., M.A.

Nursing Care Coordinator in Psychiatry
Veterans Administration Hospital of Manhattan
New York, New York

Thomas Francis Nolan, R.N., M.A.

Instructor, Nursing
The City College of New York
New York, New York

Alice Marie Obrig, R.N., B.S., M.S., M.P.H.

Certified Nurse-Midwife
Assistant Professor, Nursing
Fairfield University
Fairfield, Connecticut

Phyllis E. Porter, R.N., M.S., Ed.D.

Dean, School of Nursing
Fairfield University
Fairfield, Connecticut

Pamela A. Price, R.N., B.S.N., M.A., Ph.D.

Assistant Professor, Division of Nursing
New York University
New York, New York

Mary T. Ramshorn, R.N., B.S.N., Ed.M., Ed.D.

Associate Professor and Project Director,
Graduate Program
Mental Health–Psychiatric Nursing
Teachers' College, Columbia University
New York, New York

Lillie Ann Reed, R.N., B.A., M.A.

Assistant Professor
Maternal and Child Health
Brookdale Community College
Lincroft, New Jersey

Janice E. Ruffin, R.N., B.S., M.S.

Director of Nursing, Connecticut Mental Health
Center, New Haven, Connecticut
Associate Professor, Graduate Program in
Psychiatric Nursing, Yale University
School of Nursing
New Haven, Connecticut

Sylvia M. Schudy, R.N., B.S., M.A.

Director of Nursing Education
Norwalk Community College
Norwalk, Connecticut

Sylvia Theresa Schwartzman, R.N., B.S.N., M.S.

Staff Development Instructor
Rochester Psychiatric Center
Rochester, New York

Margretta Reed Seashore, M.D.

Assistant Clinical Professor
Pediatrics and Human Genetics
Yale University School of Medicine
New Haven, Connecticut

Barbara Flynn Sideleau, R.N., B.S.N., M.S.N.

Assistant Professor, Fairfield University
Fairfield, Connecticut
Clincial Specialist in Psychiatric–
Mental Health Nursing

Ardis R. Swanson, R.N., B.S., M.Ed., M.S., Ph.D.

Assistant Professor, Division of Nursing
New York University
New York, New York

Mary Teague, R.N., B.S.N., M.S.N.

Director of Psychiatric Nursing Services
St. Vincent's Medical Center
Bridgeport, Connecticut

Patricia Winstead-Fry, R.N., B.S., M.A., Ph.D.

Assistant Professor of Nursing
New York University, Division of Nursing
New York, New York
Therapist: Lincoln Institute for Psychotherapy
Psychotherapist, Private Practice

Laura Coble Zamora, R.N., B.S., M.A.

Assistant Professor, College of Nursing
Downstate Medical Center
State University of New York
Brooklyn, New York

Preface

Rapid, progressive, and dynamic advances in the areas of mental health legislation, treatment modalities, delivery of health care services, and in the role and responsibilities of psychiatric mental health nurses have created a demand for a current and comprehensive psychiatric nursing textbook. These advances, along with the strong belief that nurses are essential tools in therapeutic intervention with clients and that clients and nurses are constantly responding to each other, led to the conception of this project by Anita Leach. The editorial group was chosen to reflect the levels of basic nursing education and nursing service. The combined philosophies and equal efforts of this group have brought about the fruition and publication of this text.

The text reflects our belief that comprehensive psychiatric nursing care is derived from an understanding of individuals as unified wholes: that the life process is a reciprocal interaction between people and their environment; that mental health is the ability to cope effectively with the life process, while mental illness is maladaptive to this process. We also believe that the nurse's response to client behavior is a vital component in the delivery of care: that self-awareness and analysis of the mutual interaction between the client and the nurse are essential to the therapeutic process; and that application of the nursing process in the care of clients must be based on an understanding of the individual, family, and society.

Existing texts separately deal with mental illness, theoretical frameworks, and nursing care of the mentally ill; no existing source however takes a comprehensive approach. This book utilizes psychiatric mental health nursing principles to formulate an integrated approach to client care across the age span and in a variety of settings.

Issues related to both health and illness are discussed along with contemporary classical theories essential to the delivery of quality nursing care. The intention is to prepare basic nursing students to utilize principles of primary, secondary, and tertiary prevention in the delivery of health care. A knowledge base is provided and the skills needed for optimal treatment of clients with psychological, social, or biological dysfunction are identified. This text will also be useful as a resource volume for practitioners and educators already involved in professional practice.

This book is divided into six parts. Part 1 presents the conceptual framework of the book, the historical and socio-cultural aspects of mental health, and epidemiological data. It also includes theoretical models and their application to nursing practice, the exploration of personality development within the framework of crisis theory, and a theoretical examination of the nurse–client relationship.

Part 2 introduces the nursing process and presents the diverse therapeutic modalities encountered by nurses in treatment settings.

Part 3 focuses on problematic client behaviors and the responses they generate in nurses. The psycho-dynamics of these behaviors are explored, and the nursing process is used as a framework for client care.

Part 4 deals with data essential to nurses intervening with clients outside psychiatric settings. Concepts relating to health, the impact of illness and hospitalization, stress, psychophysiological disorders, the rehabilitative process, dependency on technology and life support systems, the dying process, and organic brain syndrome are explored.

Promotion of mental health within the family system is examined in Part 5. Primary prevention, the theories and principles relating to the normal family system within the childbearing cycle, is included. Secondary prevention, the assessment and early identification of emotional dysfunction in children, is examined in terms of deviation from the norm. Tertiary prevention, which meets the therapeutic needs of emotionally disturbed children and adolescents, high-risk children, and the dying child, is discussed in terms of family interaction and the nursing process.

Part 6 looks at the future of psychiatric mental health nursing practice in terms of research, legislation, education, and private practice.

The editors and contributors have attempted to provide a humanistic approach to the problems of clients and their families. They have attended to nurses and the difficulties they encounter in providing sensitive, individualized care.

The editors believe that this volume reflects their committment and that of the contributors to high-quality psychiatric mental health nursing practice. This book would not have been possible without the contributions of the many authors whose expertise has been invaluable in formulating a comprehensive textbook.

Acknowledgments

We wish to acknowledge the loving support, nurturance, and patience, of our families and friends who contributed to our continuing mental health during the many months involved in the preparation of this project. Our families: Lenny, Laurie, and Andrew Haber; the Leach family, especially Peg and Bill; George, George Jr., Cynthia, and John Schudy; Bob, Greg, Michelle, Brian, and Robert Sideleau; and Rose Flynn. Thanks also go to our supportive friends and colleagues too numerous to mention by name, and to our faithful and energetic secretaries: Rosemarie Civitella, Susan Coyne, Charlotte Folkl, Kappy McCarney, and Alice Weindorf.

Judith Haber, Anita M. Leach,
Sylvia M. Schudy, and Barbara Flynn Sideleau

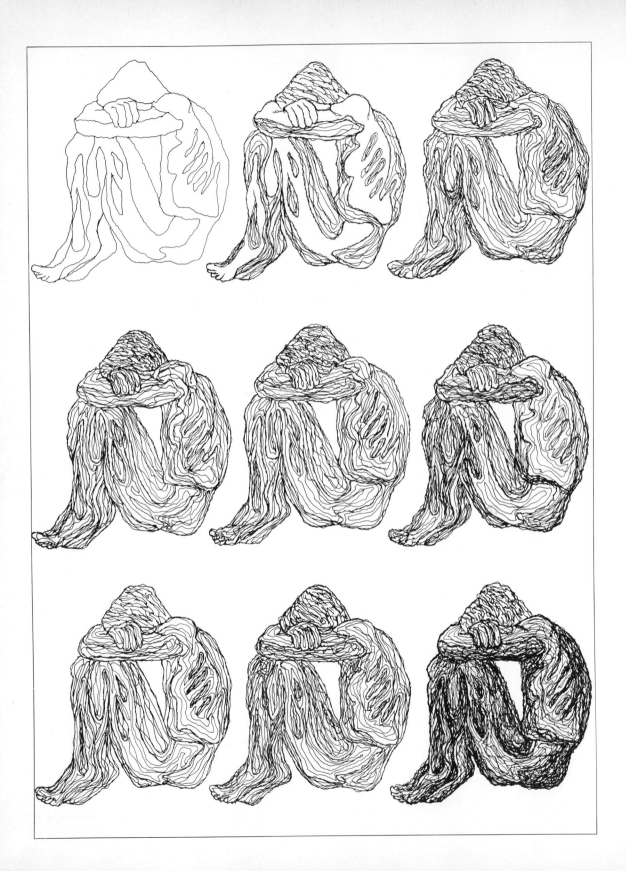

One

Theoretical Matrix

1

Conceptual Framework of Psychiatric Nursing Practice

Sylvia M. Schudy

Learning Objectives

After studying this chapter, the student should be able to:

1 Understand the conceptual framework utilized in the book
2 Define Rogers's theory of man and the principles of reciprocy, synchrony, helicy, and resonancy
3 Define Maslow's theory of motivation by describing the six basic human needs
4 Define psychiatric nursing practice
5 Know means of implementing the conceptual framework (nursing process, therapeutic use of self, self-awareness, and the nurse-client relationship).

Conceptual Framework

A conceptual framework is a set of ideas, theories, or themes, concerning a particular subject. To use a conceptual framework is to operationalize theory in the practice setting. Newman defines the conceptual framework as a system or package of ideas from which general or explanatory and predictive principles can be formulated.[1] It involves a way of thinking, conceptualizing, and intellectualizing the knowledge through which nursing grows and develops.

Nursing theory is a synthesis of theories and concepts from the natural, behavioral, and humanistic sciences which must be identified and organized, through research, into a science of nursing.[2] Nursing is also viewed as a practice discipline, and nursing knowledge can best be acquired through a systematic study of nursing practice. Both points of view are relevant, since the theory of a discipline provides the basis for its development, practice, and research.

To cope with ever-increasing knowledge and change, a conceptual framework is needed. It identifies and defines relevant theories and concepts which are an essential part of the science and art of psychiatric–mental health nursing today.

The framework of this book identifies concepts relating to nursing and health. Rogers's theory of man and the theory of human motivation or hierarchy of needs as described by Maslow provide the basis for this conceptual framework. The nursing process of assessing, planning, implementing, and evaluating provides the systematic approach to nursing practice. Included in the nursing process are approaches that involve the nurse in a human, responsive, therapeutic way (see Fig. 1-1).

Theoretical Framework

A sound theory base provides the concepts upon which to build nursing practice. Rogers's theory of man and the theory of human motivation as described by Maslow are used throughout this book. The conceptual framework focuses on interactions of people in their roles as recipients as well as caregivers.

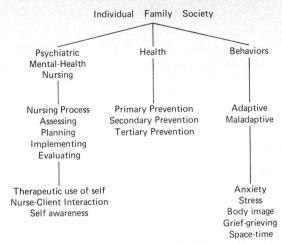

Figure 1-1 Conceptual framework of comprehensive psychiatric nursing.

Rogers's Theory of Man

According to Rogers, the individual is the core of nursing.[3] The holistic approach is the primary concern of nursing. Basic assumptions regarding this approach are identified as follows:

- Individuals are unique, unified wholes whose characteristics are greater than the sum of their parts.
- Individuals are open systems characterized by the constant interchange of matter and energy in the environment.
- The life process evolves in one direction along the space-time continuum.
- Pattern and organization identify people and reflect their innovative wholeness.
- Fundamental attributes of the humanness of the individual are abstraction and the use of imagery, language, thought, sensation, and emotion.

People and the life process are homeodynamic. Rogers identified the homeodynamic principles of reciprocy, synchrony, helicy, and resonancy which are descriptive, explanatory, and predictive, giving substance to nursing's conceptual system.[3]

The homeodynamic principles provide a

guide in assessing the client's situation and the planning, delivery, and evaluation of nursing care. They provide a way of looking at the individual and environmental interaction. These principles accommodate the multiple variables affecting health and nursing practice, including the dimensions of time and space.

Application of these principles allows for recognition of patterns which occur at specific intervals. Prediction of future occurrences which may affect health, based on recognition of factors in the past and present, is possible. Recognition and prediction of these environmental patterns and those of an individual's physical, psychological, and social behavior contribute to the determination of nursing interventions and assist clients to achieve their maximum health potential.

Reciprocy

This principle is predicated upon the basic assumption of wholeness and openness and the dynamic nature of the universe. It postulates the inseparability of the individual and the environment and predicts that sequential changes in the life process are continuous, occurring as a result of this interaction. Application of this principle guides the nurse to seek data about how this interaction is affecting the client's health. Persons, places, and things within the environment affect change. The feelings of anger, fear, or frustration generated in the nurse by the client must be assessed and considered in planning nursing care.

Synchrony

Change in the human field depends upon the state of the environmental field at any given point in space-time. The determinants of change are only what the individual is at any given moment, coupled with the state of the environment. This principle, which predicts change in human behavior, will be determined by the simultaneous interaction of the actual state of the human field and the actual state of the environmental field at any given point in space-time. Application of this principle focus-

es on the here-and-now aspect of developing a plan for care and the reality of having to engage in an ongoing revision of the care plan as each point in time presents a somewhat different problematic situation. The psychiatric nurse accepts the client at the current level of functioning in a nonjudgmental way so as to assist the client to move to an optimal level of wellness. Synchrony highlights the constantly changing dynamics and the need to revise and modify plans so they remain relevant to the client's needs.

Helicy

Further explanatory and predictive dimensions of nursing's theoretical system are suggested by helicy, which includes the principles of reciprocy and synchrony. Encompassed within this principle are the concepts of rhythm, evolution, and the unitary nature of the individual-environment relationship. This principle is concerned with the sequential, unidirectional flow, originating in the past and constantly affecting the future. Application of this principle guides the nurse to seek data on the client's previous health, coping patterns, and growth and development as well as the environmental forces that were operative. These data will provide a better understanding of the client's present situation and the extent to which previous experiences hinder or help resolution or modification of the present problem. The purpose of nursing intervention is to repattern maladaptive behavior by seeking alternative solutions at the client's pace rather than the nurse's. The rhythms of client and nurse have to be congruent.

Resonancy

This principle suggests that changes in pattern or organization of the human and environmental fields are propagated in waves. The predictive potentials of this principle arise out of a perception of the life process as an unending flow of wave patterns. Illness is caused by disruptions in the physiological patterns of the body, as well as by disturbances in psychological and social functioning, which cause changes in life-style and emotions. Disruptive changes in clients' lives, such as those arising from divorce or alcoholism, create ripple effects within a family (see Chap. 5). The mental health team determines the support systems needed, utilizing family and community resources to assist the client to return to optimum health.

Maslows Theory of Motivation

In his theory of human motivation, Maslow identified the basic human needs as physiological needs, safety needs, the need for belonging and love, esteem needs, the need for self-actualization, and the aesthetic needs.[4] These basic needs are organized into a hierarchy of relative order and predominance. As the physiological needs of hunger, sex, and thirst are satisfied, higher needs emerge. These, in turn, dominate the individual until they too are satisfied, whereupon further needs emerge. For example, no other need exists to a person stranded in the desert but to satisfy thirst. All other wants—new car, money, travel, clothes—are submerged in the desire to attain one goal, that of finding water. The hierarchy as presented by Maslow includes the levels of needs outlined in Table 1-1.

Physiological Needs

Physiological needs include the needs for food, oxygen, water, sleep, and sex. They cease to exist as active means of determining behavior when satisfied, reemerging only if they are blocked or frustrated.

Table 1-1 Nursing Application of Maslow's Hierarchy of Needs

Needs	Reactions if unmet	Nursing assessment and intervention
Physiological: food, oxygen, water, sleep, sex	Hunger, thirst, anxiety, frustration, conflict	Recognize specific needs of individuals experiencing physical or emotional illness. Develop ability to assess needs, plan realistic goals, set priorities.
Safety: security, stability, order, physical safety	Fears of separation, physical harm, pain	Provide structure, organization, boundaries, limits, familiar setting. Identify use and purpose of coping mechanisms used by client.
Love and belonging: affection, identification, companionship	Loneliness, alienation, aloneness, strangeness	Assist client to be self-directing, establish meaningful relationships, identify behaviors in themselves which interfere with goal attainment, develop positive ways of dealing with behavior.
Esteem and recognition: self-respect, self-esteem, prestige, success, esteem of others	Feelings of inferiority, worthlessness, helplessness	Utilize interviewing skills in eliciting information. Establish a caring, therapeutic relationship.
Self-actualization: self-fulfillment, achieving one's capabilities	Lack of confidence, low self-esteem	Develop increased sensitivity to feelings, attitudes, and values of self and colleagues. Utilize self in therapeutic way to meet client needs.
Aesthetic: order, harmony, beauty, spiritual goals	Feelings of ugliness, disharmony, disorder, chaos, unfulfillment, restlessness	Assist client to understand that creativity exists on many levels and can be experienced in a variety of ways. Explore spiritual striving with client. Assist the client to accept self as is and fulfill maximum potential.

Safety Needs

Safety needs include the needs for security, dependency, stability, and protection; the need to feel free from fear, anxiety, and chaos; and the need for structure, order, and limits. These needs are particularly evident in infants and children, whose reactions to danger are obvious and uninhibited. They also affect the aged, who tend to be more comfortable in surroundings that are familiar. Nursing-home clients who are allowed to keep personal belongings and their own furniture are more content than those who must accept a new, cold, impersonal environment.

Love and Belonging

Many societal factors contribute to the need for *love and belonging.* Mobility, industrialization, urbanization, the scattered family, and the generation gap all tend to separate people and groups instead of bringing them together. This helps to explain the popularity of all kinds of groups today: youth groups, singles groups, groups banding together for a common purpose or personal growth.

Maslow stresses that love is not synonymous with sex, which is a physiological need (see Chap. 12). However, sexual behavior may be motivated by the need for love and affection, which must be both given and received.

Esteem and Recognition

The need for *esteem and recognition* is concerned with the concept of self as a worthwhile person and an awareness of one's own individuality and uniqueness. Satisfaction of this need leads to self-confidence, self-respect, and feelings of importance and dignity (see Chap. 19).

Self-Actualization—Aesthetic Needs

The need for *self-actualization* involves the individual's desire for self-fulfillment. It is the expression of self in art, music, or literature, for example. A desire to be productive, to contribute, to receive satisfaction in realizing one's highest potential characterizes this need. The highest needs are the *aesthetic needs,* which include the craving for order, harmony, beauty, and truth.

Maslow identified these six basic human needs from lowest to highest. They do not necessarily occur in a fixed order, but the needs which are dominant must be met before attention can be paid to those at higher levels. The physiological needs are characterized by some deficiency such as poor nutrition, fluid or electrolyte imbalance, or lack of oxygen. The necessity of satisfying these needs produces tension or discomfort, which is unpleasant.

Basic needs must be fulfilled before attention can be paid to those growth-promoting needs which occur at higher levels. The higher needs—those involving self-actualization and aesthetic satisfaction—may never be as fully gratified as those at lower levels. Individual growth and self-fulfillment is a continuing, lifelong process of developing, emerging, and becoming. Needs are therefore a guide in setting priorities for nursing assessment and intervention (see Table 1-1).

Nursing and Health

Psychiatric nursing is defined as a specialized area of nursing practice which employs theories of human behavior as its scientific aspect and the therapeutic use of self as its art.[5] The goal or basis for nursing practice is health, which encompasses primary, secondary, and tertiary prevention. Psychiatric mental health nursing is concerned with promoting optimal mental health for the individual, the family, the community, and society. It is also concerned with early diagnosis, treatment, and rehabilitation. The role of the psychiatric nurse involves independent, interdependent, and dependent functions. There is a cooperative, collaborative relationship with members of other disciplines who are working closely with the client. Frequent interdisciplinary team meetings are required for planning quality care. Nurses practice in a variety of settings using a variety of approaches.

Implementing the Conceptual Framework

Nursing Process

The nursing process is a scientific method of problem solving applied to nursing. Nursing theories and concepts are implemented through a unified, organized progression of steps which include assessment, planning, implementation, and evaluation[6] (see Chap. 7). Among the data the nurse needs for assessment are information about clients' behavior, psychodynamics of client behavior, nurses' responses, and assessment of environmental factors. From these data, nursing diagnoses are formulated. Planning for nursing intervention is carried out through nursing goals and actions. Evaluation determines the effectiveness of the plan.

Among the therapeutic tools employed by the psychiatric nurse within the framework of the nursing process are therapeutic use of self, self-awareness, and nurse-client interaction.

Therapeutic Use of Self

Nursing takes place in an interpersonal situation. All behavior has meaning and may be seen as an attempt at communication. Understanding behavior is essential to planning nursing care. Several factors—physiological, environmental, cultural, or social—acting together may affect behavior. Responding to the individual's present behavior can have a major effect on his or her ability to behave in a mature manner in the future. Equally important is the response and behavior of the nurse in interacting with the client. Nurses respond to the humanness of the individual in the same ways that an individual responds to nurses. This added knowledge, practice, and self-awareness enables the nurse to interact therapeutically with the client.

Self-Awareness

Self-awareness is utilized when an individual examines feelings and attitudes as well as stereotyped and preconceived ideas of self and others. Ways must be developed to deal therapeutically with feelings, attitudes, ideas, and value judgments of self and others in nursing situations (see Chap 13).

Nurse-Client Interaction

An important therapeutic tool of nursing is the interaction between the nurse and the client. Nurses utilize six core dimensions throughout the initial, middle, and terminal phases of the nurse-client relationship (see Chap. 6). These include concreteness, empathetic understanding, confrontation, immediacy, genuineness, and respect. Mutual trust and respect between client and nurse is the foundation for successful, therapeutic nurse-client interaction. Appropriate nursing intervention during illness fosters learning and the development of more mature patterns of behavior. This is a growth-promoting process. As present needs are met satisfactorily, new, higher-level needs may emerge.

References

*1 Margaret A. Newman: "Nursing's Theoretical Evolution," *Nursing Outlook,* vol. 20, no. 7, p. 449, July 1972.

*2 Dorothy E. Reilly: "Why a Conceptual Framework," *Nursing Outlook,* vol. 23, no. 8, p. 566, September 1975.

*3 Martha E. Rogers: *An Introduction to the Theoretical Basis of Nursing,* Davis, Philadelphia, 1970.

4 Abraham H. Maslow: *Motivation and Personality,* 2d ed., Harper and Row, New York, 1970.

*5 Congress for Nursing Practice, *Standards of Psychiatric–Mental Health Nursing,* American Nurses' Association, Kansas City, Mo., 1973.

*6 Ann Marriner: *The Nursing Process: A Scientific Approach to Patient Care,* Mosby, St. Louis, 1975.

*Recommended reference by a nurse author.

2

Mental Health Services

Mary T. Ramshorn

Learning Objectives

After studying this chapter, the student should be able to:

1 Define mental health
2 Define mental illness
3 Appreciate the historical perspectives which influenced the care of the mentally ill
4 Define and outline the community mental health movement
5 Understand the epidemiology of mental illness
6 Grasp the principles of primary, secondary, and tertiary prevention in mental health

Societal Views of Mental Health and Illness

Definitions of mental health and illness are closely tied to the major values and institutions of society. The ways in which a society or a particular culture defines mental illness in turn influence not only the mental health services and institutions established for treatment and care but also the roles of professional workers who will be primarily involved in care. (See Chap. 3.)

Defining Mental Health

How do persons judge that they are mentally healthy or determine normality in themselves and others around them? If they are like the majority of the population, they probably have a good sense of what is normal and abnormal and under what circumstances. They have been *socialized* to that by family and community. However, formulating a definition of an abstract concept such as "mental health" or "normality" can be difficult. Practitioners and teachers alike have problems conceptualizing and explaining mental health. Some of the reasons for this follow:

1 The boundaries around mental health can be diffuse and fluid; they are defined with imprecise adjectives such as "meaningful," "self-actualizing," "fulfilling," "creative," or in terms of the competencies of a healthy person. Mental health is also defined in terms of mastery in areas of interpersonal relationships, social relationships, and role fulfillment and achievement in the realms of family, work, and community. Finally, there is a need to add the personal, experiential element to any definition that reflects ego integrity and self-acceptance: *I know I am mentally healthy because I feel good about myself and what I am doing, and because I know I can do the things I want.*

2 The major focus in the health-care system—in research, clinical work, and funding—has been directed toward diagnosis and treatment of the ill and the restoration of health and function. The curative function has been emphasized over health promotion and health maintenance; professional work with healthy populations has been more limited. Only recently have we begun to raise questions about definitions of health throughout the life span and ways of maximizing health of individuals and families. A complete departure from viewing health as merely the absence of disease, disability, or dysfunction can be found in Dunn's concept of high-level wellness. *High-level wellness* is defined as an integrated method of functioning which is oriented toward maximizing an individual's potential. It requires that one maintain a continuum of balance and purposeful direction within one's environment.[1]

3 There are cultural variations in defining mental health and labeling mental illness.[2] What is viewed as normal behavior in one culture might be considered quite abnormal in another. Further, even if different cultures label the same individual behaviors and experiences as abnormal or deviant, one culture might treat them as mental illness, another as crimes, and yet another as highly desirable mystical experiences (for example, behaviors and experiences of people under the influence of psychedelic drugs).

4 It is not uncommon for professionals to hold to one perspective of normality while clients, supported by their family and community, operate out of a different context. This difficulty is explored in the paragraphs that follow.

Views of Normality

According to Offer and Sabshin, we can view normality from four different perspectives: (1) as health, (2) as utopia, (3) as average, and (4) as process.[3]

1 Normality as *health* is defined as the absence of clinical symptomatology. This perspective is labeled the *medical model* because its major criterion is the absence of disease. In this perspective, normality may be taken for

granted. Students and practitioners alike experience difficulty responding to client families in the home or community agency when "nothing seems to be wrong" or "there's no problem." In this way, practitioners lose a valuable opportunity for preventive services to healthy, functioning families; families, in turn, receive a subtle message that health services from professionals are not available until there is a significant problem that can be diagnosed and treated.

2 A perspective that sees mental health as *utopia* does not suggest concrete health services for populations or individual clients. By definition, a utopia is an idealized place, state, or experience, one that is not to be realized in human affairs. In the field of mental health, utopia would require the ideal in human functioning and human harmony. Therefore this concept is useful more as an ideal goal or belief in human potential and evaluation than as a framework for health services.

3 The definition of normality as *average* introduces the idea of a *norm* or standard the majority accept, e.g., average behavior in a family or a community. Members who depart from these standards are deviants in the system. If normal is average and deviant members are abnormal, deviants are labeled disturbed or mentally ill. Sometimes two perspectives are combined: normality as health and normality as average. The conclusion is drawn that average behavior is health and deviant behavior is mental illness. Experience and common sense indicate that there is a potential error in such reasoning and a caution to be observed.

4 The final perspective looks at normality as *process*. This view emphasizes the individual's development over time. Situations with potential for change and growth throughout the life process are examined. The person is always developing, and the major thrust is in the direction of health and increasing capacity for self-actualization. Human personality is not arbitrarily determined at one point in infancy or childhood or by one event or relationship, however significant; rather, the developing and mature personality is a product of repeated transactions with an ever-widening environment over many years. The environment is composed of various systems having significance at different points in life, e.g., one's family of orientation, the community, play groups, school systems, health-care systems, the biologic family, and various network systems of support. *Developmental tasks* can be identified for both individuals and families; mastery and successful completion of tasks at age- and stage-appropriate periods of life enhance functioning and provide a solid foundation of learning and coping abilities for subsequent tasks. (See Chap. 5).

The validity and utility of this perspective for psychiatric nursing are increasingly apparent, since it has the following advantages:

1 It emphasizes the potential for development and change throughout the life cycle and focuses attention on the functional ability of clients. Clients may be seen at many different points in the life cycle. The nurse responds to the client's situation as it is *now* and facilitates the client's preferred change and growth.

2 Psychiatric nurses recognize that they are not the only ones interacting with the client; significant others in the family and community will also be influential, and at times their influence will have greater impact than that of any one profession.

3 Knowledge of the client's various support systems and systematic efforts to strengthen and utilize these natural systems in the service of the client can extend the effectiveness of the psychiatric nurse.

4 Short-term goals which take into account the client's developmental stage and needs can be mutually established, and both client and nurse can see them realized.

5 Strengths that the client brings to the present life situation can be utilized in moving toward

the next stage of maturity, a higher level of health and functioning, and effective coping with changing demands of the life process.

In summary then, mental health and mental illness are viewed on a continuum in a process perspective. The potential for growth and change in all individuals is emphasized. Mental health is assessed in relation to the coping abilities that the individual develops to respond and adapt to the life process in an effective and personally meaningful way. It becomes clear that there is no one final definition of mental illness. Rather, there is a *concept* formed by individuals with life experience and influenced by social and cultural norms.

Historical Perspectives in Care of the Mentally Ill
Cycles of Care and Reform

As societal values change, ways of defining mental illness and providing mental health services for clients likewise change. Cycles of care are not only discernible but also repetitive over centuries. Sometimes change develops from the impact of a major social upheaval in just one decade, e.g., a war or a period of great social unrest and reform. At other times, change can be seen as the natural progress and evolution associated with the discovery of new knowledge and the availability of new technologies. For example, the introduction of psychoanalysis in the early twentieth century and the development and effective use of psychiatric drugs in the middle of the century greatly influenced psychiatric–mental health care. Various models of mental health services have existed throughout our history; elements of each remain with us today and will undoubtedly influence future practices.

Early Traditions: The Colonial Period to the Eighteenth Century

Early care of the mentally ill in America falls into the category of the *nonmedical community-care model*. During an earlier age, the mentally ill had suffered ridicule, isolation, and persecution based

on ignorance, fear, and superstition. The colonists, in contrast, assumed a communal obligation to their poor and dependent members. Within this broad category were included not only the indigent but also the sick, physically disabled, widowed, orphaned, and mentally ill. Responsibility for their care lay primarily with the family. In the absence of a family, the mentally disturbed were supported and maintained through the charity of neighbors and community. Clearly, the mentally ill did not come within the province of medicine. Institutionalization was a last resort.

Medical-Moral Treatment: Nineteenth-Century Asylum

Little or no change occurred in the care of the mentally ill for almost forty years after American independence. In a dramatic reform movement, the asylum developed. Impelled by social forces and changing beliefs about the cause and cure of insanity in this country and Western Europe, the public embarked on the medical-moral treatment era. Within a brief period of about thirty years (1830–1860), a system of public mental hospitals spanned the country. As Rothman, writing of the cult of the asylum, notes: "Institutionalization was not a last resort of a frightened community."[4] Rather, it became—for psychiatrists, lay supporters, and finally the public at large—the first line of treatment in the cure of insanity. The structured environment with its emphasis on an orderly life, moderation in activity, and a kind but firm staff would repair disordered lives and return the newly healed to their communities. Medical superintendents of the best-known institutions reported high cure rates and received increasing public recognition and support. By 1844, they had established the American Psychiatric Association.

The original humanitarian aims of the asylum became subverted as institutions originally designed for several hundred patients were forced to house several times that number. Asylums became overcrowded with an increasing population of the poor, immigrant and chronically ill. They were understaffed and underfunded because of changes in social commitments. State mental hospitals became at best custodial institutions and at worst warehouses for the poor and unfortunate. Deteriorating conditions, reports of abuses, and questionable treatment practices led to the new elements of reform, which were incorporated in the Child Guidance Movement and the Mental Hygiene Movement founded by Clifford Beers in 1909.

Psychoanalysis and the Freudian Era: 1909–1945

Sigmund Freud, the "father of psychiatry," began to have an influence on the care of the mentally ill at the turn of the century. New approaches, new treatment, and renewed hope were supplied by him in abundance. Freud's early influence in the United States spread from the foundations of the psychoanalytic movement and training institutes throughout human development and mental health services and training programs. The psychoanalytic movement as a major force influenced American psychiatry until after World War II, and it remains significant today.

Medical-Therapeutic Model: 1945–1960

Just after World War II came the watershed years in the move to consolidate existing gains and advance mental health services. Renewed public concern for mental health and illness came from several sources:

1 A higher proportion of young Americans than would be anticipated were found to be emotionally unfit for military service during the war.

2 Psychiatric casualties returning after the war required new treatment approaches and rehabilitation (see Chap. 11).

3 Criticism of the primitive and sometimes inhumane custodial treatment of the mentally ill in large state institutions was widespread

In 1946, President Harry S. Truman signed into law the first National Mental Health Act. The act represented the first national commitment to the major problem of mental illness through research, services, and training. The National Institute of Mental Health, established in 1949, became the agency of this commitment.

Psychiatric nursing as a clinical specialty arose during this period. During the long history of custodial care in the United States, limited possibilities existed for the professional practice of nursing. Nursing's major function was one of control over ward and patients and support of any existing medical regimen. Nurses themselves expected to be primarily involved in managerial, coordinating types of activities; the art and science of therapeutic work with clients was left to psychiatrists. It is therefore not surprising to find that nurses functioned from the perspective of a *medical model* and adopted the medical ideology of their institutions. Graduate programs in psychiatric nursing that were developed during this period formed the foundation of the clinical specialist movement and made possible the practice of professional nursing in the mental health field.

Biomedical research during this period significantly influenced patient care and treatment approaches. The development and effective use of the *phenothiazines* and major tranquilizers led both clients and professionals to hope that the major symptoms associated with *psychosis* could be controlled. (See Chap. 8.) Once target *symptoms* were controlled, it was possible to reach clients who had apparently been completely cut off from reality. These clients, once medicated, were able to engage in significant interpersonal relationships with psychiatric staff. As clients' behavior became more predictable and therefore less frightening to those around them, it was possible to implement an open-door policy in the large mental institutions, to accept the concept of a therapeutic community in the hospital, and to allow visits away from the hospital to the community.

The definition of mental illness is changing, both in the psychiatric establishment and in the larger society. While the etiology of mental illness remains generally unknown, specific chemotherapeutic interventions are available for the control of symptoms. It can be argued that mental illness is quite similar to a number of physical health problems for which effective treatment is available, even if the etiology and cure are still unknown. Mental illness is no longer hopeless; nor does it require prolonged and even lifelong institutionalization. Clients are helped and can look forward to returning and functioning within their families and communities after hospitalization.

The Community Mental Health Movement: 1960 to the Present

Heralded as the third revolution in psychiatry, the community mental health movement marked a significant shift from institutional services for mentally ill individuals to comprehensive community-based mental health services for populations. The Community Mental Health Centers Act of 1963 authorized funding for the establishment of community mental health centers which would provide at least five essential services for their catchment areas: (1) emergency care, (2) inpatient care, (3) partial hospitalization, (4) aftercare, and (5) consultation. Emphasis was placed on the concepts of comprehensive care, continuity of care, innovative treatment approaches, and the use of professional and paraprofessional mental health workers in a team approach.

Critics of the community mental health movement maintain that as a system of health-care delivery, the community mental health center has not fulfilled its early promise; that it draws too heavily from a traditional medical model; and, finally, that it has not addressed the issue of defining and delivering preventive services to populations.[5] Still others point out that in practice the community mental health movement has contributed to the "revolving door" problem, in which large numbers of the mentally ill are returned too rapidly to their communities without provisions for any supportive, therapeutic aftercare services. As a consequence, community tenure is short and these clients are rehospitalized at frequent intervals.

Many of the gains of this period are still to be consolidated. Innovations in treatment still need to be evaluated over time. Roles and functions of psychiatric nursing in community-based services are still evolving.[6,7]

Epidemiology of Mental Illness

Epidemiology as a science and specialized field of public health is concerned with the health of populations—specifically, with all factors related to the distribution and control of disease and promotion of health in identified populations over given time periods. Two terms—"incidence" and "prevalence"—are significant in discussing mental health problems and levels of prevention. *Incidence* refers to the number of new cases of a disease in a specific population over a period of time. *Prevalence* refers to the rate of established or diagnosed cases of the illness in a population at a certain point of time. "Prevalence," then, would include the number of newly diagnosed cases of the disease as well as the number of old cases under treatment.

In speaking of populations, it is helpful to identify *populations at risk*. These are all members of a specific population who might, under the right conditions, be vulnerable to the disease.[8] For example, the population at risk for measles during the winter months in a given community might be identified as the school population, pupils and teachers alike. Since teachers are apt to have immunity to the disease, either natural or acquired, young children would be identified as the target population for primary prevention measures, specifically immunization. (For further elaboration of the epidemiological method, the student should refer to a basic text in the field.) Valid and reliable statistics on the incidence and prevalence of a health problem in a population at risk yield valuable information on the need for preventive health services and community programs and are one measure of effectiveness of the health-care delivery system.

Measures of Prevalence and Incidence of Mental Disorders

Research on a national level on the epidemiology of mental disorders is a relatively new endeavor. As recently as the period just after World War II, the incidence and prevalence of mental disorders for the nation as a whole were unknown. While data had been collected for individual states or communities, they were not comparable, and they commonly represented prevalence (i.e., the number of cases of mental illness under treatment at a given time). It would be more accurate to recognize the limitation of these data—that is, these statistics as showing the utilization of psychiatric services rather than as a measure of established cases of disease.

Researchers at the National Institute of Mental Health point out that studies of the utilization of psychiatric facilities (primarily state hospitals until the last 10 years) produce biased data on incidence and prevalence rates in populations. Several factors are operating:

1 Many social, community, and personal factors—including a fact as specific as what service is available in the local community —influence what clients go to which service for specific treatment.
2 Many clients are treated outside psychiatric facilities (e.g., in outpatient clinics, by private physicians) and will not be included in institutional case reporting
3 A proportion of the population suffering from mental disorders are not diagnosed or treated at all.[9]

Priorities for Research
Recognizing the limitations of our current knowledge, several priority areas can be identified in the epidemiology of mental illness:[9]

1 Accurate statistics on the rate of occurrence of mental disorders in the general population.
2 Broad-based studies of utilization of psychiatric services with follow-up of clients discharged from psychiatric services and identification of factors associated with utilization of services
3 Standardized case finding techniques which can be uniformly applied by professionals in various settings for early identification of persons in the general population with mental disorders

4 Reliable, differential diagnostic techniques to ensure that cases are assigned to a specific diagnostic classification and to provide a comparable base for national and international studies in the incidence and prevalence of mental disorders

Concepts of Prevention in Mental Health
Levels of Prevention Defined
The field of public health and the epidemiological approach have been the main source for the concept of levels of prevention in psychiatry. *Primary prevention* acts to reduce the incidence of disease in populations at risk. *Secondary prevention* aims to reduce the prevalence of the disease through early case finding and effective treatment. *Tertiary prevention* aims to reduce the disability associated with the disease through rehabilitation. All levels of prevention refer to populations over a period of time.

Primary Prevention Principles
Primary prevention emphasizes the promotion of healthy personality development, healthy families, and healthy communities through the reduction of factors considered harmful to these various systems. It applies to the population, community, and social institution rather than to the individual. Primary prevention of mental illness is *unlike* the primary prevention of physical health problems of single-agent etiology, in which one can immunize populations at risk or remove the causative agent from the environment. While research in the mental health field has associated genetic, biochemical psychological, and social factors with incidence of disease, it has not determined what necessary factors, in what relationship, at what point in the life process, and under what conditions will produce mental illiness in a relatively constant proportion of the population. Consequently, primary prevention in the mental health field aims at promoting mental health and reducing new cases of

disease generally rather than preventing any one single disease or category of disease.[8]

Crisis Intervention as Primary Prevention

Certain predictable events occur in the lives of all persons. These events influence and are influenced by our mental health and coping ability. Events such as first separation from parents, negotiating adolescence, getting married, and becoming a parent have the potential for becoming developmental crises (see Chap. 5). The demands of the transition period from one level of development to the next call for new ways of behaving and relating and can seriously disturb the individual's equilibrium. While such a period may involve great upset and tension, it also has the potential for significant growth and new learning over a relatively short time. It is also a time when individuals are most open to help from significant others. Successful mastery of the crisis period builds up a range of coping abilities which are then available for the next phase of development. Poor resolution can leave an individual more vulnerable to the next crisis.

Primary prevention, then, would be concerned with reducing the hazards of the crisis events and preparing populations for the demands of new roles and expectations. For example, young couples can be more adequately prepared for the role of new parents during the antipartum period. Adolescents can be prepared for their first job or first semester at college. This preparation might take the form of *anticipatory guidance,* a particular form of health counseling emphasizing coaching for a future experience or event in an effort to endow individuals with some of the skills and understandings necessary for new events and new roles.

Primary prevention programs would also emphasize brief, supportive services to families made vulnerable by an unpredictable *situational crisis* such as bereavement, children's separation from family due to hospitalization, or loss of job or home.

In all these situations, the emphasis is on normal healthy families who would not necessarily be seen by mental health professionals at times of crisis. Visotsky points out that the work of primary prevention is carried out in the community: first by the individual's family and significant support systems and then by physicians and various social agencies, schools, churches, and local government leaders.[10]

Secondary Prevention Principles

Programs of secondary prevention in the field of mental health aim to reduce the prevalence of mental disorder through early case finding and effective treatment. Emphasis is placed on referrals to appropriate health services, accessibility of services for clients, and rapid initiation of active treatment. Treatment might take the form of short hospitalization in the psychiatric unit of a general hospital, chemotherapy and psychotherapy on an outpatient basis, conjoint family therapy, or crisis intervention. In all these modalities, the psychiatric nurse functions as a significant member of the health team, participating in multidisciplinary team conferences, therapy activities, discharge planning conferences, and family counseling. Nursing makes a major contribution, maintaining the therapeutic milieu of inpatient services and providing a structured environment for clients in which they can try out new ways of relating to and communicating with others (see Chap. 9).

Tertiary Prevention Principles

Tertiary prevention aims to reduce the long-term disability of disease through programs of aftercare, rehabilitation, and resocialization. Emphasis is placed on preparing clients and families for the client's discharge from an institution and return to the community.[11] This preparation might include helping the family to understand and respond to the client's needs, to have confidence in the client's ability to resume activities and responsibilities in the home and community, and to recognize periods of stress and assist clients in coping with them in productive ways. The community-health nurse might well support and counsel the family on periodic home visits for health maintenance. Social and vocational agencies in the community might be utilized in helping the client resume former activities or prepare for new ones. The important element in tertiary prevention programs is *continuity of care* and modification of care as circumstances change. Too often—as many community health, social, and education agencies become involved with the client—care is fragmented. The natural support systems that exist in communities and could aid the client in rehabilitation are less effective when their programs and services are not coordinated.

References

1 Halbert L. Dunn: *High Level Wellness,* Beatty, Arlington, Va., 1961, pp. 4–5.

*2 Mary T. Bush, Jean A. Ullom, and Oliver H. Osborne: "The Meaning of Mental Health: A Report of Two Ethnoscientific Studies," *Nursing Research,* vol. 24, pp. 130–138, March–April 1975.

3 David Offer and Melvin Sabshin: "Concepts of Normality in Psychiatry," in Alfred Freedman and Harold Kaplan (eds.), *Comprehensive Textbook of Psychiatry,* Williams and Wilkins, Baltimore, 1967, p. 256.

4 David Rothman: *The Discovery of the Asylum,* Little, Brown, Boston, 1971, p. 131.

*5 Jacquelyn Murray: "Failure of the Community Mental Health Movement," *American Journal of Nursing,* vol. 75, pp. 2034–2036, November 1975.

*6 Anne J. Davis and Patricia Underwood: "Role, Function, and Decision Making in Community Mental Health," *Nursing Research,* vol. 25, pp. 256–258, July–August 1976.

*7 Jill K. Nelson and Dianne Schilke: "The Evolution of Psychiatric Liaison Nursing," *Perspectives in Psychiatric Care,* vol. 14, no. 2, pp. 60–65, 1976.

8 Gerald Caplan: *Principles of Preventive Psychiatry,* Basic Books, New York, 1964.

9 Report of the Research Task Force of the National Institute of Mental Health: *Research in the Service of Mental Health,* Department of Health, Education, and Welfare, Washington, D.C., 1975, pp. 351–357.

10 Harold M. Visotsky: "Community Psychiatry: Intervention," in Alfred Freedman and Harold Kaplan (eds.), *Comprehensive Textbook of Psychiatry,* Williams and Wilkins, Baltimore, 1967, p. 1537.

*11 Mary Bayer: "Easing Mental Patients' Return to Their Communities," *American Journal of Nursing,* vol. 76, pp. 406–408, March 1976.

*Recommended reference by a nurse author.

Chapter

3

Sociocultural Aspects of Mental Illness

Janice E. Ruffin

Learning Objectives

After studying this chapter, the student should be able to:

1 Identify the four major categories of individuals and groups who participate in differentiating those who are mentally ill from those who are not

2 Describe some relationships between culture and mental illness among ethnic minorities and racial groups

3 Describe some relationships between culture and mental illness among women

4 Identify the factors which facilitate an individual's decision to seek psychiatric help

5 Define the sociological concept of deviance

6   Identify paths or routes which may be taken by a person who needs to be admitted to a mental hospital

7   Discuss differences between social-class groups in relation to the paths which may be taken to admission in a mental hospital

8   Describe the roles played by families when a member becomes mentally ill

9   List the areas of the law pertaining to the admission and treatment of the mentally ill

10 Identify at least two implications for the role of the nurse in view of the fact that many people require but do not seek or accept psychiatric help

During 1971, approximately 3 million Americans received treatment for mental illness.[1] These people were treated in a variety of settings including federal, state, and county mental agencies; private mental hospitals; outpatient psychiatric clinics; day-night psychiatric units; and private offices. Regardless of where they sought and secured treatment and of the nature or severity of their illness, they shared the common identity of "mental patient." Or, in accord with the more precise, contemporary nomenclature, these people were "clients" of the mental health services system. The following analysis of the process of becoming a mental patient utilizes a broad perspective, giving due consideration to social, political, economic, and cultural factors. It is derived from a diversity of scientific fields and schools of thought. The disciplines of psychiatry, psychology, sociology, anthropology, and epidemiology have provided major contributions to this approach.

The Pre-Client Phase

The client who enters the mental health services system may be viewed as having a "career" which can be studied for purposes of understanding the changes which have occurred over time. The con-cept of career allows for the study of both the clients' inner lives and their patterns of interaction with others within a social network. According to Goffman (1961), the client's career falls into three main phases: the period prior to entering the hospital (the pre-patient phase), the period in the hospital (the in-patient phase), and the period after discharge from the hospital (the ex-patient phase).[2] The pre-patient phase is the period that precedes entry into *any* part of the mental health services system, hospital or other.

Becoming a Client

Five distinct assumptions about the process of becoming a client in the mental health services system may be summarized as follows:

1   *Mental illness is a psychosocial matter.* The identification and definition of mental illness occurs within specific sociocultural contexts.

2   *The definition of mental illness occurs within an interpersonal transaction between the individual and other "definers of mental illness."* Sills has coined this term to describe the people who participate in differentiating those who are mentally ill from those who are

not. Other than "the self," the three major categories are "the socially legitimated mental health professions, the legally empowered societal agents, and those who represent 'significant others' to the protagonist."[3]

3 *At any point in time, the number of people who actually become clients of the mental health services system are smaller than the eligible pool of potential clients.* The people who become clients are those who are identified by themselves or others as being mentally ill *and* who are willing to seek or accept help. The eligible pool includes two additional groups: (*a*) people who are identified by themselves or others as being mentally ill *but* who are unwilling to seek or accept help and (*b*) people who are unidentified by themselves or others as mentally ill but who would be defined as such by prevailing standards of illness (i.e., the "undiscovered ill").

4 *The individual's decision to seek or accept help for mental illness—and, accordingly, the particular paths which are taken to become a client of the mental health services system—reflect the interaction of multiple variables.* These include age, sex, income, ethnicity, education, marital status, availability of services, and the organization of services within a given community.

5 *The pathways taken to the mental health services system and the nature of the admissions process have a crucial bearing on the individual's adjustment to or rejection of an identification as "mental client."* Such an identification is based upon, among other things, congruence between the individual and clinicians on what is wrong and on what treatment is desired or needed.

The relationships between these complex processes are integral to understanding the process of becoming a client. In Fig. 3-1, these relationships are outlined. The interplay of the norms and values of society with standards of mental health and illness is illustrated. Cultural

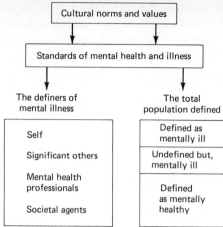

Figure 3-1 The identification and definition of mental illness. *Defined mentally ill* are those persons who identify themselves or who are identified by others as mentally ill. *Undefined mentally ill* are those persons who have not been identified as mentally ill but could be so identified by prevailing standards of illness, i.e., the undiscovered ill. *Mentally healthy* are those persons who could be identified as mentally healthy in accordance with prevailing standards.

norms shared by people in our society regulate their conduct. Values, as well, are reflected in the establishment of a variety of standards for behavior, including standards of mental health and illness. The definers of mental illness serve a regulatory function in determining what behaviors violate established standards of "normal" behavior.

Culture and Mental Illness

Culture is, in part, a symbolic organization of behavior in which the meaning of that behavior is expressed in interpersonal processes stemming from cultural traditions. Culture is a way of life. It is an organized set of customs, habits, ideas, and beliefs shared by a group of people. Culture also includes traditional systems for the transmission of methods of regulating behavior, ethics, and attitudes. Families and other social units put these traditions into operation. Since transmission does not occur with perfect regularity, the elements which ultimately are incorporated from the culture into personal functioning may produce individuals whose behavior does not conform to cultural norms and who are judged to be mentally ill or deviant.[4]

Since the study of culture and mental illness is relatively new, there are many more unanswered questions than conclusive findings. The study of the relationships of culture to mental illness falls within the province of social psychiatry. Social psychiatry is concerned with individual and collective social forces in relation to adaptation and psychopathology. It has investigated the environmental, sociocultural, transcultural, ecological, and interdisciplinary aspects of psychiatry.

Of specific interest to the pre-client phase is the question of whether culture has an impact on the incidence and prevalence of mental illness within the United States. Cultural groups have been found to vary in the amount and kinds of deviance they will tolerate. In addition, it is known that there are variations among cultural groups in the ways in which behavior is identified and defined as mental illness. Consequently, there are significant differences among cultures in their utilization of the range of facilities within the mental health services system. For example, in a study conducted by Jaco (1959) on Spanish-Americans in Texas, they were found to have a lower-than-average incidence of mental illness.[5] That is, the number of people in the Spanish-American population who had been treated for psychosis was significantly lower than the corresponding number in other ethnic groups. Madsen (1969) has interpreted these findings as evidence of cultural phenomenon: Spanish-Americans in Texas are less likely to become mentally ill because stress is shared by the tightly knit family group.[6]

Similarly, the influence of culture on mental illness has been investigated in studies of another ethnic group, black Americans. Crawford (1969), on the basis of a review of studies on blacks, concludes that while blacks and whites have similar rates of mental illness, the crucial differences are that blacks do not receive the full range of services utilized by whites, are not kept under treatment as long as whites, and use multiple sources of help less frequently than whites.[7] Others have also commented on this picture of inequality of psychiatric care for blacks and other ethnic minority groups. In recent years, attention has shifted to an emphasis on the development of services which are much more easily accessible to minority groups so as to increase the utilization of such services. In addition, there has been a marked interest in understanding the impact of racism on the mental health and treatment of minorities. Specifically, racism has been observed to be a major cause of the differential treatment afforded black clients.

Other studies which provide clarity relative to the influence of culture on mental illness have focused on family dynamics and ethnic variations.[8-11] Cultural values have been associated with differences in the definition of family roles. For example, Barrabe and Von Mering (1953) found differences in the mother-son relationships of Italian, Jewish, Irish, and Yankee (or "old American") families with psychotic children. Selected descriptions included the following: Italian mothers were observed to be oversolicitious, Jewish mothers and sons had highly emotional relationships, Irish sons were excessively dependent on their mothers and Yankee mothers were overprotective, restrictive, and moralistic with their sons. It has been hypothesized that, when viewed in the total cultural context, these variations may either have health-promoting (i.e., stabilizing) or stress-producing effects.

Interest in ethnic variations in mental illness has been at least equaled by parallel studies on the effect of cultural conditions upon women. Chesler has reviewed statistical data on mental illness and concluded that women of all classes and races constitute the majority of the psychiatrically involved population in America, Britain, Sweden, and Canada.[12] She argues that sex-role stereotypes are at the heart of what is defined as mental illness and pleads with women and all mental health professionals to simultaneously develop alternative conceptions of mental health and abolish double standards of treatment for men and women. Although these specific findings have not been validated conclusively, the effects of the women's liberation movement have prompted many others in the mental health professions to evaluate prevailing conceptions of mental illness in women more carefully.

The existence of sex-role stereotypes in judgments about the mental health of women was confirmed in a study by Broverman and her colleagues. A sample group of mental health professionals were surveyed to determine whether clinical judgments about the traits characterizing healthy, mature adults would differ as a function of the sex of the person judged. The researchers found that a double standard existed. Clinicians were less likely to attribute traits which characterize "healthy adults" to a woman than they were to attribute these traits to a "healthy man."[13]

In this discussion of culture and mental illness, it should be noted that there is a voluminous amount of literature on the effects of social class on the prevalence of mental illness and the differential treatment afforded people in various classes.

Perspectives on Illness

This society's conceptions of mental health and illness have undergone profound changes in the past two decades. Historically, the mental health movement has shifted in orientation. Initially, it devoted much of its effort to its own establishment and legitimization; now there is a greater focus on the community and its institutions. President Kennedy's support of the need for new types of mental health facilities and the subsequent passage of the Community Mental Health Act of 1963 provided substantial impetus for the intense dialogues which have ensued about the theoretical and practical problems of psychiatry. Current dialogues emphasize the prevention of mental illness. Inherent in such a new thrust is the need to reexamine and reevaluate the conceptual frameworks of psychiatry.

Perspectives of Normality

Normality was not the focus of psychiatric research until the last decade. Offer and Sabshin have provided a comprehensive review of prevailing concepts of normality as presently used in psychiatry, biology, sociology, psychoanalysis, anthropology, and psychology. Based on their reviews, four distinctive approaches to concepts of normality are proposed: (1) normality as health, (2) normality as utopia, (3) normality as average, and (4) normality as process[14] (see Chap. 2). These approaches are valuable in clarifying the difficulties inherent in achieving uniformity among the disciplines in definitions of mental health and illness.

Identifying the Mentally Ill

Assessment of the prevalence of mental illness is also related to the fundamental issue of defining mental health and illness. The results of studies which have been conducted in the past two decades have varied according to the geographical location and the particular definitions of "mental illness" used. Estimates of the need for psychiatric help have ranged from a low of 10 percent to a high of over 20 percent. Several of these studies will be summarized here with a focus on identifying characteristics of those people who needed psychiatric help.

In 1960, the Joint Commission on Mental Health and Illness published a monograph entitled *Americans View Their Mental Health*. In contrast to other studies which imposed their own definitions of "illness," the researchers surveyed their sample for the subjects' own perception of their mental health. The sample included 2,460 Americans over the age of 21, selected so as to be representative of the total population in age, sex, education, income, occupation, and place of residence. This group, therefore, constituted a miniature of the "normal" population of the United States.

Although one out of four (25 percent) of the total population said that they had *needed* help with personal problems at some time in their lives, only 14 percent reported that they had actually gone for help.[15] The group of people who had actually gone for help included significantly larger numbers of women, younger persons, and the better educated. These groups were observed to have a tendency to define their problems in psychological terms; they were inclined to be introspective and self-critical. In contrast, the group of people who recognized the need for personal help but who never went for help belonged to lower educational and income groups. In general, however, few significant attitudinal differences were observed between those who went for help and those who did not. The authors conclude that once a problem has been seen in mental health terms, the decision to go for help should be largely a function of facilitating factors rather than of psychological or motivational factors. These factors included the actual availability of resources in the community, one's knowledge and information about these resources, and the social customs and traditions with respect to help-seeking behavior.[15]

The Midtown Manhattan Study suggests that overall prevalence of mental morbidity varies inversely with socioeconomic status. The lower socioeconomic groups were found to have many more impaired people who had not sought psychiatric help than did the higher socioeconomic groups.[16] (See Chap. 2.)

The pioneering work of Hollingshead and Redlich is of major significance to this review of identifying the mentally ill. Based on a representative sample of people living in New Haven, Connecticut, a systematic relationship was identified between social class and the prevalence of treated mental illness. The higher socioeconomic groups were underrepresented in the patient population, and the lower socioeconomic groups were greatly overrepresented.[17]

Perspectives on Deviance

Theories of deviance and labeling serve to further explicate dimensions of the pre-client phase. Deviant behavior is the standard sociological concept which signifies behavior that violates a social norm in a given society. Norm violation is viewed as a function of culture. The culture of a group determines the distinctions between those behaviors which are categorized as, for example, crime, perversion, drunkenness, bad manners, and mental illness. Persons who, for instance, display withdrawn, mute behavior, talk aloud to themselves, or repeatedly provoke physical fights with others may be categorized as shy, idiosyncratic, or oversensitive. The labeling of these deviant behaviors as mental illness is dependent upon cultural norms which regulate the recognition and definition of mental illness.

Mechanic has presented a descriptive model of the definitional processes by which persons within a community are adjudged mentally ill by family, friends, and themselves. He notes that the basic decision about illness is made by community members, not professional personnel. Mechanic proposes the following components of a descriptive model:[18]

1 The frame of reference of the evaluator determines whether a deviant act is seen as mental illness, eccentricity, or criminal behavior. When the evaluator is unable to adequately empathize with the person who is behaving in a deviant manner, the behavior is more likely to be labeled sick.

2 Intervention into a situation of assumed mental illness is largely dependent upon the *visibility* of the symptoms, the *seriousness* of the consequences of the deviation for the group, and the *frequency* of the act.

3 As the vulnerability of the group increases, its tolerance for deviance decreases.

To illustrate these principles, the example of a person who is withdrawn and mute is elaborated. If the person is a Native American (Indian), such behavior may reflect a culturally sanctioned practice of communicating with spiritual beings. Those who are not Native Americans may misjudge that behavior as mental illness and force hospitalization, as happened in the reported case of a Navaho Indian male.[19] Or consider the hypothetical but conceivable situation in which a mother of several young children has gradually, over a year's period, become withdrawn and mute to a point of relinquishing all role functions as a mother and wife. If the father then becomes unemployed, the family's ability to sustain itself while also tolerating the deviance is threatened. They may no longer be able to define the mother's behavior as eccentric or deal with it in other ways which avoid a definition of mental illness. If, further, the family's vulnerability is enhanced by the need to interact with school authorities who encourage the husband to define the mother as sick, the family may shift in their definition of the behavior. In this example, the centrality of the mothering role and the intervention of others who are not members of the family both create a more vulnerable group.

Another concept employed within this sociological framework is that of *residual deviance*. Residual deviance defines the diverse kinds of norm-violating behavior for which society provides no explicit label and which, therefore, sometimes lead the norm-violator to be labeled mentally ill. For example, people who exhibit unusual behavioral patterns in their life-style or mode of dress can be labeled mentally ill. It has been hypothesized that, once labeled, these persons may establish "careers" as residual deviants in the mental health services or criminal justice systems.[20]

The essential criticism leveled against those who employ the concept of deviance is that the theories tend to exaggerate the importance of social processes while understressing individual processes. Further, there is considerable disagreement as to the validity and usefulness of the labeling perspective as applied to mental illness. Some believe that theorists have overemphasized secondary deviance (behavior *produced* by being placed in a deviant role) and underemphasized primary deviance (the behavior which leads to the labeling).[21] Others believe that there is a strong "presumption of illness" by mental health professions who assess persons appearing for evalua-

tion. Indeed, the use of the APA diagnostic classification (See appendix) can contribute to the inaccurate labeling of behavior as sick in the face of nothing more than a strong presumption of illness. In order to arrive at an accurate sociopsychological assessment of potential clients, such bias must be guarded against.

Pathways to the Mental Health Service System

Clients may be assisted by their families, friends, social agencies, or the legal system in entering the mental health services system. In discussing the paths which clients took to psychiatric treatment, Hollingshead and Redlich note that there were significant differences among classes. A majority of upper-class clients were either self-referrals or were guided by family and friends; a majority of the middle-class clients were referred by physicians.[17] By contrast, the majority of lower-class clients were referred by social agencies, the police, and the courts.[17] These differences in routes to psychiatric treatment can still be observed in many communities. The reluctance of some lower-class people to seek treatment frequently results in the use of authoritative, compulsory (legal) means to move them into the mental health service system.

Other data suggest that the readiness of persons who need help to *seek* help is aided by the prevailing view or attitude climate of their family and peers. A majority of those in the upper socioeconomic bracket would urge such a person to seek psychiatric help; conversely, a minority of those in the lower socioeconomic brackets would advise the seeking of *any* professional help.[16]

Often people do not go to psychiatrists because they are "really sick" but because they *think* they are sick. Kadushin contends that social position has a major influence on people's reactions to problems and suggests that within our culture there are basically two reactions: a "Marxian" reaction in which one blames the situation or the environment and a "Freudian" reaction in which one evaluates problems on the basis of self-analysis.[22] Kadushin's study of over 1,400 applicants to six outpatient psychiatric clinics in New York prompted him to develop a theory of "the friends and supporters of psychotherapy." Those "friends" were described as a social circle of people who knew others with similar problems, knew others in therapy, and solicited or accepted help from others in pursuing psychotherapy for themselves. Most of them were culturally sophisticated, well educated, young, and did not live with their families. Further, the decision to seek psychiatric help was composed of four steps or stages: the realization of a problem, consultation with lay persons, choice of type of healer, and choice of an individual practitioner.[22]

Family Processes and Becoming a Mental Client

Bloch has categorized the family of the psychiatric client according to the theoretical views of the relation of the family to psychiatric disorder. These categories are as follows:[23]

1 *Psychiatric Disorder as an Endogenous Stress* This was a view frequently held in earlier periods of psychiatry in which the illness was assumed to have originated from *within* the client. The family was thought of as needing to manage the stress of the illness as they managed other crises.

2 *Psychiatric Disorder as Caused by Pathogenic Relationships* This view reflected a shift in reasoning about the dynamics of mental illness. Clients' illnesses were understood to be *caused* by specific attitudes, traits, or practices of family members, particularly the mother.

3 *The Family as Pathogenic Culture Carrier* This framework utilizes sociological concepts to analyze the complex relationship between the influence of culture on the family's role in socializing children into healthy, nondeviant

behaviors as opposed to mental illness. The family is viewed as adequate or not, within a given culture, for this task of socialization and acculturation.

4 *Psychiatric Disorder as an Expression of the Systems Properties of the Family* This approach attempts to understand the family as a dynamic system which tends to maintain certain patterns of self-regulation. Illness in one member of the system is viewed as an expression of a property relevant to that system (e.g., its need to have a role of "patient" in the family or its inability to tolerate certain behaviors, such as hostility or sexuality, in a member).

It is apparent from these diverging conceptualizations that families can be viewed in strikingly contrasting ways in terms of their role in the pre-client phase. Families may be seen as consciously or unconsciously preventing the client from receiving needed help; relatively unimplicated in the unfolding of an illness in a member; victimized by the member's illness; or the unwitting purveyors of pathology within the culture in which they are embedded.

Often, evidence of severe disturbance in a family member may be minimized and rationalized as a defense against defining the person as mentally ill.[24] For example, families with a father who is becoming progressively paranoid may explain his suspicious accusations and hostile outbursts as the result of stress from his job. Or family members may become oversolicitous in the face of such paranoid behaviors, hoping to allay the father's extreme suspiciousness. Even after a family has determined that a member is mentally ill, they do not always know how to proceed to secure psychiatric help.[25] Many families do not seek professional help until their problems become unmanageable. Lower-class families have been found to keep severely disturbed persons at home for longer periods than do middle-class families.[26]

Families may also be described in terms of their ways of accommodating deviance in a member. Two typical accommodations have been described.[27] In the first situation, the future client and his or her immediate interpersonal community withdraw from each other and reciprocate withdrawal by withdrawal. In the second type, the future client and a member of the immediate interpersonal community become locked in an intense interdependence and reciprocate withdrawal by concern. In both situations, there is a high tolerance for deviant behavior.

Legal Processes and Becoming a Mental Client

The legal system articulates with the mentally ill and their families in several substantial ways. First, the law defines behavior which violates standards established by society and determines whether the violator should be considered a criminal or mentally ill. Second, the law serves to protect the civil liberties of the mentally ill and their families. Third, the laws of each state provide for the care and treatment of the mentally ill. The development of the law as it affects the rights of the mentally ill has become dependent on medical knowledge about mental illness, public acceptance of responsibility for the mentally ill, and the legal profession's awareness of the needs of the mentally ill in the safeguarding of their rights.

The areas of the law pertaining to the mentally ill in the pre-client phase are described as follows:[28]

1 Involuntary Hospitalization   The removal of a person from his or her normal surroundings to a hospital authorized to provide treatment

2 Voluntary Admission   Procedures for hospitalization which are initiated by clients or someone empowered by law to act in their behalf

3 Emergency Detention   Provisions for the temporary detention of mentally ill persons who may be dangerous to persons or property

4 Mental Disability and the Criminal Law   Provisions regarding the legal punishment of mentally ill persons accused of a criminal act

Additionally, the law provides for the hospitalized client's rights in the following areas:[28]

- Procedures for the transfer, release, or discharge of clients
- The safeguarding of clients' rights to adequate, humane, and dignified treatment and to privacy
- Declaring the mentally ill incompetent
- Personal and property rights

Each state has its own legal statutes that regulate the commitment or hospitalization of the mentally ill. Some states hold that the sole criterion for hospitalization is whether individuals are dangerous to themselves or others. Other states augment this provision to indicate that an individual's need for treatment can be an alternative basis for hospitalization. Finally, a few states provide no other basis for hospitalization than need for care or treatment.

The Admissions Process

The process of becoming a client is a complex one requiring multiple frames of reference for analysis. Entrance into the mental health services system is, similarly, a multidimensional phenomenon which varies according to the individual or subgroup seeking treatment and the agency from which service is sought. The interaction between these parties may either lead to an offer of automatic admission or to a more rigorous assessment of the client to determine his or her suitability for the agency's services. In general, the former tends to apply to hospital admissions while the latter describes many outpatient admissions. In Fig. 3-2, the process of becoming a client in the mental health services system is outlined for groups of individuals. Of significance is the fact that the process may be interrupted at any step or phase along the way.

Available data on patterns of utilization indicate that, for some services, there is often a high correlation between treatment desired and the particular facility approached. In Kadushin's

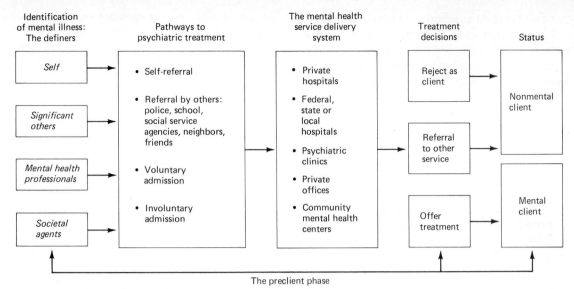

Figure 3-2 Becoming a mental client.

study, clinic applicants were found to be members of different cultures or social circles who, therefore, held different views of certain facilities: applicants to analytic clinics, religiopsychiatric clinics, or hospital clinics each chose them on the basis of their perception of what help they needed and which professional group could best help them.[22]

Other studies have found that, when service is made available to any who apply, the facility receives clients who, in effect, shape the nature of services offered. Tischler and his colleagues have explored the association between clienthood in a community mental health center and prevalence of symptomatology in the community. It was found that some groups were overrepresented in terms of service utilization: the unmarried, the unemployed, those living alone, and those without religious affiliations. The authors concluded that it was almost as though those individuals sought out and accepted the client role in an effort to compensate for the absence of viable social supports.[29]

The Mental Health Team

The members of the mental health team who have contact with the client upon admission vary greatly among the psychiatric facilities currently available. The team may function as an organized group on the psychiatric unit of a general hospital, in the outpatient unit of a community mental health center, or in a psychiatric hospital—private, local, state, or federal. The hospital team is usually composed of psychiatrists, psychiatric nurses, psychologists, social workers, and psychiatric aides. Since over 85 percent of psychiatric nurses and a majority of psychiatric aides are employed in hospital settings, the outpatient team is more characteristically composed of psychiatrists, psychologists, and social workers. As change takes place, however, psychiatric nurses in increasing numbers are participating in the widest range of functions in the mental health services system, including the assessment and evaluation of clients who seek admission.

Treatment Planning

The essential dimensions of treatment planning include arriving at an accurate diagnosis of the client's illness and deciding upon a particular treatment for that illness. Much has been written about the diagnostic process in psychiatry, including the difficulties of achieving high reliability, objectivity, and consistency among clinicians.[30-33]

The "processing" of prospective clients for admission to a particular facility can be enhanced when the psychiatric nurse conceives of this proceeding as an *applicancy*.[34] In contrast to perceiving the person who seeks help as a client from the start, this conception allows for a process of exploration. Questions asked by the nurse of the applicant may include the following:

1 What do you think is wrong with you?
2 What were some of the most recent events which led you to seek help?
3 Who were some of the people who assisted you in deciding that you needed help?
4 Do you think that you are mentally ill?
5 What are some of your ideas about the services offered here?
6 What kind of help do you think you need?

When such an approach is used, it is possible to negotiate with the prospective client around the available and recommended treatment. This principle is espoused on the basis of knowledge that clinicians and those who seek their help are often worlds apart in their assumptions about what is involved in becoming a client. For instance, many persons seeking help expect to be given medication only. If the clinician believes them to need hospitalization or a period of psychotherapy instead, the admissions process may become unnecessarily confusing for an already disorganized applicant.

Second, the potential client's cultural world must be understood in order to estimate the existence of illness, its severity, and its contextual meaning. It has been acknowledged that the greater the sociocultural distance between the clinician and the client, the less accurate diagnoses become and the more nonspecific dispositions are likely to be. White clinicians diagnosing black clients were significantly more likely to diagnose them as sicker, and as requiring more lengthy treatment than nonblack clients.[35] It is also well known that there are double standards of treatment for white, educated males and the affluent generally as opposed to females, members of minority groups, the relatively uneducated, and the poor. What is proposed here is not that any one form of treatment (for example, insight-oriented psychotherapy) is unquestionably suited to all groups but that active efforts to assure equality in treatment planning will do much to abolish this double standard.

Psychiatric nurses should give careful thought to the meanings attached to the label "mentally ill." While it is not established that labeling is the single most important variable that launches people into client careers, there is evidence that it contributes greatly. In some instances, it may be more constructive to help potential clients see their problems in the context of their social situations, thereby enabling them to appreciate the environmental stresses that can lead to a "diagnosis" of mental illness. Of course, no amount of relabeling will erase the obvious symptoms of distress which applicants present. The sensitive nurse, therefore, will do well to remain mindful of the authority implicit in the role of "definer of mental illness" and will exercise that authority with due consideration for the complexity of this society's prevailing conceptions of mental illness.

References

1 Julius Segal and Donald S. Bommer (eds.); *Research in the Service of Mental Health,* Summary Report, National Institute of Mental Health, DHEW Publication No. (ADM) 75-237, 1975, p. 3.
2 Erving Goffman: *Asylums,* Doubleday, New York, 1961, pp. 130–131.
*3 Grayce Sills: "Social Systems and Mental Health Services," in Elaine Goldman (ed.), *Community Mental Health Nursing,* Appleton-Century-Crofts, New York, 1972, pp. 187, 300.

*Recommended reference by a nurse author.

4   Marvin K. Opler (ed.): *Culture and Mental Illness*, Macmillan, New York, 1959, p. 9.

5   Gartley E. Jaco: "Mental Health of the Spanish-American in Texas," in Marvin K. Opler (ed.), *Culture and Mental Illness*, Macmillan, New York, 1959.

6   William Madsen: "Mexican-Americans and Anglo-Americans: A Comparative Study of Mental Health in Texas," in Stanley Plog and Robert Edgerton (eds.), *Changing Perspectives in Mental Illness*, Holt, New York, 1969.

7   Fred Crawford: "Variations between Negroes and Whites in Concepts of Mental Illness, its Treatment and Prevalence," in Stanley Plog and Robert Edgerton (eds.), *Changing Perspectives in Mental Illness*, Holt, New York, 1969.

8   John Speigel: "Cultural Strain, Family Role Patterns, and Intrapsychic Conflict," in John G. Howells (ed.), *Theory and Practice of Family Psychiatry*, Brunner-Mazel, New York, 1971.

9   Paul Barrabe and Otto von Mering: "Ethnic Variations in Mental Stress in Families with Psychotic Children," *Social Problems*, vol. 1, 1953.

10 Marvin K. Opler: "Cultural Differences in Mental Disorders: An Italian and Irish Contrast in the Schizophrenias—U.S.A.," in Marvin K. Opler (ed.), *Culture and Mental Illness*, Macmillan, New York, 1959.

11 E. G. Piedmont: "Ethnic Differences in Schizophrenic Development," *Psychiatric Quarterly*, vol. 11, pp. 654–658, 1966.

12 Phyllis Chesler: *Women and Madness*, Doubleday, New York, 1972.

13 Inge K. Broverman et al.: "Sex Role Stereotypes and Clinical Judgments of Mental Health," *Journal of Consulting and Clinical Psychology*, vol. 34, pp. 1–7, 1970.

14 Daniel Offer and Melvin Sabshin: *Normality*, Basic Books, New York, 1966, p. 9.

15 Gerald Gurin, Joseph Veroff, and Sheila Feld: *Americans View their Mental Health*, Basic Books, New York, 1960, pp. 299, 302–343.

16 Leo Srole et al.: *Mental Health in the Metropolis—The Midtown Manhattan Study*, McGraw-Hill, New York, 1962, pp. 248, 250.

17 August B. Hollingshead and Frederick C. Redlich: *Social Class and Mental Illness*, Wiley, New York, 1958.

18 David Mechanic: "Some Factors in Identifying and Defining Mental Illness," in Stephan Spitzer and Norman Denzin (eds.), *The Mental Patient: Studies in the Sociology of Deviance*, McGraw-Hill, New York, 1968, pp. 197–200.

19 D. P. Jewell: "A Case of a 'Psychotic' Navaho Indian Male," in D. Apple (ed.), *Social Studies of Health and Sickness: A Sourcebook for the Health Professions*, McGraw-Hill, New York, 1960.

20 Thomas J. Scheff: "The Role of the Mentally Ill and the Dynamics of Mental Disorder: A Research Framework," in Stephan Spitzer and Norman Denzin (eds.), *The Mental Patient: Studies in the Sociology of Deviance*, McGraw-Hill, New York, 1968, pp. 9–10, 21.

21 Walter Gove: "Societal Reaction as an Explanation of Mental Illness: An Evaluation," *American Sociological Review*, vol. 35, pp. 873–884, 1970.

22 Charles Kadushin: *Why People Go To Psychiatrists*, Atherton, New York, 1969, pp. 243, 309.

23 Donald Bloch: "The Family of the Psychiatric Patient," in Silvano Arieti (ed.), *American Handbook of Psychiatry*, Basic Books, New York, 1974, vol. 1, pp. 179–180.

24 Marian R. Yarrow et al.: "The Psychological Meaning of Mental Illness in the Family," *Journal of Social Issues*, vol. 11, pp. 12–24, 1955.

25 John Clausen and Marian R. Yarrow: "Paths to the Mental Hospital," *Journal of Social Issues*, vol. 22, pp. 25–32, 1955.

26 Jerome K. Myers and Bertram H. Robers: *Family and Class Dynamics*, Wiley, New York, 1959, pp. 213–220.

27 Harold Sampson, Sheldon L. Messinger, and Robert D. Towne: "Family Processes and Becoming a Mental Patient," in Stephan Spitzer and Norman Denzin (eds.), *The Mental Patient: Studies in the Sociology of Deviance*, McGraw-Hill, New York, 1968, pp. 203–213.

28 Frank T. Lindman and Donald McIntyre: *The Mentally Disabled and the Law*, The University of Chicago Press, Chicago, 1961, p. 17.

29 Gary Tischler et al.: "Utilization of Mental Health Services," *Archives of General Psychiatry*, vol. 32, pp. 411–415, April 1975.

30 B. Mehlman: "The Reliability of Psychiatric Diagnoses," *Journal of Abnormal Social Psychology*, vol. 47, pp. 577–578, 1952.

31 Ellen Langer and Robert Abelson: "A Patient by Any Other Name . . . Clinician Group Differences in Labeling Bias," *Journal of Consulting and Clinical Psychology*, vol. 42, pp. 4–9, 1974.

32 Maurice K. Temerlin: "Suggestion Effects in Psychiatric Diagnosis," *The Journal of Nervous and Mental Disease*, vol. 147, pp. 349–353, 1968.

33 Robert J. Stoller and Robert Geertsma: "The Consistency of Psychiatrists' Clinical Judgments," *The Journal of Nervous and Mental Diseases,* vol. 137, pp. 58–66, 1963.

34 Daniel J. Levinson, John Merrifield, and Kenneth Berg: "Becoming a Mental Patient," *Archives of General Psychiatry,* vol. 17, pp. 385–406, 1967.

35 Herbert S. Gross et al.: "The Effect of Race and Sex on the Variation of Diagnosis and Disposition in a Psychiatric Emergency Room," *The Journal of Nervous and Mental Disease,* vol. 148, pp. 638–646, 1969.

4

Theoretical Models

Pamela A. Price

Learning Objectives

After studying this chapter, the student should be able to:

1 Understand the theoretical basis of client behavior
2 Understand the theoretical rationale for nursing intervention
3 Define a theoretical base for psychiatric–mental health nursing practice
4 Define intrapsychic, interpersonal, behavioral, phenomenological, communication, and system theories

Many people consider theory a topic to be avoided or at best tolerated. Some tend to be adamantly opposed to theory, believing themselves to be "action-oriented." For example, practicing nurses can sometimes be heard to accuse a nurse-theoretician of living in an ivory tower, being uninvolved with real-world problems, "copping out" on the responsibility to "perform." It is a fact, however, that people spend their entire lives evolving plausible reasons and hypotheses to explain their experiences. An infant spends days learning which vocal utterance brings Mom in a hurry. Weeks are devoted to learning how to get the cup to the lip without a slip. Crossing the street safely requires much study, and a 6-year-old can tell you about the many factors to be considered before stepping off the curb. Adults cross busy streets "without thinking," but once upon a time that feat took careful deliberation. After one has achieved success, the figuring slips back into unawareness; but it still continues.

Intuition is defined as the act or faculty of knowing without using the rational processes.[1] One way to explain intuition is to see the rational processes as having occurred at an earlier time in life, having worked successfully, and now being carried out beyond conscious awareness.

Depending on one's view of the situation (or one's *theory*), decisions are made about what to do. Theory, then, is a way of thinking about and hence *seeing* an event. More formally, *theory* is systematically organized knowledge applicable in a relatively wide variety of circumstances; it is a system of assumptions, accepted principles, and rules of procedure devised to analyze, predict, or otherwise explain the nature or behavior of a specified set of phenomena.[1]

Consider the person who is drunk. One theory states that people do have control over themselves and can accomplish anything if they want it badly enough; that will power is what makes people upstanding citizens. The person who is drunk is seen by proponents of this theory as disgusting; they are furious because the alcoholic exercises so little will power. In practice, such people may put distance between the alcoholic and them-

selves; they will most certainly refuse requests for money from alcoholic beggars.

A different theory states that people are victims of unconscious forces over which they have no control, and that alcohol abuse is a symptom of unresolved unconscious conflicts. A person who accepts this theory will see alcoholics as pitiful lumps of humanity, tossed about by forces beyond their understanding and control. In practice, such a person may ignore the present behavior, since it is only a symptom, and attempt to help those suffering from alcoholism. These examples show that the action a person takes derives logically from the theory he or she holds.

Professional nursing practice is based on awareness of the theory one uses. The education of professional nurses places emphasis on increasing self-awareness through the study of theoretical frameworks. Nurses sometimes intervene appropriately when using intuition, but there is no way to communicate why a particular intervention was chosen; on the other hand, if the nurse becomes aware of the assumptions made, the beliefs held, the theories used, then the ideas behind intervention will be understood. The nurse is then able to participate in building models of human behavior unique to the nursing profession.

In this chapter, six theories utilized by nurses in psychiatric–mental health nursing practice will be explored. These are (1) intrapsychic theory, (2) interpersonal theory, (3) behavioral theory, (4) phenomenological theory, (5) communications theory, and (6) systems theory.

Intrapsychic Theorists

With intrapsychic or intrapersonal theories, the focus is within the person's mind. It is there that the difficulty is thought to exist, and the intervention focuses on the person's thoughts and feelings.

Sigmund Freud

Sigmund Freud introduced some revolutionary concepts which have had worldwide influence on the understanding of human behavior. His major assumption was that all behavior is meaningful. He considered that every thought, feeling, action, and dream is an expression of something unique and important about the individual.

Freud considered the primary motivation for behavior to be anxiety. Anxiety is an experience of tension or dread that seems to have no purpose or object. The object of anxiety is unconscious and is related to loss of self-image. This is contrasted to fear, which involves a conscious object and usually refers to some threatening environmental event (see Chaps. 14 and 15).

Because anxiety is such a distasteful experience, people have several built-in mechanisms to defend against it. *Defense mechanisms* are abilities the ego calls into play to protect against anxiety; they operate outside awareness. Anxiety is thought to be the response to unconscious material threatening to emerge into consciousness. The ego uses defense mechanisms to protect against this anxiety by keeping the material unconscious. Table 4-1 outlines the defense mechanisms, giving examples of each.

Table 4-1 Ego Defense Mechanisms

Defense mechanism	Example
Repression: A widely used unconscious mechanism. Painful experiences, disagreeable memories, unacceptable thoughts and impulses are barred from consciousness. Selfish, hostile, and sexual impulses are also usually repressed. It takes a constant expenditure of energy to keep repressed material out of awareness. Consequently, less energy is available for constructive activity.	Mrs. S does not remember having spent 6 months in a body cast at age 7. Mr. Z does not remember having sexually exposed himself on a subway train.
Regression: The ego returns to an earlier stage of development in thought, feeling, or behavior. Regression is a normal component of our developmental sequence and appears transiently during times of stress, when it is utilized as a retreat from anxiety and conflict.	Mr. B, an adult, has temper tantrums (child behavior) when frustrated. Tim, a 4-year old, is confronted with the birth of a new sister. He is toilet-trained and articulate but responds to the birth of the new baby by regressing to nighttime bed-wetting, daytime soiling, and baby talk. All this stems from his effort to regain his old unchallenged position with his mother.
Identification: A person becomes like something or someone else in one or several aspects of thought or behavior. This contributes to ego development but does not replace the person's own ego. The personality consists of multiple identifications that have been tested for their ability to reduce anxiety.	Mr. K, a young man whose father has recently died, begins to talk and act like the father. Miss Thomas, who is studying nursing, incorporates into her personality the assertiveness she admires in one of her instructors.
Introjection: A form of identification which is a symbolic taking in or incorporation of a loved or hated object or person into the individual's own ego structure. Introjection is important in the development of the superego when the child incorporates the parents' instructions, rewards, and punishments.	Paul, a 5-year-old boy tells his 2-year-old brother, "Look both ways when you cross the street."
Reaction Formation: Occurs when an individual expresses an attitude that is directly opposite to unconscious feelings and wishes.	Mr. J has unconscious feelings of hate and anger toward his boss; he covers them up by being excessively polite. Johnny, a teen-ager, has an unconscious desire to be dependent and cared for; this is masked by his independent attitudes.
Undoing: Closely related to reaction formation. A person negates an act by behavior which is the opposite of what was done before.	Miss M crosses her fingers while telling a white lie. Little Peter, who has just told his mother that he hates her, goes over to her and hugs and kisses her.

Table 4-1 Ego Defense Mechanisms (continued)

Defense mechanism	Example
Isolation: The exclusion from awareness of the feelings connected to a thought, memory, or experience. The person remembers the experience or thought but does not reexperience the emotion that originally accompanied it.	Mrs. James, an obsessive client, relates her repeated thoughts of having thrown her baby out of the window. As the woman speaks, she conveys no affective response to the content of this frightening thought.
Displacement: The discharge of emotions feelings, or ideas upon a subject other than the one to which the feelings rightly belong. This is a security operation in which the feelings are discharged away from the actual source of the emotion because it is not considered safe to express them directly.	Mrs. Green has had a difficult day at the office. A project she had worked hard on was rejected by her boss. When she comes home from work, she begins yelling at her husband and children, displacing the anger felt toward the boss onto her family.
Projection: The attribution of one's feelings, impulses, thoughts, and wishes to others or the environment in an effort to deny their existence in the self. Projection is used in a wide variety of normal situations. It is used excessively by clients with paranoid thought patterns.	David, a freshman, has failed an exam. He blames the instructor for having made a poor choice of questions on the exam. Miss K, a suspicious, paranoid client, projects hostile, aggressive feelings that are part of the self onto others when stating "I can't eat, the food is poisoned," and "I can't go to sleep, they're just waiting to kill me."
Rationalization: A coping mechanism that is universally employed. It is an attempt to make one's behavior appear to be the result of logical thinking rather than of unconscious impulses or desires. It is utilized when a person has a sense of guilt or uncertainty about something that has been done. It is a face-saving device that may or may not deal with the truth. It relieves anxiety temporarily.	Mary S, a sophomore, fails a course and says that the teacher was ineffective. Mr. W has no friends; he says people do not appreciate his efforts at friendship. Miss B says she wants to get married but has trouble with dating. Every time she goes out with a man, she refuses a second date, saying, "He's not my intellectual equal." In doing this she is probably rationalizing deep fears of sexuality.
Denial: The total failure to acknowlege the existence of an affect, experience, idea, or memory. The person simply pretends that what is painful, anxiety-provoking, or threatening does not exist.	Mr. L, who has cancer, was told that he was terminally ill and had approximately a month to live. Later in the day, the nurse hears him talking to his travel agent. He is planning a trip to Europe next summer.
Substitution: The replacement of a highly valued, unacceptable object with a less valued one which is acceptable.	Mr. E wants to marry Miss L, probably because she looks quite a bit like his mother.
Sublimation: Transformation of psychic energy associated with unwanted sexual or aggressive drives into socially acceptable pursuits. The activity or its object is changed, but the energy is discharged.	After Bobby's father forbade him to use the family car, Bobby spent a half hour punching a punching bag. Eleanor's boyfriend has left her to pursue a career as a rock musician. Now she spends much of her time writing love poems.

Freud's theoretical model has two major parts: aspects of consciousness and aspects of personality. The aspects of consciousness are the conscious, the unconscious, and the preconscious. The *conscious* includes all the elements that are easily remembered. The things that are a little difficult to remember but can be recalled with help are considered *preconscious. Unconscious* materials are those thoughts, feelings, actions, experiences, and dreams that are not remembered, very difficult to bring into consciousness, and not recognized if one is told of them.

Freud divided the personality into the id, the ego, and the superego. The *id* includes the instinctual forces and is primarily unconscious. If uncontrolled by the ego and/or superego, the id would lead people to "kill, plunder, and destroy." These unconscious forces find expression through thoughts, feelings, and perceptions. Examples of id: a person eats 2 pounds of cotton candy at a county fair; another has a temper tantrum after finding out about a low grade.

The *ego* appraises the environment, assesses reality, stays in touch with bodily and environmental changes, and directs the motor activity of the body. The *superego* contains the rigid, absolute rules that direct a person's thoughts, feelings, and actions. "Conscience" is thought to be analogous except that the superego includes unconscious as well as conscious material. The superego often directly opposes the forces of the id. The ego, with its reality orientation, maintains the balance between the id and the superego. *Ego strength* is the relative ability of the ego to maintain a sense of reality, to keep unconscious material buried, and to deal effectively with the forces of the id and superego. Whether a person exhibits neurosis or psychosis depends on ego strength. A person with

greater ego strength is better able to maintain a sense of reality when facing severe anxiety.[2]

Certain experiences, thoughts, and feelings generate tremendous anxiety; the ego defends against this anxiety by relegating these unacceptable experiences to the unconscious. The more energy required to keep these experiences unconscious, the less there is available for innovative, fulfilling life experiences. In addition, the person must avoid experiences that threaten to aid the emergence of unconscious material. These conditions result in a neurotic personality configuration (see Chap. 16).

Freud thought that sexual growth and development was the basis of many unconscious conflicts. He developed a scheme of sexual growth and development to clarify the stages and emerging conflict. Table 4-2 lists each developmental stage, the time of development, the characteristics of each stage, and examples. According to Freudian theory, if all stages of development are negotiated successfully, the person is emotionally mature. Difficulty in negotiating any of the stages makes the next stage more difficult. The unre-

Table 4-2 Freud's Theory of Sexual Growth and Development

Stage of development	Time frame	Characteristics	Examples of unsuccessful experience
Oral	Birth to 18 months	Learning to deal with anxiety-producing experiences by using the mouth and tongue	Defenses centered around oral experiences: smoking, alcoholism, obesity, nail biting, drug addiction, difficulty with trust
Anal	18 months to 3 years	Learning muscle control, especially that involved with urination and defecation	Defenses centered around holding on and letting go: constipation, obsessive-compulsive personality, fastidiousness, perfection drive
Phallic	3 to 6 years	Learning sexual identity and developing awareness of the genital area	Difficulty with sexual identity: transsexuality, difficulty with authority, homosexuality, *Oedipus complex* (erotic attachment of male child to mother), *Electra complex* (erotic attachment of female child to father)
Latency	6 to 12 years	Quiet stage during which sexual development lies dormant	Defenses centered on inability to conceptualize: Lack self-motivation in school and job.
Genital	12 years to early adulthood	Developing sexual maturity and learning to develop satisfactory relationships with the opposite sex	Unsatisfactory relationships with the opposite sex: frigidity, impotence, premature ejaculation, serial marriages

solved conflicts occurring during each stage remain part of the person's current personality structure. These conflicts are often unconscious and find expression through dreams as well as through emotions or thoughts inappropriate to a current event.

Psychoanalysis is the treatment modality based on Freudian constructs. The goal of the therapeutic relationship is to make unconscious material conscious, thereby curing the symptom. This occurs through analysis of the relationship the client develops with the psychoanalyst. The client-analyst relationship is used because it is held that unresolved conflicts are exhibited in every relationship. When a client attributes to the analyst some characteristics really belonging to a person the client knew in childhood, this is called *transference.* Two techniques are used to analyze the transference that occurs in this relationship: free association and dream analysis. *Free association* is the reporting of thoughts, feelings, sensations, perceptions, and so forth, without passing judgment or censoring anything, as one becomes aware of them. *Dream analysis* is the interpretation of the symbolism contained in the reported dream.

Resistance is expected to occur throughout the relationship because, though the symptoms are disruptive and stand in the way of a fulfilling life, the unconscious material is very threatening and anxiety-provoking. The more central the unconscious material is to personality organization, the more the client is expected to resist its disclosure. Since the material is unconscious, the client cannot simply be told about the unresolved conflicts. Working through the resistance and acquiring insight is the goal of therapy. *Insight* is the emotional recognition and acceptance of an underlying difficulty. Freud thought that all people are subject to unconscious conflicts, which exert an influence over the personality. Psychoanalysts, therefore, must undergo psychoanalysis themselves in order to qualify to offer this type of therapy.[2]

Several of Freud's theoretical constructs are used in nursing practice. The first is the notion that *all behavior is meaningful.* For example, repeated pregnancies may result from a woman's unconscious wish to remain dependent. They may also represent an unconscious need for love objects or may simply be motivated by the conscious wish for a large family.

The idea that each phase of sexual growth and development involves specific experiences and conflicts that must be successfully resolved is very important in working with children and their families. For example, in order to avoid early toilet training or rigid bathroom schedules, nurses can inform parents about myelinization of nerve tissues and about body rhythms. Offering options for toilet training may decrease power struggles between children and parents, and children may also learn to deal effectively with authority figures.

The defense mechanisms explain many of the unusual behaviors clients exhibit when anxious. If the client's behavior is counterproductive, the nurse may alter the environment in order to reduce the client's anxiety. For example, if a client develops an anxiety reaction when exposed to a noisy, chaotic environment, the nurse may take the client to a quiet place and stay there until the client becomes calm. Another way the nurse can help decrease the client's anxiety level is to accept him or her and create an atmosphere that is safe and inspires trust (see Chap. 14).

Erik H. Erikson

Erik Erikson is a psychoanalyst who added another dimension to Freud's theories: society. Erikson considers that, besides being the product of heredity and experience, every person is also influenced by society; that is, every personal anxiety also reflects societal concerns. Erikson stresses the ego and its development. He thinks that the gradual, stage-by-stage growth of ego identity, based on experiences of social health and cultural solidarity, culminates in the individual's sense of humanity.

Erikson sees the sex roles as essentially biological and hereditary rather than social. Besides the hereditary aspect, Erikson sees people as developing through eight social development stages (as contrasted to Freud's sexual development stages). These are outlined in Table 4-3. Developmental stages, time frames, developmental tasks, and examples are included. This psychosocial development proceeds in a series of crises, and a person's degree of success in passing one stage will influence his or her ability to negotiate the next. The way the tasks are negotiated is not either-or, but rather is conceptualized on a continuum (see Chap. 5).

The motivation for behavior is anxiety generated by failure to successfully negotiate the stages of development. Play therapy is used with children to help them negotiate earlier stages and to resolve present crises. Psychoanalysis is the mode of therapy used with adults. The goal of the therapeutic relationship is the successful resolution of conflicts and the expansion of awareness to include latent anxieties. The ultimate goal is a strong identity; a strong, healthy body; and a discerning and curious mind.

The therapist using Erikson's framework would be someone who is self-observant and aware of social influences—a person who is both in the world and of it, very much a participant. Psychoanalysis is a prerequisite for anyone who wants to qualify as a therapist of this school. According to Erikson, there are four dimensions of psychoanalysis:

1 The *cure-research* dimension includes studying the unique individual while both client and therapist are engaged in observation and cure.
2 *Objectivity-participation* is concerned with the therapist's participation in the relationship while objectively observing self and other's behavior.
3 *Knowledge-imagination* encompasses the therapist's use of theory and creative intervention in the therapeutic relationship.
4 *Tolerance-indignation* is considered a

Table 4-3 Erikson's Theory of Social Growth and Development

Stage of development	Time frame	Developmental tasks	Examples
Sensory	Birth to 18 months	Trust vs. mistrust	Experiences with the nurturing person are the foundations of the level of trust a person will develop.
Muscular	1 to 3 years	Autonomy vs. shame and doubt	The toddler learns the extent to which the environment can be influenced by direct manipulation.
Locomotor	3 to 6 years	Initiative vs. guilt	The child learns the extent to which being assertive will influence environment. If important others disapprove of beginning assertiveness, the child will experience guilt.
Latency	6 to 12 years	Industry vs. inferiority	The child either learns to utilize energies to create, develop, and manipulate, or the child learns to shy away from industry, feeling inadequate to the task.
Adolescent	12 to 20 years	Identity vs. role diffusion	The adolescent either integrates all life experiences into a coherent sense of self or is unable to integrate these experiences and feels lost and confused.
Young adulthood	18 to 25 years	Intimacy vs. isolation	The young adult is primarily concerned with developing an intimate relationship with another person.
Adulthood	21 to 45 years	Generativity vs. stagnation	The adult is primarily concerned with establishing a family and guiding the next generation.
Maturity	45 years to death	Integrity vs. despair	The life-style gives life meaning and the person must come to accept his or her life as fulfilling and meaningful. The lack of ego integration results in fear of death.

dimension of the therapist's work and is contrasted with the traditional analyst's attitude of detached objectivity. This attitude is displayed toward self, toward others, and toward society.[3]

Nursing uses several of Erikson's concepts. The stages of social development are important in working with children and their families (see Chap. 32). The idea that growth is a lifelong process is heartily embraced by nursing. When considering intervention plans for clients, nursing also acknowledges the importance of society's influence on health and behavior. Though Erikson continues to espouse the notion that heredity is the basis of sex-role behavior, nursing considers sex-role behavior to be culturally learned. Like the therapists using Erikson's mode, nurses also use theory as the basis of therapeutic intervention.

Interpersonal Theorists

The focus of interpersonal theories is the relationship between and among people. Interpersonal theorists consider major life events and sources of difficulty clients encounter to be the result of interpersonal relationships.

Harry Stack Sullivan

Harry Stack Sullivan assumed that mental disorders resulted from inadequate communications with others. He included in his framework the society in which people live. He saw people as gifted animals who must be socialized into people who are able to live in a social organization. Sullivan implied an inherent intolerance of anxiety; he thought that the ways people learn to cope with anxiety can interfere with their capacity to have meaningful experiences later on. The motivation for behavior, in Sullivan's view, is the avoidance of anxiety and the satisfaction of needs.

Much of Sullivan's thought about people centered around his theory of interpersonal growth and development (in contrast with Freud's sexual emphasis and Erikson's focus on social growth

and development). He thought that biological changes determine the emerging needs and directions of growth. He considered the biological changes and emerging capacities as *tools* and the directions of growth and development as *tasks*. His developmental scheme is charted in Table 4-4; it includes stage of development, developmental tools and tasks, and examples. Sullivan felt that if the tasks of all stages were accomplished successfully, the cumulative result would be a person able to fulfill the tasks of late adolescence, to become interdependent, and to learn to form a durable sexual relationship with a selected member of the opposite sex.

The therapist, in Sullivan's view, is a participant-observer in the relationship with the client. The therapist helps the client to identify areas of development that are incomplete and to increase awareness of self. *Consensual validation* is an important tool that the therapist encourages clients to use, since it helps them to develop the ability to assess reality objectively.

Sullivan calls reality orientation the *syntaxic mode* of perception. This occurs when perceptions form whole, logical, coherent pictures of reality that can be validated by others. The first kind of experience, common in infancy, is the *prototaxic mode*, the sense of self and the universe as an undifferentiated whole. In the *parataxic mode*, common in childhood and juvenile periods, the undifferentiated whole is broken into parts that are momentary, illogical, and disconnected.

Another area of therapeutic focus is the self-system. Sullivan considered the *self-system* to be an organization of experiences that exist to defend against anxiety and to secure necessary satisfaction. One aspect of the self-system is known as *good-me, bad-me, not-me*. The child learns those behaviors approved of by parents and identifies them as good-me. For example, an adult will identify cleanliness as a positive quality if this behavior was regarded as good by his or her parents. Behaviors receiving disapproval generate anxiety and are identified by the child as bad-me. For example, an adult who was, as a child, punished for such behavior, may talk about the bad

Table 4-4 Sullivan's Theory of Interpersonal Growth and Development

Stage of development	Developmental tools	Developmental tasks	Examples
Infancy: Birth to the emergence of speech, about 1½ years	Mouth Ability to cry Satisfaction response Empathic observation Autistic invention Exploration Emergency reactions: fear, rage, anxiety	Learning to count on others to gratify needs and to satisfy wishes	During this period, an infant cannot be spoiled. Meeting an infant's needs lays a firm foundation for the development of trust.
Childhood: 1½ years to the emergence of the need to associate with peers, about 6 years	Language Anus Self Autistic invention Experimentation Manipulation Identification Emergency reactions: anxiety, anger, shame, guilt, doubt	Learning to accept interference with wishes in relative comfort, to delay gratification	The child must have realistic limits set during this time. The limits must be consistent if the child is to develop a sense of reality about the environment.
Juvenile period: 6 years to the beginning of the capacity to love, about 9 years	Competition Compromise Cooperation Experimentation Exploration Manipulation	Learning to form satisfactory relationships with peers	The child learns to attend to peers' wishes in order to have needs met. Family rules may be ignored in deference to friends' ideas.
Preadolescence: 9 years to the first evidence of puberty, about 12 years	Capacity to love Consensual validation Collaboration Experimentation Exploration Manipulation	Learning to relate to a friend of the same sex	More allegiance to friends than to family marks this era. The opposite sex is shunned and "best friend" knows all secrets, dreams, and fantasies.
Early adolescence: 12 years to the completion of primary and secondary changes, about 14 years	Lust Experimentation Exploration Manipulation Anxiety	Learning to master independence and to establish satisfactory relationships with members of the opposite sex	Rebellion and dependence mark this era. Sexual relationships and peer mores are more influential than family allegiance.
Late adolescence: 14 years to establishment of durable situations of intimacy, about 21 years	Genital organs Exploration Manipulation Experimentation	Developing an enduring intimate relationship with one member of the opposite sex	During this period, a deep love relationship is established and marriage follows.

habit of eating between meals. Behaviors generating an extreme level of anxiety are denied and identified as not-me. For example, an adult who was strongly conditioned in childhood against showing hostility may say, "I never hate anybody, that's not me." The self-system is dynamic, changeable, and positively directed; it must be reorganized if substantial change is to be effected.

The goal of treatment is to correct developmental deficits, to replace inadequate, inappropriate responses with adequate, healthy ones and to develop the syntaxic mode of perception. The process of treatment based on Sullivan's formulations is focused on anxiety. The appearance of anxiety shows where the developmental deficits have occurred. The problem causing the anxiety—rather than symptomatic behavior—is the focus of treatment. The dynamic changes in the client-therapist relationship provide opportunities for the client to live through and to correct developmental deficits.[4]

Hildegard E. Peplau

Hildegard Peplau, a nurse, developed the notion of therapeutic relationships with clients. She based much of her theoretical framework on Sullivan's formulations, sharing with Sullivan the assumption that human beings have an innate drive toward health. She and Sullivan thought that behavior is goal-directed and that prolonged and/or severe anxiety can result in personality disorganization.

Peplau's view of humanity is optimistic and respectful. Clients are thought to know what they need, although they may need help to become aware of their needs. The nurse intervenes by helping the client recognize these needs.

Peplau states that the nurse as well as the client are objects of scrutiny in a relationship. The relationship itself assumes importance, since both parties have needs, emotions, thoughts, and motivations that must be examined. The client is the focus of the time spent relating. Nurses consider their own dynamics at other times. Several roles emerge as a relationship is begun, worked through, and terminated. Each role has its set of expected behaviors and can be distorted by both client and nurse. The nurse must examine self needs and motivations and not allow them to distort perceptions of the client or of the relationship. In the chapters that follow, the focus is on the nurse's response to clients and the therapeutic use the nurse makes of self.

Peplau sees needs as the motivation for behavior. People behave, think, feel, and dream in order to meet needs, and a primary motivating need is freedom from anxiety. Peplau developed Sullivan's idea that anxiety can be thought of as falling along a continuum ranging from mild anxiety to panic.[5] (See Chap. 14.) Anxiety has no specific object and is experienced as a discomfort. Each level of anxiety influences people differently. These levels include the following:

1 On the *mild* level, the person is alerted and perceives more than when he or she is not anxious. Awareness, attention, and the ability to make connections are heightened.

2 The *moderate* level of anxiety narrows the perceptual field, but one can pay attention if directed to do so. With mild and moderate levels, the person can solve problems fairly effectively.

3 With the *severe* level of anxiety, the perceptual field is greatly reduced and the person focuses on scattered details. With both moderate and severe anxiety, selective inattention prevails.

4 With *panic*-level anxiety, one's ability to observe narrows until only the object of anxiety is noticed. With severe and panic-level anxiety, the person tends to dissociate in an effort to escape; learning and adaptation are focused on relief. Automatic protective behaviors are used to prevent and reduce anxiety (see Fig. 14-1).

Relationships are goal-directed and go through four phases:

1 During *orientation,* the nurse explains the nature and purpose of the relationship, the role of the nurse, and the responsibilities of the client.

2 During *identification,* the client identifies the problem to be explored.

3 During *exploitation,* the problem and underlying needs are explored in the relationship with the nurse.

4 During *resolution,* the events in the relationship and the growth occurring in the process of exploitation are summarized by the

client and the nurse. The relationship is then terminated.

The phases of the relationship often overlap as the problem is explored and refined and underlying needs are identified.

The goal of the nurse-client relationship is to find a solution to the presenting problem and to further the growth of the participants in the relationship. (See Chap. 6.) Both the nurse and the client are involved in the process, and learning theory is used as a basis for intervention. It is very important to be consistent in the relationship so that the client may develop trust in the nurse. A nurse offers to serve clients as a sounding board and a listener. Empathy, nondirective listening, and unconditional acceptance are the tools of the therapeutic use of self (see Chap. 13). The exploration of the nurse's own attitudes toward clients is essential to the therapeutic use of self.

Respect for and belief in the client is inherent in interpersonal theory. Nurses in all specialty areas are able to utilize these constructs. All nursing practice takes place in, and is effective because of, the relationship developed with the client. It is not what the nurse does to or for the client that is the focus but rather the way the nurse uses self as a therapeutic tool.

The anxiety continuum is helpful in understanding the constructive and destructive effects of anxiety on behavior in relationships. Likewise, it provides a basis for understanding conflict resolution at each point on the continuum.

Behavior Theorists

Behavior theorists hold that the difficulties people suffer are neither intrapsychic nor interpersonal but behavioral. They believe all behavior is learned, and since it is learned, can be unlearned and replaced with more adequate, appropriate behavior.

Joseph Wolpe

Joseph Wolpe uses B. F. Skinner's principles of behaviorism and applies them to people. Wolpe states that problems are behavioral, while therapists using other modalities consider maladaptive behavior as symptomatic of underlying problems. He holds that sometimes maladaptive behaviors do not extinguish themselves. These behaviors are the realm of behavior therapy. Wolpe considers psychosis organically based and deals only with neurotic behaviors.

Wolpe does not expound a view of people. Rather, he deals exclusively with behavior, which he defines as a *conditioned response*. Therefore, behavior is a response to a stimulus, and this response has been rewarded. The motivation for behavior is habit, or responding to stimuli in established, long-standing patterns. Maladaptive behaviors are thought to have begun in response to uncomfortable levels of anxiety and to have been rewarded by the decreased anxiety level.

The behavior therapist, in contrast to practitioners using other therapeutic approaches, takes total responsibility for the cure of the client. The client has the maladaptive behavior, and the therapist has the tools to correct this behavior. The goal of treatment is to *decondition* anxiety and to alter maladaptive behavior. Each person has an individually designed program which is based on a clinical history. The behavior therapist is interested in the history of maladaptive behavior, since it is unique to the individual client in focus. Therapists using other modalities consider behavior only symptomatic and are interested in the underlying motivation.

Three learning principles underlie Wolpe's behavior therapy:[6]

1 *Reciprocal Inhibition* When a response inhibiting anxiety occurs in the presence of an anxiety-provoking stimulus, the bond between the stimulus and the anxiety weakens. For example, a child being held by its mother will not be as frightened by a barking dog as when facing the dog alone.

2 *Positive Reconditioning* The undesired behavior is not rewarded, while the behavior that is to replace the undesired behavior is rewarded every time it is exhibited.

3 *Experimental Extinction* Undesired behavior

is evoked but never rewarded; therefore it becomes progressively weaker. Mechanisms of experimental extinction are still being developed by behavior therapists.

The deconditioning of anxiety is central to the success of behavior therapy.[6] Four methods are used:

1 *Assertive behavior* is the expression of emotion appropriate to the current situation rather than an expression of anxiety. Expressions of normal emotions are rewarded. However, clients are warned not to act assertively when it is likely to evoke punishment from the environment.

2 *Systematic desensitization* is a step-by-step use of a counteracting emotion to overcome an undesirable emotional habit. This technique occurs in four steps: (*a*) training in deep muscle relaxation, (*b*) use of a scale of subjective anxiety, (*c*) construction of anxiety hierarchies, and (*d*) use of relaxation techniques in conjunction with anxiety hierarchies. Imagery is often used in conjunction with desensitization.

3 *Evoking strong anxiety* is used as another way to decondition anxiety. Two techniques are used: (*a*) *Flooding* uses real or imaginary situations to evoke strong anxiety responses. For example, a girl with a phobia about automobiles was kept in the back seat of a car in which she was continuously driven for 4 hours. Her fear soon reached panic proportions and then gradually subsided. At the end of the ride she was comfortable and henceforth was free from this phobia. (*b*) *Abreaction* is the process of stirring up distressing memories to evoke anxiety. These techniques are used repeatedly until the client no longer responds with fear or anxiety. The ability of the situation to elicit fear or anxiety is diminished and finally exhausted.

4 *Operant conditioning* refers to conditioned responses of motor and cognitive behaviors versus autonomic behavior. The point of operant conditioning is to elicit adaptive motor and cognitive behaviors. There are five operant techniques: positive reinforcement, negative reinforcement, differential reinforcement, extinction, and punishment. The techniques, definitions, and examples are shown in Table 4-5.

The major criticism of Wolpe's behavior therapy is that, since behavior therapy treats only the symptom and not the underlying problem, *symptom substitution* will occur. Another maladaptive behavior will replace the extinguished behavior. Wolpe, on the other hand, states that the behavior is the problem and not a symptom. In his clinical experience, there have been no symptom substitutions.[6]

Behavior therapy principles are being researched extensively by nurses. Establishing self-feeding in nursing-home residents[7] and body positioning of patients with spinal-cord injuries[8] are just two examples of the uses of behavior therapy principles in nursing. Nurses are using learning principles to help patients and their families alter many forms of behavior, for instance, enuresis and alcoholism.

Neal E. Miller and John Dollard

Neal Miller and John Dollard combined the Freudian outlook with Pavlov's learning theories to develop their behaviorist theory. They think, as Freudians do, that behavior is symptomatic of underlying personality. Also, like the behaviorists, they hold that behavior is learned and can be unlearned. They accept Freud's description of neurosis, defense mechanisms, and treatment. They advocate the use of learning theories as the basis for treatment. There are four fundamentals of learning: drive, cue, response, and reinforcement. *Drive* is motivation; it can be *primary* (biological) or *secondary* (learned). *Cue* is a stimulus, a push to respond. *Response* is a thought, feeling, or action caused by the cue. *Reinforcement* is a reward for the response. Miller and Dollard consider a decrease in fear-anxiety to be the major reinforcement in neurotic behavior. The object of fear is

Table 4-5 Operant Conditioning Techniques

Technique	Definition	Examples
Positive reinforcement	Use of reward to increase the rate of response	When a child picks up the toys, praise and a piece of candy are given.
Negative reinforcement	Removal of tension or pain to increase the rate of response	As the examination approaches, the student becomes more anxious. The evening before the examination, the student develops symptoms of a cold. After the student decides to call in sick, the anxiety level decreases markedly.
Differential reinforcement	Combination of positive and negative reinforcement	A person experiencing a chronically uncomfortable level of cervical pain begins meditating. This decreases the anxiety. The person reports the results to the nurse, suggesting this option, and the nurse responds with delight to the person's efforts.
Extinction	Lack of reinforcement of behavior patterns, designed to decrease the rate of response	A nurse has noticed that Mr. Jones talks constantly about his psychosomatic symptoms when she listens and asks questions (positive reinforcement). She changes the subject to avoid focus on his symptoms (lack of reinforcement).
Punishment, or aversion therapy	Giving an obnoxious reward to inhibit an undesired response	A man guilty of child molestation is given a moderate electric shock each time he looks at a picture of a child.

repressed and is called *anxiety.* Four learning principles are based on these fundamentals.

1 *Extinction* is a decrease in the rate of neurotic behavior when the behavior is not reinforced.
2 *Spontaneous recovery* is the tendency for neurotic behavior to recur periodically, even in the absence of reinforcement.
3 *Generalization* is the tendency to transfer the learnings in one situation to other similar situations.
4 *Discrimination* is the ability to notice the similarities and differences in like situations.

Miller and Dollard state that one sign of neurosis is the inability to solve one's own emotional problems. This occurs primarily because of repression, a defense mechanism rendering the person unable to remember thoughts, feelings, actions, and perceptions. Miller and Dollard hypothesize that anxiety-provoking situations must be either unlabeled or mislabeled in order to be repressed. Consequently, there is no method by which to recall them. Since the problem is uncon-scious and undefined, the patient is unable to use problem-solving processes.

Miller and Dollard submit that conflict is the basis of neurosis. Drives build up, like the drive for water (primary drive) or for money (secondary drive). If the ways to decrease the drive generate fear, the behavior is blocked. Conflict between drive and fear occurs. The result is neurotic behavior that slightly decreases the drive and avoids the fear-anxiety.

There are two kinds of conflicts. The *avoidance-avoidance conflict* occurs when one must choose between two undesirable alternatives. For instance, a person may not want to suffer with cholecystitis but may not want surgical intervention either. The *approach-avoidance conflict* occurs when one has ambivalent feelings toward the same object. One wishes, simultaneously, to approach and to avoid the object. For example, a nurse may want an administrative position but may not want the responsibility. The conflict theory revolves around the assumption that fear-anxiety is one of the strongest sources of avoidance.

In this view, people are seen as learners.

When rewarded, people learn adaptive as well as maladaptive behaviors. Neurosis is defined by behaviorists as the result of having learned maladaptive behaviors. It is characterized by the manifest difference between the opportunity for enjoyment and the capacity for it. Conflict, stupidity, and misery portray the neurotic's behavior. Behavior is motivated by primary and secondary drives, including the drive to reduce anxiety-fear.

The therapist is seen as a teacher who listens, accepts, and does not punish or condemn. The therapist has four characteristics: (1) mental freedom from repressions and fears, (2) empathy with the client's fears, (3) restraint from talking too much or giving too many rewards, and (4) positive belief in the person's capacity to learn and to unlearn.

The goal of therapy is to remove repressions and to restore the use of higher mental processes for problem solving. The processes of therapy are primarily analytic. The therapist creates an atmosphere conducive to openness and trust, one that decreases anxiety-fear. Free association is a primary technique used to uncover repressed material. The principles of learning are used. The therapist aids the client in increasing the ability to discriminate between old and new situations. The client is helped to look at childhood behaviors that have been generalized to adult situations. The therapist rewards only the attempts at constructive new behaviors and encourages the client to seek major rewards outside the therapy situation. The therapist attempts to construct graded social situations that will help the client to overcome anxiety-fear and to reach the goal: constructive new behavior. There are two aspects to treatment: talking with the therapist and changing behavior in the real world. The client must be encouraged to take risks, to develop connections between the plan and the action. Without behavior change, therapy is a failure. For instance, a person may develop insight into the reasons for distrust of others. However, if relationships based on trust are not developed after insight has been gained, therapy is a failure.

Nurses utilize several of these concepts. The principle of discrimination has been used to help clients describe cognitive, physiological, and psychomotor changes. For instance, the nurse encourages the client to describe thoughts, feelings, and actions that were associated with new situations in the client's childhood. Then the thoughts, feelings, and actions associated with beginning a new job are elicited. Finally, the nurse aids the client in identifying the aspects of the situation that are different *now*.

The principle of generalization is used to transfer learning from therapeutic relationships to the situation at home (see Chap. 6).

Graduated learning situations are helpful in teaching clients about procedures that may generate fear-anxiety. For example, expanding teaching to include preadmission, presurgery, and postdischarge helps the client deal with anxieties associated with these situations. Having the client identify, in rank order, what aspects of a given technique generate least anxiety to most anxiety helps the nurse set priorities. The nurse will not move on to the next aspect of learning until the client is comfortable with what has already been learned.

The concept of labeling encourages nurses to share information about anatomy, body functions, and emotions with their clients. Understanding the dynamics of conflicts increases the nurse's understanding of clients' ambivalence and the very real misery they feel.

Phenomenological Theorists

Phenomenological theories focus on the person's thoughts, feelings, experiences, and perceptions; they are not concerned with "reality."

R. D. Laing

Laing feels that one has to study more than behavior to understand people. Laing is interested in three modes of human experience: perception, memory, and imagination. He is certain that, if a disturbed person's perceptions, memories, and fantasies were known and understood, that person's behavior would make sense.

Laing's view of the individual includes his or her environment, especially the family. Laing sees experiences as being filtered through rules taught by the family and imposed by the culture. This experience, then, becomes an image. Thus one would not experience a family but an image of the family. The rules can distort the actual experience. It is difficult to know whether an experience has been distorted, because there are often rules about the rules, called *metarules.*

One's behavior is a reflection of the images of the true experience. Laing states that self-identity is learned in the same way as other experiences are perceived. *Identity is the story one tells oneself of who one is* [9] *and is the part of self that seems unchanging.* Laing says we become who we are *told* we are. Children may be told they are mean, witty, or intelligent, and they proceed to become what they have been told. Their identities are reflected by what they do, which is what they were told to do. *Attribution* is the process of telling another person what he or she is. *Induction* is the process of getting others to act the way one wants them to act. *Complementarity* is the relationship with another in which both people achieve actualization of their self-images; one fulfills or completes self in the other.

The therapist in Laing's framework is a detective. In order to understand a person, one must discover what is actually going on in that person's social situation. The therapist discovers the rules and the metarules in order to understand what determines the person's perceptions and memories. The goal of therapy is to help the person authentically experience self, others, and the world without the restrictions imposed by rules and metarules. This is accomplished through *demystification,* or defining issues properly and getting rid of the images.

Another mode of treatment is to let people be, to treat them as normal, involved human beings, respecting their rights to behave as they seem to feel compelled to behave. *Regression,* or acting as though one were younger chronologically, is accepted as normal behavior for the client. When they are allowed to live through this process uninterrupted, Laing says people feel reborn, unencumbered with the rules and metarules learned earlier. He holds that regression, rather than being the beginning of psychosis, may be the beginning of the healing process. Consequently, Laing's therapy goes on in communities where the rules and metarules are discovered, studied, and discarded. People learn to be themselves. One experiences the real self when an act is genuine, revealing, potentiating, and felt to be fulfilling. The therapist does not collude with the members of the social situation to continue the illusions and images of experience. Instead, the therapist articulates the underlying fantasy systems so as to expose them. The therapist gives *confirmation,* true positive or negative information relevant to the current situation. It often takes a long time to find out what is really going on, since the energies of the social system are used to prevent anything from happening. A static, unchanging reality versus a dynamic, ever-changing reality exists and is often difficult to analyze.

People in social situations join in *collusion,* which is self-deception among two or more people. *Disjunction* occurs when one refuses to collude with the group or sees a different image from the group's collusive image. If one's image threatens to dissolve the collusive image, one is thought to be crazy, psychotic, and unable to recognize reality.

By using *transpersonal defenses,* one can regulate the inner life of another person in order to preserve one's own inner life. An example of transpersonal defense is *mystification,* or misdefinition of the issues. For example, a parent may say to a child, "I know what you're really feeling. You're not angry. You're tired." Another example of transpersonal defense is *disconfirmation,* the act of denying the truth and confirming false images. This is often carried out through a tangential response. *Tangential responses* fit the initial statement inadequately, have a frustrating effect, and/or emphasize a part of the statement that is incidental. [9]

Nurses have utilized the confirmation response to validate a patient's experience of the current situation. Family systems, rather than individuals, are the focus of treatment among nurses. It is necessary for nurses to become aware of the rules and metarules governing their perceptions. For example, a nurse must recognize what rules govern the response to people like alcoholics, unwed mothers, and the aged. Professional education should be examined as carefully as the family context to discover rules that distort true experience. For example, students may be taught that the professional knows, better than the client, what the client needs. If the rule is learned, the nurse will be inattentive to the client's identification of needs.

Carl Rogers

Carl Rogers assumes that people see themselves as the center of a continually changing world of experience and that they respond to the world as it is perceived. The person responds as a whole to the perceptions of the world, and the response is in the direction of actualization and enhancement. Rogers believes that the best vantage point for understanding behavior is from the internal frame of reference of individuals themselves. He states that psychological maladjustment occurs when people deny significant experiences, which consequently do not become integrated into the experience of self. This circumstance is reflected by the presence of tension.

Rogers views people as able to direct their lives in healthy, forward-moving ways. If the therapist holds unwaveringly to an attitude of respect for and confidence in the client's capacity to direct self, the client will develop self-confidence and self-respect. Rogers feels that in a climate of unconditional acceptance, people are able to become aware of the unconscious material that is controlling their lives. As clients come to know and accept that material, perceptions and behaviors change.

Behavior is goal-directed and motivated by needs. Unlike the intrapsychic and interpersonal theorists, Rogers states that current needs are the only ones the person endeavors to satisfy.

The therapist offers unconditional understanding and acceptance to the client. It takes work and self-development to achieve change in attitude and the locus of evaluation must always lie with the client. The outcome is a more broadly based structure of self, involving the inclusion of a greater proportion of experience and a more comfortable, realistic adjustment to life. This is reflected in lasting behavior and personality change. These changes are accomplished by creating an environment in which unconscious material can emerge. In this environment, attitudes are explored, concerns are addressed directly, and the client finds the answers. Clients face difficult periods as they discover denied attitudes, face repressed feelings, and reorganize perceptions. The major therapeutic tools are reflection, nondirective participation, and empathic identification. The point is to understand the client so well, through empathic identification, that the therapist becomes a reflection of the client. During this process the therapist continues to accept the client and to forfeit evaluation, encouraging the client to accept self and look at self objectively. The technique of reflection helps the client hear the perceptions and attitudes more objectively. Reflective statements are not evaluative. For example, the client says, "I hate myself and I'd be better off dead." Using reflection, the nurse may say, "You hate yourself so much you want to die."

Communication Theorists

Communications theories are based on the idea that behavior disorders result from the effects of human communication.

Eric Berne

Eric Berne assumed that all human behavior could be categorized into three states: *parent* ego state, *adult* ego state, and *child* ego state. These are often confused with Freud's superego, ego, and id. However, Berne's states are all functions of the ego, and no aspect of the theory deals with superego and id. No ego state is considered more valuable than another at any time. Six-month old infants exhibit adult ego-state behaviors, and the spontaneity, creativity, and joy of the child ego state are hallmarks of healthy people throughout life. Healthy people are thought to respond to the current situation with ego-state behaviors that promote personal growth, effective relationships, and efficient problem-solving. Ego states are presented in Fig. 4-1.

The clients are thought to be capable of deciding on what they need, their directions of growth, and how to live their lives. Clients are thought to be in full control of themselves rather than at the mercy of unconscious libidinal forces. This entails much more than an exercise in self-control.

Berne developed *script theory* to explain the control people exercise over their lives. At an early age, based on the integration of childhood experiences—including fairy tales, comic books, television, and experiences with significant people—children decide how the world is and choose their places in that world. This happens even though the child has undeveloped assessment skills, thinks very concretely, and has inadequate information. People live according to those early decisions, which are like lifelong self-fulfilling prophecies. When stuck with early script decisions, people feel they have no choices, even though the decision is obsolete and the resulting behavior is troublesome.

Much of the theory of *transactional analysis* uses language that appeals to the child ego state. Since the child decided the life script, it is the child in the person who must be addressed. The parent and adult ego-state efforts are sabotaged by a neglected, stroke-starved child ego state.

Motivation for behavior is the need for gestures of personal recognition called *strokes.* Strokes can be *positive* ("I love you"), *negative* ("I wish you were never born"), or *plastic,* which means that they sound positive but feel negative. One of the first (implicit) questions children ask is "How do I get strokes around here?" The answer depends on the people in the child's life who give recognition. They may stroke feelings such as happiness, anger, or depression. They may reward behavior such as helplessness, helpfulness, or rebelliousness. The child may decide that the exhibition of the stroked behavior is the way to get strokes, now and forever. People act out those behaviors, fearing that the strokes will stop and they will shrivel up and die. One motivation for change is the realization that one is no longer dependent on the childhood sources of strokes. One has many other options now.

The therapist using Berne's theories is a resource person who is able to offer potency, protection, and permission to the client. Since it is the child in the person who decided how things were, the child must be addressed. The therapist must be seen by the client as potent enough to protect the child when rules that are thought to be sacred are broken. In addition, the child often needs permission from this potent therapist to break the rules governing perceptions, feelings, and life plan. The process of therapy usually occurs in groups, and each person develops a *contract*, a behavioral objective, with the therapist. The client knows what would make his or her life more fulfilling, more interesting, or more fun. This knowledge is stated in concrete terms and discussed with the therapist. The therapist decides whether to work with the client to fulfill the contract statement. When the goal stated in the contract is completed,

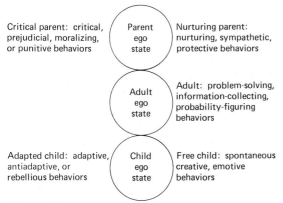

Figure 4-1 Berne's ego states. (*Adapted from E. Berne, Transactional Analysis in Psychotherapy, Grove, New York, 1961.*)

the client opts to terminate therapy or to develop another contract. At all times, the decision is in the hands of the client. The therapist uses five kinds of analysis to help clarify the client's difficulty:

1 *Ego-state analysis* aids the client in determining what ego state certain behaviors come from, thus helping the client to detect problematic behaviors in each ego state.
2 *Transactional analysis* is the analysis of communications between two people. A *transaction* consists of a stimulus from one agent and a response from another. The three kinds of transactions are explained in Fig. 4-2.
3 *Script analysis* is the discovery of the client's life plan, since the client is often not aware of this.
4 *Game analysis* is the discovery of recurrent behavior patterns that are problematic.
5 *Stroke-economy analysis* is an analysis of the kinds of strokes that are acceptable to the client. Increasing the available strokes helps to change one's life plan. The idea here is that the script was determined in order to maintain the source of strokes.[10,11]

Nurses utilize the concept of strokes by acknowledging the client's need for recognition. Some client behaviors are bids for personal recognition. Meeting the need for recognition and attention becomes positive and health producing when the nurse works within Berne's framework. The notion that people may need permission to take care of themselves, to slow down, or to have fun rather than killing themselves is being utilized effectively by nurses. Game theory is helpful in understanding the interpersonal relationships in families. It is also useful in understanding the collegial relationships among nurses, physicians, and administrators. Understanding that misunderstandings occur in crossed transactions is helpful in almost all situations.[12]

Paul Watzlawick

Paul Watzlawick worked with Janet H. Beavin and Don D. Jackson to evolve a communications theory. This theory assumes that there is no difference between a normal and a disturbed person's communication if both are stuck in a situation and are unwilling to communicate. The circumstance dictates a certain response which may be considered disturbed. For example, when a client is given no pain medication, is told not to move or scream, and undergoes a painful procedure, the client may kick the physician. While this is considered disturbed behavior, the client has been given no avenue through which to express emotion.

This theory focuses on the relationship between two people. Relationships are characterized by dynamic communication patterns which are recognized by their redundancies. The topic changes but the pattern remains the same. Relationships are dynamic by virtue of the *feedback loop*. Every piece of communication is at the same time a response to a stimulus and a stimulus designed to elicit a response, establishing a circular pattern of communication. The feedback loop is shown in Fig. 4-3. *Positive feedback* is any communication that leads to change in the relationship. *Negative feedback* is any communication that maintains the status quo in the relationship. The behavior of each person affects and is affected by the behavior of the other person. Because of the continuous, circular nature of the communication, any distinction between beginning and end or cause and effect is purely arbitrary.

Watzlawick and his colleagues proposed five tentative axioms underlying communication:[13]

1 *A person cannot not communicate.* There is no such thing as nonbehavior. The attempt to avoid behavior results in confusing, unorthodox messages denying that communication is occurring. For example, as a mother says, "I love you, son," she backs away from his embrace.
2 There are two levels of any message: the content and the relationship. The *content level* conveys information verbally, and the *relationship level* conveys information about the relationship between the people sending messages. There are three possible classes of relationship messages: the relationship can confirm, disconfirm, or reject the other

A *complementary transaction* occurs when a person responds from the ego state addressed.

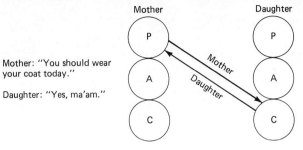

Mother: "You should wear your coat today."

Daughter: "Yes, ma'am."

Diagram of a complementary transaction

(a)

A *crossed transaction* occurs when a person does not respond from the ego state addressed.

Mother: "You should wear your coat today."

Daughter: "You probably shouldn't go out at all with your cold, mother."

Diagram of a crossed transaction

(b)

An *ulterior transaction* occurs when the interaction seems to occur on one level, but really occurs on another.

Mother:."You should wear your coat today." (Ulterior: "You're too stupid to know what to do.")

Daughter: "Yes, ma'am." (Ulterior: "I'm smart enough to agree with you.")

Mother Ulterior

Daughter Ulterior

Diagram of an ulterior transaction

(c)

Figure 4-2 Crossed, complementary, and ulterior transactions. (*Adapted from E. Berne, Games People Play, Grove, New York, 1964.*)

person's message about the relationship. *Confirming messages* agree that the other person's message about the relationship is correct. *Rejecting messages* state that the other person's message about the relationship is wrong. *Disconfirming messages* tell the

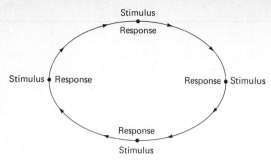

Figure 4-3 Feedback loop. Every response is at the same time a stimulus, evoking another response. (*Adapted from P. Watzlawick, J. H. Beavin, D. D. Jackson, the Pragmatics of Human Communication, Norton, New York, 1967.*)

receivers that they do not exist. The relationship aspect demands a response from the receiver. This aspect is called *metacommunication,* or communication about communication (Laing's concept). Problems occur when there are confusions, contaminations, or contradictions between the levels. In the mother-son example above, there is a contradiction between the content and the relationship levels.

3 Though communications appear uninterrupted to the outsider, the participants identify arbitrary beginnings and endings in the sequence. These arbitrary decisions are called *punctuation.* Punctuation organizes communication patterns and is vital to ongoing relationships. Problems occur in a relationship when two people punctuate the communication sequence differently. For example, a husband may say he drinks because the wife nags, while the wife says she nags because the husband drinks.

4 Two kinds of communication occur: analogic and digital. *Analogic communication* is all nonverbal communication, including such variables as voice tone, inflection, posture, and the choice of words. *Digital communication* is verbal communication and is more logical, complex, and abstract than analogic communication.

5 There are two possible interactions: symmetrical and complementary. *Symmetrical interactions* are characterized by equality, with a minimum of difference between the two partners. When problems occur in symmetrical interactions, then the two people compete with each other and escalate behavior. The relationship aspects of the message reject the other's view of the relationship. *Complementary interactions* are based on a maximum of difference between the two partners; they are sometimes called "one-up, one-down" interactions. When problems occur in complementary interactions, the relationship becomes rigid and the one-up person is always *one-up* while the partner is always *one-down.* In rigid complementary interactions, the relationship aspect of the message disconfirms the other's view of the relationship. Both complementary and symmetrical interactions are found in healthy, dynamic relationships.

People in a relationship form a unit, a system with rules guiding the behavior patterns. Sometimes the pattern established in a relationship goes awry. The therapist is considered an outsider who can help the system do what it cannot do by itself, that is, change its rules. A primary tool in this endeavor is metacommunication. The goal of treatment is to teach systems—families, groups, dyads—how to communicate about their communication, interactions, and relationships. The process of treatment includes a search for the communication pattern, here and now, in the system. The entire system is treated, since a change in one person will alter the behavior of the others. Problematic communication patterns are often treated in brief psychotherapy.

There are two other tools unique to this modality: prescribing the symptom and using the therapeutic double bind. When *prescribing the symptom,* the therapist suggests that the client increase or in some way manipulate the manifestation of symptomatic behavior. The client discovers that the behavior believed to be out of control is controllable. The *therapeutic double bind* is based on the naturally occurring double bind which leads to disturbed communication. (See Chap. 11.) The therapeutic double bind uses the importance of the psychotherapeutic relationship to give the client an injunction in which the two messages are mutually exclusive. There are three components to a double bind:

1 An interpersonal situation exists which is meaningful to at least one person.
2 A message is given in which the content and the relationship aspects are mutually exclusive.
3 The recipient is prevented from leaving the situation.

The person in a double-bind situation feels "damned if he does and damned if he doesn't." Therapeutic double binds are difficult to create, but if well constructed, they will force the client to step out of the frame set by the dilemma. The client will "change if they do act and change if they don't." This technique forces the client to communicate about the communication verbally and/or nonverbally. Whatever the clients do, behavior different than the usual has been forced. This is a form of metacommunication. The therapist then works with the system to increase digital metacommunication rather than allowing the metacommunication to remain analogic, or nonverbal.

The application of this theory to nursing practice defines the client within the context of family and society. This emphasis will drastically alter nursing practice as nurses increasingly offer autonomous service.

Since the context of communication determines the communication, nurses can examine the present relationship, here and now, to clarify the relationship and the content levels of the communication. For example, the hospital setting dictates that the physician is responsible for the clients' treatment. This places the physician in a one-up position in relation to the nurse. When the nurse makes a decision concerning nursing care, a conflict may occur in the usual one-up, one-down relationship.

Metacommunication is an important tool for nurses. Because nursing services are delivered via relationships, nurses must develop the ability to talk about what is happening in their relationships with clients. Communication becomes much richer with this theory. Nurses realize that communications consist of relationship as well as content aspects.

Systems Theorists

Systems theory is based on the idea that *wholes* should be the object of study. To study a part is misleading, since the answers pertain only to the part and not to the whole. For instance, focusing on the mind does not say anything about the person. Systems theorists propose that there are abstract laws applying to all systems. A system is a person, a family, a hospital, the ecological system, the economic system, etc.

Ludwig von Bertalanffy

Ludwig von Bertalanffy is a biologist who became concerned about personality theories that reduced human beings to the equivalent of rats, dogs, and robots. He thought that taking into account only a person's mind led to a mechanistic picture of people and a dehumanized society. He developed an *organismic* concept. He deals with a living system as a whole, as opposed to using an analytical and summative approach. A *system* is defined as a complex of components in interaction.[14] People are thought to be more than and different from the sum of their parts. Systems research is the study of wholes as entities rather than as conglomerations of parts.

Von Bertalanffy was one of the first theorists who considered the world as an organized system. He discovered several abstract laws guiding the behavior of all systems, including people.

1 *Systems are organized complexities.* This is contrasted with the idea of a cause-effect relationship, in which too few variables were considered. An example of the cause-effect view: When children undergo stringent toilet training (one variable), they will have

obsessive-compulsive traits (the effect) as adults. An example of the systems view: Behavior traits are the reflection of hundreds of variables, including family, culture, and individual factors. Systems theory is nonmechanistic in holding that behavior is not determined by structural conditions but by relationships among forces. The interplay among various forces and the patterns of these interactions identify the uniqueness of a system.

2 *No system repeats its interactions.* There are no feedback loops or stimulus-response-reward loops in systems theory. Instead, there is a dynamic interaction among the variables currently present in the situation. Every moment is a unique situation, never having occurred before and never to be repeated.

3 *Evolution proceeds from a less to a more differentiated state.* The changes occurring with the person and environment proceed from simple to complex. The interaction between the person and environment results in a more complex person and environment.

4 *There are regular changes in the evolution of all systems.* For example, all children are expected to undergo changes in growth and development within certain parameters. If the development is too fast or slow, too much or little, the child undergoes diagnostic testing to discover abnormalities. The evolution of systems toward states of higher improbability, order, and differentiation is included in this principle. This negates the "survival of the fittest" idea. All systems change in surprising directions, not in the direction of simplicity. Von Bertalanffy states that adaptation is an incorrect view. It is precisely the lack of adaptation that has made it possible to conquer the planet and explore the universe.

5 *People are living, open (metabolizing) systems,* exhibiting self-differentiation, providing energy, and having a stored information system (genetic code) to steer the process. Two factors do not apply to all living systems but are unique to humanity: the evolution of symbolism and an active personality system.

Symbolism is the product of evolution. There are four criteria of symbolism:

1 Symbols are representative; the symbol stands for the thing it symbolizes. Language and art are examples.
2 Symbols are transmitted by learning processes rather than by innate instinct.
3 Symbols are freely created. There is no biological connection between the symbol and the thing symbolized. This contrasts with Freud's concept that all symbols have biological derivations.
4 Symbolism is the impetus in human evolution. The symbol of country has led to the national anthems, flags, armies, wars, war-making machinery, arms escalation, and detente. Symbolism is a stronger motivating force than organismic drives. Symbolism leads to behavior that directly contradicts biology and individuality. Symbolism makes it possible for people to starve themselves as a form of protest, to remain passive while being assaulted, to risk dying in the face of war.

The *active personality system* is the second characteristic unique to humanity. This system is the result of the fact that people are open systems, able to maintain states distant from equilibrium and to use the potential inherent in their humanity.[14] Spontaneous activity is the primary ability. The person participates fully in evolution, in the relationship with the environment. This contrasts with the stimulus-response model, which cuts out a small piece of behavior, ignores many important variables, and arbitrarily decides what is stimulus and what is response.

Von Bertalanffy's view expands the time and space frame and looks at a more complex picture. It is this totality that maintains the dignified, complex understanding of humanity.

Reality, in von Bertalanffy's system, has three levels: inanimate, living, and symbolic. Each level has its own laws which cannot be derived from or reduced to another level.[14] However, the behavior of one level often resembles that of another. An example of this is the pattern of growth and development found on all three levels. Studying the growth and development of the inanimate level will not explain the growth and development of symbolism.

Von Bertalanffy was concerned with explaining the behavior of the human system as a whole and did not concern himself with pathological behavior and its treatment. His theories indicate that pathological behavior must be viewed in light of current culture and time. Hundreds of variables participate in the formation of current behavior, therefore one cannot look for one cause.

Nursing takes into consideration the wholeness of people. Many disciplines are studied in order to arrive at an understanding of the complex nature of humanity. Nurses learn that one part does not add up to the totality of a person. For instance, people are not treated as gallbladders. The attempt to reduce the whole person to a part is incorrect and dehumanizing.

Treating the parts of a person as structures that change only under pathological conditions is also misleading. Nurses focus on the relationship and on the interaction of all the parts to understand the uniqueness of the individual. Nurses also look at the relationship of one family member with the family as a whole to understand behavior in the family. This applies to the relationships among all systems, for instance, between family and community or between a nation and the world. It is the pattern of interaction that is important when one utilizes systems theory.

Kurt Lewin

Kurt Lewin applies systems theory to the individual. He sees the person as a totality of systems. It is the way the systems are integrated that makes a person unique. The field Lewin chooses to study is the person-environment field.

Behavior in Lewin's framework is the result of all the forces in the person and the environment acting together. The environmental forces are not purely physical. Rather, there are *psychobiological forces*—quasi-physical, quasi-social, and quasi-mental forces—which are dynamic. The psychobiological environment consists not only of those facts that are actually perceptible but also a range of past and future events.[15] Each force in the psychobiological environment has a positive, negative, or neutral *valence,* the strength of attraction or repulsion. A force also has a direction, called a *vector.*

The totality of forces present in the psychobiological field controls the direction of the process. All forces are changed by the process, and the changed forces yield different processes in an ongoing, dynamic relationship.

Lewin's ideas of reality are similar to the phenomenological view. The way the person perceives the environment is important. For instance, an underground newspaper has a neutral valence for the person who is neither attracted nor repelled by it, while it has a positive valence for the person who thumbs through it. The newspaper has a negative valence for someone who is upset and repelled by it.

In Lewin's framework, the individual is seen as a relatively closed system. That is, the individual does not simply respond to the environmental forces like a billiard ball. People choose their objects of interest and initiate activity.

For Lewin, the motivations for behavior are needs or needlike tensions. It is the person's needs that make objects, people, or events take on a positive, negative, or neutral valence. Once the tensions accompanying the needs are decreased, other tensions arise and the objects in the environment take on different valences. The past is only one of many factors influencing a person's needs and the way in which the environment is perceived. The energies of a psychic process do not flow from momentary perceptions or from distant, past developmental events. Instead, the whole person, the current needs, and the psychobiological environmental forces determine the direction of the process.

Lewin considers the development of the child an important influence on the person. The total milieu in which the child is raised is more important than particular factors. Some theories state that factors such as one-parent families, poor nutrition, or domineering mothers warp children's personalities. Lewin states that consideration of particular features confuses the understanding of development. Only consideration of the total situation over time will yield an understanding of the person's development. During the first months of life, forces of the psychobiological environment are determined primarily by the infant's needs. As a child grows, possibilities and difficulties arise primarily because the child lives in the field of other people's social forces. The child's sense of reality must include an awareness of his or her needs. When not based on recognition of one's needs, the assessment of reality is flimsy and easily collapses.

The present will influence future situations. A person learns the content of an experience and also the rules that guide the experience. The content of a situation may be completing an arithmetic problem, making a new friend, or figuring out how a compass works. Accompanying each of these experiences is a set of rules that can be learned and generalized to similar experiences. These rules are rarely discussed but are required to complete the experience successfully and to repeat a similar experience more quickly. For instance, to make a new friend, a child must learn the rules: don't stand too close, learn the name and say it several times, find out what interests the person, do not speak too loudly or too softly, approximate the other in quality and intimacy of speech, find something to like in the person. If the rules are learned incompletely, the task may take on a negative valence and the solution may be inferior. The next time the experience is approached, the negative valence becomes stronger, which compounds the difficulty of the task and compromises the quality of the solution. According to Lewin, the vicious cycles often seen in mental retardation, behavior problems, and learning disorders are the result of the person-environment interaction.

The future is also important in the present. A person must learn temporal displacement of goals in order to function effectively. In other words, the future must have some reality in the present if the person is to be motivated to delay gratification.

Problem solving for Lewin consists of assessing the total situation. The totality of the valences, vectors, and barriers in the situation are assessed before problem-solving behavior begins. Movement toward the goal will alter the view of the total situation and may encourage continuation of behavior or call for different behaviors. For example, a child sees a ball on the other side of a bench. The first view of the situation may create a positive valence of motivation toward the ball, generating a vector directly toward the ball. The child moves toward the ball and finds the bench in the way. The bench takes on the character of a barrier, necessitating a new assessment of the situation. The child may decide to climb over the bench, maintaining a straight vector toward the ball. If the child finds the bench impassable, another look at the situation is required. Once the child has decided that the bench is impassable, the bench takes on a negative valence—stronger than the positive valence of motivation toward the ball—and the child will give up and turn away. On the other hand, if motivation maintains a positive valence toward the ball, the child may try other behaviors. In this process, the assessment of the total situation may change. The child may discover that the way to get the ball is to move away from it first, to move around the barrier, and then move toward the ball. Problem solving, therefore, requires restructuring one's view of the total situation in order to discover feasible alternatives.

Barriers are psychological as well as physical. Parents' injunctions are real barriers to a child. Every rule a parent gives a child decreases the child's life space. *Life space* consists of all the facts that have existence for the individual at a particular time, the physical-psychological room in which a person feels free to move. Physical barriers temporarily decrease life space and eliminate only the space beyond the barrier. Psychological barriers permanently decrease life space and are often generalized to other areas as well, depending on the total situation over time. For example, a child is told, "Don't touch me." The child may figure that the parent does not ever want to be touched or to be touched only under certain circumstances. The child may also decide that any loved person should not be touched or should be touched only under certain conditions.

Punishment is one way a rule can be reinforced. In Lewin's view, punishment adds a negative valence to the situation. For instance, a woman is told that if she takes a job, her marriage will end. Taking a job takes on both a positive and a negative valence because of the punishment. It must be remembered that the total valences in any situation alter the individual's perception of every factor present.

Another example of punishment influence: Graduates think that if they do not study for State Nursing Board examinations, they will fail. The situation results in an avoidance-avoidance conflict.

The threat of punishment involves three possibilities:

1 The threat may be inherent in the situation, like thorns on a rose stem.
2 The threat can be made by one person to another, for example, by a teacher to a student.
3 The threat may be learned and may later arise from within the learner. Adults often punish themselves for behavior their parents once punished.

The difficulty with punishment is that the threatening person and the person receiving the threat become adversaries. The person who threatens takes on a negative valence; he or she will be avoided, feared, and hated. If people threaten themselves with punishment, they become enemies to themselves. The threat of punishment in a situation leads to six possible solutions:

1 The person may choose to close off from the task, the punishment, and the threatening person. The threatened person becomes insensitive to the threatening person and other forces in the situation.
2 The person may choose punishment and become disillusioned. The person finds that, though he or she is punished, the task must still be completed. This often leads to docility.

3 The person may attempt to avoid the task as well as the punishment by using flattery, defiance, or deceit.
4 The punishment may lose its aspect of disgrace. Failure to perform a task comes to seem more worthy of pride than does its completion.
5 The threatened person may choose to challenge the power of the threatening person by tracing all the vectors and barriers to the latter. If that power can be successfully challenged, the whole situation disintegrates.
6 The person may opt out of the field entirely. The ultimate physical method of leaving the field is suicide. The ultimate psychological method is psychosis.

Lewin advocates the use of valences and vectors present in the situation to induce wanted behavior. For instance, natural curiosity and inclination to learn may be utilized. The person's natural wish to please a loved one is more effective than a threat of punishment.

Since Lewin developed a theory of behavior based on the total person and the environment, he did not focus on pathology and treatment. Nurses utilize his concepts in several ways. The nurse realizes the importance of helping people recognize their needs in order to develop a strong sense of reality.

Utilizing natural curiosity and interest is important in deciding when to teach a client. Discovering the ways clients learn best is also important. Allowing the client to choose the direction and pace of learning derives from Lewin's concepts. The difficulties inherent in the use of punishment help nurses understand how they become adversaries rather than advocates. It is also clear how clients become enemies to themselves. The concept of life space helps the nurse understand what happens when clients seem unable to undertake necessary activities. For instance, if, as a child, a person has been taught, "Never play with your feces," it is difficult to teach him or her ileostomy care until that person's life space has been enlarged.

References

1 William Morris (ed.): *The American Heritage Dictionary of the English Language,* Houghton Mifflin, New York, 1969, pp. 688, 1335.

2 Sigmund Freud: *A General Introduction of Psychoanalysis,* Pocket Books, New York, 1972.

3 Erik H. Erikson: *Childhood and Society,* 2d ed., Norton, New York, 1963, pp. 423–424.

4 Harry Stack Sullivan: *The Interpersonal Theory of Psychiatry,* Norton, New York, 1953.

*5 Hildegard E. Peplau: *Interpersonal Relations in Nursing,* Putnam, New York, 1952, p. 126.

6 Joseph Wolpe: *The Practice of Behavior Therapy,* 2d ed., Pergamon, New York, 1973, pp. 16–20, 83, 95, 192, 205–215.

*7 Margaret M. Baltes and Melissa B. Zerbe: "Reestablishing Self-Feeding in a Nursing Home Resident," *Nursing Research,* January–February 1976, pp. 24–26.

*Recommended reference by a nurse author.

*8 Barbara C. Rottkamp: "A Behavior Modification Approach to Nursing Therapeutics in Body-Positioning of Spinal Cord-Injured Patients," *Nursing Research* May–June 1976, pp. 181–186.

9 R. D. Laing: *Self and Others,* Penguin, Baltimore, 1975, pp. 93, 103.

10 Eric Berne: *Games People Play,* Grove, New York, 1964.

11 Eric Berne: *Transactional Analysis in Psychotherapy,* Grove, New York, 1961.

*12 Pamela Levin and Eric Berne, "Games Nurses Play," *American Journal of Nursing,* March 1972, pp. 483–487.

13 Paul Watzlawick, Janet H. Beavin, and Don D. Jackson: *The Pragmatics of Human Communication,* Norton, New York, 1967.

14 Ludwig von Bertalanffy: *Robots, Men and Minds,* Braziller, New York, 1967, pp. 33, 69, 89.

15 Kurt Lewin: *A Dynamic Theory of Personality: Selected Papers,* McGraw-Hill, New York, 1935, pp. 79, 87.

5

Problem Resolution versus Crisis

Judith Haber

Learning Objectives

After studying this chapter, the student should be able to:

1 Identify the elements of a crisis
2 Define "maturational crisis"
3 Identify the developmental issues of the stages of growth and development throughout the life cycle
4 Define "situational crisis"
5 Identify the components of crisis intervention
6 Formulate a plan of intervention for clients based on a crisis-intervention model

A crisis is a turning point in a person's life, when a conflict or problem of basic importance is perceived as threatening and not readily solvable by means of previously successful coping mechanisms. The person is in a state of psychosocial disequilibrium. As a result, anxiety and tension increase, effective cognitive functioning decreases, behavioral disorganization follows, the person becomes less able to find a solution to the problem, and feels helpless to deal with it effectively.[1]

In the course of the life cycle, many experiences arise which have the potential for provoking conflicts and problems. Death of a significant other, marriage, parenthood, leaving home for college, and retirement are among such events. Rapaport states that in each of these situations emotional strain is generated and stress experienced. When such situations arise, a series of adaptive behaviors are activated which lead either to mastery of the situation or to the emergence of a crisis.[2] Aguilera states that when solutions are not forthcoming, such events become crises for those who by personality, previous experience, or other factors in the current situation are especially vulnerable to this stress and whose emotional resources and problem-solving abilities are taxed beyond their usual capacity.[3]

Crises have an inherent growth-producing potential. People who master the crisis situation independently or with professional assistance develop a new, broader repertoire of coping skills that help them deal effectively with life situations. Crises are limited by time and are generally resolved positively or negatively within 1 to 6 weeks.[4]

Two types of crises have been identified; the anticipated developmental or maturational crises of the life cycle and the unanticipated or situational crises. Nurses in a variety of occupational and health-care settings are in daily contact with people in crisis. People who are physically or mentally ill may be in crisis because their life-style has been disrupted, because of the uncertainty of the outcome of their illness, or because of the illness's financial cost. A couple who are approaching parenthood for the first time are facing a potential crisis revolving around role changes, expanded emotional investments, and changes in life-style. Because they confront these situations so often, nurses need to have a sound theoretical base from which to make nursing diagnoses and plan intervention for individuals and families in crisis.

Maturational Crisis

Maturational or developmental crises are predictable life events which normally occur in the lives of most individuals. A person's life is continuously changing because of the ongoing process of maturation. Aguilera states potential crisis areas are the periods of physical, social, and psychological change which are experienced during the normal growth process. These changes occur during periods of biological and social role transition between infancy, childhood, adolescence, young adulthood, marriage, parenthood, middle age, and old age.

The onset of a maturational crises is gradual and occurs over time as the person moves through a period of change.[5] Such transitional periods are characterized by internal disequilibrium and disorganized behavior. The person may experience mood swings and variations of normal behavior in terms of roles and relationships. Resolution occurs gradually—as the individual experiments with new feelings, roles, and behaviors—until a "comfortable fit" is achieved. The person then moves onto a new level of mastery and maturity.

Maturational crises are predictable and therefore can be anticipated and prepared for. However, hazardous situations such as physical illness, job loss, or divorce are unpredictable and may act to compound the stress and disequilibrium experienced during a maturational crisis. The goal of intervention is to decrease the crisis experience and utilize it as an opportunity for internal growth and mastery of the environment. New coping skills are learned in order to deal with maturational tasks. For example, expectant parents have three coping skills to learn in relation to parenting: role modification, expanding the relationship, and energy redistribution.

Negative resolution of a transition period may result in a developmental stall. The stall may interfere with the person's self-concept, relationships with others, and control of the environment. The theoretical concepts relating to maturational crises will be divided into the generally acknowledged stages of growth and development.

Infancy

During the first year of life, the developmental crisis revolves around helplessness and dependency. The infant does not view the self as separate from others or the environment. The state of helplessness and fusion forces the infant to trust that the nurturing figure will gratify basic physical and emotional needs. Predictability and continuity are internalized by the infant through the developing olfactory, visual, auditory, and tactile senses.[6]

The symbiotic relationship with the mother forms the foundation for the development of the self-concept. The infant whose nurturing needs are met in a positive way will experience the mother as good and the self—a fused part of mother—as good. This forms the basis for trust and confidence in self and others.[7] As a result of varied interchanges between the nurturing person and the child, confidence is developed.

In infancy, the oral zone is the primary one through which gratification is obtained. Feeding becomes an important activity. Prompt feedings accompanied by ample amounts of tactile stimulation increase the infant's confidence that needs will be met and that the environment can be trusted. Sporadic feedings and inconsistent feeling tones communicated by the mother will lead to uncertainty, anxiety, and a sense of mistrust in the infant. The anxious behavior of the infant may generate further inadequate or inconsistent nurturing patterns and perpetuate a cycle of anxiety and mistrust of others and the environment. Maladaptive behavior patterns emerge quickly in an infant. The cycle of protest, crying, withdrawal, despair,

and death can appear within 4 to 6 weeks of inadequate mothering and stimulations.

A gradual decrease in symbiosis and the beginning of separation occurs as the infant explores self and external environmental boundaries through sensorimotor learning.[8] If the child does not develop a positive sense of self and trust in others, the stage is set for problems in later life such as mistrust, depression, superficial relationships, and dependency.

Early Childhood

During the second and third years of life, the developmental crisis revolves around the shift from dependence on others to self-reliance and independent activity. The beginning sense of "I" marks the initiation of autonomy. The child begins to learn socially acceptable behavior by abandoning needs for self-gratification to some extent and incorporating parental demands, which are representative of the larger society. At this period, sexuality and gratification center around the anal zone of the body. Issues of control, which contain the ingredients of a power struggle, are exemplified by the child's need to coordinate "holding on and letting go." Toilet training, or the "battle of the pot," exemplifies this and is resolved when the child complies with the parents' wishes in order to retain parental approval and love and to maintain minimum levels of anxiety.[6,7] The child develops other areas of control relating to activities of daily living as well as interpersonal and cognitive tasks. Mastery of words such as "no" and primitive conceptual abilities[8] help the child to manipulate the environment.

Basic concepts regulating a balance between love and hate, cooperation and willfulness, self-expression and suppression are developed. Failure to negotiate the tasks of this stage is manifested by feelings of shame and doubt, fear of self-disclosure, and ritualistic behavior. In adulthood, lack of autonomy is exhibited in the individual who has an excessive need for control, order, and approval, which may be manifested in overconforming behavior and irrational rituals.[6]

Preschool

During the preschool period (ages 3 to 6) the developmental crisis revolves around the issues of initiative and identity. Children use initiative to further explore self and the environment. They consider what kind of people they are going to be and move about the environment to explore play, language, and relationships. Play offers an opportunity to utilize imagination and fantasy and to experiment with gender and role identity. Language expands and children ask many questions to cognitively substantiate their expanding world of imagination and fantasy. Sexual identity is developed via identification with the parent of the same sex and infantile sexual strivings toward the parent of the opposite sex are renounced. Fantasy, imagination, and preoccupation with the body result in normal guilt about dreams, wishes, and thoughts relating to self and parents. The conscience develops as external prohibitions are *introjected* and become part of the self. The child develops *signal anxiety,* which is the ability to anticipate wrongdoing by connecting a wish with its consequence. Anxiety is controlled through play, fantasy, and pride in accomplishment. Work is goal-directed and learning occurs quickly. The child begins to share as the circle of significant others expands. Networks for positive feedback increase via nursery school, peers, and relatives.

Children who are adjusting well will talk about the future and their possible roles in it. Children who have encountered developmental blocks, on the other hand, may feel that they have no right to dream. The secure child feels worthy and competent even though small.[3] Failure to successfully negotiate the issues of this developmental stage results in a child who suffers psychosexual confusion and displays rigidity and guilt in interpersonal relationships. Such children experience loss of initiative in the exploration of new skills.

School Age

During the school-age period (ages 6 to 12) the developmental crisis revolves around the issues of industry and learning. The child feels that "I am what I learn"[6] and learns to win recognition by producing things. There is pride in mastery and feeling useful. The child feels good when diligence produces a completed task. Sexual fantasy is repressed and sublimated into industry. Gender identity is solidified through work and play.

The cognitive phase of development is characterized by mastery of skills in manipulating objects and understanding relationships. This enables the child to begin problem-solving processes; by age 11 abstract deductive problem solving should be present.[8]

Self-esteem is derived from accomplishment and chumships. As peers and other ego ideals, such as teachers, become the center of the child's universe, the parents' influence decreases. Through cooperation, compromise, and collaboration, children take their place in their peer group, which is the core of their social life. Peers of the same sex are sought out and "best friends" develop. Secret societies, gangs, and team sports offer opportunities for playful aggression and acceptable sublimation of hostility.[6,7]

Failure to develop self-esteem and a sense of mastery at this stage may lead to feelings of inadequacy and inferiority which pervade later life. Earlier failures to develop a sense of initiative lead to lack of preparedness for school, or the school itself may fail to assist the child in developing the necessary skills for competency. The child feels, "I'll never be good at anything," and may increasingly display reluctance to explore the environment and relationships.[6]

Adolescence

During the years from 12 to 18 the developmental crises revolve around issues of individuation and differentiation. It is a time of rapid growth equaled only in early childhood.[9] Biological, psychological, social, and cognitive changes occur simultaneously; nothing is the same, everything is changing. There is a heightened vulnerability to stress because all the changes are occurring at once. Conflict is the instrument by which the individual learns the complex differences between self and the environment.[9]

Biologically, the child has to adjust to hormonal shifts, height-weight changes, and the development of secondary sex characteristics. As a new body image is being incorporated, feelings of discomfort, awkwardness, and self-consciousness predominate. The child wonders, "Am I normal? I feel so weird." Psychologically, a sense of personal identity is being forged. The child is coping with ambivalence centering about autonomy. Until a personal adjustment is arrived at, adolescents swing back and forth between covert dependence and independence. For example, one minute they may be borrowing a parent's clothes and the next minute they will accuse their parents of trying to run their lives and of not knowing anything. Rebelliousness against authority and the establishment is another way in which ambivalence is exhibited. Adolescents begin to blend the "wants" and "oughts" of significant others with their own. Judgments of self by significant others determine feelings of self-worth.[6] Feelings of sexuality must be dealt with and discharged in an acceptable way. This is a problem for the adolescent, who is often overwhelmed by sexual feelings and has no outlet for them other than self-stimulation. The adolescent needs to know that these feelings are completely normal.

Socially, adolescents are in transition. A concept of an acceptable social role identity is arrived at through experimentation. An inner lack of trust in self is manifested in group conformity. Peer-group cliques and gangs often show intolerance of those who do not belong. Rigid clothing styles, mannerisms, fetishes, and codes of behavior reflect a need to be accepted, wanted, and loved. If the person experiences acceptance in a group social situation, then individual heterosexual relationships will be sought. On the basis of these, a more or less enduring relationship with a member of the opposite sex will develop.[3,7]

Contemplation of the future—"Who I want to be and what do I want to do"—begins. Occupational identity becomes an issue of concern at this time. The adolescent is continuously bombarded by questions about career plans. Uncertainty is compounded since people of this age have not participated extensively in the world of work, and have observed only fragments of work situations and job roles. Consequently, they find it difficult to commit themselves to full-time job responsibility or to identify career choices.[3] Cognitively, the stage of formal operations is in progress. The adolescent can carry out abstract thought processes and is capable of complex deductive reasoning.[8]

Failure to negotiate the tasks of this stage result in the adolescent's failure to consolidate an idea of "who I am," which leads to deficits in assuming self-responsibility, a sense of inadequacy in controlling self, and an inability to compete successfully.[6]

Young Adulthood

Equipped with a provisional sense of identity, the young adult between the ages of 18 and 22 is coping with the developmental task of mastering the future versus the urge to remain directed and sheltered by others. Not all people become independent at this point. Many are not emotionally ready and need a moratorium to continue exploring the world and themselves. Others are educationally and financially dependent. However, most young adults do locate themselves in a peer group, a sex role, and an anticipated or actual occupation. They also develop an ideology or world view.

Young adults exercise their own power and choices; they have arrived at a degree of personal uniqueness which shows itself in a consistent way of feeling and behaving. Marriage and parenthood may be considered at this time. A healthy, intimate relationship with a significant other reflects interdependence. Minimal amounts of fusion should be exhibited in the relationship (see Chap. 11). Conflict can arise between parental values and identities and what the young adult can and wants to become. Inability to resolve the conflict results in low self-esteem which, in turn, often leads to reluctance to reach out to others, inability to form significant relationships, or failure to enter the career world with confidence.[10]

Adulthood

Adulthood includes the years between 22 and 38, during which developmental crises revolve around taking hold in the adult world.[10] Multiple role changes occur. The individual assumes new roles as a worker, lover, spouse, parent, and social participant in the community.[10,11] In the world of work, adults in their twenties are busy shaping their dreams, hoping to help bring about significant change. A mentor who can guide them in their careers is sought. Hope and energy abound. Demonstrating competence in mastering external tasks such as one's job is of great importance. An alternative to job commitment is to continue to explore and experiment with career options throughout one's twenties. At this time the person begins to build for a safe future, but decisions are not viewed as irrevocable.

Other major life choices are made at this time. When a lover or spouse is selected, an opportunity for intimacy and consolidation of sexuality without loss of differentiation is created. Options for parenthood are considered and implemented. At this point people make decisions about their future roles as spouses, career people, and parents. For women, the question of combining roles arises. Some women opt to stay home and be mothers for a number of years. Others decide to postpone parenthood indefinitely (see Chap. 32). The decision that the couple arrives at will result in role and identity shifts. The decision to postpone parenthood will shift a career role and identity into high gear, whereas the decision to stay home and parent will bring the parenting role and identity to the forefront. Conflict can occur when both roles are desired. This requires role modification for both partners so that marriage, family, and career can be successfully combined.[10,12,13]

Adults in their thirties are usually preoccupied with the question, "What do I want out of life now that I'm doing what I *ought* to do?" It is a time of greater introspection. There is often a feeling of restlessness and restriction accompanied by an urge to expand one's horizons.[10] This is an outgrowth of commitments made during the twenties. Important new choices which start people on the road to a new vision are made, and commitments are altered or deepened. A review of career plans takes place. Many people are eager to convert their dreams of success into concrete goals. Branching out into one's own business is not uncommon as job slots become constricting. People feel that they still have time to achieve, that things can still change. There is a sense of impatience but not urgency.

The marriage relationship is examined by both partners, and qualities to be retained or discarded are evaluated. Men and women alike are making decisions regarding their lives. At this point, for example, many women want to expand their horizons because their children are in school. They have more free time, and the total role of mother and wife no longer fits. Decisions regarding their future directions have to be made. Often, previous career choices are no longer appropriate or desirable and a return to the job market will require a return to school. Many women question their identity as persons, wives, and mothers. They want to reject their shadow role of living on the basis of a husband's identity. However, they may not feel confident about leaving the home and returning to an adult world. Can they cope? What do they have to offer?[10]

Many husbands are intent on pursuing their own career goals; they want to be free to do so with minimal interference from marital and family responsibilities. They want their wives to expand their horizons but do not want to contribute to a marital division of labor that would facilitate their partners' plans.

The sexual relationship is another area for renegotiation. Women are usually experiencing an increase in sexuality that may or may not be congruent with the sexual interest of their spouse. Men experience a constancy in their sexual desire or a decrease due to preoccupation with business interests and other tensions. Increased self-confidence and openness for both partners in other areas of life can lead to the desire for exploration of new levels of sexual satisfaction within the relationship. On the other hand, couples may begin to grow apart if—intellectually, emotionally, and socially—they progress at different rates. They may have varying levels of personality development, different values, and different role expectations (see Chap. 11). Unless commitments are renegotiated, the couple's relationship may dissipate to the point where it is nonviable.

The Middle Years

The middle years represent the midpoint in most people's lives. They ask "Where have I been? What have I accomplished? How am I going to spend the future?" The period from the late thirties through the fifties represents a time when people must try to adjust to the gap between what they wanted to accomplish in their life, what they actually have accomplished, and what they still can accomplish before time runs out. People in their early forties may feel that this is their last chance and will therefore examine their inner selves. It is a time when one feels prompted to examine past accomplishments and renew previous commitments.

Multiple role changes occur. Children leave the home and active parenting is completed. The former molds of meaning are gone. Women whose lives have been bound up in mothering and keeping house feel that they have lost their purpose in life. The *"empty-nest syndrome"* stems from the sense of purposelessness many women experience at this time. Children are given up and allowed to lead their own lives. The woman's former identity no longer fits. She is confronted with the question, "Who am I?" and asks, "What is my purpose for the rest of my life?" Every woman needs to develop a sense of individual importance and a means of independent survival, otherwise she will continue to depend on the well-being and largesse of her husband and children.

Men in middle life may feel that their opportunities for advancement are limited, that younger people are crowding their field with better knowl-

edge and skills. Men also question what their purpose will be for the rest of their lives. Many men and women must confront the choice of a second career or obsolescence. Even people who have attained their dream need new ideas to renew their zeal.

The marital relationship also changes. The couple are alone together as they have not been in years. They may find that they no longer share mutual interests or values or that they have been in the habit of communicating through their children. They may find that they need to renew their relationship and develop new interests which will enrich their lives. Role reversals occur. Adults become parents to their own parents as they age and become infirm. The last shreds of childhood dependence are severed. The adult realizes that "I am alone." This is often a moment of terror.

Physical changes occur which reflect changes in body image. Men and women experience a moving apart in sexual capacity. Men find that they are unable to perform as frequently as in previous years, while women, on the other hand, experience no drop in sexual ability and may actually feel increased desire due to freedom from fear of pregnancy; freedom from the responsibilities of earlier years; and a positive redefinition of self, particularly if they return to work. However, menopause and the accompanying physiological changes may contribute to emotional disequilibrium and reconfirm a woman's sense of loss and depression.[14,15]

The capacity for love and intimacy is not decreased for men or women, and sexuality in the middle years can be most fulfilling if creative approaches to sexual activity are utilized. The general physical process of aging, however, confronts people with their own mortality and finitude. Illness and death among friends and relatives make it difficult to deny a decrease in endurance and physical capacity. But in a youth-oriented culture, many people do try to hold on to a youthful self-concept. They look back at the past to evaluate whether or not they have had enough "kicks" and question whether or not they want to pursue such youthful pleasures now. They may seek the exclusive company of people younger than themselves, have extramarital affairs with younger people, or maintain a frantic pace of life. They may dye their hair, have cosmetic surgery, or dress in a very youthful way. All these activities may be attempts to deny the aging process and to maintain a sense of vigor and self-esteem.

The basic crisis of the middle years is one of introspection and self-confrontation. The process of peeling away the layers is often painful because feelings which have been buried for years emerge. People are not sure they like what they see. However, this is a unique opportunity to put things together and come to accept oneself. At this stage, many people are no longer preoccupied with pleasing others. They utilize this as a time in which to enrich their lives and to do what they themselves *want* in order to discover the unique answers they need.

If these issues are not confronted in the forties, they crop up again during the fifties. Failure to negotiate these tasks and accept one's own finitude results in denial, depression, psychosomatic symptoms, and stagnation.

Old Age

The developmental crisis of old age revolves around the concept of change. There is no specific point of entry into old age. It appears to depend on a complex interrelationship of physical, emotional, and social events. Older adults do have specific organic problems in relation to aging, but many of these develop as generalized reactions to loss of influence, unfulfilled life goals, onset of interpersonal isolation, and threats to economic security.[3] Old people are not revered in our culture as they are in others. In our youth-oriented society, older adults may feel angry about their physical decline, dependence, and helplessness. They may cope with these feelings through withdrawal and isolation.

Adjustment in old age appears to be a direct consequence of ego development in earlier years. Most people who have, in old age, a high level of

ego integration and self-differentiation have cultivated independent life-styles in their earlier lives. While they may have become less flexible about problem solving, they rarely spend their older years doing nothing. This capacity to remain active enhances their ability to cope with the stresses and conflicts that confront them.[14,16]

Fear of death is not unique to this age group, but for them its proximity is undeniable. Peer groups of old, close friends grow smaller as friends die. Opportunities for social contacts shrink. Those who respond to the aging process with a sense of integrity will reach out and form new relationships. Those who respond with despair tend to withdraw from social situations and isolate themselves in their own loneliness. People *are* living longer, but life does not continue indefinitely. Some people deal with the prospect of death through denial, while others seem to accept it, saying that they have lived full lives and have no fear of death. Cultural norms avoid the subject of death and thus make it difficult to verbalize positive or negative feelings on the subject. This often leads to the suppression of fear, increased anxiety, and maladaptive behavior[3] (see Chap. 31).

The greatest loss in old age is loss of independence. Physical disability results in a measure of dependence on others for care, support, and security. The presence or absence of environmental and situational supports will determine the individual's ability to overcome these disabilities. People who are economically secure may be able to overcome the social attitude that old age means obsolescence and continue to exert influence over their lives and society. Otherwise, they may be forced to accept the obscurity that our society inflicts on the aged.

Emotional and social changes occur as a result of retirement, which brings with it a loss of economic security, social role, peer group, and identity. For example, men often do not have many interests or social contacts away from their work and thus find it difficult to feel purposeful after they retire. For a woman, the loss of her spouse deprives her not only of a significant other but also of the identity which she achieved through her husband's social and economic position. If a woman has not developed an individual identity in previous years, she must now redefine herself socially and economically. These are crucial experiences because they conclude the central tasks of adulthood.[3]

Despite the losses sustained, the undercurrent of grief running through their lives, and the potential crises that exist, members of this older age group are at the same time concerned with actualizing their remaining potential and maintaining their integrity and dignity. By developing new leisure patterns and educational skills, these people can enhance their self-concepts.[15] The extent of involvement with others will determine the degree to which boredom and stagnation occur. There is a desire to leave a legacy, to pass something personal along to others, to make a gesture that enables one to feel a sense of immortality and connectedness with the future. This represents an active effort to make life more meaningful or better for those who follow. Such a legacy can be transmitted through younger people, relatives, or the community.[16]

Those who do not cope effectively, who do not reach out to actualize their remaining potential, become bored and stagnant. Many become bitter and withdrawn, feeling themselves to be victims of their age. Because the processes of decline and growth occur concomitantly but not in equal balance, it is of utmost importance for the caretaker to examine the symptomatology before making judgments about the client.[3] More than with any other age group, it is necessary to be aware of stereotyped attitudes toward the aging process and the effectiveness of intervention within this age group. Additionally, crisis symptoms must be evaluated for an organic component. Frequently, a sudden onset of bizarre behavior can be precipitated by a cerebrovascular accident or other organic syndromes associated with older age (see Chap. 30). Behavior that can be ameliorated with treatment must be separated from organic damage that is irreversible and not amenable to treatment. The

family or friends who bring the client to the treatment setting may also be in crisis and should be evaluated simultaneously. They may need intervention so that they can effectively support the parent or spouse in question.

Situational Crisis

Situational crises occur when unanticipated events threaten the individual's biological, social, or psychological integrity.[3] There is an accompanying degree of disequilibrium. The person's coping mechanisms become ineffective or chosen solutions prove to be impractical. The stressful event involves a fundamental loss or deprivation which threatens the person's self-concept. Williams states that a situational crisis is precipitated by the loss of a systematized support which enhanced the person's feelings of security and control and is essential to maintaining the integrity of the self-concept.[5]

Situational crises are life events involving overwhelming threats to a person's physical or psychological integrity. Such events may stem from three areas: the environment, the family, or the self. Environmental hazards include natural disasters such as fires, floods, and earthquakes; national disasters such as wars, riots, and racial persecution; and violent crimes such as rape and murder. Family hazards include death of a family member, divorce of parents, change in financial status, birth of a premature or defective child, and emotional problems such as alcoholism, schizophrenia, and depression. Self-related hazards include physical illness such as a heart attack or amputation, job loss, failure in school, juvenile delinquency, or becoming involved with drugs.

Caplan states that the unpredictable nature of these events introduces an element of hazard that does not exist in the anticipated maturational crises.[17] The element of unpreparedness increases the disruptions in life-style that people will experience. This will influence a person's control and ability to cope in such a situation.

One's perception of situational events influences the point at which a hazardous situation becomes a crisis. Additionally, situational crises can either disrupt many related areas in an individual's life-style or promote growth and change. Crises create ripple effects, like stones tossed into a pond. The total configuration of disruptions become the concern of crisis intervention, as in the example below.

Case Study: Family Financial Crisis
John F, age 45, was offered a vice-presidency in a California engineering firm that had just secured a large government contract. The offer was too good to refuse. The family, consisting of his wife and three children, ages 12, 15, and 17, reluctantly moved from their lifelong Connecticut home to Los Angeles. After 6 months of work, the contract fell through; John's firm went bankrupt and he was out of a job. At the same time, John's wife was depressed and lonely, 3000 miles from family and friends. Now she was faced with financial insecurity as well. The children were having difficulty adjusting to a different academic program and making new friends. The financial crisis led John to begin drinking heavily, as he was embarrassed to call his old firm in Connecticut, had few business contacts in the area, and was not making any new job connections. The family's savings were rapidly being depleted. The job change and geographic move initiated a sequence of personal and financial crises which would have to be confronted before resolution could take place.

Crisis Intervention
People are constantly faced with the need to solve problems in order to maintain a homeodynamic state. There is usually a relatively even balance between the stress experienced and the available coping mechanisms. If there is an imbalance between the problem (as perceived by the person) and the available repertoire of coping skills, a crisis may be precipitated.[17] If solutions cannot be found or if problem solving takes more time and effort than usual, disruption of the homeodynamic state occurs. Tension rises and discomfort is experienced, along with such feelings as anxiety, depression, fear, guilt, shame, and helplessness.[3] As the anxiety increases, coping skills become less available and less effective. The precipitated crisis is not the result of the event itself but of the person's inability to cope with it.

Crisis intervention utilizes a problem-solving approach. During the 4- to 6-week crisis period, a person is psychologically less defended and is consequently readier for and more amenable to change. The distress experienced during this period of crisis serves as a motivating factor, enabling the person to engage in an active problem-solving partnership.[18] The goal of crisis intervention is to reestablish a level of functioning equal to or better than that of the precrisis level.

Morely, Messick, and Aguilera have identified four phases of crises intervention: assessment of the individual and the problem, planning for therapeutic intervention, intervention, resolution of the crisis and anticipatory planning.[19]

Assessment
Assessment of the problem involves three areas of consideration: the client's perception of the problem, situational supports, and the client's coping skills.

Perception of the Problem
The nurse must explore the client's perception of the crisis-precipitating event and identify the factors which are affecting the client's ability to solve the problem. Questions like these are asked of the client:

> Why did you come for help today?
> What effect is this problem having on others around you?
> How do you see this affecting your future?

What do you see as the solution to your problem?

The nurse assesses how realistically or unrealistically the client perceives the problem and what factors are influencing the client's perceptions. An important factor which can influence perceptions is where the client stands in terms of the developmental cycle.

Situational Supports

The next area for consideration is that of situational supports. The client is part of a social system. Those identified as significant people in the client's life should be involved to maximize the effectiveness of the intervention. Who in the environment supports the client? With whom can the client communicate? With whom does the client live? Who can the client trust? What is the client's social network? Who from the social network has responded to the client's problem?

Coping Skills

Coping skills involve the ways in which an individual behaves when confronted with a problem that cannot be solved. Coping skills are very individual, so the client must be asked: "Has anything like this ever happened before? What have you done to deal with anxiety, tension, or depression? Have you tried the same thing this time? Has it worked? If not, why not? What else do you think might work?"[3] Many people cope by playing a musical instrument, jogging, or yelling at somebody. Coping mechanisms such as projection, displacement, and others that we use unconsciously are identifed in Table 4-1.

Planning Intervention

After data have been gathered from the individual and the social network such as family, school, or other professional agencies, intervention is planned from an analysis of the above areas. The therapist must be able to answer several questions:

Question	Example
1 At what level is the client functioning?	1 I can't go to work, school, play, or care for my family. I can't think.
2 How is this state of disequilibrium affecting others?	2 My wife, husband, mother, father, brother (etc.) are upset. They're angry at me because I'm acting peculiar.
3 What do significant others think you should do?	3 Study more, get some help, have different friends.

The crisis must be identified as self-related, family related, environmentally related, or a combination of these. For example, a young couple experiencing the normal stress of first-time parenthood would also be precipitated into a situational crisis with the birth of a retarded child.

Preliminary hypotheses are advanced about why the problem exists. When the dynamic issue is explored, more than one cause may emerge. Alternatives are considered and evaluated as past events are contrasted with present experience.

Intervention

Crisis intervention can take place in a mental health clinic or in the home. Intervention is characterized by goal directedness. It focuses on the problem at hand and usually consists of six to eight structured interviews. Other times crisis work is completed in 48 to 72 hours and the client is referred to another agency for ongoing therapy. The nurse conveys an attitude of authority, responsibility, and concern, keeping the client focused on issues relating to the problem that is causing the current disequilibrium. Several steps are taken in resolving the problem. *First,* the nurse labels her perception of the problem, checks it out with the client's perception of the problem, and then both nurse and client explore their mutual perceptions of it. Connections are made between the meaning of the event and the resulting crisis. *Second,* the multiple feelings accompanying the crisis are observed and acknowledged. This helps the person to sort out feelings and thoughts, to express them, and to have them validated as normal and acceptable. *Third,* the nurse and client explore alternative problem-solving behaviors and coping skills such as reaching out to others and verbalizing feelings and expectations. *Fourth,* the nurse and client test or rehearse new approaches to problem solving in order to arrive at a comfortable fit. This will reinforce new behaviors and give the client positive feedback. Throughout the process, the therapist acts as a role model for open, direct communication, innovative thinking, flexibility, and self-awareness.[18]

Resolution and Anticipatory Planning

Evaluation is made to determine the effectiveness of the planned intervention. The goals should be compared to the behavioral outcomes. If the intervention has been successful, the client will experience a decrease in distress and will return to a precrisis level of functioning. The client will be able to identify the events and feelings that caused the disruption, evaluate changes in life-style, and implement these changes to the satisfaction of client and nurse. This provides an opportunity to consolidate learning that has occurred to date, identify emerging unmet needs, and test the client's capacity to initiate activity to meet these needs. All learning may not take place within the 6 to 8 weeks of the crisis therapy; true integration may occur only after the actual sessions are completed. Then, although the contract time is over, the nurse should remain available for future consultation. Clients with additional areas of concern are often referred to other agencies for long-term counseling once the current crisis has been resolved.[3,18]

Case Study: Intervention in a Maturational Crisis—Old Age

Mr. W, age 75, called the crisis unit of the mental health clinic after finding their number in the phone book. He asked whether the unit could help him and his wife. At the first interview, Mr. and Mrs. W related their problem.

They live in a small apartment in a five-story walk-up building in what has become a transitional neighborhood. The incidence of crime in the neighborhood has reached epidemic proportions, and they are afraid to go out alone. Most of their old friends have died or—if financially able—moved away. Mr. W was a tailor for many years until failing eyesight forced him to retire. He is now supporting himself and his wife on a small pension and social security. Their two married children have moved to the suburbs, have their own problems making ends meet, and visit only occasionally. Mrs. W has a heart condition; she is increasingly unable to climb the stairs and clean their apartment. Mr. W helps her, but his near blindness makes it increasingly difficult for him to go out and do the necessary errands. They are feeling trapped by their aging bodies, lack of money, and inadequate living quarters.

Just when they were feeling very blue, they got a phone call from their daughter-in-law telling them that their son had been laid off from his job. Mrs. W said, "Oh my God. What is happening? We can't help ourselves, much less our children." She sat crying for days, refusing to get out of bed. At the interview, the nurse identified that the W's were experiencing feelings of inadequacy, powerlessness, helplessness, and hopelessness. The crisis-precipitating event for the W's was their children's disaster, which accentuated their own helplessness and generated guilt because they were unable to help themselves, much less their children. They felt that their situation could not be altered in any positive way and were unable to identify any situational supports.

Intervention was directed toward assisting the W's to express their feelings, examine their expectations of themselves, look at the problem realistically, and arrive at alternative solutions. First, it was necessary to help the W's examine their feelings of responsibility for their children. Once they acknowledged that their middle-aged children's financial status was not their responsibility, they were able to begin focusing on their own needs and problems. They identified the liabilities—such as blindness, heart condition, financial strain, etc.—that were interfering with their ability to cope. Their strengths were their solid marital relationship, their willingness to socialize, and their independence.

By the third week, Mr. and Mrs. W, with the assistance of the nurse, had located an apartment in a senior citizens' housing project with a senior citizens' center attached to it in a safer part of the city. Medical services were also found, and Mr. W was scheduled for a cataract operation to correct his eyesight. Mrs. W was being evaluated for a medical regimen to monitor her heart condition. The W's felt more hopeful about their future but were apprehensive about making a move to a new neighborhood and about Mr. W's impending surgery. The children were contacted, and their son agreed to stay with Mrs. W during her husband's hospitalization. He said he did not realize how difficult life had become for his parents. The W's were assured that they could return to the crisis clinic if help were needed in the future.

Case Study: Intervention in a Situational Crisis—Divorce

Marie, age 34, arrived at the mental health clinic crying and saying that she felt she was losing control of her life. During the first session, she gave the following information:

She and her husband Don, age 36, are planning to divorce following her recent discovery that he had been having numerous extramarital affairs. Don had not denied the involvements but simply said, "So what. All I get from you is nagging. I have to have fun somewhere." A fight ensued, and Marie told him to get out.

In the month since Don left, their two children,

ages 6 and 9, have been having nightmares and problems at school. The younger child does not want to let Marie out of her sight. Marie is having money problems and should be out looking for a job, but she finds herself crying when she looks at the job ads. In addition, she says that she still loves Don. She feels that they had gradually grown apart. They seemed to be moving in two different worlds, hers at home and his at business. She felt increasingly unable to play a role in his more dynamic life. Don's acknowledged infidelity—which Marie had suspected for a while—was the crisis-precipitating event.

Marie was experiencing feelings of depression, worthlessness, and guilt, believing that she had been a "bad" wife and now was also incompetent as a mother because her children were having problems. Although her family lived in another state, Marie had several situational supports, including a number of neighbors and friends who had reached out to her. But she had reacted to her problem by giving up and becoming immobilized.

Intervention was directed toward helping Marie to express her feelings and look at the problem in a more realistic way. It was necessary to diagram the relationship to see the points at which it went awry and to define how each partner had contributed to the discord. Once Marie could acknowledge that she was not completely at fault, she was able to begin identifying her strengths. She had been a good mother and homemaker; her children had friends and did well in school; she had been an effective worker in community activities; she had a number of good friends. She also had a professional skill, teaching. As she began to see her strengths objectively, she began to feel less depressed. She was able to talk with the children more and help them explore their feelings about the separation.

By the fifth week Marie had applied for a job as a substitute teacher and had been called for a job. She was considering a reconciliation with Don, and alternative behaviors in the relationship were explored. Don was contacted and plans were made for couples therapy at the center. At termination, Marie was teaching part time, had joined an evening book discussion club, had had her hair restyled, and had found that the children's symptoms had decreased. Marie and the therapist reviewed the adjustments she had made, the insight she had gained, and her needs regarding future plans. She felt more confident that even if the divorce went through, she would be able to cope more effectively with her life.

References

1 Gerald Caplan: *An Approach to Community Mental Health,* Grune and Stratton, New York, 1961.

2 Lydia Rapaport: "The State of Crisis: Some Theoretical Considerations," in Howard J. Parad (ed.), *Crisis Intervention: Selected Readings,* Family Service Association of America, New York, 1965.

*3 Donna C. Aguilera and Janice M. Messick: *Crisis Intervention: Theory and Methodology,* Mosby, St. Louis, 1974.

4 Howard J. Parad and Gerald Caplan: "A Framework for Studying Families in Crisis," in Howard J. Parad (ed.), *Crisis Intervention: Selected Readings,* Family Service Association of America, New York, 1965.

*5 Florence S. Williams: "Intervention in Maturational Crises," in J. C. Hall and B. R. Weaver (eds.), *Nursing of Families in Crisis,* Lippincott, Philadelphia, 1974, pp. 43–50.

6 Erik H. Erikson: *Childhood and Society,* Norton, New York, 1963.

7 Harry S. Sullivan: in Helen S. Perry (ed.), *Interpersonal Theory of Psychiatry,* Norton, New York, 1953.

8 J. Piaget: *The Child's Conception of the World,* Littlefield, Adams, 1963.

*9 Helen Dylag: "How Difficult the "I": The Adolescent Maturation of Critical Identity," in J. Hall and B Weaver (eds.), *Nursing of Families In Crisis,* Lippincott, Philadelphia, 1974, pp. 51–63.

*10 Gail Sheehy: *Passages,* Dutton, New York, 1976.

*11 Nancy L. Diekelman: "The Young Adult: The Choice Is Health or Illness," *American Journal of Nursing,* vol. 76, no. 8, pp. 1272–1277, August 1976.

*12 Mardelle K. Wuenger: "The Young Adult Stepping Into Parenthood," *American Journal of Nursing,* vol. 76, no. 8, pp. 1283–1285, August 1976.

*13 Gail J. Donner: "Parenthood as a Crisis: A Role for the Psychiatric Nurse," *Perspectives In Psychiatric Care,* vol. 10, no. 2, pp. 84–87, 1972.

14 Theodore Lidz: *The Person: His Development Throughout the Life Cycle,* Basic Books, New York, 1968.

*15 Hildegard Peplau: "Mid-Life Crises," *American Journal of Nursing,* vol. 75, no. 10, pp. 1761–1765, October 1975.

*16 Irene M. Burnside: *Nursing and the Aged,* McGraw-Hill, New York, 1976.

17 Gerald Caplan: *Principles of Preventive Psychiatry,* Basic Books, New York, 1964.

*18 Lorna M. Barrell: "Crisis Intervention: Partnership in Problem-Solving," *Nursing Clinics of North America,* vol. 9, no. 1, pp. 5–17, 1974.

*19 Wilbur E. Morely, Janice M. Messick, and Donna C. Aguilera: "Crisis: Paradigms of Intervention," *Journal of Psychiatric Nursing,* November–December 1967, pp. 531–544.

*Recommended reference by a nurse author.

6

The Nurse - Client Relationship

Judith Ackerhalt

Learning Objectives

After studying this chapter, the student should be able to:

1 Describe a personal reason or motive for entering into a helping relationship with a client

2 Describe personal fears or concerns which are related to the nurse's participation in a helping relationship

3 Identify goals of the helping relationship

4 Describe ways in which helping relationships may pose a threat to a client's self-image

5 Define the core dimensions which lead to positive change in a helping relationship

6 Cite instances of the core dimensions in communication with clients throughout each phase of a relationship

7 Describe the purposes of planning, describing, and analyzing helping relationships

Historical Perspectives

Historically, efforts to comprehend and explain in writing the significant aspects of the one-to-one nurse-client relationship have been fragmented and lacking in clarity. Diverse opinions have been expressed regarding the desirable personality characteristics of psychiatric nurses, the kinds of knowledge upon which their practice ought to be based, the actual activities of helping, and the criteria of effective psychiatric nursing practice. In the past, nurses appeared to be primarily concerned with custodial and managerial functions. Up until the early 1950s, the notion of professional use of self remained ill defined and dimly understood.[1]

The publication of Hildegard Peplau's book *Interpersonal Relations in Nursing*,[2] brought to a close a period marked by confusion and theoretic impoverishment. Dr. Peplau presented a theoretic rationale for psychiatric nursing practice, clarified the various roles of the psychiatric nurse, and explained the goals and activities associated with the counseling role (see Chap. 4).

Initially, advances in the conceptualization of psychiatric nursing practice stimulated controversy about the therapeutic use of self. Nurses labored over the question, "Can nurses maintain their nursing identity while assuming the helping role in the one-to-one relationship?" Out of this inquiry, there gradually evolved a concern about *how* the nurse does psychotherapy.[1]

Today, many psychiatric nurses are diligently studying the concepts, principles, and theories which help to explain human experience. These same nurses are looking at, analyzing, and interpreting helping interactions. The goal is to make rational modifications of their methods of helping and to extend the scope of their technical ability.

In a sense, the historic and often arduous journey of psychiatric nursing is repeated by each nurse in a unique way. The maturation and refinement of a professional self-image requires an inner effort of great intensity. When a nurse chooses to explore a new role, reexamination of professional ideals, values, and responsibilities is essential. Beliefs about the therapeutic use of self are sub-jected to review. A deeper understanding of the nurse-client relationship begins with commitment to the acquisition of greater technical ability.

Definition of the Nurse-Client Relationship
Participants' Subjective Experiences

A study of the nurse-client relationship derives its impetus and direction from the actual clinical practices and direct experiences of professional nurses. A grasp of the true significance of this interpersonal helping process requires recognition of the familiar concerns, well-known dilemmas, and real purposes and accomplishments of nurses engaged in one-to-one relationships with clients. Nurses, as well as clients, each have a distinctive way of experiencing and responding to the specific situations which form the helping process. These idiosyncratic experiences, which illuminate the meaning of the nurse-client relationship, include the following:

1 The forces which have brought the nurse and the client together; i.e., what each initially hopes and expects to gain from the collaborative effort
2 The participants' resultant fears, concerns, and reservations
3 The participants' resources for coping with these experiences

Much of what happens when nurses attempt to enter a therapeutic relationship with clients is a product of the complex interaction between these various personal elements.

Process and Goals

The nurse-client relationship can also be viewed and understood as an interpersonal process, an organized sequence of activities or events leading toward some goal or objective. While the terms "goal" and "objective" suggest a determined future, in reality, these images of the future are used only to suggest and legitimize the events which take place throughout the helping relationship.

Facilitative Interpersonal Processes

It is impossible to draw a sharp distinction between the anticipated outcomes of the nurse-client relationship and the way in which these goals are accomplished. For the past two decades, investigators have been attempting to identify and operationally define the helper behaviors which enable clients to fully experience, explore and resolve problems and to become self-actualized. A number of facilitative interpersonal processes have been conceptualized. Each describes a way of being with a client so that healing takes place. These "core dimensions" or "facilitative dimensions" include the following: (1) empathic understanding, (2) concreteness, (3) respect, (4) genuineness, (5) confrontation, and (6) immediacy.[3] These six core dimensions, each of which has the potential for demonstrating the interconnection between actual helping transactions and specific outcomes, are outlined in Table 6-1. These concepts are discussed in depth throughout this chapter.

Nurses' Concerns at the Outset of the Helping Relationship

It seems to be a characteristic of human nature that, having committed themselves to a course of action whose outcome is uncertain, individuals fall prey to an assortment of doubts and fears. When the step that these persons have decided to take brings them face to face with the necessity of revising their self-image or exposes them to real or imagined threats to self-esteem, their determination may waver. Each nurse-client relationship, like any promising new venture, is not without its attendant risks and impediments. Typically, the novice helper is fearful and uncertain; yet each nurse interprets and responds to these experiences in a distinctive way.

Nurses frequently have difficulty making the transition to and picturing themselves in the counseling role. One nursing student, a mature 40-year-old mother of three children, summed up her experience in this way: "I felt like a fish out of water . . . so very awkward. I was certain that the client would see right through me, that he would see how incompetent and ill-qualified I was." During the early stages of the helping relationship, novice helpers are often uncertain as to how to conduct themselves. Lacking a clear role defini-

Table 6-1 Core Dimensions

Core dimension	Definition
Empathic understanding	The temporary experiencing of another individual's feelings: expressions which convey the nurse's accuarate recognition of the feelings, motives, and meanings underlying a client's communications.
Concreteness	The clear, direct expression of personally relevant perceptions, values, and feelings as they exist in the present relationship.
Confrontation	Communications which call attention to significant discrepancies in the client's experience; verbal messages which are intended to help a client to recognize information which is not consistent with the self-image.
Immediacy	A dimension of communication which deals with the relationship-building element of the helping process; expressions emphasizing immediacy draw relationships between clients' overt communications and their underlying impressions of what is going on between client and nurse in the here and now.
Respect	Communication of acceptance of the client's ideas, feelings, and experiences; recognition of a client's potential for self-actualization.
Genuineness	Spontaneous expressions conveying an individual's inner experience.

tion and a sense of direction, they are likely to perceive themselves as unskillful or, what is worse, as bungling and inept.

Fear of Rejection

A common fear of novice helpers is that the client will detect that they are unaccustomed to the counseling role and reject their efforts to help. No one likes to be rejected, and the possibility that this will occur exists in each new relationship.

Regardless of how one really feels about it—whether one is secretly relieved or truly disappointed—each nurse ponders the client's motives for withdrawing from the relationship. Questions such as "Did I do something wrong?" and "Could I have acted to prevent this from happening?" reflect the nurses' recognition that a client's termination can be understood only if it is viewed in relation to the helpers' actions. Unfortunately, all too often nurses and nursing students blame themselves for a client's premature departure. Sometimes, students fear that others on the health team will think less of them because they did not maintain an alliance with their client. Nurses sometimes rationalize a rejection by claiming that a client is unable to accept help or is hopeless. Frequently, those nurses whose efforts have been rejected fear that it will happen again and again. A nursing student who had succeeded in establishing a firm alliance with a client noted, "During the first 2 weeks of the semester, I lost two clients. They just didn't want to see me anymore. I began to think that I was the only one who couldn't hold onto a client. It seemed like all the other students were doing OK. Boy, was I jealous. We are really relieved when our clients want to see us again."

Fear of Exploiting the Client

Nurses who at the outset of a nurse-client relationship regard themselves as novices are apt to negate the value and usefulness of previously acquired helping skills. In so doing, their view of what they might have to offer a client is obscured. That nurses might exploit clients or use them for their own purposes, selfishly, becomes a pressing concern for some. When a client who has come to mistrust human kindness and warmth asks, "Are you using me as a guinea pig?" the nurse is at a loss as to how to respond. In such instances, an empathic instructor or supervisor and/or a group of understanding classmates or peers might be called upon to help the nurse make a rational assessment of the situation. Nurses might pause to reflect upon earlier personal achievements; they might be reminded that the clients having made a commitment to the relationship, have the right to express their needs and to expect help. The client also has the responsibility for indicating to the nurse when help is not being given.

Fear of Helplessness

Generally speaking, nurses hope to effect some change in clients' life situations. When clients exhibit extreme forms of maladaptive behavior but appear to be satisfied with the status quo, when clients' sources of support are minimal, and when the treatment environment is viewed as having many shortcomings, nurses become disheartened. At first glance, it would appear that it is impossible for the nurse to have an impact on the client or the client's milieu. Such an assessment is frequently accompanied by feelings of helplessness, powerlessness, and frustration. Small inroads made by the helper are then apt to go unnoticed.

Fear of Mental Illness

Many individuals, though deeply troubled, do not exhibit overt forms of maladaptive behavior. Initially, nurses wonder why these people have been assigned to the client role. Nurses are likely to compare themselves and aspects of their own lives to those of a client who appears to be "normal." When similarities are noted, nurses may begin to question their own mental health. Questions such as "Am I mentally ill?" or "How am I different from my client?" are anxiety-provoking. Some nurses may have initially entered the field of mental health to avoid the client role. These poignant questions compel nurses to probe deeply into the significance of their personal experiences as well as those of the client. Out of this inquiry, a new meaning of mental health and mental illness may emerge.

Fear of Physical Assault

Fears of being physically assaulted or verbally abused are common experiences among nurses. A student who had been working with a client who had little control over sexual or aggressive urges described the situation in this way. "I didn't want to do anything to upset my client's balance. It was like walking on eggs. I was terrified of making a mistake." Clients' potential for losing control is but one reason why students fear harm. Other factors contributing to students' feelings of vulnerability to assault include stereotyped images of the "violent" mental patient; physically intrusive, contact-seeking behavior of some clients; and feelings of alienation and powerlessness which students occasionally experience when, as strangers, they enter a psychiatric unit for the first time.

Many nurses have sustained these fears; however, few have realized that these apprehensions were the natural attendants of risk taking. Acts requiring courage are facilitated when we recognize and accept the appropriateness of being afraid. The misinterpretation of fear as cowardice places an additional burden on nurses. Failure to come to grips with ever-present fear poses one of the most serious barriers to the development of the nurse-client relationship. Misunderstood and borne in secret, fears are intensified and generalized. Brought out into the open—shared with an instructor, classmates, peers or supervisors—fears can be named and understood.

Clients' Fears and Concerns

As the helping relationship gets under way, both nurse and client live through moments of fear and uncertainty. Like the nurse, persons seeking help may not readily recognize, understand, or own up to their misgivings. As clients become more deep-

ly involved in the helping process, the outcome of which is unknown, they must grapple with a number of threats to their self-image. Getting help has different meanings for clients with low self-esteem. It may imply that they are helpless, that they are not competent to handle their own problems, or that they are inadequate as individuals. These impressions may then engender fear, anger, resentment, or guilt.[4]

When clients recognize that the nurse is listening and that they are understood better than they understand themselves, they begin to develop transference feelings. The client begins to project onto the nurse past or present attitudes toward loved ones or persons in authority.[5] Thus clients experience nurses as they might have experienced other persons who have played significant roles in their lives. Clients form an image or a multiplicity of images of the nurse. Accordingly, clients anticipate the roles that both they and the nurse will play in the helping relationship. They contemplate the specific techniques that the nurse will employ, and perhaps they think about the duration and outcomes of the interpersonal helping process. The client may repeat interaction patterns which were characteristic of earlier relationships. Transference accounts for both the positive and the negative expectations which clients have of nurses. It evokes feelings of fear that nurses will treat clients with disrespect, that nurses will control, punish, stereotype, manipulate, humiliate, or abandon them. These feelings usually originate in the transference. Previous experiences in the client role or stories told by friends or family members regarding their encounters with nurses may reinforce these emergent fears.

Expectations of Nurses at the Outset of Helping Relationships

One suspects that there are innumerable reasons why individuals are drawn to the study and practice of nursing. A broad range of interests, values, expectations, and aims have motivated nurses to participate in helping relationships with clients.

The wish to actualize humanitarian values, to maintain self-esteem, to find diversion, or to control another are motivating impulses which find expression in the nurse-client relationship. Frequently, however, nurses do not readily recognize or understand these inducements which operate prior to meeting clients and throughout the relationship itself. Therefore a brief discussion of each of these is indicated.

Humanitarian Ideals

Nurses sometimes perceive helping another as an act of generosity. Those who have succeeded in overcoming internal conflicts or external obstacles may wish to help others find inner peace and satisfaction. Experiences with friends and loved ones who have supplied support and guidance may inspire nurses to share themselves with clients. Feeling fully aware and alive, many nurses would like to introduce their suffering clients to what life has to offer. Studies of the character traits of effective helpers indicate that these individuals hold strong humanitarian values.[6]

Value Clarification

The nurse-client relationship may be viewed as an opportunity to actualize any one of a multitude of prized beliefs or values. An example is the inner conviction that it is worthwhile to explore and to grasp the deeper meaning of one's conscious experience. Through participation in the helping relationship, nurses may enable themselves, as well as their clients, to attain greater self-understanding, self-acceptance, and self-actualization.

Maintenance of Self-Esteem

For some, the maintenance or enhancement of self-esteem is a pressing need. Not infrequently, nurses experience increased status when clients perceive them as helpers. Through helping, nurses may hope to gain confidence in their personal well-being. They are capable of sustaining a client, therefore they may be reassured that they are "OK."

Diversion

Nurses who are troubled by personal problems may wish for a respite. Focusing upon the clients' problems, rather than one's own, may provide needed diversion. The helpers are thus able to get their minds off themselves.

Control

Sometimes, the actions that individuals take are motivated by the wish to exert power or control over others. Such impulses may be operating when a nurse approaches a helping situation. The nurse may find a client who needs to cling or lean upon someone. Other hopes and expectations are associated with nurses' concepts of themselves as students or professionals.

Performance Evaluation

Nurses are often concerned about performance evaluations. They feel pressured to demonstrate competence. They want clients to move rapidly toward some designated goal and may be disheartened when this does not occur. When the ability to describe and to analyze the helping interaction is valued over and above the client's progress, nurses are less pressured and are able to revise their expectations.

Nurses who are struggling to picture themselves in the helping role enter into the nurse-client relationship with numerous expectations. They hope to acquire knowledge of the helping process, a repertoire of helping skills, and, perhaps, an opportunity to try out various kinds of nursing interventions. When nurses recognize the self-enhancement motive underlying their participation in the nurse-client relationship, they have a tendency to chastise themselves. Underlying their self-accusations is the assumption of opposites;

i.e., one is either *out for oneself* and hence *self-seeking* or one is acting in the best interest of the other. This *either-or* assumption is nonrational. Most often, the generous impulse and the self-enhancement motive are intertwined. To deny either would deprive the nurse of a significant aspect of self-experience.

Expectations of Clients

Clients have expectations of the helping relationship. What do clients hope to gain by collaborating with nurses? Do clients know what they want? These are questions which are sometimes raised by nurses. Research findings suggest that clients are capable of identifying and making accurate statements regarding their needs and the treatment that they think will help to bring about desired changes.[7] The numerous and diverse ambitions which lay the foundation for all nurse-client interactions are known as client goals.[5] These goals, each of which represent the clients' image of their personal future, include control, reality contact, confession, ventilation, advice, clarification, psychological expertise, psychotherapy, social intervention, referral, and medical treatment.[8]

Control

Some clients are besieged by thoughts of doing violence to themselves or to others. They may be nearly exhausted by the struggle to control powerful aggressive or sexual urges. Disabled by severe anxiety, intense guilt feelings, or paralyzing depression, these clients frequently claim that they are unable to "pull themselves together," that they are "cracking up," "falling apart," or "going crazy." They foresee and fear a complete loss of self-control and require help in keeping a rein on the direct expression of frightening impulses. Such individuals hope to find, in the nurse, a protector, someone who will set firm limits upon their behavior or "take over" until they have reestablished a sense of balance and control.[8]

Reality Contact

Severe anxiety, social isolation, physical trauma, or unexpected physiological changes may lead to a feeling of unreality or personal estrangement. On occasion, the often terrifying experience of being out of touch with oneself or the world motivates a client to attempt to establish rapport with the nurse. The clients' aim is to make contact with a representative of the real world and to get back in touch with themselves. Such aspirations may be the source of the incessant demands of the individual recovering from a myocardial infarction, the lonely, aging widow, or the psychiatric client who has spent an afternoon in seclusion.[8]

Nurturance

Clients who have sustained the loss of a significant other person upon whom they were dependent for support may feel needy, deprived, or empty. Such individuals are frequently prompted to look for a caring, sympathetic helper. They hope that the nurse will listen, respond in a kind, supportive way, and perhaps "fill them up." This expectation is frequently held by clients in the older age group who may recently have lost a spouse.[8]

Administrative Request

Professional helpers have certain administrative and legal powers which are delegated to them by institutions or by society at large. Not infrequently, clients want nurses to exercise authority in helping them to acquire an honor card, to obtain a weekend pass or hospital discharge, or to secure legal or financial assistance. Usually, these clients will not acknowledge other concerns until these initial requests are addressed by the nurse.[8]

Institutional Contact

A client may not want anything from any one particular person. Instead, the client who lives in the community may wish to make contact with the institution where help has been received in the past. Recently discharged clients may not yet be certain of their ability to survive outside the hospital and may need to feel that the institution will always be there. They will be reassured and comforted by just walking past the building or sitting in the reception area. Occasionally, such clients will drop in to visit one or all of the nurses; they are "touching base," not seeking intimate personal relationships.[8]

Confession

Individuals will look for a nurse who will listen in a nonjudgmental way rather than moralize when they wish to confess real or imagined transgressions. Often clients hope to be told that what they have done is not as terrible as they believe it to be. They wish to be rid of guilt or shame and desire respect, forgiveness, and self-acceptance.[8]

Ventilation

Some individuals have problems which they do not seek to resolve. Clients who claim that they just want to "get something off their chest" mean exactly what they say. They want to unburden themselves to a nurse who will listen. They do not expect the nurse to help them examine or solve the problem.[8]

Advice

Frequently, clients hope that the nurse will have the answers to what is troubling them. They may want the nurse to come up with solutions to a particular problem or to make a decision for them. Seeking direction, they would like to be told what to do or which way to go. The nurse needs to keep in mind that directive counseling is sometimes appropriate. Assessment that the client is in crisis is a clue to nurses that they must give advice and be directive.[8]

Clarification

A client who hopes to clear up some confusing thoughts, to crystallize an idea, or to better under-

stand the meaning of a critical event anticipates brief contact with the nurse. Getting things into perspective may be the person's sole motive for seeking help.[8]

Psychological Expertise

Clients who wish to know why they feel or act as they do may hope that the nurse, whom they see as an expert, will have the answers. When the expected answers are not forthcoming, these persons may claim that the nurse is "holding out" on them. The role of the nurse is to allow clients to grow in insight and recognition of their motivating dynamics. The nurse must be wary of falling into the "expert trap" and making premature interpretations.[8]

Psychotherapy

Hoping to discover the relationship between current experiences and past events, clients may wish to engage in an ongoing relationship with the nurse. Usually, these individuals believe that by subjecting their experiences to careful scrutiny over a period of time they will acquire greater self-understanding and self-acceptance. They hope to get more satisfaction out of life. Often clients will express their feelings by stating "All I want is to be happy."[8]

Social Intervention

Frequently clients underestimate their ability to fend for themselves. Consequently, their initial request from nurses is to have them contact a relative, friend, landlord, or employer. In these instances, the clients' expectation is that the nurse will actively intervene in some problematic situation on their behalf. Anger is often the response when the nurse attempts to assist clients to make the contact themselves.[8]

Referral

Sometimes, individuals only hope to get information about where to go to get various needs satisfied. An example of this is the client who requests information regarding how to secure an appointment with the medical clinic.[8]

Medical Treatment

Occasionally, clients are unwilling to share their concerns with anyone but a physician. These individuals may hope that a physician will provide a diagnosis, medication, electroconvulsive therapy, or even surgery. These hopes are reinforced in some institutions where clients' problems are viewed as somatic in origin or where the nurse's role is defined as custodial rather than therapeutic.[9]

Evolution of Client Goals

During the evolution of the nurse-client relationship, clients' anticipated outcomes decline in significance. As clients encounter new aspects of themselves, their values and images of what is possible for them in the future changes. Frequently, as goals are revised, the one-to-one relationship becomes a way of helping clients to strengthen or to acquire those qualities essential for self-realization. Independence, spontaneity, living in the present, trust, self-awareness, honesty, and responsibility are qualities which will enable clients to grow and to realize their potential. Eventually these qualities or actualization goals may become the transformed purposes of the relationship.[5]

Stages of the Nurse-Client Relationship

The helping relationship is, in fact, a manifestation of a historical or temporal process, interweaving expectations and concerns of nurses and clients with the unfolding core dimensions. Three distinct yet interrelated phases of this evolving process can be identified: the *initial phase*, the *middle phase*, and the *termination phase*. Each core dimension undergoes a transformation as the nurse-

client relationship evolves. For example, at the outset of a helping relationship, a nurse uses empathic understanding to help a client overcome feelings of isolation and alienation and to determine how well clients understand their problem. Later, deeper levels of empathic understanding enable clients to extend their understanding of those problems.

The Initial Phase of the Nurse-Client Relationship

The initial phase of the nurse-client relationship has been referred to as the orientation phase,[9] the establishing phase,[10] or the downward or inward phase.[11] During the initial phase, the crucial tasks to be accomplished are the establishment of a working partnership between nurse and client and the identification of the client's chief problem or area of concern.

During the first phase of the relationship, nurse and client, who are strangers to one another, meet. Neither knows much about the events which are about to take place. The things that will happen throughout the relationship can, at best, only be anticipated.

Identification of Client Goals

Identification of client goals is one of the initial steps in the helping process. A nurse solicits discussion of clients' concerns by asking them to clearly and directly state their wishes and expectations.

The following questions are intended to convey the nurse's willingness to consider the client's requests and the expectation that personally relevant problems will not be dealt with in an abstract, highly intellectual fashion:

- What, specifically, is bothering you?
- What do you see as the cause of your difficulties?
- Why are you looking for help now?
- What do you think I can do for you?

- What do you think is the best help for your difficulty?
- What do you think will happen if you are not helped with your problem?

Nurses must evaluate the feasibility of the clients' requests and share their impressions regarding what might be considered a reasonable goal. Confusion and the feeling that one is lacking direction and purpose result when the nurse fails to clarify and evaluate client goals. When nurse and client come to a mutual understanding of the purpose to be served by the relationship, much of the confusion and uncertainty which so frequently characterizes the experiences of both participants at the outset of their relationship is checked.

Structuring

"Structuring" is the term used to describe those activities aimed at establishing a working partnership with a client. From the outset, the nurse must carefully outline the roles and responsibilities of both participants in the helping process. Structuring procedures—which include indicating the focus, duration, frequency, times, length, and location of meetings—give clients an idea of what they can expect and tend to reduce anxiety engendered by ambiguity.

Interviewing Skills

Knowledge of interviewing skills further assists nurses to structure their meetings with clients. Nurses and clients alike bring to the interview their many concerns. The use of basic techniques helps allay some of the anxiety associated with initial interpersonal contacts. One technique the nurse can use is to *make an observation:* "You appear tense." "Are you uncomfortable when . . . ?"

Encouraging a description of the client's perceptions and *encouraging comparisons* are other skills which can be utilized. *Placing events in time sequence* is very useful when the nurse deals with a confused client: "Was this before or after . . . ?" "When did this happen?"

Nurses may *offer self* with statements like "I'll sit with you a while," or "I'm interested in your comfort."

Giving broad openings often facilitates conversation in the early part of an interview. For example: "Is there something you would like to talk about?" "Where would you like to begin?"

Silence is a most effective technique. When the nurse remains silent, clients react spontaneously, often revealing a great deal about the meaning they have attached to silence in past situations.

The following example illustrates the technique of *restating:*

Client: I can't sleep, I stay awake all night.
Nurse: You have difficulty sleeping?
Client: The fellow that is my mate died at war and is pending me yet to marry.
Nurse: You were going to marry him but he died during the war.

Reflection is another useful technique for soliciting information during an interview.

Client: Do you think I should tell the doctor?
Nurse: Do you think you should?
Client: My brother spends all my money and then has the nerve to ask for more.
Nurse: This causes you to feel angry.

There are many *techniques* which will make the initial stages of new relationships less anxiety provoking and more productive. Nurses must, however, develop their own style. It is counterproductive and inhibiting to the therapeutic use of self to continue to use stereotyped responses or techniques without making them part of a comfortable self.

Nursing students or nurses wishing supervision for their interviews frequently utilize a mechanical device to record sessions or maintain a written running narrative of their interchanges with clients. On occasion, a client will object to the recording of an interview. When this occurs, it is essential that helpers determine the exact nature of the client's misgivings. Some individuals feel as if they were losing part of themselves when they see their thoughts put down on paper. Others, who are uncertain as to how this data will be used, fear that hospital personnel or family members will use it against them. Generally, instructors, supervisors, peers, or classmates are the only persons who are privy to this data. Nevertheless, it is considered unethical to record or share the contents of interviews without a client's knowledge or permission. A simple and clear explanation of the purposes, routine nature, and confidentiality of these recordings will help to eliminate clients' suspicions.

Core Dimensions in the Initial Phase

The core dimensions outlined in Table 6-1 occur during each phase of the helping relationship. Knowledge of these core dimensions and their vicissitudes will guide nurses who are concerned with ways of being with clients that promote growth and healing.

Empathic Understanding

People who are unable to solve their current problems frequently feel cut off or isolated from potential helpers who occupy a place in their everyday environment. It is not hard to understand why individuals often feel as if they were "losing ground" as they struggle, alone, to find the right answers to perplexing problems. Sometimes, crucial information which might shed light on a problem and in so doing pave the way for its resolution is simply unavailable to the troubled persons. Forces operating within them prevent them from recognizing ideas, feelings, or behaviors which are not consistent with their image of themselves. Constructive problem solving often requires that a person come face to face with previously unacknowledged and hence threatening elements of personal experience. When nurses convey sensitivity to the client's inner world, their intention is to help the clients overcome feelings of alienation and to see themselves more clearly. From the beginning of the therapeutic relationship, when the helper's emphasis is upon accurately perceiving the client's experience, the nurse pays close attention to the client's verbal and nonverbal behaviors,

facial expressions, voice tones, and postural changes. Entering into the client's world, the nurse attempts to share in and comprehend the client's feelings, though not to the same degree. Grasping the reality of another requires that nurses act as participant observers, alternating between direct experience and objective recognition of the other's feeling state. While nurses' personal memories may supplement their understanding of the client, recognition of their separateness and individuality is essential.

After reflecting upon clients' experiences, the nurse formulates a response which is similar in content and feeling tone to that which they have expressed. This is what is meant by the communication of empathic understanding. The clients' response to the nurse's communication enables the nurse to determine their readiness for examining ideas, feelings, or actions which may be inconsistent with their self-image and hence threatening. The following excerpt illustrates the application of empathic understanding during the initial phase of helping:

Client: (*Sounding irritated.*) My wife always criticizes me and threatens to leave me.

Nurse: You resent your wife for the things she says to you and the threats she makes.

Client: No. That is not so. In some ways, my wife is right. (*Brief pause.*) I feel guilty for talking about her this way to you.

In this instance, the nurse's simple interpretation of the client's resentment is probably correct. However, the client's response is an indication of his lack of readiness to acknowledge the feelings he harbors toward his spouse.

A typical error of nurses during this early stage of helping is the premature rendering of penetrating interpretations of the client's feelings or behavior. Consider this illustration:

Client: We have only been married 3 months and already my wife is beginning to nag me. (*Pause. Client rocks back and forth in his seat.*) She wants too much from me. In some ways she is just like my mother. (*Sounding angry.*)

Nurse: You have angry feelings toward your wife which are similar to those you had toward your mother. These forbidden impulses are upsetting to you. What is even more disturbing is your fear that you will be a disappointment to your wife.

Client: I don't understand what you are getting at. I love my wife. She is the one who is a little scared about taking on a lot of new responsibilities.

High levels of empathic understanding may have a disruptive effect upon the helping relationship when they are ill timed. These reflections are apt to be experienced by clients as threatening and intrusive. Hence, they may arouse anxiety, resentment, and mistrust of the nurse.

Concreteness

In the initial phase, concreteness is used by nurses when they are attempting to directly influence clients to focus on specific problems, to sharpen their observation skills, and to recall the significant details of past or current experiences despite the discomfort that might be felt. Storytelling or the recitation of irrelevancies is discouraged. The following excerpt illustrates the nurse's use of concreteness during the early stage of helping:

Client: The people here bug me. I'm at a loss about how to deal with them.

Nurse: Name one person here who disturbs you.

Client: Mr. Mills, the attendant, always bothers me.

Nurse: What specifically, does Mr. Mills do that bothers you?

Client: He always wants me to go to those group therapy sessions. I never know how to respond.

Nurse: Tell me about one time when Mr. Mills asked you to attend a session and you were bothered.

The client's discovery of solutions to critical life problems is generally preceded by a thorough examination of personally relevant perceptions, ideas, feelings, and behaviors. When the nurse's verbal communications are concrete—that is, pre-

cise and relevant—the client's direct expression of significant personal experiences is facilitated. Peplau's operational definition of the concept of learning[12] provides nurses with a step-by-step guide to collecting personally relevant clinical data. Learning is an active process that utilizes thought, perception, and knowledge for three major purposes: (1) acquiring new knowledge to explain events, (2) facilitating change, and (3) solving problems.[12] This learning process is outlined in Table 6-2.

Confrontation

Confrontation is an interpersonal process which is used by the nurse to facilitate the modification and extension of the client's self-image.[3] Self-image is a ubiquitous concept denoting a multiplicity of perceptions which may be consciously experienced or exist on a preconscious or unconscious level. These perceptions include the following: (1) the image of value or belief system; (2) one's life goals; (3) the cluster of roles that one enacts: (4) one's sense of worth; and (5) perceptions and feelings about one's body.[13] Information or input which is not harmonious with one's self-image is experienced as threatening.

Individuals tend to avoid anxiety by seeking input which maintains their self-image; therefore, confrontation by the nurse is often perceived initially as painful by the client. Individuals who ignore or suppress potentially threatening information about themselves engage in a form of self-deception which impedes problem solving. Troubled individuals may wish that someone would help them to perceive reality with greater accuracy, but when nurses call attention to significant discrepancies in the client's experience, there is often a defensive response. The intention of communications emphasizing confrontation is to enable the client to see what is real, that is, to perceive internal and external reality with greater precision and clarity. The initial stage of the nurse-client relationship may be viewed as a preparatory phase with regard to confrontation. The nurse attempts to discriminate between the real person that the client is and the client's wishful

Table 6-2 Learning Process[2]

Learning	Operations of the Nurse	Nurse statements
Steps in learning as a concept and as a process	Operations, performances, behaviors separate skills, associated with each step in learning. (Major use of the perceptual processes—seeing, hearing, smelling, touching, etc.)	Examples of statements by the nurse to facilitate development of each step in a patient in the total sequence of the process of learning
1 *To observe:* The ability to notice what went on or what goes on now.	To see with one's eyes To hear To feel using empathic observation To feel using tactile senses	What do you see? What is that noise? Are you uncomfortable? Do you have something to say to me? Could I share the thought with you or is it private? Tell me about yourself. What happened? I don't follow. Tell me, what did you notice? You noticed what? Did you see this happen? Who was with you? When did this occur? What is the color? Where were you? Tell me. Then what? Go on. Give me a blow-by-blow description. Tell me every detail from the beginning.
2 *To describe:* The ability to recall and tell the details and circumstances of a particular event or experience.	Increased verbalization Greater recall Enumeration of details Focus on details of one event	Tell me about the feeling. What name would you give to your feeling? Tell me more. Then what? Go on, . . . Give me an example. Who are they? What about that? For instance? Describe that further. Give me a blow-by-blow account of that. What did you feel at the time? What happened just before? Which was it? Who was the person? What did you say? What did your comment evoke in the other?

Source: (Adapted from Hildegard Peplau: "Process and Concept of Learning," in Shirley Burd and Margaret Marshall (eds.), *Some Clinical Approaches to Psychiatric Nursing*, Macmillan, New York, 1963, pp. 333-336).

Table 6-2 Learning Process (continued)

Learning	Operations of the Nurse	Nurse statements
3 *To analyze:* The ability to review and to work over the raw data with another person.	Identify needs Decode key symbols Distinguish literal and figurative Sort and classify 1 Impressions 2 Speculations 3 Thematic abstractions 4 Generalizing Compare Summarize Sequence Application of concepts Application of personality theory as a frame of reference	Explain. Help me to understand that! What do you mean? What do you see as the reason? What was the significance of that event? What are the common elements in these two situations? What is the connection? Boil this down to the one important aspect. What caused this? What was your part in it? In what way did you participate?
(Step 3 may occur simultaneously with step 4)	Formulating relations resulting from the foregoing: 1 Cause and effect 2 Temporal 3 Thematic 4 Spatial	In what way did you reach this decision? What caused this feeling? (I expected you at 8:30; you were late; that caused my anger.) Have you had this feeling before? Is there anything similar in this situation to your previous experience?
4 *To formulate:* The ability to give form and structure, to restate in a clear, direct way, the connections resulting from step 3. (Analysis.)	Restatement of data in light of step 3 Verbal or written result of analysis of data	State the essence of this situation in a sentence or so. What did you feel? What did you think? What did you do? Tell it to me in a sentence or so. Tell me again. Was there a discrepancy between what you felt, thought, and did? What would you say was the problem? What name would you give to the patterns of your behavior as you interacted with another person?
5 *To validate* (by consensus): The ability to check with another person and to reach agreement as to the result of step 4 (formulation) or to state the issue clearly if there is divergence in the formulations of the two persons.	Checking with, comparing notes of, two or more people	Is this what you mean? Let me restate. Is this what you were saying? Do you go along with this? Is this what you believe? Is this the way it appears to you? Is it that you feel angry when people tell you what to do? Am I correct in concluding that . . . ? Are you saying . . . ?

Table 6-2   Learning Process (continued)

Learning	Operations of the Nurse	Nurse statements
6 *To test:* The ability to try out the result of step 4 (formulation) in situations with people, things, etc., for utility, completeness		(Set up situations where patient can try out new behavior patterns.) Now that you have thought about this and come to this conclusion, why don't you try it out? What would you do if a situation like this came up again? In what way can you use this conclusion to prevent repeating this mistake? In what way will this conclusion help you in the future? What difference will it make now that you know this?
7 *To integrate:* The ability to see the new in relation to or as an integral part of the old; to add to previously acquired usable knowledge for active use by the person.	Enmeshing the new with the old	
8 *To utilize:* The ability to use the result of step 4, (formulation) as foresight.		(Set up situations where patient can use new behavior patterns.)

self-image. In addition, the nurse attempts to gauge the clients' readiness to look at the ways in which they have failed to live up to an idealized image of themselves. During this phase of the therapeutic relationship, the nurses' success in confronting clients is contingent upon their ability to question or reflect upon the clients' behavior without directly pointing out contradictions between their wishful and actual selves.[3]

For example, a nurse might reflect upon a client's unsuccessful attempts to dominate and control others in this way: "You wish to always be on top on things, but sometimes this isn't possible." During later stages of helping, clear and direct communication of behavioral discrepancies is appropriate. In the middle stage of a relationship, the nurse might observe, "You would like to always be in control of yourself and the situations with which you are involved; sometimes, things get out of hand and you become anxious and frightened; at these times, you may tend to behave inappropriately."

Confrontations are anxiety-provoking. Calling clients' attention to selected facets of their self-images or behavior is the initial step in the lengthy process required to enable clients to face themselves and their problems in a straightforward manner.

Immediacy

As individuals move through various stages of their lives, they recast their impressions of acquaintances and of those with whom they are intimate. In her memoirs, the noted writer Anais Nin revealed the highly subjective nature of this process.[14] As her needs changed, so did her images of others. No doubt clients' ever-changing perceptions of significant others shape and reshape their relations with them. Interpersonal relationships are rarely fixed and immutable. Individuals witness the strengthening or diminution of familial ties, the intensification or erosion of bonds of friendship. Individuals are conscious of and sensitive to relationship changes.[3]

Nurses strive for partnerships with clients that are vital and productive. It is because nurses have this desire that they so frequently find themselves subjecting facets of their relationships with clients to close and careful scrutiny. While nurses are forming and reacting to their impressions of the relationship, so too is the client. Throughout the entire interpersonal helping process, clients' behaviors are determined, in part, by their varying images of the nurse as well as their personal impressions of the relationship. The clients' perceptions reveal much about their earlier experiences with helpers and persons in authority, their beliefs about the helping process, their expectations, wishes, and fears. Most clients, however, do not initially feel free to disclose or react directly and openly to their impressions. Instead, clients tend to convey their impressions in more indirect ways, more specifically through the use of metaphor or behavioral expressions.

Prerequisite to the establishment and maintenance of a vital working alliance is the sensitivity of nurses to the client's perception of them and their adroitness in eliciting the direct expression of these immediate and relevant interpersonal themes.

The following vignette illustrates the use of immediacy to establish a working alliance between a nursing student and a client.

The client, a 38-year-old woman, rarely uttered a word to the nurse who had been seeing her twice weekly for 2 months. One day, in a desperate effort to transcend the communication barrier which existed between herself and the client, the nurse placed before the silent woman a drawing pad and some crayons. "Draw a picture of whatever is on your mind," the nurse suggested. Much to the nurse's surprise, the woman picked up a crayon and proceeded to sketch the outline of a house. Notably, the house had no door, the windows were shut tightly, and the shades were drawn. The nurse asked the client to explain the picture. The woman indicated that she lived in this house with an imaginary female companion. "The shades," the client explained, "are meant to keep people out."

"Perhaps it is difficult for you to let people know what is going on with you in lots of situations," the nurse stated, tentatively.

"Yes, this is true," was the client's response.

"And perhaps you keep me out," the nurse continued. *"Even now, you may be telling me with your drawing that it is difficult for you to let me know what you are thinking and feeling."*

Looking directly at the nurse, the woman smiled and said "Yes, it is very hard for me."

"Most of the time," the nurse explained, "it is hard for me to get to know what is on your mind. I want very much to help you but it is difficult when you don't let me in."

The statements in italics illustrate the core dimension, immediacy. These statements are intended to explain the relationship between the client's behavior—in this instance, silence—and her perceptions of the helper and the helping situation. The client's response suggests that it is hard for her to disclose her inner thoughts and feelings and that at the moment she views the nurse as an outsider intruding on her private world. The discussion affords the nurse an opportunity to convey to the client her wish to serve as a helpful ally. It is critical that the nurse explicitly convey support, particularly at the outset of the relationship.

Some clients are prevented from immediately recognizing the nurse as a sensitive and caring collaborator. They presume that the nurses bear malice toward them, that they are going to be judgmental or perhaps overly friendly.

Some clients perceive current situations in the

light of earlier experiences which have taught them that disclosure of their observations may destroy a relationship or cause resentment.

Clients often fear exposing their secrets. Shame and concern about the social acceptability of certain ideas are powerful deterrents to self-disclosure. A client who feels love or hatred, sexual or aggressive urges, dependency longings, or perhaps suspicion may be loathe to share personal impressions with the nurse. Other clients may conceal these thoughts because they view them as signs of weakness.

Sometimes, clients' hesitation to reveal their perceptions is rooted in the belief that their impressions, beliefs, or wishes are unimportant. These individuals often think that they are not really entitled to feel or see things as they do. For example, a male client reluctantly told the nurse that he had the impression that the nurse was not really paying attention to what he was saying. After sharing his perception, he immediately added, "But I really shouldn't feel that way!"

Clients require repeated permission to express their thoughts and feelings. Nurses need to give this permission and, at the same time, focus on clients' resistance or withdrawal.

That clients' perceptions of the nurse account for many of their actions throughout the helping relationship is a noteworthy assumption. Many of the client's behaviors are calculated or unknowingly intended to induce a mood in the nurse or to elicit a response which will minimize a perceived threat or gratify a wish. Sometimes a client's actions are motivated by a need for approval or a wish to be liked. Other times, a client may act out of a desire to control certain aspects of a relationship.

Cultural differences frequently explain the diversity in clients' mood- or response-inducing behaviors. Thus, a male Jewish client may think that he must display intense emotion if he wishes the helper to take him seriously. Englishmen, on the other hand, may understate their case, fearing that an emotional display will evoke scorn and rejection.[15]

The following questions, intended to elicit the client's impressions of the nurse, will facilitate the expression of immediacy:

1 How do you think things are going with us?
2 Perhaps you are trying to tell me something about yourself in relation to me?
3 Are you trying to tell me that you see me as (specify attribute)?
4 Are you saying that you feel that I am (specify attribute)?
5 Sometimes clients see nurses as (specify attribute); could this be the case with you?

These statements are aimed at helping clients to examine relationships between overt behavior and inner experiences:

1 Perhaps your (specify client's behavior) is a way of telling me indirectly that you wish me to (specify nurse's behavior).
2 Perhaps your behavior is meant to tell me that you see our relationship as (specify characteristic of relationship).

Expressions of immediacy are intended to explain connections between overt behavior of clients and their underlying impressions of the nurse and/or the helping relationship. By drawing attention to the relationship itself, these expressions sometimes have the effect of intensifying the clients' anxiety and magnifying their distorted perceptions of the nurse. Nevertheless, there are critical times when communications of immediacy are necessary for the development and maintenance of a viable working partnership. These critical times are listed below.

1 The initial phase of the helping relationship, when nurse and client are strangers to one another
2 Before and after a temporary separation between nurse and client. For example, a vacation taken by either person
3 Prior to or after the occurrence of some unusual event, such as a change in the fee schedule or location of sessions

4 After the nurse has committed a technical error such as the premature rendering of advice

5 When, for unexplained reasons, the client is unable to share inner experience with the nurse

6 Prior to termination of the relationship[16]

Respect

Individuals who possess self-respect view themselves as worthy people who are capable of solving their problems and acting constructively. When nurses convey their acceptance of clients' ideas, feelings and experiences and when they recognize clients' potential for self-actualization, they provide the conditions necessary for the development and maintenance of self-respect.

Respect is expressed in diverse ways as the helping relationship evolves. During the early stages of helping, nurses convey to clients their intentions to hear them out. Nurses' responses lead clients to believe that they will listen without judging them, depreciating them, telling them how they ought to act, or demanding their compliance with some expectation. The nurse's responses suggest confidence and trust in clients' ability to act on their own behalf and to come to a successful resolution of their difficulties. Within this climate of acceptance and trust, clients will feel free to engage in deeper levels of self-exploration.

Genuineness

Throughout the interpersonal helping process, the nurse experiences feelings toward the client and/or the relationship. Genuine expressions which convey the nurse's personal reactions to the client can be used by the nurse to further the client's self-exploration. To facilitate the expression of genuineness, nurses need to look inward. During the initial stage of the relationship, emphasis is upon noticing personal reactions to the client. Nurses can use the self-administered checklist in Table 6-3 to help them recognize their responses.

Countertransference

Countertransference is the term used to describe all the feelings which nurses experience toward clients.[5] Feelings of attraction, warmth, and concern are common countertransference reactions; negative responses to the client—such as discouragement, resentment, boredom, guilt, or anger—are equally typical. Unanticipated changes in the nurse's behavior take place when countertransference feelings go unrecognized or when they evoke anxiety. In these instances, the overt communication of nurses may be unrelated to their inner feelings. Thus, while nurses may appear to be attending to the client's concerns, their energies are in fact being diverted toward efforts to recapture a feeling of personal security.

Major indications of a discrepancy between the overt communication of nurses and their inner experience are outlined below:

1 Nurses respond to clients as a parent would to a child, conveying a tone of superiority.

2 Nurses react the way they think they *should*, in a rehearsed, "professional" fashion.

3 Nurses convey opinions in a rigid, dogmatic way.

In each instance, nurses fail to provide clients with any indication of how they truly feel. Incongruent expressions generally have the effect of eliciting

---

Table 6-3 Self-Examination Checklist[17]

1 Today I felt that we had a pretty relaxed, understanding relationship. _____
2 Today I was at a loss as to how to respond to this client. _____
3 Today I couldn't get close to this client. _____
4 Today I resented the client's attitude. _____
5 Today I felt I am doing a pretty competent job with this client. _____

defensive responses from clients. Genuine expressions, on the other hand, further the spirit of inquiry. Honest, spontaneous communications, regardless of their emotional content, are usually liberating and contribute to a feeling that one is more oneself.

The Middle Phase of the Helping Relationship

The gradual transition to the middle phase is accompanied by the client's willingness to assume a more active role in self-exploration. In view of the client's accomplishments during the initial phase, nurses and clients can, during the middle phase, pursue activities aimed at enabling clients to cope with or profit from a problematic experience. The main tasks to be accomplished during the middle phase are the in-depth exploration of significant themes and the discovery and testing of solutions which are most appropriate to the clients' life situations.

Stalls or blocks occur at any time in a relationship. When they do occur, "work" stops. The nurse and client must remain alert and aware of their existence and take steps to explore them. Table 6-4 lists common stalls and solutions for each.[18]

During the middle phase, the core dimensions continue to serve as a guide for nursing practice.

Core Dimensions in the Middle Phase

Empathic Understanding

The mutual recognition of the client's troubled world, acquired during the initial phase of the nurse-client relationship, provides a foundation for deeper inquiry. During the middle phase, nurses' empathic expressions are intended to help clients clarify and extend the meaning of their experiences. When the problem is better understood by nurses than by clients themselves, nurses make tentative statements aimed at calling attention to relevant though previously unexplored thoughts and feelings. The nurse conveys feelings which transcend those initially expressed by clients. Thus, the nurse prepares the way for clients to experience and fully express feelings which were,

up to this time, unacknowledged. The following conversation is an illustration of empathic understanding as expressed during the middle phase of a relationship.

Client: I'm afraid to talk about what is going on between my wife and me.

Nurse: It is difficult for you.

Client: Yes. It's just that sometimes I get so mad that I'm ready to walk out.

Nurse: It really bothers you to get so angry with someone you care for.

Client: I shouldn't be so furious with my wife. I love her and have made a commitment to our relationship.

Nurse: You seem to think that it is not acceptable for a person to have both loving and angry feelings toward another and that you must always be devoted to your wife.

Client: Yes. Isn't that true?

Nurse: No. Most people experience a whole range of intense feelings toward their marital partners. However, you tend to feel guilty about this.

Client: I think that I may have some unrealistic expectations.

Nurse: Yes. And when you fail to live up to them, you blame and condemn yourself.

Client: Yes. That is exactly what happens to me.

Nurse: Perhaps it is time to stop this self-condemnation and to begin looking at the situations which evoke your anger.

Clients frequently derive benefit from hearing the nurse's impressions of their life situation. Communications which are intended to convey the nurse's perceptions of the clients' experience need to be differentiated from the premature giving of advice. Often, an astute nurse will quickly "size up" a client's situation and suggest a course of action. When advice is not based upon the client's thorough self-understanding, it tends to steer the client away from self-exploration and to impose directionality upon the helping process. As the nurse and the client acquire deeper comprehension of and insight into the client's problem, the real but limited number of available alternatives

Table 6-4 Stalls in the Nurse-Client Relationship[18]

Stall	Solution
Judgmental feelings	• Autodiagnosis • Acceptance and realization
Ambivalent feelings	• Realization of its normality • Acceptance and understanding in self and others
Rescue feelings	• Avoid secret alliances with client • Share responsibilities and goals with others
Pessimistic feelings	• Look for client assets, not just problems • Set realistic goals • Develop optimism about goals of the relationship • Give supportive encouragement
Omnipotent feelings	• Realize human limitations • Realize achievement in a relationship is a partnership • Develop humility • Develop respect for self and for the client • Consult with colleagues and supervisors when necessary
False reassurance	• Be supportive rather than reassuring • Be honest
Misuse of confrontation	• Stay with here-and-now issues • Be aware of "timing" when making interpretations
Misjudging independence	• Acknowledge the misjudgment • Ask what clients *can* do for themselves • Reassess client and family capabilities • Do not infantilize
Labeling	• Acknowledge feelings and reason for label • Describe rather than label • Remember that diagnostic labeling is only a small part of the client's behavior
Overidentification	• Acknowledge the existence of overidentification • Talk over and assist client to look at the problem from all perspectives
Overinvolvement	• Recognize that the reason for hospitalization of a client is serious • Maintain a therapeutic involvement • Do not allow client to deny reality of illness • Avoid discussing personal life • Avoid social invitations from the client • Avoid calling the client at home
Painful feelings	• Explore the possible sources of painful feelings (anger, etc.) • Avoid isolation and withdrawal when confronted by the client • Utilize autodiagnosis • Learn to accept and adjust own feelings with other people
Misuse of honesty	• Avoid failure to fulfill promise • Answer questions directly and honestly; avoid "hedging" • Avoid omissions in conversations with the client
Listening pitfalls	• Autodiagnosis • Avoid excessive verbalization • Avoid giving advice and making decisions for the client • Avoid faking attention, interrupting, and asking clients to repeat what they have said • Maintain eye contact • Avoid introducing "intolerable" words • Avoid changing the subject; keep the client focused • Be alert to repetition • Make efforts to clearly understand what is being said

open to the client become apparent and true directionality emerges.

A theoretic understanding of empathy, experience, and supervision helps nurses to gauge the timing of empathic communications.

Concreteness

Problem solving requires that nurse and client speak in concrete terms about the client's future. When clients' plans and expectations are formulated and reviewed in specific terms, rather than in generalities, clients are likely to sense the active role they play in determining their experiences in the time to come. When, on the other hand, nurses and clients fail to communicate clearly about clients' plans, clients may get the impression that the future is, in fact, governed by fate.

Throughout the nurse-client relationship, misunderstandings by clients frequently stem from nurses' ambiguous responses to clients' inquiries. When clients do not receive concrete answers to their questions, they tend to pursue the inquiry in a more indirect fashion or to "invent" explanations which may or may not be valid. Sometimes, clients will interpret the ambiguity or evasiveness of helpers as an indication that they are withholding some terrible bit of information. In such instances, clients come to anticipate the worst.

Concrete responses to clients' inquiries are essential. Pokorney[19] has noted that professional helpers tend to become vague and evasive when clients ask them questions which arouse their anxiety. The basic mechanisms which nurses sometimes use for the purposes of evasion are illustrated in Table 6-5.

Confrontation

Communications conveying high levels of empathic understanding tend towards confrontations. Clients who seek perfection in themselves and others are frequently resistant to confrontations; they anticipate that confrontations will evoke pain, guilt, or anxiety. Clients' efforts to maintain self-deception are generally proportional to their expectations of discomfort. The following statements, made by nurses, are intended to diminish clients' resistances to confrontations during the middle phase of the helping relationship:

1 No one is all good or all bad. People cannot be perfect; neither can the world be a perfect place to live in.
2 You are a human being. Human beings are fallible and make mistakes.
3 It is not possible to be always good, loving, lovable, or kind. Trying to be this way uses up too much energy and requires that you sacrifice who you really are.
4 Our behavior is often influenced by thoughts and feelings of which we are not aware.

Table 6-5 Evasion Strategies

Evasion strategy	Evasive response	Direct response
Nurse confuses who is acting by switching to passive tense.	The idea *was expressed* that. . . . The question *was posed*. . . .	*You asked* whether. . . . *You wonder* if. . . .
Nurse uses unnecessary qualifiers.	*Apparently*, some confusion exists. . . . *At this time*, it looks like. . . . *From my standpoint*. . . .	You seem confused. This is how I see it. I think that. . . .
Nurse broadens the subject.	*Many nurses* claim that. . . . It has been noted by others that. . . .	*I* think that. . . . *I* have noticed that. . . .
Nurse uses analogies or figures of speech.	It is *like a three-ring circus*. We are playing a *cat-and-mouse game*.	It is chaotic. We are being evasive with each other.
Nurse delays answering question.	I first want to discover how an answer will help you.	(Nurse answers question.)
Nurse completely changes subject.	Let's look at something else first.	(Nurse pursues subject at hand.)

Recognizing these inner experiences gives us more control over our lives; we are less the "victims of fate."

5 The pain that accompanies self-discovery is temporary. It won't last forever and often is short-lived.

6 Feelings are simply feelings, not facts.

Immediacy

Efforts to discuss the nurse-client relationship openly frequently must originate with the nurse. The nurse can start out by listening to the hidden messages, the feelings or thoughts which lurk beneath the surface of the client's manifest concerns. These central ideas underlying clients' overt communication are called *content themes.*[9] In the following example, the client experiences the pain of separation. An alert nurse can determine the underlying theme and confront it.

As the summer months approached, the client, an elderly woman, was becoming increasingly apprehensive about the nurse's impending vacation. Not wishing to appear overly dependent or clinging, the woman made a conscious decision to refrain from discussing her anxiety. When the nurse tried to elicit discussion of the client's reactions to the impending separation, the client initiated a broad and lengthy monologue on stoicism. At no point did she speak plainly of her resolve to remain calm and tough in face of sadness and fear. This underlying theme could only be inferred by the nurse.

Sometimes, *how* clients convey concerns imply how they are perceiving the nurse and/or the relationship. For example, Mr. J, a client who feared being dominated by the nurse, was guarded and defensive when he informed the nurse that he had decided to terminate their relationship. Clients' interpersonal needs frequently determine their impressions of the helping situation. In this instance, the client's need was to maintain control of himself and the situation. On occasion, nurses assume roles which are complementary to those of clients. An example of role complementarity is the situation where nurses find themselves making numerous decisions for the client who refuses or seems unable to make choices. The assumption of a role which is complementary to that of the client may obstruct further development or stall the nurse-client relationship. Identification of these interaction patterns is an initial step in exploring with clients their images of and reactions to the nurse.

Ujhely uses the term "interaction theme"[9] to describe clients' behaviors toward the nurse and nurses' responses to these behaviors. Analysis of clinical data and the use of supervision can help nurses to recognize and label significant interaction themes.

Respect

The more clients reveal their inner life and personal adventures, the greater is the nurse's opportunity to appreciate the characteristics which differentiate them from other human beings. Nonjudgmental recognition of and positive regard for the particular ways in which clients perceive and respond to various situations constitutes a higher form of respect. This form of respect is characteristic of the middle phase of the helping relationship.

Messages which convey high levels of respect reduce anxiety and heighten clients' feelings of personal security. Under these conditions, clients are less likely to respond defensively when the nurse directs their attention to the ways in which they are not living up to their fullest potential. Many individuals suppress needs for human contact, smother or conceal vital emotions, kill spontaneity, evade responsible action, and eschew self-sufficiency. By the time the nurse and the client have reached the middle phase of the helping relationship, the nurse sees quite clearly the ways in which the client makes choices which tend to be stifling. As the middle phase unfolds, the nurse conditionally conveys positive regard. This means that clients are commended only when they choose a vitalizing course of action. The nurse strives to help the client recognize the incapacitating consequences of restrictive behavior patterns and to appreciate the value of self-realization.[3]

Genuineness

As the helping relationship evolves, the nurse comes to recognize countertransference feelings evoked by clients' verbal and nonverbal behaviors. Nurses can utilize these personal reactions to discover clients' impressions and suppressed feelings about the one-to-one relationship and to facilitate this helping process. The following exerpt illustrates the communication of genuineness during the middle phase of the nurse-client relationship:

Client: It's just no use. Things are never going to change. And all you ever give me is a meaningless bunch of words.

Nurse: You're telling me that you are feeling hopeless. Even though we have shared a great deal, you are not experiencing me as helpful.

Client: No, its probably my fault that I haven't solved my problem. I should have been more open with you. I always ruin everything.

Nurse: Look, at this very moment, I'm feeling frustrated and useless. I have the impression that, in truth, you are angry with me. You want to show me how much you are suffering so that I too will suffer.

Client: I guess I've been afraid that you would punish me in some way if I told you how annoyed I've been with you lately.

The Termination Phase of the Nurse-Client Relationship

The period of time preceding the permanent separation between nurse and client has frequently been referred to as the *termination phase* of the helping relationship. Clients' reactions to termination are determined by the meaning they ascribe to this event.

As termination approaches, nurse and client are becoming part of each others' past and, at the same time, each moves into a future in which the other will have no part. The future brings change, and if this change is not known to be harmless, both nurse and client experience anxiety as they ready themselves for the events to come. While anxiety is a response to the danger which a loss entails, grief is the reaction to a specific loss. Anticipation of ending and the realization that reunion with the nurse in unlikely activate the grieving process. This process has as its aim separation from the nurse (see Chap. 31). The end point of grieving is the client's internalization of the helping relationship itself.[20]

The onset of grieving is often marked by the client's preoccupation with the nurse and the experiences shared during their relationship. Grieving clients may begin to experience a variety of somatic symptoms. They may become depressed and preoccupied with guilt. They may wonder whether it was something that they did that *caused* the nurse to leave. A stiff manner, designed to hide anger, often emerges. For a while, the client may lose the capacity for initiating or keeping up with organized patterns of behavior.[21]

In a study of psychoanalytic treatment of adults who had experienced losses of significant others during childhood, it was noted that the treatment situation itself, particularly the situations occurring during the last phase, activated interrupted grieving work and helped clients resume the process.[22] Observations of nurse-client relationships correspond with these findings.

It is clients' terror of facing grief which deflects their ability to find meaning in the relationship as it nears conclusion. To reduce anxiety, clients may use coping mechanisms such as acting out, dependency, resignation, denial, or reaction formation.

Acting out occurs when clients cannot readily control or contain their anxiety. During the termination phase, some clients leave the hospital on a pass and fail to return. Others sign themselves out of the hospital precipitately, "against medical advice." Some clients abruptly end the relationship by refusing to participate in any more meetings with the nurse. On occasion, clients "sabotage" discharge plans or behave inappropriately so that they can remain in the hospital.

Adult clients who sense their dependency upon the nurse for feelings of wholeness feel, at times, that they have been absorbed or have become part of the nurse. This leads to a fear of loss of identity. For some clients, loss of personal identity is the danger which separation from the nurse entails.

Clients who fear that they will not survive without the nurse may use guile or adopt ruses to demonstrate their helplessness. They may regress, reexperiencing former symptoms.

Frequently, clients disassociate any thoughts regarding the danger which the nurse's leaving may entail, along with the anxiety that has been stirred up. Instead of concern, these clients report disinterest in the nurse and the impending termination. Clients who cope by resigning themselves have, in a sense, "withdrawn from the battlefield."

Denial is a defense mechanism in which the external reality is rejected and replaced by a wish fulfilling fantasy.[23] The content of denial ranges from a lasting distortion of individuals' perceptions of themselves and their world to a limited avoidance of reality during a particularly stressful period. The denial of the reality of termination may be manifested by clients' negation of the importance of the nurse, an insistence on repeating with the nurse, a fictional relationship with another who was lost in the past, or a refusal to talk about termination. During the termination phase, the clients' use of denial may have both negative and positive aims. The negative aim is to increase the perceived distance between themselves and the danger. A positive aim is to effect a necessary change while preserving personal integrity.

Sometimes, clients who are experiencing painful feelings attempt to find fault with the nurse and everything in the setting. Using reaction formation, clients may complain about the food, the services, or hospital personnel. They avoid feelings of warmth and attachment at any cost.

Core Dimensions during the Termination Phase

It has been noted that the single most important nursing intervention during the termination phase of the helping relationship is that of alerting the client to the impending separation.[24] The most

critical *attitude* of the nurse, which must underlie any intervention taken, is the following: *Leaving is not something the nurse is doing* to *the client, but rather, something the nurse is doing* with *the client.* Summarizing the situations which occurred throughout the relationship, exchanging memories, and evaluating the relationship are experiences which nurses *share* with clients to help them to cope with the ending of the helping relationship.

During the termination phase, nurses continue to convey high levels of each of the core dimensions: empathic understanding, concreteness, confrontation, genuineness, immediacy, and respect.

Nurses' ability and willingness to spontaneously disclose their inner experiences to clients and their capacity for conveying to clients their concern for what is transpiring between themselves and clients in the here and now are particularly critical as the helping relationship draws to a close. The core dimensions of immediacy and genuineness play key roles during the termination phase.

Immediacy

Frequently, clients are aware of the impending termination but will not come right out and initiate discussion of the subject. Nurses need to be on the alert for verbal and nonverbal communications from clients which indicate that they are thinking about the nurse's leave taking. In addition to the aforementioned coping behaviors, clients may reveal their concerns by alluding to the length of the nurse-client relationship or by introducing material which relates to separations from significant others.

One interesting reason why clients may be reluctant to introduce the subject of termination has to do with the expectation that they should be able to make with relative ease the transition from being with helpers to no longer seeing them. This expectation may be related to the American lifestyle, which leads individuals to anticipate sudden and often shocking changes. The ability to accept rapidly and continually changing conditions is a prevailing American value.[25]

When clients fail to initiate discussion of termination, the nurse can broach the subject by indicating the date of the last meeting, the number of interviews remaining, and the reasons for ending them. Once the subject of termination has been introduced, the nurse may discover how, in fact, the client views the chain of events which have occurred. Clients may have trouble recognizing and labeling these situations; therefore it is suggested that the nurse begin to reminisce with clients. With the nurse's encouragement and support, clients can be helped to remember significant past events and to clarify the significance of the helping relationship.

Genuineness

Sometimes, clients refuse to talk about the feelings and thoughts related to termination of the therapeutic relationship. At other times, clients open up and barrage the nurse with expressions of despair and accusations of abandonment or rejection. Clients' reactions to termination can wreak havoc with nurses who are out of touch with their own feelings and responses to the ending of the relationship. During the final phase of the nurse-client relationship, nurses' unrecognized countertransference feelings preclude genuine communication.

It has been noted that there is a correlation between helpers' attitudes toward their next clinical assignment and their ability to handle termination adequately. Helpers who regard future assignments with displeasure or anxiety have more difficulty handling termination. Supervision can facilitate nurses' examination of their perceptions of the present and the future.[26]

During the final phase of the relationship, nurses tend to look back upon the situations which occurred. They may recognize factors which have influenced their behavior throughout the relationship. For example, nurses frequently get in touch with their therapeutic zeal, their need to cure a client, or the wish to perpetuate a client's dependence.[9] Observations made by a nursing student during the termination phase of a helping relationship illustrate this point.

If I had done everything right, my client would have gotten better. During the initial and middle phases of the relationship, I made a few mistakes. But there was time left to try and correct these. I could look at my client's suffering and try to alleviate it. Now, if I make a mistake, there is no time left to fix it up. I'm powerless. My client will soon be gone and he hasn't been cured. I will be able to do nothing more to ease his suffering.

Nurses who have plunged headlong into a relationship hoping to cure a client are in trouble during the termination phase. However, recognition of this unrealistic motive and its impact upon the relationship may give the nurse a new sense of clarity and relief.

Discovering that one has acted to perpetuate a client's dependency is, perhaps, a more painful experience for the nurse. Nurses who need to be needed[9] sometimes discourage clients' efforts to move out from the refuge of the relationship. It is likely that these helpers never seriously acknowledged clients' goals. Likewise, they may have failed to draw attention to goals which were attained. These nurses probably neglected to urge clients to become aware of their growing selves and may have presented themselves as necessary factors in clients' adjustment. During the termination phase, nurses who need to be needed sense the loss of a gratifying relationship. Often, these helpers would like to think that clients cannot tolerate living without them. Having trouble "letting go," such nurses may experience guilt over deserting their clients. Consequently, they may discourage clients from venting responses to the impending separation. Genuine expressions of pain, sadness, anxiety, or perhaps anger are thus discouraged. When nurses minimize or avoid dealing with their clients' experiences, the clients' pain and anger is often intensified, thereby increasing the nurses' guilt.

Looking back over the relationship, nurses may recognize what has been described as the inevitable distortion of the therapeutic process. Throughout the one-to-one relationship, nurse and client may tend to underestimate a client's strengths and overestimate weaknesses. Each may devalue the significance of the relationship and may harbor unrealistic fears regarding the client's ability to cope with loss or to confront the future without the nurse. An initial assessment which includes clients' strengths as well as problems will help to avoid this pitfall.

During the termination phase, progress cannot be measured only in terms of attainment of concrete goals which nurse and client originally planned. Progress can also encompass a deeply felt experience of growth and forward movement which derives from the extension and clarification of the meaning of the events or situations which occurred throughout the helping relationship. The extent to which nurses can help clients find meaning is dependent, in part, upon their own ability to find meaning in the events which have transpired and upon their capacity for conveying high levels of each of the core dimensions.

Supervision can enable nurses to recognize and resolve termination problems. Travelbee has noted that a nurse's decision not to seek guidance or commit oneself to the task of resolving issues of termination, is, in fact, an act of self-betrayal.[27]

The Planning, Description, and Analysis of a Helping Relationship
The Value of Theory
There is a growing body of evidence to suggest that persons designated as helpers may have beneficial or harmful effects on persons seeking to be helped.[28] While the wish to be facilitative provides a base for nurses' interactions with clients, they do not always attain this end. The fact is that, on occasion, the fears of nurses and those of clients do become painful realities. How do nurses ensure and evaluate their effectiveness as helpers? For the most part, nurses' reactions to clients are spontaneous. Rapidly occurring events render it impossible to think out or thoroughly plan responses. Nurses can never anticipate everything that will transpire, nor can they plan all their actions in advance. Thus, most nurses do what they *"feel"* or intuitively *"know"* is right.

Much of nurses' behavior which is quite rele-vant to the helping process is carried on outside of the nurse-client relationship, when nurses focus on improving their helping efforts by means of planning, describing, and analyzing actual helping transactions. Since helping interactions are truly complex, nurses must rely on theories to enable them to think about their relationships in a systematic way (see Chap. 3). Theories explain relationships between events which occur during helping interactions. They serve as a guide to observation and provide nurses with a framework for organizing vast amounts of clinical data. The use of theory requires specialized knowledge and skill. One of the primary roles of the clinical supervisor is to teach novice helpers this skill in order that they may better understand and advance their clinical practice.

The Value of Clinical Supervision
Clinical supervision is an interpersonal process which is aimed at helping nurses to understand and advance their practice through the acquisition of professional knowledge and skill.

The complex psychological interaction between nurses and clients constitutes a major part of the helping process. Empathic understanding, concreteness, confrontation, genuineness, immediacy, and respect are concepts which have been used to describe and explain this psychological interaction. An essential function of the psychiatric nursing supervisor is to enable novice helpers to overcome barriers to the full expression of each of these core dimensions. With the aid of more knowledgeable and experienced helpers, nurses can objectively look at their practice and increase their repertoire of therapeutic skills. In addition, each can hope to attain a higher level of knowledge of the facilitative interpersonal processes.

The extension of one's professional self-image and the understanding and advancement of professional nursing practice are the objectives of the supervisory relationship. It is noteworthy that, although the supervisor functions not as a psychotherapist but as a teacher, the most effective supervisors are those who convey high levels of each of the core dimensions.

References

*1 Suzanne Lego: "Psychiatric Nursing: Theory and Practice of the One-to-One Nurse-Client Relationship," paper presented at a conference titled *"The State of the Art of Psychiatric Nursing,"* April 1974.

*2 Hildegard Peplau: *Interpersonal Relations in Nursing,* Putnam, New York, 1952.

3 Robert R. Carkhuff: *Helping and Human Relations,* Holt, New York, 1968, vols. 1 and 2.

4 Lawrence Brammer: *The Helping Relationship: Process and Skills,* Prentice-Hall, Englewood Cliffs, N.J., 1973, p. 3.

5 Lawrence Brammer and Everett Shostrum: *Therapeutic Psychology,* Prentice-Hall, Englewood Cliffs, N.J., 1968, pp. 72, 234, 246.

6 Arthur Combs: *Florida Studies in Helping Professions,* University of Florida Press, Gainesville, Fla., 1969.

7 L. Hornstra, Bernard Lubin, Ruth Lewis, and Beverly Willis: "Worlds Apart: Patients and Professionals," *Archives of General Psychiatry,* vol. 27, pp. 553–556, October 1972.

8 Aaron Lazare, Frances Cohen, Alan Jacobson, Melvin Williams, Robert Mignone, and Sidney Zisook: "The Walk-in Patient as a Customer," *American Journal of Orthopsychiatry,* vol. 42, pp. 873–883, October 1972.

*9 Gertrud Ujhely: *Determinants of the Nurse-Client Relationship,* Springer, New York, 1968, pp. 103–108.

*10 Frances Monet Carter: *Psychosocial Nursing,* Macmillan, New York, 1976, p. 145.

11 Bernard Berenson and Robert Carkhuff: *Beyond Counseling and Therapy,* Holt, New York, 1967, p. 132.

*12 Hildegard Peplau: "Process and Concept of Learning," in Shirley Burd and Margaret Marshall (eds.), *Some Clinical Approaches to Psychiatric Nursing,* Macmillan, New York, 1963, pp. 333–336.

13 Silvano Arieti: *Interpretation of Schizophrenia,* Basic Books, New York, 1974, p. 88.

14 Anais Nin: *Diary of Anais Nin,* Harcourt Brace Jovanovich, New York, 1976, vol. 6, pp. 17–18.

15 John Spiegel: *Transactions,* Science House, New York, 1971, p. 316.

16 Robert Langs: *The Technique of Psychoanalytic Psychotherapy,* Jason Aronson, New York, 1973, vol. 1, pp. 124–125.

17 William Snyder and June Snyder: *The Psychotherapy Relationship,* Macmillan, New York, 1960, pp. 377–379.

18 Ann Burgess and Aaron Lazare: *Psychiatric Nursing in the Hospital and the Community,* Prentice-Hall, Englewood Cliffs, N.J., 1973, pp. 130–150.

19 Alex Pokorney: "When to Talk Fuzzy," *Psychiatric News,* vol. 71, p. 4, 1971.

20 Hans Loewald: "Internalization, Separation, Mourning, and the Superego," *Psychoanalytic Quarterly,* vol. 31, p. 488, 1962.

21 Erich Lindemann: "Symptomatology and Management of Acute Grief," in Howard Parad (ed.), *Crisis Intervention: Selected Readings,* Family Service Association of America, New York, 1966, p. 20.

22 Joan Fleming and Sol Altschul: "Activation of Mourning and Growth by Psychoanalysis," *International Journal of Psychoanalysis,* vol. 44, pp. 419–431, 1963.

23 Leland Hinsie and Robert Campbell: *Psychiatric Dictionary,* Oxford University Press, New York, 1960, p. 117.

*24 Barbara Sene: Termination in the Student-Patient Relationship, *Perspectives in Psychiatric Care,* vol. 7, p. 43, January–February 1969.

25 Jurgen Ruesch and Gregory Bateson: *Communication: The Social Matrix of Psychiatry,* Norton, New York, 1968, p. 147.

26 Eugene Pumpian-Mindlin: "Comments on Techniques of Termination and Transfer in a Clinical Setting," *American Journal of Psychotherapy,* vol. 12, p. 456, July 1958.

*27 Joyce Travelbee: *Intervention in Psychiatric Nursing,* Davis, Philadelphia, 1969, p. 175.

28 Robert Carkhuff and Bernard Berenson: *Beyond Counseling and Therapy,* Holt, New York, 1967, p. 4.

*Recommended reference by a nurse author.

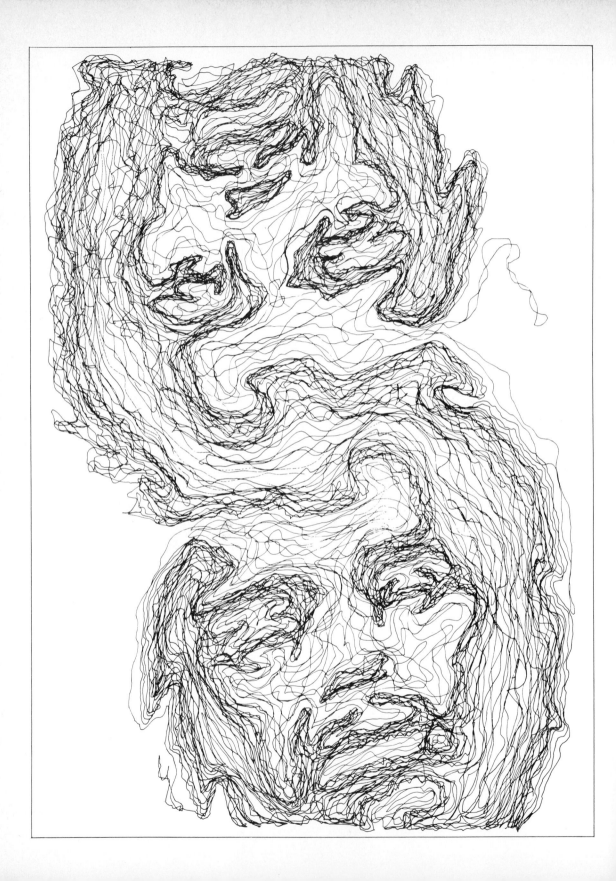

Two

Entry Into Psychiatric Treatment

Chapter

7

The Nursing Process

Elizabeth M. Maloney

Learning Objectives

After studying this chapter, the student should be able to:

1 Identify the components of the problem-solving process
2 Identify the components of the nursing process
3 Define the assessment process
4 Utilize the assessment process to collect a client data base
5 Define and formulate nursing diagnoses
6 Define and formulate client goals
7 Define and formulate nursing interventions
8 Define the evaluation process
9 Formulate criteria for evaluating client care
10 Identify the components of the problem-oriented record
11 Formulate a care plan utilizing the components of the problem-oriented record

One of the vital attributes or benchmarks of a service profession is a consensus on what constitutes the core of the practice. The comprehensive analysis of the core of clinical nursing practice is the set of operations called nursing process. The various tools that are used to communicate and summarize the actions and interactions comprising the entire process are problem-oriented records and nursing audits.

General Discussion of Process

The use of the word "process" to describe the sum total of the actions formerly assembled under the rubric "nursing care" is an evolutionary phenomenon. The phrase is commonly accepted throughout nursing as the central way in which the occupational goals of the particular health group are achieved. The tools which are associated with it are in widespread use throughout almost every care system in the nation.

Interestingly enough, while the term "interpersonal process" has been a common one in psychiatric nursing since the early 1950s, the term "process" or "nursing process" did not seem to gain much ground in other areas of nursing until well over a decade later. At present, the term "nursing process" and the operations associated with it are accepted by nurses and are viewed as the core process by which the purposes of nursing are fulfilled.[1]

Nursing as a Professional Process

The range of activities traditionally known as problem solving lie at the heart of any helping or service profession. Among the occupations so designated, a universally shared set of operations or a common framework can be discerned. These operations are strikingly alike in the literature of social work, law, and medicine.[2,3]

It is well known that *a frequent preliminary to seeking professional assistance is to try to cope with the problematic situation by oneself.* Exhausting the obvious means of aid at hand is a general preliminary to seeking professional assistance. Most of us will try to deal with new problems by seeking solutions that are familiar or that have worked before. Failing to deal with the situation alone, we turn to family, friends, and neighbors for advice. Only if no other workable solution emerges do we call for professional assistance. There are few clients who arrive at any helping professional's door without at least a beginning assessment of what their problem(s) might be. This is as true of the psychiatric problem as it is of a painful fracture. The importance of the client's assessment is self-evident.

The foregoing comments could be summarized operationally as follows: (1) A situation exists where individuals encounter a problem or difficulty in daily living. (2) They make abortive attempts to solve problems on their own. (3) They find that they do not have the necessary knowledge or skill for a solution. (4) Therefore they turn to one designated by society as an expert in the specific class of difficulty. (5) By so doing, they have instituted a specialized helping process. These steps are the usual preliminaries to the initiation of any professional process.

"Process," then, implies something in the course of being done; a state which is never static or completely at rest but which proceeds systematically, logically, and in serial order to some previously defined end. Process is characterized as having a beginning and an end. To that extent it can be described as having temporal or time-bound qualities. When it occurs in a particular geographic or social and psychological space, the spatial dimension becomes of marked importance. For example, human growth has been called a process. It has a clearly defined beginning and end, proceeding in its broad outlines in a predictable, orderly fashion from cradle to grave. Some participants in this process enter life for only a brief moment, while others exceed the biblically allotted three score and ten. Any process, then, can have a number of ramifications as to length of time and surrounding circumstances.

Clinical Art and Professional Process

The importance of selecting the proper abstractions, propositions, theories, and facts which can then serve as guides to concrete action cannot be overemphasized. However, sooner or later, the question of nursing as an art needs to be discussed. It can be speculated that the clinician's art is derived from increasing experience in looking at the available data base of assembled evidence. Selecting the relevant explanatory concepts for the appropriate class of problem, developing working propositions for solution of the problem, testing them out in concrete action, and evaluating them does or does not lead to their modification or rejection.

Reliance on experience, while acknowledged as important, can, if carried to extremes, lead to stereotyped solutions of problems. Essentially, experience is useful only when the practitioner is presented with the same situation over and over again and where the same knowledge can be applied without risk. Sometimes *the art* consists of disregarding experience and structuring innovative strategies in response to client problems that are not ameliorated by the usual solutions. For example, nine times out of ten an admission procedure for clients can be carried out without deviation. During the nurse's first experience admitting a psychiatric client the focus tends to be as much on the mechanics of the admission as on the individual client. Much later, after experience, the focus shifts so that the mechanics of the admission procedure become second nature and the client is of paramount importance. Theoretical and practical expertise facilitates rapid decision making in which a deliberate problem-solving approach may apparently be lacking. Consequently, an experienced nurse faced with an anxious client who is swiftly moving into panic will omit *all* admission procedures and move the client directly to the service unit. This rapid decision-making process does not entirely rule out what we know as the inspirational or procedural leap which illuminates a particularly trying problem from time to time. Such leaps are based on knowledge lying just out of the moment's awareness, knowledge that is processed unconsciously and emerges to constitute an unquantifiable part of the art. Feeling, talking, empathy, and a sound knowledge base *is* the effective core of the psychiatric nursing process.

The nursing process as defined by Yura and Walsh is divided into four areas: (1) assessment of client and family needs; (2) formulation of nursing diagnoses; (3) planning, which is subdivided into goals and interventions; and (4) evaluation.[1] The practitioner proceeds through these stages sequentially. However, since these operations extend over varying time frames, new data continuously emerge which may require returning to a prior step and revising either the data base or the plan.

Assessment

Assessment can be defined as the collection of data about an individual's and family's mental health status so that the client's concerns and problems can be identified. Analysis of the data leads to the development of a conceptual formulation of the client and the nurse's perception of the problems.[1] Data are collected from the client, the family, the physician, and the social network, which includes significant others, neighbors, religious advisers, teachers, and employers. Data collection takes place in a formal interview setting and through informal observation and talking with family and health-team members.

The two sources of informational input are subjective and objective data. *Subjective data* consist of verbal statements made by the client or other informants. Perceptive use of interviewing skills by the nurse facilitates the articulation of the client's perception of the problem, the contributing factors, and the possible solutions. When respectfully interviewed, a suspicious client may be able to verbalize the belief "my children are poisoning me." Exploration of vague statements will clarify the client's perceptions of reality.

Some clients are unable to contribute subjective information because they are psychotic, deeply depressed, or intoxicated. In this case, the nurse has to move from the primary source of information, the client, to secondary sources,[4] such as the family and social network, to obtain essential data. The secondary sources may become primary sources in certain areas of the assessment process, such as those relating to family perceptions and environmental support systems.

Objective data consist of those aspects of information which are obtained and verified by thorough observation. Included are measurable data such as laboratory tests; vital signs; nonverbal data conveyed by the client, such as tone of voice, facial expressions, gestures, posture; and process data about client actions and decisions. The objective data base also involves the environment: the home, employment setting, and school setting. The list is almost infinite. The nurse correlates subjective data (if available) and objective data, checking one out against the other to identify discrepancies and to determine the validity of the information.[4]

The initial data base is expanded as the relationship with the client and family expands. Assessment is an ongoing process. Priorities are set according to data available based on primacy of needs.

Assembling the Data Base

The nurse is often the staff member present at the time of admission and is most available to the client and family. At this time an assessment is made which becomes the basis for the initial plan of care. In some situations, a record of previous interviews provides initial information about the client's problems and past history. Home visits by the community-health nurse can also serve as an initial source of information about client and family problems. Subsequent or additional home visits can contribute to expansion of the data base about client and family if the community-health nurse acts as a liaison between the treatment setting and the community.

A *total* assessment is completed through the efforts of the entire mental health team (see Chap. 9). One member of the team is selected to act as a liaison between the client, family, and hospital. This approach immediately involves the family in the treatment process and assists them in sharing responsibility for successful implementation of the treatment program.

In addition to securing data from the client and family, the team initiates the family's involvement with social service and other supportive services. This communicates concern for family problems and indicates the expectation of involvement in the decision-making process. Openness and honesty regarding the process of admission, the goals of treatment, and the plan of action minimize the fears and stereotypes of the client and family regarding the staff, hospital, and treatment regimen and prepare them to work with the mental health team.[5]

How the Individual Comes for Help

Once the decision to enter treatment is made, clients arrive at the care setting—the emergency room of a general hospital, the psychiatric hospital, or the outpatient clinic—in a variety of ways.

Howard L, age 21, was brought to the emergency room of the general hospital by his parents. He had been in bed in a fetal position for 2 weeks, refusing to eat or get dressed. They could do nothing to change his behavior. He kept muttering, "They want to kill me, they're out to get me," as he was carried into the emergency room.

Barbara G, age 31, was referred to the outpatient clinic by her priest. She arrived weeping, stating, "My husband just beat me and took away my money. What can I do? I don't know how to handle him."

Ronald S, age 49, was brought to the emergency room of the general hospital by the police and admitted to the psychiatric unit. He had been spotted by a neighbor standing on the edge of the roof of a twelve-story building, talking to himself. The neighbor called the police and they coaxed Ronald off the roof. Ronald stated that he had been depressed following a job layoff and thought his family would be better off without him.

Rita W, age 70, recently widowed and living alone, arrived at the state mental hospital where she had formerly been a client saying, "I have nobody, I'm so lonesome, please talk to me."

People may initiate ntry into a care setting in a self-directed way, they may come as a result of referral, or they may be brought to the facility by another individual.[5,6] The manner in which they arrive depends on the nature of the precipitating event and the social network. The person who accompanies them provides important clues as to whose aid the client is able to enlist in times of stress.

Client's Perception of the Problem

Psychiatric clients are frequently unable to see that they present any problem. Awareness of the problem may come from a social definition of mental illness originating in the individual's immediate life-space or from intrapsychic distress felt and defined by the person without outside intervention. Often it is a combination of factors operating simultaneously. This is especially true for those persons who themselves define their problem as existing in the psychiatric area and who at the same time have family, friends, and employers who reach the same conclusion (see Chap. 3). For example, people who become increasingly obsessive about their getting-up routines in the morning, expanding them gradually from a tidy, organized hour to an increasingly ritualistic 3 hours, are aware of their problem themselves. Although they may have given reassuring explanations to their families, they find themselves compelled to extend their obsessive behavior into their social lives and then, despite careful and rational explanations, into their lives at work. This is a brief picture of one sort of psychiatric problem which confronts clients whose inner lives are invaded by illness almost at the same time as those closest to them begin to perceive the problem. Many cases such as this are seen in what is loosely called the *outpatient psychiatric system.* Such clients approach the care system at one of its several points and solicit assistance or relief from the disruption in their lives. They may see a private psychiatrist or family physician, or they may turn to an outpatient clinic. The psychiatric social worker and psychiatric nurse-clinician are also among the persons they may encounter. At this point, such clients have loosely defined what they think is their difficulty. Once defined by the client, the problem will be defined again and redefined through the therapeutic work in the psychiatric setting.

Clients will vary in their ability to accurately perceive their problems. On the one hand, there will be the clear self-recognition described above, and, on the other, the contention that the client's problems are being caused by others. There are people who believe they have no problem at all.

For example, the police of a large city pick up John Doe, who has assaulted a fellow shopper in a department store. There is no discernible explanation for this behavior other than the one John provides. The customer, he believes, has been following him for several days and is a member of a gang out to kill him. This is his view, which he presents along with a lot of other material of sufficient irrationality to cause him to be admitted to the city psychiatric ward. This is an instance where others—the customer and the police—have identified the behavior as a problem. The professional then has to deal with a client who defines the situation in a way that is totally at odds with reality. This is one of the knottiest problems that the psychiatric worker has to face, since, under these circumstances, it is difficult for client and caretaker to agree that a problem exists. The nurse is confronted with a unilateral definition of the problem or at least one which the client does not share.

Similar situations arise when people enter a treatment setting because they have been advised or convinced by others to come. Here too, it is not the client but others who define an existing problem. For example, a client may say, "I'm here instead of going to jail on a drug rap," or "My father says I have to come if I ever want to live at home again." Such clients, like John Doe described above, often enter the treatment setting via community agencies—such as the courts, police, school, family, or family physician—who have convinced or advised them to seek help.

Between the extremes of self-recognition and denial fall those people who enter the treatment setting because of a stated inability to control thoughts, feelings, and actions. When such clients are interviewed, they make statements like the following: "Those voices keep talking to me. I can't make them disappear." "I want to kill myself and I'm afraid I'm going to do it." "I got so mad at my husband that I picked up a knife and was about to go at him with it." "I stole a car last night; I had the strangest feeling something was wrong with me, but I couldn't stop myself."

Also within this range are relatives who bring the client because *they* cannot control the client's behavior. Peter, age 18, was brought to the mental health clinic by his parents, who complained that they could not do anything with him. He simply would not listen. He was off until all hours of the night drinking with his friends and riding his motorcycle. He would come home at 5 or 6 A.M., go to sleep, and refuse to get up to go to school in the morning. The parents complain that he stays in his room and refuses to speak to the family. Peter says, "They're so straight, it's sickening."

Other clients enter the treatment setting for safety and protection, wishing to escape a threatening environment. These clients may say that they cannot stand it and have to get away from the family's constant fighting and nagging, that they are terrified of a wife or husband and fear bodily harm, or that they want to end a drug habit and cannot do it alone. In summary, people define their problems in various ways, ranging from self-recognition through partial recognition of a problematic area in their lives to complete denial.

Family's Perception of the Problem

The family's perception of the problem may or may not agree with that of the client, or the family members may disagree among themselves. On interview, Ann and her parents expressed *similar* perceptions about her problem:

Ann: I'm so scared. The only place I feel safe is in my room.

Parents: Ann is so fearful about everything that she just sits cowering in a corner of her room all day.

On interview, Howard and his parents expressed *dissimilar* perceptions of the problem:

Howard: I have no problem, it's the FBI that has the problem. They're after me so I have to hide.

Parents: Howard has quit his job and has been curled up in bed for the past 2 weeks talking to himself.

On interview, Mary's parents each have a *different* perception of the problem, and Mary herself contributes a still different view of the situation:

Mary: I'm not crazy. I just do what my friends do.

Father: She's a no-good junkie. She belongs in jail!

Mother: She has problems we've never wanted to acknowledge. Now that it's out in the open, maybe we can change things.

It is important for the team to identify agreement or conflict in terms of family perceptions. The degree of congruence will affect the way in which goals are negotiated so that therapeutic blocks can be avoided.

Family members who have a realistic perception of the problem can be utilized to enhance a therapeutic alliance. The family members who utilize denial or disinterest to perpetuate noninvolvement need to feel accepted despite their feelings, and they must be given time to explore their feelings and perceptions with a member of the health team before mutually agreeable goals can be negotiated.

What the Client Sees as the Solution to the Problem

When clients enter the treatment setting, they have expectations about *what is going to happen and how their problems can be solved*. The team explores client expectations about what they want or expect to have happen in treatment. Specific goals need to be identified. These include the following:

- I want to either strengthen my marriage or dissolve it.
- I want to stop drinking.
- I want to be more comfortable speaking in a group.
- I want to be able to get through the day without feeling that I'm falling apart.
- I want to be able to understand why I get depressed.
- I want to be able to live normally without being afraid to go out.

It is also important to identify client expectations about *what is going to solve the problem.* Caretakers may not agree with the stated expectations and must help clients to redefine solutions and seek other alternatives. For example, Barbara G came to the clinic stating "My husband just beat me up. I can't handle him. You have to make him stop." Responsibility was placed on the clinic and caretaker for improving the situation. However, the caretaker could not make the husband stop beating her. The caretaker could assist in helping the couple to establish more effective patterns of communication but could not take total responsibility for creating change. Thus it is important to ascertain the goals the client has in terms of desired therapeutic outcomes and how the clinical setting will assist in the attainment of these goals.

What the Family Sees as the Solution to the Problem

Families also have expectations about *what is going to happen and what they would like to see happen in treatment.* It is essential to assess the *congruence* of client and family goals. Are the goals and desired outcome similar or dissimilar? Are family members aware of the discrepancies among the desired outcomes? Does the family want the client to change? How do they want the client to change? Does the family want to change?

Often it is only after making a complete assessment, and after the treatment regimen is in progress, that discrepancies become evident. For example, many times parents complain about their child's repeated schizophrenic episodes; how the illness drains the family's resources financially and emotionally, and how they wish the child were well and independent. However, each time reintegration is attained and an independent life-style is discussed, the parents will find ten reasons why the child should continue to live at home and not work.

Another example concerns spouses of alcoholics. These husbands and wives may complain bitterly during the course of the addiction, but they will frequently leave or divorce their mates once rehabilitation is achieved. Despite overt protests, the illness seems to meet underlying emotional needs. Recovery brings with it changes in role relationships and communication, giving rise to new and sometimes intolerable demands[5] (see Chap. 17).

Families also have notions about what will solve the client's problem. For example, they may say, "Stop drinking," "Grow up," "Stop fighting," or "Act like a man, not like a mouse!" They often see the problem as lying entirely with the client and not only deny their own role in it but refuse to become involved in the treatment program.

An important aspect of assessing the validity of expressed family goals is to identify significant family members. Burgess and Lazarre highlight important questions to consider:[5]

1 Who comes to the hospital with the client?
2 Who visits the client?
3 Who participates in the treatment program?
4 Who sabotages the treatment program?
5 Are the missing people important to implementation of the treatment program?

For example, Susan L, age 20, arrived at the mental health clinic with her father. Susan said, "My mother is not here because she had a bridge party and luncheon. She cares more about her friends and card game than she does about me." The preexisting relationship between mother and child as well as the angry feelings expressed at the admission interview will remain unresolved as long as the mother continues to absent herself from the treatment setting.

Psychological Assessment

Psychological assessment includes data collection about the client's emotional status, communication style, interaction patterns, psychodynamic issues, and coping patterns.[5,6]

Emotional Reactivity

1 Is the client emotionally controlled or is there appropriate expression of feeling?
2 Is the client's affect congruent with subjective statements and behavior?
3 Are there discrepancies in the client's affect and emotional reactivity?
4 Are current affects and emotional reactions consistent with the client's usual emotional response pattern or are they being influenced by the stress of the interview?

Communication Style

1 Is the client's verbal style quiet, loquacious, or guarded?
2 Does the client spontaneously offer information or respond only when questioned?
3 Does the client refuse to respond?

Interaction Patterns

1 To whom does the client respond?
2 With whom does the client communicate?
3 Who is important to the client?
4 Whom does the client seek out for help?

Psychodynamic Issues

A component of the psychological assessment process is determining the meaning of the precipi-tating cause or events that led the client to seek psychiatric help. When the nurse listens to and observes the client's verbal and nonverbal communication, recurrent feelings or themes emerge which enable the nurse to understand why the client is experiencing distress.

Psychodynamic issues are always present and underlie every situation. They relate to unfulfilled expectations and lack of basic need fulfillment, such as loss of love and security; loss of power, self-esteem, and mastery; loss of control and acceptance.

Coping Patterns

It is important to differentiate between coping patterns used over a long period of time and those which predominate during the crisis period (see Chap. 5). Coping patterns relate specifically to ego defenses and reflect the person's ability to struggle against the thematic issues that underlie the psychodynamics of client behavior. The major factor to consider is the relationship of the coping mechanisms to internal or external stress. For example, John became suspicious about poison in his food and felt that people were spying on him. Here the coping mechanism of projection is utilized to minimize unacceptable *internal* feelings of aggression. The blame is projected onto others and difficult feelings are dealt with in an acceptable if not an appropriate way.

Other clients react to *external* stress, such as impending surgery, by exaggerating the normal coping patterns. An accountant who is normally meticulous and orderly may ritualistically organize his bedside environment and react with anger if his meal trays come late or diagnostic tests are delayed. This ritualism is an attempt to order an environment that is losing its normal boundaries of control and predictability. The previous patterns of coping and maintaining order are exaggerated when the client is experiencing external stress.

Other coping patterns take on symbolic meaning for clients attempting to deal with internal or external stress. For example, conversion symptoms represent a physical way of dealing with feelings. A client who reported a loss of sight had earlier witnessed the violent murder of a neighbor and good friend. Blindness may symbolically represent this client's inability to acknowledge and accept the witnessed event.

Client strengths must also be assessed. This is the core of health that needs to be addressed by the team to ensure the therapeutic program's maximum effectiveness. Such an approach avoids excessive regression, dependency, helplessness, and hopelessness. Every client has some area of strength which can be drawn upon. For example, Stanley was very verbally withdrawn, but he played the piano well. He would go to dances to play dance music; initially, this was the only time he would verbally interact with others who came up to talk to him. Gradually, that verbal behavior generalized to other situations. Other client strengths might include occupational, social, recreational, or artistic skills. Such strengths are assessed by observing how successful the client has been in various aspects of life. The staff must be careful that the client does not overutilize a strength and consequently avoid confronting other problem areas.

The number of strengths identified will in part determine the client's prognosis. Usually, a good number of strengths indicates that despite regressions, the therapeutic outcome will be positive. Even a minimum number of strengths—such as little education, poor work history, no friends, no kin network—does not doom a client to failure. However, in such cases the therapeutic advances may be more limited.

Social Assessment

The assessment factors in this area include socioeconomic, religious, and cultural background. These data are obtained from the client, the family, friends, and the occupational and educational history. Assessment of the above factors indicates the client's relationship to family, friends, and the community; it points toward the factors in the family or larger social system that contribute to the problem.

Socioeconomic Factors

A client who left school at age 16 and has worked as an unskilled laborer may be at a greater disadvantage in terms of being able to effect a vocational adjustment following discharge than a high school or college graduate would, or a person who has worked at a skilled trade or in a professional capacity. This will depend upon the status of the job market as well as the client's value as an employee. Bob H left college following his first psychotic episode. After discharge from the hospital, he began to work for a printing firm. His skill at his job is highly valued and his boss holds his job for him during his periodic hospitalizations. His job and his employer's understanding are important links to the community, ensuring independence and self-esteem. This may be a motivating force in Bob's returning to health. Social and financial resources are important support systems in helping the client and family to obtain and utilize effective treatment services.

An assessment of the client's social network identifies important environmental support systems.[6] Who visits the client and what types of patterns may be determined in part by cultural and religious norms. Do family members visit singly or does the whole clan involve itself in the treatment and visiting program? Do they demonstrate understanding of client behavior or do they view the client's mental illness in terms of cultural or religious stereotypes? Mary C's grandmother, her guardian, could not understand why Mary was hospitalized. She felt that the voices Mary was hearing were indicative of special powers being conferred on her. Support from religious advisers, peers, and other community people may also take on cultural or religious overtones.

It is important to observe the family and other visitors in terms of interaction patterns as well as the affective and behavioral reactions of the client before, during, and following visiting hours. Pat G would become very agitated on the day prior to her parents' Sunday visit. Her behavior would become increasingly inappropriate and difficult to control. While her parents were visiting, she was fine; but after they left, she would again become agitated. Mike L, on the other hand, apparently looked forward to his parents' visits but became argumentative and hostile as soon as they arrived and remained so for several days following their visit.

Sometimes limits must be set on visiting, restricting who visits, when, and in what setting. Clients can make it difficult to terminate a visit; they may make the visitors feel guilty about departing and leaving the client in the hospital. Mary C would hold her grandmother's hand and beg her not to leave. The grandmother would become very upset at this request, knowing that she had to go. The nurse must frequently intervene and set limits on such behavior, for example, by stating, "Mary, it's time for dinner and grandmother must leave and get back to the rest of the family. She'll be here again on Wednesday."

The staff should observe nonverbal communication between family members:

1 Seating pattern—close together or far apart?
2 Physical contact—kissing, touching, embracing
3 Eye contact, tone of voice, gestures
4 Conversation patterns—talk among visitors, with client, with other clients

Jill A, aged 26, was frequently observed during family visits to be sitting on her father's lap; Mike B, on admission, sat with his head cradled in his mother's lap; while Diane C and her parents sat holding hands and watched television during visiting hours.

Such behaviors are indicative of the extreme dependency of the client on the family and the role enacted by the client in the family system. Ways of dealing with such behavior are discussed in the chapters on management of client behaviors (Chaps. 13–22).

The family history must be obtained so that factors relating to the client's current status can be clarified. Communication patterns emerge which identify family roles, rules, alliances, myths, and channels of communication. Relationships between peers (such as parent-parent, friend-friend, and brother-sister interactions) and intergenerational relationships (such as parent-child, grandparent-parent, grandparent-child, relative-child) must be identified.

It is important to identify communication styles, that is, who talks to whom and when. Communication patterns between family members are often clouded and indistinct (see Chap. 11 for an extensive discussion of family dynamics). For example, as Mike B lay with his head in his mother's lap, she talked about how she wished he would grow up, get a job, and get married. This double-bind communication, like other types of disordered communication, makes it impossible for the client and family to respond to one another successfully.

The family history can further elucidate dynamic factors contributing to the distress and disequilibrium of both client and family.

Brenda M, 19 years old, was brought to the mental health center by her stepmother, who said, "We can't do a thing with her. Can't talk to her or make her listen to reason. All she does is hang around with those bums and booze it up. My husband and I can't understand her, much less begin to deal with her."

Brenda's mother died when she was 7. Her father traveled frequently, leaving her in the care of a succession of housekeepers and then her maternal grandmother. Brenda states she felt lonely and unloved most of the time. Her father remarried and had two children with his new wife. Despite a semblance of family life, her stepmother's natural children were perceived by Brenda as receiving most of the attention. She began to drink to make herself more sociable at parties; a few drinks and she "loosened up." Many sexual encounters resulted in an out-of-wedlock pregnancy, which led Brenda's father to throw her out of the house. Following an abortion, Brenda was brought home by her parents, who she feels continued to ignore her. This morning her stepmother found her on the bathroom floor with her wrists slashed, moaning, "He doesn't want me anymore."

Brenda's difficulties revolve around feelings of rejection and low self-esteem. She has never had consistent nurturing from a single significant other. Her parents and parent surrogates have either departed at will or have been indifferent to her needs. They have either failed to care or to demonstrate caring. Her suicide attempt was a result of what she felt was one more rejection.

One of the major goals of therapy for this client is to strengthen family bonds and improve channels of communication. Additional significant others in the client's environment need to be involved, and appropriate interpersonal skills must be directed toward establishing new, effective, and enduring relationships.

Behavioral Assessment

It is important to assess the appropriateness of the client's behavior. Is there a discrepancy between what the client says and does? The nature of relationships needs to be examined. Are they egalitarian, domineering, manipulative, or passive? Is the client the victim or the aggressor? To people of which sex does the client relate best? When maladaptive behavior occurs, it is important to identify the antecedent of the event, the event itself, and the reinforcer of the event.[5]

Medical Assessment

The mental health team is always aware of the significance of the client's physical and medical needs. A thorough physical examination is completed upon admission. The data obtained provide a baseline for the evaluation of physical changes. This may be useful in determining choice of psychotropic drugs, identifying side and toxic effects of psychotropic drugs, and identifying withdrawal syndromes from drugs or alcohol.[5,6]

Nursing Assessment

The nursing history is a component of the total assessment process. It relates to the way the client structured space, time, tempo, and style of life before entering the hospital.

Personal habits and general ways of life provide a baseline for making an assessment of a client's adjustment to unit life. An example would be an 18-year-old woman, unemployed, whose customary bedtime before admission was anywhere between 2 to 4 A.M. If this fact is not known, it can easily enter the clinical picture as a symptom when the woman does not comply with hospital rules for an earlier bedtime.

A nursing history of the psychiatric client, whether in the home or clinical service, can be summarized as *most useful when focusing on the daily life of the client.*

Case Study

An example of a client whose appraisal of his problem is realistic, both as he perceives it and as he communicates it, will illustrate the initial phase of a nursing assessment. The time is the first week in May, 10 o'clock in the evening. The place is the health-service psychiatric clinic of a university medical center. The person is a young man enrolled in his third year at the engineering college. He is accompanied by a member of the general emergency staff who introduces him, hands over a summary sheet, and departs.

Nurse: What brings you here?

Client: I was studying for a final exam and all of a sudden I thought I would pass out—heart beating so fast, dizzy—couldn't breathe right. For a minute I thought I was going to die.

Nurse: Has this ever happened before?

Client: Yes, twice. Both times I was admitted but they didn't find anything after a lot of tests. Probably pressure builds up around the end of the year, a stress syndrome. What I need is some sleep for a few days, something to calm my nerves, and I'll be OK.

This, then, is the client's story or view of how he happened to be admitted to the psychiatric unit. As the information base is later expanded and verified, several things will probably emerge. First, a description of how the client attempted to deal with this episode himself will undoubtedly develop. The nurse's initial, immediate, or first stage of assessment has begun. One useful way of proceeding is to ask several questions as guides to the initial assessment; other possible questions follow (see Table 7-1).

Results of Action

The nature of the care setting usually dictates which member of the interdisciplinary team assembles which pieces of the information. In a small community hospital, one person may do almost all the assessment—soliciting admission complaints, requesting standard laboratory work, and taking a standard admission history. In a large medical center, where a great deal of teaching and research goes on, the procedure may be infinitely more fragmented. Regardless of the setting, assessment is an ongoing process from admission or first encounter to termination. Out of it comes the problem identification and the goals to solve the problems. The final assessment is an evaluation of how useful the professional has been to the client. It will be considered under "Evaluation," below.

Nursing Diagnosis

Defining and Framing the Problem

After the initial assessment, the next step is a nursing diagnosis. *A nursing diagnosis is the formulation of a list of problems which emerge from analytic consideration of objective and subjective data gathered previously.* It is also a list of the strengths or specific functional abilities of the individual. In other words, the nurse develops a working description of the problem. As more information is obtained, it is likely that some elements, at least, of the original problem definition will shift. A seemingly minor problem may be identified as the major difficulty and what appeared to be the primary difficulty will turn out to be part of a complex network of several interrelated difficulties.

The competent clinician works back and forth between a data base, tentatively stated problems, relevant or appropriate theory, newly gathered information, and possible revision of the formulations. Let us outline a way of dealing with the information collected in the clinical observation of a client over a period of 2 weeks. The problem is with Mr. Smith, who fears that his close relatives are about to die, yet smiles while outlining his

Table 7-1 Nurse's Initial Assessment

Assessment Factor	Action
1 Client tells reason for seeking psychiatric help. Client describes logically, coherently, and in a reasonable amount of detail why he is there.	Nurse listens without comment, interjecting only two informational questions.

2 Circumstances of client's arrival:
  a Client's appearance. (Pale, tremor of the hands, perspiration, inability to sit still, rapid breathing, very rapid speech.)
  b Manner of client's arrival; person accompanying client, if any. (Admitting team member accompanies client, leaves admission sheet with the following notes: "Anxiety state, severe. administer Valium, admit for observation.")
	Nurse makes note of physical appearance; coherence, manner, logic, and delivery of speech; orientation.

3 Behaviors observable during this initial contact. (Took Valium without question; remained restless and walked about rapidly; gradually became quieter and went to bed at midnight.)	The nurse administered the drug and supported client by staying with him; walking with him until relaxation appeared; suggesting he might sleep and turning out room light.
4 Recurrent themes in client's remarks. (Loss of control, helplessness, powerlessness.)	

anxiety. Mr. Smith's records may include the following notations:

> Mr. Smith expressed concern that the nurse assigned to his care would be hurt on a weekend trip he was planning. When discussing this with Mr. Ash, the nurse involved, Mr. Smith appeared to be smiling slightly.

> A client in Mr. Smith's therapy group is described as being angry because Mr. Smith talks about "death and doom" all the time in the group and how worried he is about his father's health. However, when the father visits, Mr. Smith leaves him and goes off to the ballgame.

As this type of information is collected over time, recurrent patterns or themes can be pulled out and problems validated by the nursing staff and others. In the instance described, the discrepancy between the expressed feelings and the behavior is immediately obvious. In each instance, Mr. Smith is concerned about a significant authority figure in his life, one old and one new. Staff could then begin to draft possibilities based on their knowledge of such concepts as guilt, hostility, transference, and repressed rage. They could then project a possible strategy. Since Mr. Smith has repeatedly expressed fear of the death of male authority figures while also unconsciously showing that this idea amuses him, his behavior is paradoxical. It might be decided that the open expression of verbal hostility might be a valid goal for Mr. Smith, and that the male nurse, Mr. Ash, might be the logical target for the aggression.

Initially, Mr. Smith's problems would be defined in terms of:

1 Discrepancy between expressed feelings and behavior
2 Inability to acknowledge feelings of hostility
3 Inability to express hostile feelings toward authority figures verbally
4 Anxiety about dependence on others

This leads, with some areas of overlap, to the next problem-solving step: the formulation of goals.

Planning
Goals

Once the data base has been established, the initial problem or problems defined, and the appropriate theory identified, appropriate nursing goals may be outlined.

A nursing goal is the expected or end result of an action. It is an objective to be gained; a planned change to be achieved in a current condition or behavior. In the psychiatric situation, it almost always involves a change in some behavior or set of behaviors that is deemed desirable for the client. Thus, goals should be stated in relation to expected outcomes (e.g., "The client will brush his teeth 3 times daily, once after each meal.").

The first step in goal formulation is to work within the interdisciplinary effort so that the nursing goals are not at odds with those of the psychiatrist or other members of the staff. Let us speculate that Mr. Ash is to be given the responsibility of helping Mr. Smith recognize and express his fear of male authority figures. This goal has been identified and validated; it is theoretically sound. The overall plan has been set up through joint planning involving various members of the psychiatric team. Mr. Ash will then set up the nursing problems, define the goals, and make decisions and actions to carry them out within the larger therapeutic plan. The goals are (1) to increase awareness of daily situations where the problem emerges, (2) to have Mr. Smith recognize his problem and express it in words, and (3) to have Mr. Smith test his responses and feelings in graduated interpersonal settings.

> Goal 1: Increase Mr. Smith's awareness of everyday situations in which the problem occurs.

> Example: Medications are being given by one of the "floating" or temporary nurses. The nurse is an older man who says very little to any client. When it is Mr. Smith's turn, Mr. Smith becomes very anxious and drops the pill in his agitation.

> Activity: Mr. Ash raises a question: "Is there anything about this new nurse that

bothers you? You seemed uncomfortable, and dropped your pill."

Goal 2: Assist Mr. Smith to express recognition of the problem area in words.

Example: The recreation teacher is about 40 years old, talkative, and cheerfully aggressive. As Mr. Smith misses the ball, he shouts loudly, "That's it, butterfingers!" Everyone laughs, but Mr. Smith walks out of the game and is depressed all afternoon.

Activity: Mr. Ash makes it a point to see Mr. Smith in his room and says, "You're really down. Want to talk about it?" When Mr. Smith says no, Mr. Ash pushes the point tactfully: "Well, the medication nurse upset you yesterday and the recreation teacher upset you today. What's the story?"

Using the material of everyday encounters, Mr. Ash starts out to achieve the goal of connecting Mr. Smith's daily life with nonproductive, interpersonal responses until Mr. Smith makes a connection with the problem.

At times, goals have to be more palliative than curative, since there are people for whom the most therapeutic environment does little. Most practitioners learn to be realistic about what they can hope to accomplish with a given client.

Intervention

Intervention is the nursing action that is taken after the assessment, problem identification, and goal formulation have been made from the data base. Following that, activities that are designed to change behavior begin (see Chaps. 13–22).

Evaluation

At some point the nurse's efforts to help a given client will come to an end and the client will, it is hoped, have learned to live with whatever problems remain. For example, a specific siege of depression may lift, but the underlying dynamics may persist for a lifetime. It may be that if depres-

sions are punishing in their effect, the client will learn to recognize early symptoms and find ways of averting them, such as becoming involved in hard, unpleasant work. A nursing goal might well be to help the client substitute an active hour in the gymnasium for what begins to be a depressed morning. Recognition of factors which precipitate depressions and the means of substitution are subject to evaluation. The recognition of what clients have learned about their disorders and what they are able to do to remain free from their disabling effects is part of evaluation. A successful period of residence outside the psychiatric settings is an evaluation in itself, provided that the client is functioning comfortably. (This is a social criterion, of course, and is commonly referred to as *community tenure.*) It is an evaluation process posthospitalization. In summary, one can focus on a more specific definition: Evaluation is an analytic process that continues as long as the nurse is active with the client. It includes strengths as well as failures to produce change.

Sometimes putting the plan into action is, as the old saying goes, easier said than done. Constant monitoring of the plan, with fine tuning at every necessary point, is part of the individual, evaluative, clinical role. Again, the role of monitor and evaluator may fall to a group in which daily reports are shared. It may also be a matter of discussion with clinical supervisors or other knowledgeable professionals.

For example, Mr. Ash (Mr. Smith's nurse in our earlier example), may receive advice from the group on the best way to handle his client's depression. When dealing with the "butterfingers" incident at recreation, for instance, Mr. Ash might be cautioned against asking direct questions. He might be encouraged to help the client work out his depression nonverbally instead.

These, then, are the generally accepted steps in problem solving. They have been presented as the core of any professional service, not solely the service presented by nursing. These processes, as intellectual operations, cannot be sidestepped. No matter what actions or activities are decided upon and eventually carried out, there are logical, intellectual steps which are in a constant process of evaluation.

All these steps, taken as a sequential whole, comprise the nursing process. That these steps overlap at various stages is not argued. Many of them occur over and over again in circular fashion. Thus all the steps in the process are just that, in process, progress, and motion (see Figure 7-1).

Problem-Oriented Records

The primary record keeping in psychiatric agencies has generally followed that of the medical-surgical or more generalized medical institution. Thus charts, histories, progress notes, and diagnostic summaries constitute the major tools or records in psychiatric hospitals as well as in less specialized institutions.

Foremost among current forms and written devices are the *problem-oriented records.* The nomenclature varies from place to place and one finds superficial differences in terminology in the literature. For example, there are problem-oriented hospital records, problem-oriented medical records, and problem-oriented nurse's notes, but it is

immediately clear that the common concern is a problem orientation to the health situation. Perhaps, as one source[7] has indicated, the whole process ought to be referred to as a "problem-oriented system for client-centered care"; the term will be used in that general sense here. Since these problem-solving systems are in common use with general hospital populations, their application to the psychiatric client is the primary focus.

In a time when many disciplines are in the client-care arena, some method of coordinating information becomes vital. It is evident many times that each of these groups are collecting the same material from a single client, albeit for a different purpose. The very unwieldiness of older systems became visible as increasingly complex data were collected from more people and more levels and kinds of specialists became involved in the health field. The story may be apocryphal, but one client is said to have counted at least fifteen strangers in search of data in one 8-hour day in the unit. These were over and above the regular unit personnel. It becomes obvious that there is a distinct gain for the client when several parallel data-collection sources are combined into one pool to which each discipline contributes. The problem-oriented record also becomes a device for auditing professional performance in relation to each client's care.

In the past, the keeping of various records has become, as Kramer points out, an end in itself rather than a means to an end, a final goal rather than a way of contributing to the attainment of nursing goals.[8] The decline and fall of the Kardex system in many situations is a case in point. It remains physically present, but its usefulness is often diminished by the large number of clients to be served. The problem-oriented record system, however, will probably hold up longer than some of its predecessors for several reasons. First, it is, as one source says, "based on scientific method and designed for problem solving and for preserving the logic used in arriving at solutions of patient problems."[9] Second, the record helps to provide the careful documentation that is needed for third-party health insurance payments. Third, the record

Figure 7-1 Components of the Nursing Process.

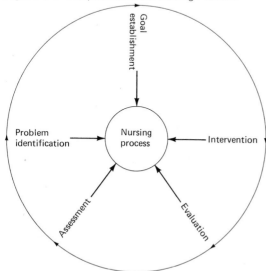

serves as a precise chart in a legal sense, for malpractice suits do regrettably exist.

The first substantial contribution to the problem-oriented system of record keeping was made by Weed.[10] There are four basic structural components of the problem-oriented record which appear to be universal and which *parallel the nursing process.* Although the language is slightly different in some instances, the following elements are always present:

1 Data base.
2 Comprehensive problem list.
3 Initial plans (goals) with numbered and titled entries. Included are diagnostic factors, therapies, and client participation factors, such as teaching and informing clients.
4 Numbered and titled progress notes which are narrative and include flow sheets and discharge summaries.
5 Evaluation summaries.

The data base is collected through the various components of the assessment process, either in a formal interview setting or during informal observation periods. Formulation of the problem list is determined by the center's mental health team or that team member who is responsible for this task. Behaviorally stated problems demonstrate verification of goal achievement or lack of it. For example, one aspect of a series of identified problem behaviors is that of eating habits in the clients' dining room on the treatment unit. A client who throws and spills food is engaging in inappropriate social behaviors which are documented in progress notes on a sample day:

Eating Behavior, J. Smith

Monday: No spilling, throwing, or stealing when older client ate with Mr. S at breakfast; Mr. S ate alone at lunch, stole Mr. D's plate; ate with attendant at dinner, no spilling or throwing of food.

The extent of the problem can be further clarified through a counting procedure which would indicate the actual incidence of throwing, stealing, or spilling of food during a sample week. (See Fig. 7-2.) In this way, initial performance levels of problem behavior can be established and compared to the *goals* or terminal outcome criteria (i.e., to eliminate throwing, stealing, and spilling of food and to establish appropriate eating habits in the clients' dining room).

Nursing interventions are identified based on observations of client behavior and theoretical rationale; they are designed to decrease or resolve the problem behavior. During a week of observation, the staff notices that when Mr. Smith eats alone, his eating behavior is at a distinctly disruptive level; when someone older or in "authority" is at his side, his eating habits become socially acceptable. The problem-oriented process would consequently be outlined as in Table 7-2.

Out of the preceding would come a reassessment, a new goal might be set, and new interventions identified until the client's changed eating habits fit into the larger goal: to teach him living habits acceptable to his community.

Nursing intervention can readily be evaluated because the problem and goal have been behaviorally identified and quantified. This process lends itself to determining whether or not this client's behavior changed and whether the client received the best care possible.

Figure 7-2 Occurrence of stealing, throwing, and spilling of food.

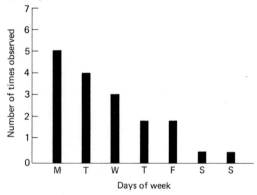

Table 7-2 Mr. Smith's Eating Behavior

No.	Problem description: Asocial eating habits	Goal: Restore socially acceptable eating habits	Intervention
1	Throws food	Eliminate throwing food	Have someone sit with him each meal
2	Steals food	and stealing food	Reward verbally when meal is eaten
3	Spills food upon clothing		without spilling, throwing, or stealing

SOAP

SOAP notes are the written communication tool of the problem-oriented record. The components include:

> *S:* Subjective data consist of verbal information from client and significant others which may or may not be congruent with objective data.
>
> *O:* Objective data consist of information obtained about the client through observation or measurement. They include nonverbal behavior, laboratory data, and other measurements such as vital signs, height, and weight.
>
> *A:* Assessment is an analysis of the subjective and objective data and includes (*a*) rationale for problems, (*b*) the effect of medication and nursing intervention, (*c*) progress, and (*d*) prognosis.
>
> *P:* Plan of action includes specific plans for gathering further data and implementing diagnostic studies, treatment approaches, and client/family education.

A sample SOAP note follows:

SOAP Note
Problem: Client eats poorly, especially at night.

> *Subjective:* "I ate well at all meals today."
>
> *Objective:* Ward reports that client ate nothing at lunch and dinner.
>
> *Assessment:* Client is conveying inaccurate information.
>
> *Plan:* A staff member will (1) continue to observe client at mealtimes and (2) point out the discrepancy between the reality (not eating) and the reporting (what the client sees as the situation)

Audit—A Tool for Evaluation

"Audit," a term derived from the world of business and finance, is used in the health-care field to describe an operation of maximum accountability to the consumer of health care. It includes any thorough examination and evaluation of a problem which summarizes all the key events in a given client's health care. An audit, then, "accounts" for action and decision making by liable and responsible professionals. The appearance of terms like "nursing audit" and "flow sheet" to describe client care and progress is probably not accidental, since accountability for professional action is tied most firmly to the economic structure of the American health-care system. It is this commitment and need to be accountable that is at the bottom of any health-care audit. However, the audit, no matter who uses it, is likely to suffer from subjective distortion unless criteria for certain outcomes in any nursing intervention are well defined beforehand. Even then, two professionals looking at the same client behavior can arrive at varying appraisals. This problem does not exist when the criteria are set up to include highly quantitative, objective aspects. Evaluation criteria take two forms:[7]

> *Process Criteria:* These involve operations in progress at any given time and are usually evaluations of the ongoing actions or care given by the nurse.

Terminal Criteria: These refer to the changes which occur in the clients' condition as a result of their contact with the health-care system.

Mary Anderson, a schizophrenic, may develop a viral infection. Process or terminal criteria for evaluating her condition can be set up as in Table 7-3.

The chart or the flow sheet is the communication tool for determining whether these actions were carried out (process criteria) and whether they were successful (terminal criteria).

Although data in the world of medicine and surgery are more highly quantifiable, those relating to psychiatry can also be expressed quantitatively. For example, measurable goals can be established in relation to the central dynamics of a specific psychiatric illness.

Factors for Concern

Of vital importance in psychiatric nursing is the identification and maximum use of the client's strengths and assets.

One of the things that the phrase "problem-oriented record" tends to do is to focus nursing activities on the problems. There is also a tendency to reductionism involved, in that there may be a push to reduce an extremely complex psychiatric disturbance to a neat list of problems. Thus, there is a need to be sure that the problem list is complete and that the assets duly noted in planning intervention are always to be kept in the foreground. The system employing the problem-oriented record should be viewed as the best that we have to date for humanizing client care and for coordinating the work of various professional disciplines through improved reporting and communication as well as the structuring of accountability systems, so that psychiatric clients today may receive higher-level care than was given in the past.

The Future

It might be interesting to speculate about how the problem-oriented record system will operate in another three decades. Since, today, even many relatively isolated hospitals are tied into computers in larger urban medical centers and since it is possible to store, analyze, retrieve, and use all kinds of diagnostic data in many different ways, the future would seem even more open in this regard. Certainly the cumbersome handwritten forms we now use will be replaced. Probably the basic process will not change unless our main method of coping with the world changes from problem solving to some other as yet unspecified process. As computers become more and more available for what we might call "home" use, there is no reason why all the up-to-date data on a given client could not be available instantaneously to all health disciplines from some central control area in each hospital. Surely if small computers can be carried in checkbooks to obtain rapid, accurate balances, the next step is to codify information and

Table 7-3 Audit Process

Problem: Elevated temperature due to viral infection	
Symptoms: Temperature, sleeplessness, joint pain, anorexia	
Process criteria	Terminal criteria
Ongoing nursing interventions aimed at relieving client symptoms:	Changes which occur in the client's condition as the viral infection is reduced:
1 Client's temperature is taken every 4 hours.	1 Temperature returns to normal.
2 Aspirin is administered.	2 Joint aches disappear.
3 Frequent fluid intake is encouraged.	3 Anorexia decreases.
4 Restful environment is promoted.	4 Inability to sleep disappears.

use computer screens in nurses' stations for an instant summary of available test results, problem listings, and actions taken.

References

*1 Helen Yura and Mary Walsh: *The Nursing Process,* 2d ed., Appleton-Century-Crofts, New York, 1972, pp. 22–23.

2 Martin Bloom: *The Paradox of Helping,* Wiley, New York, 1975, pp. 100–113.

*3 Shirley Burd and Margaret Marshall: *Some Clinical Approaches to Psychiatric Nursing,* Macmillan, New York, 1963.

4 J. B. Walters, G. P. Pardee, and D. M. Molbo: *Dynamic Problem-Oriented Approaches: Patient Care and Documentation,* Lippincott, Philadelphia, 1976.

*5 Ann C. Burgess and Aron Lazare: *Psychiatric Nursing in the Hospital and the Community,* Prentice-Hall, Englewood Cliffs, N.J., 1975.

*6 Lucille A. Joel and Shirley M. Davis: "A Proposal for Base Line Data Collection for Psychiatric Care," *Perspectives in Psychiatric Care,* vol. 11, no. 2, pp. 48–57, 1973.

*7 Mary Woody and Mary Mallinson: "The Problem-Oriented System for Patient-Centered Care," *American Journal of Nursing,* vol. 73, no. 7, pp. 1168–1175, July 1973.

*8 Marlene Kramer: "Nursing Care Plans . . . Power to the Patient," *Journal of Nursing Administration,* September–October 1972, pp. 29–34.

9 Jacques Sherman and Sylvia Fields: *Guide to Patient Evaluation,* Medical Examination Publishing Co., Flushing, N.Y., 1974, p. 13.

10 Lawrence Weed: *Medical Records, Medical Education and Patient Care,* The Press of Case Western Reserve University, Cleveland, 1969.

*Recommended reference by a nurse author.

Chapter

8

Therapeutic Modalities - Somatic

Loretta Kawalec Guise

Learning Objectives

After studying this chapter, the student should be able to:

1 Identify the four major drug groups included under the heading of psychotropic drugs

2 Know the classifications, actions, extrapyramidal effects, complications, contraindications, and usefulness of major tranquilizers

3 List the side effects of the major tranquilizers and the nursing interventions for each

4 Know the classifications and actions of minor tranquilizers

5 List the side effects and dangers of minor tranquilizers

6 Outline the nursing interventions necessary during the administration of minor tranquilizers

7 Describe the antidepressants, their side effects, and appropriate nursing interventions

8 Discuss the use of lithium as a psychotropic drug

9 Understand the use of convulsive therapies

10 List the theories of actions of ECT

11 Outline the nursing care of clients receiving ECT

12 Describe psychosurgery

13 Understand orthomolecular therapy and hydrotherapy

Somatic therapy is the treatment of emotionally ill or incapacitated clients by physiological means. Major and minor tranquilizers, antidepressants, lithium, and megavitamins are among the drugs used in treatment. Electroshock, psychosurgery, and hydrotherapy are other treatments which supplement the use of psychotherapy or psychopharmatherapeutic agents.

Psychotropic Drugs

The synthesis of chlorpromazine in the 1950s had a revolutionary impact on the treatment of mental illness. The major benefit of treatment was the alleviation of disabling symptoms, making clients more amenable to other forms of treatment. Anxiety was decreased without producing a loss of consciousness. As a result, custodial care in hospitals was no longer necessary for many clients and a greater number of people returned to their communities. Many clients who would formerly have been hospitalized are now cared for at home. Four major drug groups are included under the heading of psychotropic drugs. These are major tranquilizers, minor tranquilizers, antidepressants, and lithium carbonate.[1]

Major Tranquilizers

The major tranquilizers, also called neuroleptics or ataractics, reduce anxiety and substantially decrease psychotic symptoms such as hallucinations, delusions, distorted thought processes, and disturbed affect (either agitated or withdrawn). Over time, a large number of chemically related drugs have been synthesized in an effort to produce an antipsychotic agent which is more effective than the original chlorpromazine and/or which has fewer side effects. As a result, there are currently on the market many phenothiazine derivatives and antipsychotic compounds which are similar in actions and effects to the phenothiazines, namely, the thioxanthene and butyrophenone derivatives. The trade names of the drugs in each of these groups, their method of administra-

tion, and the usual psychiatric dosage are outlined in Table 8-1.[2]

Actions

There are four significant pharmacologic *characteristics* of the phenothiazine drug group:

1 Antipsychotic activity (normalize overactive or withdrawn behavior)
2 Production of extrapyramidal side effects (both reversible and irreversible)
3 Absence of deep coma and anesthesia with the administration of large doses
4 Absence of either physical or psychic dependence

The exact way in which these drugs work is not known. They are thought to depress the central nervous system, having a major effect on the thalamus and hypothalamus. Anxiety, irritability, and apprehension are decreased. These drugs are known to have antiemetic and anticonvulsant effects, although these are not the intended actions. Body temperature and blood pressure are lowered. The actions of opiates, sedatives, and anesthetics administered with the major tranquilizers or close to the same time are potentiated (intensified). Phenothiazines act like local anesthetics on sensory nerve endings, clouding out stimuli. They decrease contractions of skeletal muscles. They (except Mellaril) also relieve nausea and vomiting by depressing the chemoreceptor trigger which activates the vomiting center.[3]

The metabolism of the phenothiazines is not known. They are found at the highest level in the liver. The rate at which the major tranquilizers leave the body is very slow; breakdown products have been found in the urine several months after medication has been discontinued.

Extrapyramidal Effects

Extrapyramidal effects are seen quite commonly in clients taking major tranquilizers. These effects are dramatic and may occur after the first dose or only gradually after prolonged usage. Some

Table 8-1 Major Tranquilizers

Drug	Trade name	Method of administration	Usual daily Psychiatric dose, mg
	Phenothiazines — dimethylamine subgroup		
Chlorpromazine	Thorazine	Oral (tablets, spansules, syrup, concentrate) IM IV Suppositories	30–1500
Promazine hydrochloride	Sparine	Oral (tablets, syrup, concentrate) IM IV	50–1000
Trifluopromazine hydrochloride	Vesprin	Oral (tablets, concentrate) IM	20–200
	Phenothiazines — Piperidyl subgroup		
Thioridazine	Mellaril	Oral (tablets, concentrate)	100–800
Mesoridazine	Serentil	Oral (tablets, concentrate) IM	30–400
	Phenothiazines — Piperazine subgroup		
Perphenazine	Trilafon	Oral (tablets, repeat-action tablets, syrup, concentrate) IM Suppositories	6–64
Carphenazine maleate	Proketazine	Oral (tablets, concentrate)	40–400
Fluphenazine dihydrochloride	Prolixin Permitil	Oral (tablets, concentrate) IM	0.5–20
Trifluoperazine hydrochloride	Stelazine	Oral (tablets, concentrate) IM	2–50
Acetophenazine maleate	Tindal	Oral (tablets)	40–80
Piperacetazine	Quide	Oral (tablets)	10–180
Thiopropazate hydrochloride	Dartal	Oral (tablets)	10–150
Butaperazine maleate	Repoise	Oral (tablets)	5–100
Prochlorperazine maleate	Compazine	Oral (tablets, sustained-release capsules, syrup, concentrate) IM IV Suppositories	15–150
	Thioxanthene derivatives		
Chlorprothixene	Taractan	Oral (tablets, concentrate) IM	30–600
Thiothixene	Navane	Oral (capsules, concentrate) IM	6–60
	Butyrophenone derivatives		
Haloperidol	Haldol	Oral (tablets, concentrate) IM	2–40

drugs—such as Prolixin, Stelazine, and Trilafon—cause a higher incidence of these effects, whereas a lower incidence is associated with Mellaril. Extrapyramidal reactions include the following:

1 *Pseudoparkinsonism* Symptoms usually associated with parkinsonism, such as tremor, shuffling gait, drooling, rigidity, and loose movements of arms

2 *Akathisia* Continuous restlessness, fidgeting, and pacing

3 *Akinesia* Fatigue and muscular weakness

4 *Dystonia* Bizarre, involuntary movements of the face, arms, legs, and neck; often, difficulty in talking and excessive salivation

5 *Oculogyric Crisis* Uncontrolled rolling of eyes

6 *Tardive Dykinesia* (Less common but far more dramatic because of sudden onset) All symptoms of dystonia plus bizarre facial and tongue movements, stiff neck, and difficulty swallowing

Extrapyramidal symptoms are controlled by lowering the dosage or changing the medication to one with a lower incidence of these side effects and/or by the use of antiparkinson drugs such as Congentin, Artane, Akineton, and Kemadrin. Nurses should consider the occurrence of these symptoms a crisis and take the necessary emergency measures. Reassurance and protection should be provided for the client until symptoms subside.[4]

Complications

Liver and hematologic complications sometimes occur as a result of phenothiazine therapy. Fortunately, such complications are rare. Liver disease manifested by obstructive jaundice usually appears within the first 5 weeks of treatment. Initially, a flulike syndrome develops, consisting of fever, general malaise, diarrhea, abdominal pain, and vomiting. The nurse will recognize these symptoms and alert the physician to order liver function tests; these will indicate whether there is bilirubinuria and/or icterus. Medication should be discontinued. The forcing of fluids together with sympto-

matic treatment will result in recovery from jaundice within a few weeks.

Hematologic conditions such as leukopenia, agranulocytosis, purpura, and granulocytopenia occur rarely, but the mortality resulting from them is high. The initial symptoms are sore throat, fever, or generalized weakness. A white blood cell (WBC) count and differential should be done regularly on clients receiving phenothiazine treatment. The most important aspect of the treatment of clients with this diagnosis is to prevent them from being exposed to infections. Careful observation of clients and routine monitoring of blood and urine studies are important preventive precautions which the nurse can take in anticipation of these two major side effects.

Contraindications

The major tranquilizers should not be given to clients with glaucoma or prostate problems. Extreme caution should be observed when administering them to clients with cardiac problems, since autonomic blockade may result in circulatory collapse. These drugs are likewise contraindicated in convulsive disorders, because they significantly decrease the convulsive threshold.

Phenothiazines potentiate the effects of other drugs, especially hypnotics, analgesics, and anesthetics. Clients should be cautioned against using these drugs and alcohol simultaneously because of the resultant depressive affects on the central nervous system. Since all the phenothiazines except Mellaril possess secondary antiemetic properties, their use may obscure nausea and vomiting.[2]

Usefulness

Conditions such as schizophrenia, the manic phase of manic-depressive psychosis, involutional psychosis, and certain toxic psychoses respond well to these medications. Excessive psychomotor activity, hostility, panic, anxiety, and antisocial behavior can be significantly minimized in the agitated individual, whereas other clients who are withdrawn and apathetic can be stimulated into become more alert, communicative, and sociable.

The effects should not be overestimated. Psychotropic drugs do not "cure" mental illness. They alleviate the symptoms that interfere with normal functioning, thereby allowing the client to become more involved in treatment. It is an individual's ability to interact in a positive and meaningful way with the environment that will provide for any significant and enduring improvements in his or her condition. Both the medications and the environmental interaction processes work hand in hand in potentiating or detracting from the effectiveness of the client's treatment program.[5]

Side Effects and Nursing Intervention

In general, the major tranquilizers are safe compounds, although dangerous side effects do occur occasionally. There are a number of relatively mild but nonetheless annoying side effects which could possibly interfere with the effectiveness of these medications, especially if resistance to taking drugs is heightened by a client's annoyance or discomfort. Minor side effects and discomforts which occur as a result of effects on the *autonomic nervous system* include blurred vision, dry mouth, constipation, nasal congestion, inhibition of ejaculation, decreased libido, and postural hypotension. Photosensitivity and dermatitis are *allergic* reactions. Behavioral effects include impaired psychomotor functions and drowsiness. Weight gain, edema, irregular menstruation, amenorrhea, and decrease in sex drive are the result of endocrine action. Table 8-2 lists client side effects and discomforts[2] (assessments) and appropriate nursing interventions for each.

Nursing care is essential in minimizing side effects and helping clients to develop positive attitudes toward taking medications. Careful observation and knowledge of client behavioral patterns prior to drug administration can help the nurse assess the possibility that serious complications of side effects may exist. A careful nursing history should be documented in the record. Allowing clients to ventilate fears, misgivings, misconceptions, and resistances about medications will help ensure that they will continue to take medications after their discharge from the hospital. Careful education and observation of the client is essential nursing intervention when major tranquilizers are being administered.[6]

Minor Tranquilizers

Minor tranquilizers are substances that relieve the mild or moderate anxiety usually associated with psychoneurotic and psychosomatic conditions. However, they are generally not considered to be effective in treating psychoses. Pharmacologically they are similar to the barbiturates but cause less cortical depression and are less addicting than the latter. They act as central nervous system depressants, causing sedation and relaxation of muscle tension. They are used primarily as antianxiety agents.

The minor tranquilizers are grouped as benzodiazepines, diphenylmethanes, and propandiols. Table 8-3 lists the drugs in each group with their trade names, method of administration, and usual psychiatric dosage.[2]

Side Effects and Nursing Intervention

Side effects may be seen with certain minor tranquilizers. These include dizziness, gastrointestinal complaints, urticaria, nervousness, blurred vision, dry mouth, headache, and mental confusion. There have also been a few reports of insomnia, rashes, fatigue, ataxia, genitourinary complaints, diplopia, palpitations, irritability, slurred speech, depression, and decreased blood pressure. Intervention includes decreasing the dosage and treating the symptoms.

Sedation is an expected side effect. The nurse has an important responsibility in assessing whether an antianxiety level has been reached or if the client has been oversedated. Clients should be informed that, because of the sedative action of the minor tranquilizers, activities requiring mental alertness should be avoided.

Because of the depressant effect on the

Table 8-2 Major tranquilizers—Side Effects

Assessment (side effect or discomfort)	Nursing intervention
Blurred vision	Reassurance (generally subsides in 2–6 weeks).
Dry mouth	Frequent rinsing of mouth. Lozenges.
Constipation	Mild laxative. Roughage in diet. Exercises. Fluids.
Nasal congestion	Nose drops. Moisturizer.
Decreased libido and inhibition of ejaculation	Prepare client for effect. Reassurance (reversible). Ask physician about change to less antiadrenergic drug.
Postural hypotension	Frequent monitoring of blood pressure during dosage adjustment period. Advise client to get up slowly. Elastic stockings if necessary.
Photosensitivity	Protective clothing. Dark glasses. Use of sunscreen.
Dermatitis	Stop medication. Request physician to change order and prescribe systemic antihistamine. Initiate comfort measures.
Impaired psychomotor functions	Advise client to avoid dangerous tasks.
Drowsiness	Give single daily dose at bedtime.
Weight gain	Caloric control; exercise-diet teaching.
Edema	Reassurance. Request physician to prescribe diuretic.
Irregular menstruation and decreased sex drive	Reassurance (reversible). Have physician change class of drugs.
Amenorrhea	Reassurance and counseling (does not indicate lack of ovulation). Instruct client to continue birth control.

central nervous system, clients should also be advised *against* simultaneous use of other CNS-depressant drugs and alcohol. Tolerance can develop and physical addiction can result from use of these drugs. Symptoms similar to barbiturate withdrawal have been seen when these drugs are discontinued abruptly after prolonged usage. Withdrawal symptoms may include ataxia, tremors, muscle twitching, vomiting, hallucinations, confusional states, and convulsions. The prescription of minor tranquilizers for individuals considered to have a psychological potential for drug dependence—such as those who have overlydependent personalities or a history of alcoholism—should be given careful consideration and avoided when possible.

Paradoxic reactions of excitement, rage, hostility, confusion, and depersonalization can occur, particularly when these drugs are administered to severely disturbed psychotic clients or the elderly. Intervention includes withholding the drug and providing for the safety and comfort of the client. In

Table 8-3 Minor Tranquilizers

Drug	Trade name	Method of administration	Usual daily psychiatric dose, mg
		Diphenylmethane group	
Hydroxyzine hydrochloride	Atarax	Oral (tablets, syrup)	50–400
Hydroxyzine pamoate	Vistaril	Oral (capsules, suspension)	50–400
Hydroxyzine hydrochloride		IM only	50–100 every 4–6 hours
Benactyzine hydrochloride	Suavitil	Oral (tablets)	3–10
		Benzodiazepine group	
Chlordiazepoxide hydrochloride	Librium Libritabs Librax	Oral (capsules, librium; tablets, libritabs) IM IV	10–100
Diazepam	Valium	Oral (tablets) IM IV	2–40
Oxazepam	Serax	Oral (capsules, tablets)	30–120
Clorazepate dipotassium	Tranxene	Oral (capsules)	7.5–60
		Propanediol group	
Meprobamate	Equanil Miltown Meprospan	Oral (tablets, capsules, suspension) Oral (tablets) Time-released capsules)	400–1200
Tybamate	Solacin Tybatran	Oral (capsules)	250–1000

the event of overdose, induced vomiting and gastric lavage is recommended. Supportive care is given in the form of careful monitoring of the vital signs. Hypotension is usually controlled with Levophed or Aramine. Caffeine and sodium benzoate is usually used to counteract the depressant effects on the central nervous system.

Continuous assessment by the nurse of the client's behavior is necessary in order to determine if a medication's expected results are being seen. Dosages may need to be increased, decreased, or discontinued and other medications substituted. Areas such as social interaction or withdrawal, reactions to stress, overactivity or underactivity, physical condition, sleep and eating patterns, physical complaints are all to be considered in making these assessments. The role of the nurse as observer is crucial in the effective management of clients who are taking minor tranquiliz-

ers. Knowledge of the expected actions, adverse reactions, normal side effects, and the effect of the interplay between interpersonal and environmental components is needed in the continuous evaluation process.[6–8]

Antidepressants

Antidepressants are used in the treatment of depressive states. They have an energy-producing action which stimulates clients into becoming more involved in themselves and their environment and less withdrawn.

Depressive states, both endogenous and reactive, have been treated successfully with antidepressants (see Chap. 18). The drugs used—both the monoamine oxidase (MAO) inhibitors and the tricyclic compounds—along with trade names, methods of administration, and usual dosages are listed in Table 8-4.[2] The tricyclic compounds and the MAO inhibitors treat the symptoms related to depression and not the underlying causes. Results which would indicate that these drugs were effective would include elevation of mood; improved appetite and sleep patterns; increased physical activity; improved mental functioning; a decrease in the client's feelings of inadequacy, worthlessness, guilt, and ambivalence; and possibly a decrease in delusional preoccupation. On the other hand, it has been reported that antidepressants increase tension, cause agitated behavior, intensify a psychotic state, or cause clients to become disoriented and possibly to hallucinate. A decrease in dosage will usually control these situations.[9]

Monoamine Oxidase (MAO) Inhibitors

MAO inhibitors inhibit the enzyme monoamine oxidase, which is found in the liver, spleen, kidneys, brain, and blood platelets. This enzyme destroys certain neurohormones such as epinephrine, norepinephrine, and serotonin, which are responsible for stimulating physical and mental activity. MAO inhibitors are believed to be responsible for maintaining an equilibrium within the body by increasing the life span of the neurohormones.

Careful education of the client is needed when these medications are used. A severe adverse reaction—known as hypertensive crisis or a *Parnate-cheese reaction* (Parnate being the name of one such drug)—can occur when any MAO inhibitor interacts with certain foods, beverages, or other drugs. Clients should be very wary of such foods. The hypertensive reaction is signaled by the presence of a headache (either generalized or occipital), diaphoresis, increased restlessness, palpitations, pallor, chills, stiff neck, nausea, vomiting, muscle twitching, and chest pain. A severe hypertensive crisis is considered an emergency, since it can lead to intracranial hemorrhage and possibly even death. Among the substances that should not be taken concurrently with MAO inhibitors are cheeses (especially aged cheeses), liver, yogurt, herring, yeast products, sour cream, beer,

Table 8-4 Antidepressants

Drug	Trade name	Method of administration	Usual daily psychiatric dose, mg
Monoamine oxidase inhibitors			
Isocarboxazid	Marplan	Oral (tablets)	10–30
Nialamide	Niamid	Oral (tablets)	12.5–200
Phenelzine sulfate	Nardil	Oral (tablets)	15–75
Tranylcypromine sulfate	Parnate	Oral (tablets)	20–30
Tricyclics			
Imipramine	Tofranil	Oral (tablets) IM	75–300
	Tofranil PM	Oral (capsules)	
Amitriptyline hydrochloride	Elavil	Oral (tablets) IM	50–200
Desipramine hydrochloride	Norpramin	Oral (tablets)	75–150
	Pertofrane		
Nortriptyline hydrochloride	Aventyl	Oral (capsules, liquid)	20–100
Protriptyline hydrochloride	Vivactil	Oral (tablets)	15–60
Doxepin hydrochloride	Sinequan	Oral (capsules)	25–300

wines, caffeine-containing beverages (coffee, tea, cola), cold remedies (cough syrups, nasal sprays, etc.), diet pills, and psychomotor stimulants.

In addition, alcohol, barbiturates, and certain analgesics are potentiated by MAO inhibitors. Likewise, it should be remembered that there is a lag period of 3 or 4 weeks before the expected results are achieved. This knowledge will prevent premature discontinuance of the medication.

MAO inhibitors can be fatal if an overdose is taken. Initially clients might be symptom-free for as long as 6 hours. They may then progress from restlessness to coma and finally death. Close medical supervision is indicated for the 48 hours immediately following an overdose.[9]

Tricyclics

The various tricyclic drugs all have a significantly high success rate in the treatment of depression. The most common reason for failure of treatment has been inadequate dosage. The mechanism of action of the tricyclics is not precisely known, but it is hypothesized that they affect brain amine levels by interfering with amine binding ability. A wide spectrum of side effects is seen with this category of drugs, most of which can be controlled by reducing the dosage. These side effects are similar to those seen with the phenothiazines.

The most common side effect of the tricyclics is sedation. Some tricyclics, such as Elavil and Sinequan, are more sedating than others. Other common side effects involving the autonomic nervous system include blurred vision, dry mouth, palpitation, postural hypotension, dizziness, profuse diaphoresis, urinary retention, constipation, nausea, and vomiting. Generally speaking, these symptoms are mild and the client usually develops a tolerance to them after several days to a few weeks. CNS effects are usually minor and include tremors, ataxia, paresthesias, and convulsions. A decrease in dosage usually is all that is needed to control these side effects.

With the administration of tricyclics, there is little risk of hypertensive crisis. Only a very few cases of liver damage or blood dyscrasias have been reported. Nevertheless, the nurse should be careful to check vital signs on a regular basis as well as to see that liver function tests and blood counts are done frequently, particularly when these drugs are given in large doses over a prolonged period. Education about side effects and methods for relieving them is essential nursing intervention. There is a lag period of 1 to 4 weeks between the initiation of tricyclic therapy and control of symptoms.

MAO inhibitors and tricyclic compounds usually interact and cause muscle twitching, restlessness, convulsions, hyperpyrexia, delirium, and possibly death. Therefore, these two categories of drugs should not be given simultaneously. Furthermore, when changing a client's medications from an MAO inhibitor to a tricyclic, at least 10 days to 2 weeks should elapse between discontinuing one and beginning the other, since it takes that long for an MAO inhibitor to become synthesized.[10]

Nursing Intervention

Nurses need to be realistic about the benefits antidepressant drugs offer clients. They assist in the psychotherapeutic treatment of depression rather than substituting for it. Education of clients and evaluation of their learning is essential. Motivating clients to take medication and continue with psychotherapy is also a nursing function. Furthermore, alert nurses will recognize that the depressed client is always a potential suicide risk. Although the administration of medication may elevate clients' moods, it may also give them enough physical energy to decide on and act out suicidal plans. Any sudden change in behavior, however subtle, is a clue to possible self-destructive behavior (see Chap. 20).

Lithium

The main use of lithium is in the treatment of the manic phase of manic-depressive psychosis. Studies have shown that 70 to 80 percent of manic clients show marked improvement after 2 weeks of lithium administration. It also appears that lithium exerts a preventive action against both manic and depressive relapses of the manic-depressive cycle. It is unclear, however, whether lithium is of any use during a depression; the clinical results have been extremely varied.

Action

Lithium's mode of action is not clearly understood. Studies indicate that it interferes with norepinephrine and serotonin metabolism and that it may also affect the electrolyte balance within the brain. It is speculated that certain amines, involved in both mood and motor activity, increase during mania and decrease during depression. There is also speculation about the role of lithium in interfering with ion exchange and nerve conduction and also about the role of electrolytes and monoamine metabolism within the brain.

Lithium is an alkali metal found in minerals, sea water, plants, and animals. It is a natural component of human blood serum. About 95 percent of the ingested lithium is excreted through the kidneys. Consequently, it is important that the kidneys be functioning adequately or else the lithium will accumulate and cause lithium toxicity. Diuretics should not be given simultaneously, since they may potentiate sodium and fluid depletion, causing lithium toxicity. The tricyclics should also be avoided with lithium administration, since they interfere with prophylactic effects, lead to hypomania or mania, and potentiate antithyroid effects.[11]

Client Work-up

The nurse should see to it that, prior to beginning lithium administration, the client has a complete history and physical examination. Vital components of this examination are blood pressure determination, blood studies (hematocrit, WBC count, WBC differential, blood urea nitrogen or serum creatinine, and electrolyte levels), urinalysis, serum thyroid function tests, and an electrocardiogram. A careful history is essential, because lithium is contraindicated in clients with cardiovascu-

lar disease, renal disease, decreased sodium intake, or febrile conditions or with clients who are pregnant. Any condition that involves either sodium or water depletion may lead to eventual lithium intoxication. Lithium should be used with caution with the elderly client.

Preparation and Dosage

Lithium carbonate is available for oral ingestion in 300-mg scored tablets (Lithane, Lithotabs) or 300-mg capsules (Eskalith, Lithonate, lithium carbonate).

The dosage depends on the severity of the illness. The therapeutic dose given during manic episodes is usually 600 mg t.i.d., or 1800 mg/day. The prophylactic, or maintenance dose is given during remission and is usually 300 mg b.i.d. or t.i.d., or between 600 mg and 900 mg/day. Once the proper maintenance dosage is established, it can be left unchanged. Serum lithium levels should be done three times a week while establishing the dosage, weekly when first beginning maintenance dosage, and monthly once a stable maintenance dosage is established.[11]

Serum lithium levels for adequate dosage during acute mania range from 1.0 to 1.5 meq/liter and should never exceed 2.0 meq/liter. For long-term control of manic symptoms the serum range is 0.6 to 1.2 meq/liter and should never exceed 1.5 meq/liter.[12] Moderate-to-severe toxic reactions are seen in individuals having serum levels from 2.0 to 2.5 meq/liter.

Side Effects

Side effects include feelings of generalized discomfort, nausea, vomiting, diarrhea, abdominal pain, thirst, fatigue, fine hand tremor (which will not respond to antiparkinson drugs), and muscle weakness. Some of these symptoms are related to peak lithium concentrations or appear early in treatment but gradually disappear. Others continue for months or years, and the client usually becomes accustomed to them.

Lithium intoxication, although infrequent, is a

side effect which can be fatal. It develops when more lithium is administered than can be excreted by the kidneys. Treatment is mainly supportive and is aimed at the prevention of complications and the removal of lithium from the system. Lithium intoxication may last for several weeks and is generally reversible. The best way to deal with it is to prevent its occurrence through careful, individualized dosage regulation, serum lithium screening, and client education.

Lag Period

It is important to note that a lag period of 1 week to 10 days exists between the initiation of lithium therapy and the control of manic symptoms. During this time symptoms can be controlled by concurrent administration of major tranquilizers (usually the phenothiazines or Haldol) and/or electroconvulsive treatment.[12]

Nursing Intervention

Before lithium therapy is begun, nurses should see to it that an accurate history and complete physical is completed on the client. Nurses responsible for the administration of lithium must be alert to the signs and symptoms of lithium intoxication. They must also have an awareness of the side effects of the drug. Physicians depend on nursing observation of client behavior when they are regulating dosages. Accurate assessments of behavioral patterns are invaluable during the initial stages of drug administration.

Nurses assume a major role in educating clients about lithium and thereby assist in motivating them to continue treatment after they leave the controlled setting. Because of a limited safety range, clients need to know that serious damage to themselves can result from misuse of dosages. Knowledge that the medication helps only as long as it is continued and that it can be taken indefinitely without altered tolerance is reassuring to the client who wishes to prevent a relapse.

Clients should be made aware of side effects and the need to maintain adequate salt and fluid intake. Counseling and education should be ongoing and include repeated instruction about *why* a client needs to take lithium. The teaching of self-observation, not only of side effects but of the symptoms of the illness, is essential to nursing intervention.

Convulsive Therapies

Ladislaus von Meduna attempted in 1933 to induce convulsions in schizophrenics, believing that this would cure their psychosis. Since that time convulsive therapy utilizing a variety of agents has been used in the treatment of certain forms of mental illness.

Insulin Coma Therapy

In 1933, Sakel induced hypoglycemic coma in schizophrenics by administering increasing amounts of insulin to fasting clients. His technique was called insulin coma therapy. Initially, the amount of insulin was small; it was gradually increased until an amount was given which produced coma. This occurred over several days. Coma was terminated by the administration of carbohydrates, given either intravenously or by tube feedings. The average client received between 40 and 60 hours of coma. Advocates of the treatment believed that the sleeplike state of coma "rested" the brain and cured the illness. Because of the many complications involved, the highly specialized personnel and equipment needed, and the extreme length and expense of this treatment, insulin coma has gradually become obsolete—much to the regret of some psychiatrists, who felt strongly that the early stages of schizophrenia could be arrested by this technique.[13]

Electroconvulsive Therapy

Electroconvulsive treatment (also referred to as electroshock therapy, ECT, or EST) was introduced in 1933 by two Italian psychiatrists, Cerletti and

Bini. They used an apparatus which produced alternating currents of electricity to induce convulsions. A similar apparatus is utilized today.

Theories of Action

Theories related to the action of ECT are speculative. One psychological interpretation is that the treatment serves as a symbolic punishment for the client, who feels guilty and worthless. Another theory proposes that ECT is seen by clients as a life-threatening experience and they therefore mobilize all their bodily defenses to deal with this "attack." It has also been suggested that clients are able to release their inner aggressive impulses through the convulsions associated with the treatment. Still another theory holds that the electric shock produces minimal brain damage which destroys the specific area containing memories related to the events surrounding the development of the psychotic condition. Another, more complex physiological theory views the brain as consisting of multiple electric circuits and sees mental illness as stemming from a malfunction of the circuits. An internal self-corrective system assisted by ECT is thought to clear the brain of whatever material has interfered with proper functioning.

Bilateral or standard electroconvulsive treatment calls for electrodes to be applied to both the client's temples. To avoid skin burns and ensure maximum electrical conductivity, the electrodes must be firmly held in place and moistened with either a saline solution or electrojelly. No fixed number of treatments are necessary before positive results are seen. Usually, to begin with, treatments are given on 3 alternate days a week. Anywhere between 5 and 30 treatments might be indicated, depending on the client's condition. Depressive conditions may begin to improve after 6 to 12 treatments. Hyperexcitable clients may need between 8 and 16 treatments.

Nursing Intervention

Prior to treatment, written permission must be obtained from the client and a thorough physical examination—including complete blood count, urinalysis, electrocardiogram, and x-rays of the chest and the lateral aspects of the spine—must be completed and recorded on the client's chart. The client is treated in the morning and should have an empty stomach. Verbal preparation and reassurance is given as necessary to allay anxiety. The client should void, be dressed in sleepwear or loose-fitting clothing, and remove dentures (if any). Atropine is generally given to decrease secretions and to interrupt the vagal stimulation effects of ECT.

Once in the actual treatment room, the client lies in a supine position on a stretcher. The anesthesiologist administers a *short-acting barbiturate,* such as sodium methohexital, intravenously. This is followed immediately by an intravenous injection of the *muscle relaxant* succinylcholine (Anectine), given in a separate syringe. Clients are preoxygenated with 95 to 100 percent oxygen, and their chins are supported to prevent dislocation and provide a more effective airway. A soft mouthbite is sometimes used. Electrodes are put in place and the client's arms are held down close to the body to minimize movement. The psychiatrist initiates treatment by pushing the button on the ECT machine. A tonic seizure, lasting 5 to 15 seconds, then occurs; this is followed by clonic movements, which last from 10 to 60 seconds. Oxygen is administered and suctioning occurs as necessary. The client's head should be turned to the side to prevent aspiration of saliva.

Most clients awaken almost immediately after treatment. However, since they are extremely confused and lightheaded at this time, very careful nursing supervision is necessary. Some clients become extremely restless and agitated during this period of confusion and can, if not watched, possibly injure themselves by thrashing about or attempting to get out of bed too soon. The client should remain lying down for at least a half hour. Often, but not always, the client will sleep soundly for an hour or more. During this time, careful monitoring of vital signs, maintenance of adequate respiration and reassurance and orientation to surroundings are necessary. Clients do not experience physical pain nor are they aware of the actual seizure, but they are often very upset by temporary memory loss. A supportive attitude on the part of the staff which encourages the client to participate in interpersonal activities and orientation to reality are particularly important once the actual treatment is over.

Side Effects of ECT

Prior to the use of muscle relaxants, compression fractures of the vertebrae and the long bones of the arms and legs were common. The current use of the muscle relaxant succinylcholine has virtually eliminated this problem. The two most common side effects of electroconvulsive therapy are loss of memory and confusion. The intensity of these side effects is related to the number of treatments received and the age of the client. In any case, they will eventually abate and the client's memory and orientation will be restored. In the interim, the nurse needs to provide much reassurance and support. Clients may also be apprehensive about losing consciousness and control or about experiencing a convulsion, even though they are not aware of the convulsion when it actually occurs.[13-15]

Other Somatic Therapies

Psychosurgery

In 1935, Moniz received the Nobel Prize for pioneering psychosurgery, and frontal lobotomy became for a time the treatment of choice for chronic psychotic clients. However, its use has been sharply curtailed since the discovery of tranquilizers and the use of other rehabilitative measures. It is still advocated by some treatment centers for refractory chronic clients and for those with severe tension that stems from fear, worry, depression, anxiety, or agitation. Its use is recommended only after all other methods have failed.

Persons undergoing a frontal lobotomy experience a personality change. After surgery, the client usually lacks initiative and is lazy and apathetic. Psychic energy is markedly reduced, although some clients recover vigor after time. Feelings have less depth and cannot be sustained. Intelligence may be diminished.[16] Nurses generally do not encounter clients who have had recent lobotomies but rather must care for those who have been institutionalized and are chronically unable to function without custodial care.

Orthomolecular Treatment

Orthomolecular therapy is aimed at providing an optimal molecular environment for the mind—of providing it with ample supplies of substances that are normally present within the body. Linus Pauling, the founder of orthomolecular treatment, believes that mental illness is due to excessively low concentrations of specific vitamins in the brain. This condition is believed to be due to a client's genetic makeup and diet.

Orthomolecular practitioners treat schizophrenic clients with massive doses of vitamins and minerals as supplements to psychotropic drugs, psychotherapy, and electroconvulsive therapy. Megadoses of vitamin B_3, vitamin B_6, vitamin C, and trace metals as well as an antihypoglycemic diet are considered to be vital components of this regimen.[17]

Hydrotherapy

Hydrotherapy has been used for centuries as a treatment modality for agitated clients. It is defined as the use of water in the treatment of disease. Formerly, the application of wet packs was a popular treatment; however, the advent of psychotherapeutic drugs and more convenient and less expensive treatments has eliminated their use. Today, hot baths and showers have value as comfort measures, contributing to a feeling of well-being and thus having an indirect therapeutic effect. Swimming pools and whirlpool baths in some settings provide comfort and relaxation for clients.[18]

References

*1 Betty S. Bergersen: *Pharmacology in Nursing,* Mosby, St. Louis, 1973, pp. 337–371.

2 AMA Department of Drugs: *AMA Drug Evaluations,* 2d ed., Publishing Sciences Group, Acton, Mass., 1973.

3 Lawrence C. Kolb: *Modern Clinical Psychiatry,* Saunders, Philadelphia, 1973, pp. 620–638.

4 Allen J. Enelow: "Psychotropic Drugs," *Medical Insight,* May 1970, pp. 41–47.

*5 Joseph F. Krivda: "Major or Minor Tranquilizers for Relief of Common Symptoms of Psychoneurosis?" *JPN and Mental Health Services,* July–August 1974, pp. 28–33.

*6 Lisa Robinson: *Psychiatric Nursing as a Human Experience,* Saunders, Philadelphia, 1972, pp. 213–243.

7 Nathan S. Kline and John M. Davis: "Psychotropic Drugs," *American Journal of Nursing,* vol. 73, no. 1, pp. 54–62, January 1973.

*8 Dorothy Mereness: *Essentials of Psychiatric Nursing,* 8th ed., Mosby, St. Louis, 1970.

*9 Carolyn Adams Kicey: "Catecholamines and Depression: A Physiological Theory of Depression," *American Journal of Nursing,* vol. 74, no. 11, pp. 2018–2020, November 1974.

10 Oakley S. Ray: *Drugs, Society, and Human Behavior,* Mosby, St. Louis, 1972, pp. 136–156.

11 Joe P. Tupin: "The Use of Lithium for Manic-Depressive Psychosis," *Hospital & Communinity Psychiatry,* vol. 21, no. 3, pp. 73–78, March 1970.

12 Robert Prien, Eugene M. McCaffrey, and James C. Klett: *Lithium Carbonate in Psychiatry,* American Psychiatric Association, Washington, D. C., 1970, pamphlet, 15 pages.

13 Lawrence C. Kolb: *Modern Clinical Psychiatry,* Saunders, Philadelphia, 1973, pp. 639–655.

*14 Roberta Cohen: "EST and Group Therapy Equal Improved Care," *American Journal of Nursing,* vol. 71, no. 6, pp. 1195–1198.

15 Lewis R. Wolberg: *The Technique of Psychotherapy,* 2d ed., Grune & Stratton, New York, 1967, pp. 91–101.

16 Alfred M. Freedman and Harold I. Kaplan (eds.): *Comprehensive Textbook of Psychiatry,* Williams & Wilkins, Baltimore, 1967.

17 David N. Leef: "Megavitamins and Mental Disease," *Medical World News,* August 11, 1975, pp. 71–82.

18 Richard I. Shader (ed.): *Manual of Psychiatric Therapeutics,* Little, Brown, Boston, 1975.

*Recommended reference by a nurse author.

Chapter

9

Environmental Management

Anita M. Leach

Learning Objectives

After studying this chapter, the student should be able to:

1 Define "environment" and its implications for nursing practice
2 Understand the roles of the members of the mental health team
3 Know the essential components of a therapeutic environment
4 List the various therapies conducted in mental health treatment settings
5 Define "therapeutic community"
6 Describe characteristics, goals, and problems of a therapeutic community
7 Describe the role of the nurse in a therapeutic community

Environment Defined

People of all ages are influenced by their environment. When clients enter into relationships with nurses, they bring with them the effects their environment has had over time, and they are influenced by the environment as it exists in the here and now.

The environment is the patterned wholeness of all that is external to an individual. People and the environment are continuously exchanging matter and energy with one another. They interact as an integrated whole with the totality of the environment. The environment consists of a set of objects, a change in which affects the total system. These objects can be persons, places, or things and can be changed by the behavior of the total system.

Everyday life is filled with experiences that validate the concept that individuals are affecting and are being affected by the objects around them. These people-environment transactions are characterized by continuous repatterning of both the person and the environment.[1] Persons, places, and things are part of the environment of clients and nurses and consequently effect change in each of them.

Therapeutic Environment

A therapeutic milieu is based on conscious application of the knowledge that everything that happens to clients in their environment has the potential of being therapeutic or antitherapeutic.[2] Clients quickly respond to the emotional climates of the settings in which they find themselves. Their emotions are reflected from the environment. To make an environment useful and helpful, nurses need to keep certain specifics in mind.

- Clients should be assured that they are safe from physical danger and needless emotional trauma.
- Clients should have the freedom to express their feelings and to do so in ways that will be acceptable to both themselves and others in the environment.

- Clients should have the opportunity to use their own abilities to solve problems. They should have the support of nursing personnel in the tasks they undertake.
- Clients should have behavioral expectations explained to them. One of the most common concerns of newly admitted clients is a fear of violating the "rules."
- Clients should not be exposed to staff tensions or staff needs for approval. These tensions and needs are easily transmitted to clients in unconscious, nonverbal ways and should, therefore, be dealt with outside the client setting.
- Clients should expect to be treated with respect and dignity. Their right to privacy should be ensured.

In psychiatric mental health settings, a friendly, warm atmosphere which maximizes individualization of treatment, one which provides continuity of care and a feeling of security, is essential to the client's recovery. Opportunities for clients to take responsibility for themselves—as well as for the well-being of those around them—does much to create a therapeutic milieu. Perceptual stimulation, activity to prevent regression, adequate food, rest, and comfort, and a program of resocialization help create an air of optimism about the prognosis of treatment.[2]

Nurses are the key persons in assuring a therapeutic atmosphere. The 24-hour-a-day presence of nursing personnel is a major factor in the management and positive change of client behavior. In assessing environmental needs of clients, nurses need to be alert to the persons, places, and things a client will encounter and the effect they will have on the clients' total care and recovery.

Persons in the Environment—The Mental Health Team

The psychiatric mental health team consists of psychiatrists, nurses, nursing assistants or technicians, social workers, clinical psychologists, and cooperating adjunct therapists. Adjunct therapists are those who utilize the arts when doing therapeutic work. Among those specialists who may be on the team are the art therapist, occupational therapist, psychodrama therapist, and recreational therapist. Individuals have also been trained to utilize pets, poetry, and other literature as therapeutic adjuncts. Vocational and educational therapists also make valuable contributions to clients, particularly adolescents, young adults, and children. The dietician contributes to the team in the treatment of food-related illnesses and by providing a wholesome daily menu. Table 9-1 lists the many persons who contribute to a mental health treatment team and gives brief descriptions of their functions and educational backgrounds.

In addition to the many persons who are part of a client's present treatment milieu, family members who are or will be part of the client's past and future environment need to be considered in the treatment plan. Family therapy is essential to the restoration of client and family equilibrium (see Chap. 11). Nurses should realize that persons in the client's environment effect repatterning and change as part of the therapeutic process. Likewise, the persons on the mental health team are responsive and affected in their contacts with clients.

Places in the Environment—Settings for Therapy

Treatment of clients takes place in a variety of settings, both formal and informal. Some of these are prisons, child-care institutions, locked wards, day hospitals, night hospitals, community mental health centers, private-practice offices, inpatient halfway houses, sheltered workshops, schools, general-care hospitals, intensive-care units, and emergency rooms.

Nurses are usually the persons responsible for creating a therapeutic milieu in the settings where they work. Since most treatment occurs in hospital settings, these facilities should include space for meeting basic needs. An ideal atmosphere for meeting these needs is outlined in Table 9-2. The reason for providing this therapeutic setting is to allow clients to test alternate behaviors which will contribute to their future life-style.

Objects in the Environment—Sensory Perceptions

The senses provide input from objects in the environment. *Sensory overload* and *sensory deprivation* can cause distortion of this input. Clients in an intensive-care unit, for example, may begin to have visual hallucinations because of the great number of stimuli present in their environment.

One of the major roles of the nursing staff in the care of hospitalized clients is the maintenance of a safe environment. Clients who are suicidal, for example, can hurt themselves readily on objects that are often seen as harmless. Sharp objects such as razors—and in some cases mirrors—need to be limited in psychiatric treatment settings. Furniture purchased for a psychiatric setting should be sturdy and have curved edges, since some disturbed patients are often destructive to and with objects in their environment.

Color, lighting, and sound have significant effects on the behavior of clients. Nurses manage disturbed clients, for example, by isolating them in a quiet room away from sensory stimuli. Lighting in such a room should be subdued and sound should be reduced to a minimum. Pale blues, greens, and shades of purple, because of their soothing effect, are often chosen in the decoration of "quiet rooms." Harmful objects should be removed and furniture should have blunt edges. Visitors should be kept at a minimum. Staff working in these areas should not try to engage clients in conversation but rather maintain a silent protectiveness. In the absence of excessive sensory input, a disturbed client is more likely to regain self-control.

Clients and staff alike are sometimes noisy. Nurses should be mindful that a quiet, calm, and orderly manner will modify client behavior and add to the clients' comfort. Loud noises, therefore, should be avoided whenever possible. Nurses should also be alert to odors in a unit and take steps to eliminate them when they occur.

Table 9-1 Members of the Mental Health Team

Team member	Educational preparation	Team function
Psychiatrist	M.D. with residency in psychiatry.	Physician who specializes in the treatment of mental diseases. Considered the leader of the team. Has both administrative and care-planning responsibilities—diagnostic and medical functions are the psychiatrist's main tasks.
Clinical psychologist	Ph.D. in clinical psychology.	Specializes in the study of mental processes and treatment of mental disorders. Utilizes diagnostic testing to assist the team in differentiating the causative factors of client behavior. Treats clients, using both individual and group methods.
Psychiatric social worker	Master's degree in social work (M.S.W.).	Evaluates families; studies the environment and social causes of the client's illness. Practices family therapy as a natural outcome of assessment. Works in the intake office and admits new clients.
Psychiatric nurse	R.N. (diploma), A.A., B.S.; advanced preparation at the master's level for independent practice.	Environmental management and 24-hour-a-day care. Carries out individual, family, and group psychotherapy; coordinates team activities. Supervises technicians or psychiatric assistants.
Psychiatric assistant or technician	High school education, special on-job training in setting of employment.	Works under the direct supervision of a professional nurse. Assists nurses in providing for the basic needs of clients. Carries out nursing functions, including maintenance of a therapeutic environment. Supervises leisure-time activity. Assists with individual and group psychotherapy.
Occupational therapist	Advanced degree in occupational therapy.	Assesses clients' skills for rehabilitative planning. Encourages clients to perform useful tasks. Responsible for socialization therapy and vocational retraining.
Art therapist	Advanced degree and specialized training in art therapy.	Utilizes procedures that make use of spontaneous creative work of clients. Works with groups, encouraging members to make and analyze drawings which are often expressions of their underlying problems. Adjunct to a mental health team in diagnosis and treatment of children.
Recreational therapist	Advanced degree and specialized training in recreational therapy.	Provides leisure-time activities for clients. Teaches hospitalized clients useful pastimes which can be utilized when they return to the community. Participates in pet therapy, psychodrama, poetry and music therapy.
Dietician	Advanced degree and specialized training in dietetics.	Provides attractive, nourishing meals for clients. Involved in direct treatment of such food-related illnesses as anorexia nervosa, bulimia, pica, rumination, and eating-control disorders.
Auxiliary personnel (housekeepers, volunteers, clerks, secretaries, etc.)	Various backgrounds and on-job training	When properly educated, invaluable in assisting the client to enter into and participate in the therapeutic program.

Table 9-2 Atmosphere Needed to Meet Basic Needs

Needs	Atmosphere to be created
Physiological: Food, oxygen, water, sleep, sex	*Dining Room:* Cheerfully decorated, arranged for maximum socialization, noise factor at minimum, background music *Bedroom:* Cheerfully decorated, subdued lighting and colors, reading light, desk, quiet, arranged for maximum privacy, planned for client individualization, *Outdoor Space:* Planned so client can enjoy fresh air, can walk or sit *Snack Kitchen:* Snacks and coffee available, arranged for informal socialization *Bathroom:* Provide privacy without using locks
Safety: Security, stability, order, physical safety	*Seclusion or Quiet Room:* Place for restricting clients, controlled space confinement, subdued lighting, subdued color, safe room free from objects that can do physical harm *Locked Space:* To protect clients from themselves and others *Boundaries:* Knowledge of limits of a client's personal space *Bulletin Boards:* For posting schedules, notices and client assignments
Love and Belonging: Affection, identification, companionship	*Common Room:* Homelike, comfortably furnished Furniture groupings conducive to socialization—tables for game playing, etc. Bright, cheerful color scheme
Esteem and Recognition	*Interviewing Rooms:* Conducive to establishing a caring, therapeutic relationship, quiet, conducive to uninterrupted time with clients *Group Rooms:* Chairs in round circle, no table in center, quiet, conducive to uninterrupted time with clients
Self-Actualization: Self-fullfillment, achieving one's potential, realizing one's capabilities	*Occupational Therapy Room:* Background music, woodworking and crafts equipment, freedom to explore interests, supervised and secure *Art Therapy Room:* Background music, supervision, ample supplies of oil paints, water colors, tempera paints, clay, and finger paints *Music/Entertainment Center:* Equipped with records for all types of listening, television set *Library:* Quiet, comfortable chairs, reading lights, variety of books, newspapers, magazines
Aesthetic: Order, harmony, beauty, spiritual goals	*Chapel:* Quiet, nondenominational, meditative atmosphere, place to be alone

The Therapies
Occupational Therapy

Occupational therapy is a specialty that encourages clients to develop interests which may either reestablish old skills and knowledge or initiate new learning. These interests serve as a hobby or as a basis for developing other, more challenging interests. Creative skills also serve to develop the client's self-esteem and self-confidence. Nurses should fully understand the opportunities provided by occupational therapy and how important it is for clients to accomplish something through their own efforts. Often the nurse's understanding can be influential in initiating the client's participation in the occupational therapy program.

In many settings, nurses take an active part in the activities that are carried out within the psychiatric unit. Close working relationships exist between the nurses and the occupational therapist. It is often nurses who carry out plans prepared by occupational therapists.

Activities are sometimes carried out directly on the unit so as not to remove clients from the environment that has become meaningful and secure to them. Nurses have an opportunity to give guidance, encouragement, and support to those who are participating in these activities. The walls of some hospital units, for example, have been decorated by artistically gifted clients at the suggestion of nurses. Unit activity likewise brings occupational therapy to clients in acute periods of illness as well as during convalescence.[5] Occupational therapy projects can be brought to clients who may be physically unable to go to the activity room or may be retained in the unit for reasons of behavioral modification.

Recreational Therapy

In some settings, the role of recreational leader falls to nursing staff. In some, however, an individual with advanced education in recreational leadership is designated to carry out these responsibilities.

In assessing client needs, nurses must be aware of the age of the group with which they will be working. For example, teen-age clients will be interested in very different types of recreation than will adults. Teen-agers enjoy physical activity such as bowling, basketball, or swimming. Elderly patients require quieter leisure-time activities to fulfill their needs; card games and Bingo are often of interest to this age group. Mixing both age groups can be done through having a dance at which different kinds of music is played or by taking clients on a picnic or to a theatrical performance.

If recreation is to meet client needs, the client must be actively involved in planning and initiating activities. Recreation must be included in the clients' lives if they are to develop an interest in reestablishing a balanced life away from the therapeutic setting.[5]

Dance Therapy

Dance is a form of nonverbal communication. Marion Chase, in 1940, pioneered the use of rhythmic body movements to rehabilitate people with emotional or physical disorders. This method is currently used in both individual and group therapy.[6]

Body posture and movement often gives the nurse valuable insight into the dynamics of a client's behavior. Fostering freedom of body movement also helps clients to express, in a nonthreatening way, feelings they are otherwise unable to share therapeutically. Dance and movement therapists are often recreational therapists who have chosen to specialize in these areas.

Poetry/Literature Therapy

Task-oriented groups, meeting for the purpose of studying literature or poetry, have been most effective in providing therapy for some clients. The nurse can often be the initiator of such a group. The leader proceeds by reading short passages from works selected by the clients. Group members are then asked to share the feelings and insights which they experience as a result of the reading. Exploration of the meanings the poetry has for clients often provides, both to the clients and to the nurse, new insights into the dynamics of their behavior.

Play Therapy

In this type of treatment, clients are encouraged to perform imaginative play with various toys or other materials furnished by the therapist. Play therapy is a technique most often utilized with children. It makes it possible for clients to express themselves in a nonverbal manner and in a nonthreatening atmosphere. In addition to its use with children, play therapy may be used in the psychotherapy of psychotics who have regressed to the point where verbal communication is impossible. Play therapy has also been used successfully with regressed older adults. Play therapists are generally members of another mental health discipline who have chosen to specialize in this area. Pediatric and psychiatric nurses are among those skilled in the use of play therapy.[7]

Education Therapy

Education therapy involves formal instruction that is made available to clients as part of the total treatment effort. Such instruction is given by a qualified teacher in a specific subject; it serves to enhance clients' self-esteem and to help them adjust to the treatment setting. However, for children with school phobias, education therapy serves a more essential and immediate therapeutic goal.

Pet Therapy

In work done with elderly people and autistic children, it has been found that pets have often stimulated responses that these clients do not show in relation to humans. This observation has led some therapists to utilize pets to facilitate therapy. A withdrawn schizophrenic may well respond to a nonthreatening animal but shy away from human contact. Pets can also be used as a springboard for teaching healthy relational pat-

terns. Nurses can informally introduce pets into the therapeutic milieu either as a form of recreation or as therapy.

Socialization Therapy

Socialization therapy is therapeutic work done in informal groups or clubs. Its purpose is to provide a means whereby clients can develop social skills which will lead to their being able to leave their protective environment and function socially in the community. These clubs are found in a variety of settings but most commonly in halfway houses. Other treatment centers have clubs or groups for ex-clients.[6] Clients learn to bridge the gap between the therapeutic setting and the community by their participation in social groups whose tasks may be cooking, gardening, or attending the theater. Nurses often provide the leadership, guidance, and structure for these informal task-oriented social groups.

Psychodrama

Psychodrama is primarily a form of group psychotherapy. It involves the structured, directed, and dramatized acting out of a client's personal, emotional, and interactional problems. It was originated by Moreno and has since been modified by him and others.[6] It is based on the principle that dramatic psychotherapy permits the development of greater awareness than is obtainable from merely verbal means. It includes such procedures as catharsis, abreaction, free association in acting, and encounters between persons. Interpretations may be used but are not often needed. The goal is not only insight but also spontaneity, total perception of unhealthy responses, a more accurate perception of reality, involvement with other persons, and learning through experiencing.[6]

The director or therapist leads the production in accordance with clues provided by clients, instructing all the performers in their roles. The role of the director varies with the dramatic situation. Therapists constantly change roles to bring out and correct the clients' maladaptive patterns. The relationship between the client and the therapist is not only transferential but also based on reality. The client is encouraged to express direct intuitive feelings about the immediate behavior of the therapist.

Utilization of auxiliary egos is a common element of psychodrama. Special areas of functioning such as delusions or hallucinations are the focus of the script. Soliloquy, role reversal, use of an auxiliary ego, and mirror techniques are common tools used by the therapist leading a psychodrama. Nurses are most frequently involved as participants, playing supportive, facilitative roles for the group.[6]

Social Network Therapy

Gathering together the members of a disturbed person's social community or network, all of whom meet in group sessions with the client, is referred to as social network therapy. The network includes all those with whom clients come into contact in their daily lives: not only immediate family but others such as more distant relatives, friends, tradespeople, teachers, coworkers, etc. This is a modification of traditional family therapy.[6] (See Chap. 11.) It is utilized as a means of assessing clients' interactions with persons in their environment, planning for reentry back into the community, and facilitating clients' socialization with significant others.

Gestalt Therapy

Gestalt therapy emphasizes the treatment of persons as *wholes*. Clients' biological component parts—their organic functioning, perceptual configuration, and interrelationships with the environment taken as a whole—are the focus of therapy. Gestalt therapy was developed by Frederick Perls and is used in both individual and group therapy settings. It focuses on the client's sensory awareness in the here and now rather than on recollections of the past or expectations for the future. The technique employs role playing to promote clients' growth and the development of their full potential.[8]

It might be said that gestalt therapy is a kind of environmental therapy. Nurses employ its techniques when they practice reality orientation with clients. Learning to take each day as it comes and being aware of the moment are types of focus on the here and now and could be considered part of gestalt therapy.

Milieu Therapy

Milieu therapy involves those aspects of the sociology and culture of a treatment setting which can be influential in reducing the behavioral disturbances of clients. Behavior is modified by structuring the environment to provide human relationships that satisfy emotional needs, reduce psychological conflicts and deprivation, and strengthen impaired ego functions. The concept of this type of therapy is based on the assumption that the *social milieu itself* can be the instrument of treatment.[9]

The realization that people change, learn, and mature as the result of their interpersonal and social relationships and experiences has lead to the creation of the *therapeutic community* in which the total environment or milieu is used therapeutically for the benefit of the client.

The Therapeutic Community

A therapeutic community is a complex system whose primary goal is to provide therapeutic experiences for its clients, students, or staff. It is based on a view of emotional illness as an interpersonal and social phenomenon. Manifestations of mental illness are looked at in the context of the client's relationships with other people. Emphasis is laid on the interpersonal aspect of a person's functioning. It has been stated that the ego develops as a result of crisis resolution. A therapeutic milieu is achieved when staff skills are applied to helping clients through a series of crises in a structured treatment setting.[10]

Jones, who originated the concept of therapeutic community stated that

. . . in some but not all psychiatric conditions, there is much to be learned from observing clients in a relatively ordinary and familiar social environment so that their usual ways of relating to other people, reactions to stress, etc., can be observed. If at the same time clients can be made aware of the effect of their behavior on other people, and helped to understand some of the motivation underlying their actions, the situation is potentially therapeutic.[11]

He believed this to be the distinctive quality of the therapeutic community. He also thought that the possibility always existed for an interpersonal relationship to be therapeutic or antitherapeutic. Jones's concepts involved the introduction of trained staff into a group situation. This fact, together with planned collaboration of clients and staff in all aspects of unit life, made it possible for the social experiences to become therapeutic.[11]

Characteristics of a Therapeutic Community

In a therapeutic community, the staff learn to share responsibility with clients. Client inclusion in a democratic process is considered part of treatment.[12] Clients participate in practically all information-sharing processes of the ward. Their opinions are included in decisions about other clients' readiness for such things as passes and discharges. The fact that both staff and clients are granted coequal rights as human beings in such a community in no way implies coequal function or role status. Hospitals are not democracies run by elected representatives. Rather, authority remains necessary and inescapable. Responsibility for the care of clients remains with the staff. No amount of persuasion, group decision, consensus, joint consultation, or freedom of expression can obscure this or excuse nurses from exercising the authority necessary for the responsible actualizing of their role.

In a therapeutic community, emphasis is placed on socialization and group interaction. The focus is on communication as an opportunity for living and learning. All aspects of the clients' lives are seen as presenting opportunities for growth toward wellness. The emotional climate should be one of warmth, friendliness, acceptance, and optimism. This positive group feeling is enhanced in the community that is functioning well. Group members, as individuals, feel themselves to be participants in active and productive group endeavors. Nurses play a major role in providing and maintaining a safe and conflict-free environment through role modeling and group leadership.

Community Meeting

A prime characteristic of a therapeutic community is the large unit group or *community meeting*, which is held at regularly scheduled intervals. It is attended by all staff and clients who work and/or live on a specific unit.[12]

Jones and Cummings[10,11] see the community meeting as a means of implementing the therapeutic community or therapeutic milieu approach.

The community meeting has multiple functions. It provides the setting in which the group deals with social and behavioral problems using techniques such as exposure, shaming, and reality confrontation. Role examination is another component of community meetings. Administrative matters, activity planning, and housekeeping functions are also agenda items. The meetings in a broad sense are used to inculcate values, norms, and attitudes deemed therapeutic by the leaders of the group.

Characteristically associated with the community meeting itself is the staff "rehash." Staff meets in order to discuss and clarify the social barometer, plan therapeutic strategy, interpret the covert and overt content and processes of the meeting, and learn about therapeutic community practices.[12] For members of all the mental health disciplines, work in a therapeutic community requires a reexamination of the traditional roles for which they have been trained. Training frequently has not prepared them for the jobs in which they find themselves. The therapeutic community, and especially the community meeting, lends itself especially well to a continuing process of in-service training.

Goals of a Therapeutic Community

The goal of a therapeutic community is to return its clients to the community successfully. This purpose is best served by the establishment of close relationships between the therapeutic community and the outside community. The use of community facilities such as recreation centers, libraries, general hospitals, and churches prevents the treatment facility from becoming isolated. An active volunteer group can be an invaluable resource in bridging the gap between treatment center and community.[10]

Problems of a Therapeutic Community

There are many problems inherent in a therapeutic community. To begin with, there is no clear-cut conceptual base by which to justify the operation of a therapeutic community. Role blurring between staff and staff, client and staff, and client and client is a conflict area which inevitably exists. It requires a special talent to maintain the delicate balance between exercising staff authority and at the same time sharing decision making with clients. Group responsibility can easily become no responsibility. This can be avoided by making the leadership lines clear to both staff and clients and by utilizing limit setting as a therapeutic tool.

The possibility that an individual's needs and concerns may become lost because of concern for the group is another problem. If the therapeutic milieu teaches values that, while appropriate to the controlled setting, are not always applicable elsewhere, the client may find the transition to the community difficult.

Other problems include the extreme complexity of doing research and program evaluation in a therapeutic community. Likewise, the setting must train its own staff, since educational programs suitable to personnel functioning in a therapeutic community are seldom available. Staff in a well-run therapeutic community will be aware of the many problems which exist and will take steps to anticipate and prevent them when possible.

Role of the Nurse in a Therapeutic Community

Nursing in a therapeutic community reflects the characteristics of the setting. Nursing roles are not often viewed as being different from those of other disciplines but are determined by individual nurses and the settings in which they find themselves. Nurses have the uniqueness of being in the environment 24 hours a day. They, therefore, are in contact with clients more than any other team members providing structure and continuity to the group. The task of developing the therapeutic milieu consists largely in exploiting this central role of nurses to the utmost.[9]

Nurses who plan to work in a therapeutic community need an awareness of their own humanity, energy, and spontaneity. Some knowledge of cultural anthropolgy will be helpful in assisting the nurse to tolerate a wide range of behavior.[9] In the therapeutic community situations of living are managed by the nurse. All aspects of the client's life in the social milieu are seen as presenting opportunities for a living-learning experience. The role of nurses is to use their various skills to exploit these opportunities to the fullest. The culture then becomes one in which there is a favorable climate for helping clients to gain an awareness of their feelings, thoughts, impulses, and behaviors. Such an environment helps clients to try their new skills and at the same time achieve a realistic appraisal of their social and interpersonal behavior. Nurses in a therapeutic community, therefore, lead each client to an increase in self-esteem.[13]

Nurses carry out functional duties. These involve appropriate medication of clients, limit setting, observations of behavior, and the care and observation of physical symptoms. Comfort measures are also the responsibility of the nurse.

Some nurses function in a supervisory capacity, coordinating, organizing, and evaluating team functioning. Nurses often run the unit and client-government meetings. They share responsibility with clients, encouraging them to participate in the decision-making functions of the community. This serves to prepare the client to function similarly outside the hospital and to combat the feeling of helplessness from which hospitalized clients so often suffer. It is frequently the nurse who is most influential in assisting clients to assume leadership roles in the government of a unit. Theoretically, clients and staff share equally in the responsibility for smooth environmental control; however, it is actually the nurse who encourages and supports clients in this function. A major factor involved in effective client government is the staff's trust in the ultimate good judgment of the client group and the staff's willingness to delegate real decision making to them.[13]

References

*1 Martha E. Rogers: *An Introduction to the Theoretical Basis of Nursing*, Davis, Philadelphia, 1970, pp. 49–55.

2 Arthur P. Noyes, William P. Comp, and Mildred Van Sickel: *Psychiatric Nursing*, Macmillan, New York, 1967, pp. 258–264.

*3 Charles K. Hofling, Madeline M. Leininger, and Elizabeth A. Bregg: *Basic Psychiatric Concepts in Nursing*, Lippincott, Philadelphia, 1967, pp. 501–526.

4 Abraham H. Maslow: *Motivation and Personality*, 2d ed., Harper and Row, New York, 1970.

*5 Dorothy Mereness and Louis J. Karnosh: *Essentials of Psychiatric Nursing*, Mosby, St. Louis, 1966, pp. 47–57, 83–91.

6 Alfred M. Friedman, Harold I. Kaplan, and Benjamin J. Sadock: *Modern Synopsis of Psychiatry*, Williams & Wilkins, Baltimore, 1972.

7 Virginia M. Axline: *Play Therapy*, Ballantine Books, New York, 1969.

8 Frederick Perls, Ralph F. Hefferline, and Paul Goodman: *Gestalt Therapy*, Dell, New York, 1951.

9 Alan M. Kraft: "The Therapeutic Community," in Silvano Arieti (ed.), *American Handbook of Psychiatry*, Basic Books, New York, 1966, vol. 3, pp. 542–551.

10 John Cumming and Elaine Cumming: *Ego and Milieu*, Atherton, New York, 1962.

11 Maxwell Jones: *The Therapeutic Community*, Basic Books, New York, 1953.

12 David N. Daniels and Ronald S. Rubing: "The Community Meeting," *Archives of General Psychiatry*, vol. 18, pp. 60–75, January 1968.

*13 Marguerite J. Holmes and Jean A. Werner: *Psychiatric Nursing In A Therapeutic Community*, Macmillan, New York, 1966.

*Recommended reference by a nurse author.

10

Group Dynamic Theory and Application

Suzanne Lego

Learning Objectives

After studying this chapter, the student should be able to:

1 Outline the basic principles of small-group theory
2 Understand the interrelationship between group content and process
3 Identify leadership styles
4 Describe common problems of beginning group leaders
5 Discuss phenomena occurring in small groups
6 Recognize the signs of group cohesiveness
7 Discuss the principles of group psychotherapy
8 Describe the role of the leader in group psychotherapy
9 List the phases in group development
10 Understand the concepts of transference, countertransference, resistance, acting out, and insight
11 Know the criteria for termination of a group

Nurses almost always work in groups; staff groups, faculty groups, and community teams are a few examples of such groups. In addition, work with clients is frequently done in groups, whether these be clinical groups, teaching groups, or groups that are created by accident, as in an assignment to a four-bed hospital room. For this reason it is important that nurses grasp the rudiments of group process, so that they may understand their own patterns of group behavior as well as those of their clients. The group is often used as a therapeutic tool, as in group psychotherapy sessions, therapeutic community meetings, and work and recreation groups.

Small-Group Theory
Brief History[1]

Sociologists first developed what is known today as small-group theory. Durkheim in the 1890s talked of the group as a "collective representation" which had an identity of its own; Simmel wrote of the importance of group "belongingness"; Cooley pointed out that the origins of group structure are rooted in the family; while Lewin observed that group and individual factors are merely different aspects of the same phenomena in constant interaction with one another. A very important development in the history of group theory came in 1920 with the publication of Freud's *Group Psychology and the Analysis of the Ego*.[2] While Freud was actually writing about the crowd or mob, many of the observations he made about group psychology were seen to have application to small groups.

Content and Process of Group Interaction

In the dynamics of small-group interaction, there is the phenomenon of the relationship between group content and group process. Group content refers to that which is *said* in a group, while group process refers to that which is *done* in the group or that which is implied through actions. These actions include nonverbal behavior, the tone of voice of members, the order in which topics occur, who

speaks to whom, and other kinds of group actions. Thus, group interaction continues on two levels, that which is said and that which is done. Even when there is no content (no one is speaking), there is always process. This is due to the axiom that one cannot *not* communicate. Even when group members are not speaking out loud to one another, they are communicating.

Content and process, the two levels of interaction, are constantly interweaving and giving the group its fabric. Some examples will clarify this matter. In early group meetings, when a group is forming, the members often feel uncertain and anxious about their place in the scheme of things. While this is what is *happening* in the group, what is *said* might be something about the confused state of the world today. Another example is that in early sessions, members experience feelings about the leader but are either unable to voice these or actually are unaware of them. Instead, they might discuss other "authority figures" at great length, for example, the President of the United States. In one group session Mary, a member, was accused of constantly defending her friend Ann. Upon hearing this accusation, Mary replied, "Ann needs no defending!" The members broke into spontaneous laughter, since Mary was saying in content what she was doing in process. Later in the same session, she was accused of acting too sweet and "Pollyanna-ish" at times when she "should" have been angry. She replied to this, "Thank you, that is very helpful to me!" Again, the content and process were the same.

The group leader must constantly be alert to the relationship between content and process, because it is the content that gives constant clues to what is actually happening in the group.

Phenomena of Small-Group Interaction
Leadership

Certain phenomena occur in all small groups, regardless of the purpose of the group. One of these phenomena is leadership. In most groups formed for a purpose, there is an appointed leader. This leader's behavior has a profound effect on the other members of the group and on their productiveness. The most effective leader is one who does not lead in a heavy-handed way but rather stimulates the group to develop its own direction. The following poem states this well:

A leader is best
When people barely know that he exists,
Not so good when people obey and acclaim him,
Worse when they despise him.
"Fail to honor people,
they fail to honor you;"
But of a good leader, who talks little,
When his work is done, his aim fulfilled,
They will all say, "We did this ourselves."

Lao Tzu, "Leadership"

Geller, a group psychoanalyst, has devised a chart which shows the effect of three different kinds of leaders—the boss, the guide, and the stimulator—on the group phenomena found and on the production range of the group (see Table 10-1).

It is important to note that the leader who acts as a boss severely inhibits the natural process of the group, while the leader who is a stimulator helps the group to develop beyond the leader's own individual capacities. Group leaders do not always predict the capacity of a group accurately. This is particularly true of psychotherapists who are leading groups of schizophrenic clients. Here there is a tendency on the part of leaders to do far more "for" clients than is actually necessary.

In addition to the assigned or appointed leader, there are always emergent leaders in groups. These are group members to whom the others turn for guidance. Homans has referred to the leader as the person who best embodies the group norms.[3] It is the emergent leader who has observed the needs and wishes of other members and is able to help the group move in the direction of these wishes. These norms occur in two different areas of group life; therefore, two different emergent leaders often appear in a group. The first is the task leader who helps the group to accomplish its tasks. If the group is a psychotherapy group, the task leader may seem to be a kind of "cotherapist" or assistant therapist. The second emergent leader is the social leader. This group member is usually the most popular due to his or her ability to relieve tension. When it is necessary to structure a group

Table 10-1 Relationship between Leadership of Group and Group's Development

Type of leader	Group interaction phenomena	Production range of the group
Boss: Plans, controls, directs, and decides autocratically.	Group submits, conforms when told what to do, has little influence on things except in a passive way.	From nothing useful to support of leader's irrational needs.
Guide: Plans, controls, and steers, usually subtly and indirectly.	Group can register differences, initiate complaints, and make requests.	Limited to leader's capacity.
	Group participates in thinking and forming opinions; makes minor decisions.	
	Group has some active influence but little responsibility.	
Stimulator: Educates, facilitates production and communication, balances group forces, and shares leadership.	Group generates ideas, sets limits, and establishes methods.	Can be expected to go beyond leader's capacity to members' maximum potential.
	Group sets no limits on productivity and development of members.	
	Group has primary responsibilities, uses self-evaluation, has healthy group spirit, is creative and productive.	

to accomplish a task—for example, when forming an ad hoc committee—it is a good idea to choose two people who possess the typical qualities of task and social leaders. This usually helps the committee to function smoothly. However, even without this prior planning, two such leaders will emerge as any group develops.

Attractiveness and Approachability

Blau has written about another phenomenon that occurs early in the life of a new group and also to most new members coming into an ongoing group.[4] There is the tendency of members to appear attractive first and later to appear approachable. The initial attractive behavior is designed to make a positive impression on other group members. However, this does not have the effect of producing true integration of members. Instead, it produces competition, tension, and defensiveness on the part of others. After a time, one or more members take the risk of allowing the attractiveness to give way to approachability. The member presents to the group a problem, weakness, mistake, or other evidence of "humanness." This allows the others to relax, to feel a kind of bond to the member, and to begin to relate to this person in a less defensive manner. Usually other members follow suit and begin to show their own approachability. This eventually leads to social integration.

Rank, Status, and Role

There are a number of concepts which have to do with the group member's position in the group. The first is *rank*. Rank is the position of a member relative to the evaluation of other members of the group. If all members were asked to rank one another according to some dimension such as "the person I like best," a rank order of popularity among members would then arise. While this is seldom done so explicitly, members are indeed ranked by others implicitly. The rank order of a member has influence on group behavior. Members who rank high in participation tend to have

more communications addressed to them, while those who rank low in total participation tend, after a time, to be ignored.

The second phenomenon having to do with position in the group is *status*. Status has been called, by Homans, a collection of rights and duties.[3] Status may, in part, come from the world outside the group and be brought to the group by the member. If the group is impressed by these qualities, the person is granted status in the current group. For example, in a group of schoolmates, senior students come into the group with status. In a psychotherapy group, an example of this occurred when a new member "happened" to bring along to the group a grave rubbing from the tombstone of a Revolutionary soldier who was his ancestor. This member was unconsciously attempting to create a position of status for himself inside the group that was comparable to the one he believed he occupied outside the group. Status is also attributed to a member as a result of behavior within the group. The social leader, who has exhibited the ability to relieve tension, is given the right and duty to do so as well as the status of social leader.

Role has been called the dynamic aspect of status. When group members perform a role, they are putting into effect the rights and duties granted by the other group members. When the social leader mentioned earlier performs a behavior using the status earned, the role of social leader is being acted out. In a psychotherapy group, the role acted out by a client may not be useful for growth. The status of a client may, for example, be that of group "baby." The rights and duties that go with this status may include childlike, dependent behavior. It is important to note and explore such behavior when it is acted out as a role.

Norms

Group norm has been defined as an idea in the minds of members that can be put in the form of a statement specifying what the members should do, ought to do, and are expected to do under given circumstances.[3] People often confuse group norms with group goals. Goals are explicitly stated outcomes which the group expects. For example, in a therapy group, the goal may be to be open about oneself. Everyone may agree verbally that this is a worthy goal. However, in this same group, the norm may be quite different. The point is that the norm is *in the minds* of the group members. Inside, they may fear being open, so that when it comes right down to it, they do not relate to each other openly but tend instead to be polite. The norms in a group change subtly as the group evolves, and all members are involved in this process of development and change. Neither the leader nor a member can set a norm for the group.

Subgrouping

It is not uncommon for small groups or even pairs of group members to find more satisfaction in the interaction among themselves than they find with the group as a whole. When this occurs, it is known as *subgrouping* or clique formation. Members of subgroups tend to think of themselves as better than members of other subgroups and often compete with other subgroups or with the leader. Subgrouping can be constructive when members of a pair are able to see, through exploration, how their attraction to one another constitutes a reenactment of unconscious wishes.

An example of this occurred when two group members, Joy and Betty, paired, constantly defending each other and acting as allies in all situations. Joy's behavior in the group was that of a "tough guy," often making caustic, stinging remarks to others. Most members feared her and kept their distance. Betty, however, endlessly pointed out to others that there was a heart of gold under Joy's tough exterior and that her toughness was merely a defense. She used as an illustration the fact that Joy was consistently kind to her.

Through exploration and analysis, it became evident that Joy represented, to Betty, Betty's own mother, who had been very cruel and frightening to her as a child. Betty had attempted to comfort herself throughout her childhood by telling herself that under the cruelty was a "heart of gold." She

had also acted this out outside the group by choosing men she called "diamonds in the rough" whom she tried to rehabilitate. Her relationship with Betty was also useful to Joy, as it allowed her to explore her tender side, which she felt obliged to hide from most people. While this is an example of a positive use of subgrouping, it would be destructive to group growth if it were to go unexplored, for this "mutual admiration society" excluded others and put Joy and Betty out of the other members' reach.

Cohesiveness

Another group phenomenon is *cohesiveness*. Festinger has defined cohesiveness as "the resultant of all forces acting on members to remain in the group."[5] These forces may come from a variety of sources, the first of which is the group itself. As groups develop, a kind of "belongingness" arises which leads members to want to be together. When they learn that one member wants to leave the group, they will invariably urge this member to stay. When members tell the leader that they wish to leave, the leader should encourage them to discuss the matter in the group. This is done not only to increase the pressure on the member to stay but also to promote exploration of the reasons why the member wants to leave.

A second source of pressure on members to stay is their tie to the leader. For this reason, it is a good idea for group psychotherapists to see group members individually as well as in group sessions. Then their tie to the leader helps members to remain in the group and also to be more open and comfortable in group sessions.

A third source of pressure to remain in the group may come from outside the group. The members may feel, as they compare groups, that they would rather belong to this group than any other. Or significant others may be encouraging each member to remain in the group, as in the case of a psychotherapy group.

There are a number of stages of group development which must occur before true cohesiveness appears. The group members must be free to expose *positive* as well as *negative* feelings toward each other. Simmel has written that a group does not attain unity through harmony alone but rather through a combination of conflict and harmony.[6] Members must experience both love and hate toward one another and toward the leader before true cohesiveness arises. Table 10-2 lists the signs which indicate that a group is becoming cohesive.

The more cohesive a group is, the more likely its members will be to express hostility in a direct manner.[7] It is important to keep this fact in mind, as often group leaders who fear hostility themselves will subtly prevent such direct expressions of feeling and instead promote a kind of pseudocohesiveness based on mutual "love."

Cohesiveness cannot be produced artificially, nor can its appearance be hastened. Group members must come to know and appreciate each other for their own uniqueness and in spite of their faults. This is part of the natural evolution of the group. Ways to promote cohesiveness are listed in Table 10-3.[8]

Group Psychotherapy

Group psychotherapy has evolved through many phases. Today, there are as many different schools of group psychotherapy as there are schools of personality development. They range from conservative long-term group psychoanalysis at one end of the spectrum to wild, exciting, nude weekend marathons at the other.

Types of Group Psychotherapy

All the various kinds of group psychotherapy can be categorized under four general headings formulated by Armstrong and Rouslin[9] as follows:

Activity Therapy
This is generally employed with children age 7 to 14. Its focus is on the acting out of impulses, conflicts, and deviant behavior in a group setting.

Lecture-Discussion or Didactic Therapy
In this method, the leader presents fixed content in the form of lectures or written material which is then discussed by the clients. Fairly large numbers of clients can be reached at one time using this method. Individual needs, however, cannot usually be met. Another disadvantage is that some clients use the intellectual sophistication gained as a defense against relating in a more human way.

Repressive-Inspirational Therapy
This therapy uses clients' present ego strength and further strengthens it through inspiration in order to

Table 10-2 Signs of Group Cohesiveness

Sign of cohesiveness	Example
Meetings outside the group	Members go for coffee after meetings.
Resentment of new members	Old members act closer than usual and discuss, without an explanation, matters which are unknown to new member or that are sexually or highly emotionally charged.
Rescuing the leader when under attack	When one member is critical of the leader for giving "bad advice," other members point out that it was not advice but rather exploration.
Control of monopolizers	When one member monopolizes, the others point this out and do not permit it to continue.
Looking down on those outside the group	Members state how lucky they are to be in this particular group.
Acceptance of other members even though they are disliked	One member is domineering. The others work around her bossiness and, without strong hostility, cheerfully tease her about it.

Table 10-3 Ways to Promote Cohesiveness and Examples

Ways to promote cohesiveness	Examples
Make group personally rewarding.	Clarifying observations about group or individual behavior which help members to understand themselves better.
	Pointing out to members that they seem healthier or different.
Promote usefulness of other members whether they are liked or not.	Pointing out that an unpopular member is only a symbol of a significant other or oneself and therefore useful in helping work out one's own conflicts.
	Pointing out the "good" qualities of an unpopular member.
Make activities attractive.	Subtly rewarding clients for helping others to recognize distortions or clarifying issues by saying, "Mary has a good point," and so on.

help clients repress problems more successfully than they have done previously. This type of therapy, which requires a minimum of specialized training on the part of the leader, is widely practiced by lay persons and paraprofessionals. The disadvantages are that (1) no effort is made to reach the client's specific dynamics; (2) relatively good ego strength is required on the part of the client; and (3) neurotic defenses are reenforced, making the clients more vulnerable, in some respects, to future life crises.

This is probably the most common type of group psychotherapy practiced both in inpatient facilities and with members of the general public. Weekend marathons, joy groups, and encounter groups fall into this category. These groups tend to offer members a "high" but do not have a lasting effect because of their failure to deal with individual personality characteristics.

Analytic or Intensive Therapy

In this method, intervention is based on exploration and analysis of both individual intrapsychic structures and the group process. The advantage of this type of therapy is that individual and group characteristics are explored in depth with a view toward permanent change in the individual. Each member's behavior within the group is constantly examined, keeping in mind the idea that the group is a microcosm of the larger world. By bringing to light the members' secret wishes, conflicts, and motivations of members' behavior in the group, it is possible to help them understand more about their total mode of being in the world.

Selection of Members *

There are many differing opinions about whom to select for a psychotherapy group. In general, members of an adult group range in age from 21 upward. In intensive psychotherapy, group heterogeneity is an advantage. That is, gender, age, and personality dynamics should vary as much as possible. The advantage to this is that members will be stimulated to react on a deeper, more emotional level. In a homogeneous group where all the clients are, for example, alcoholics, homosexuals, or obsessionals (as in groups of professionals), there is a tendency for the members either to discuss common problems or to support one another's defensive systems. Many psychotherapists believe that certain types of clients, such as schizophrenics, cannot be treated in groups of this kind. This is certainly not the case, as many schizophrenics respond very positively to group treatment, though it may take a very long time to notice such a response.[10] It is generally agreed, however, that certain types of clients should not be included. These are the brain-damaged or severely retarded clients and those who are destructively paranoid.

*All the remaining material in this chapter refers to intensive group psychotherapy.

All prospective members should be seen at least once before being admitted to a group. The more times they are seen individually before entering a group, the better. In general, clients should never be in group therapy only but should be seen in individual therapy as well. Clients who have not had previous psychotherapy tend to hold back the group or become so threatened by the group sessions that they leave shortly after beginning. Therefore it is best to see future members individually for some time before they enter the group and to continue to see them individually while they are in the group. This will cut down a great deal on attrition.

When entry into the group is discussed between client and therapist, as little as possible should be revealed about the specific composition of the group. This is to allow for spontaneous and often irrational responses to occur and be explored. If the member knows who will be present, his or her reaction upon meeting the other members will be controlled. For example, a new female member might exclaim upon entering the group, "I had no idea *men* would be here!" This might then lead into her exploring her feelings about men. (The same is true about bringing new members into an ongoing group. The group should not be prepared, as this prevents spontaneous reactions.)

The new member should also not be told how to behave in the group, as this again will undermine spontaneity. Therefore the leader should not say, for example, "You will be expected to tell the group about your difficulties." Instead, the leader might say, if asked what group therapy is about, "It's a chance to relate and react to people, and to explore your behavior with them." This answer is vague enough to allow spontaneous responses.

Creation of the Group

There are a number of factors to consider in creating the group. The number of members should be ten to begin with, and not more than ten. Research has shown seven to be an ideal number, and there should never be less than five. Since there is frequently attrition, ten is a good beginning

number. If four or less members appear for a session and the group is not a well-established, ongoing one, the session should be canceled. There is too much pressure on the members to talk when so few attend. As for physical setting, no table should be used, for a table sets up a physical barrier. When no such barrier exists, members feel more exposed, are more anxious, and are more likely to act irrationally. Furthermore, a table blocks some nonverbal communication, which is useful to note and explore at times.

The leader should change seats at each meeting, so that members are forced to take different seats. This helps to prevent any client from finding a comfortable niche where he or she can "blend into the furniture." Each session should last for $1\frac{1}{2}$ hours, because it takes about 45 minutes for members to loosen up. Sessions should always begin and end on time. Members pace themselves, and this pacing is in itself interesting to note and explore. It is sometimes tempting to run overtime when something valuable is happening, but the leader should avoid the temptation.

Outpatient groups and groups in long-term institutions should meet once or twice weekly. Groups held on short-term inpatient units should meet daily. Since group leaders are not interchangeable, the same person should lead the group each day. Group productivity is reduced when a different leader appears each session or when outside professionals are permitted to sit in on the group. If, as in teaching centers, students must observe groups, they should do so through a one-way mirror or on closed-circuit television with the group's knowledge. The presence of a mirror or camera is less inhibiting than that of a person.

In intensive group psychotherapy, open-ended groups are preferable to time-limited ones. An open-ended group is structured so that when one member leaves, another enters. This creates anxiety and evokes irrational responses from members that often lead to important exploration. For example, the introduction of a new member often stimulates a client to recall the birth of a new sibling.

Role of the Leader in Group Psychotherapy

At present, the qualifications desirable in the leader of an intensive psychotherapy group are governed by standards set by the American Nurses' Association. The ANA suggests that the function of group psychotherapist be limited to nurses with master's degrees in psychiatric nursing. Additional criteria include further didactic preparation, ongoing supervision as a leader of a psychotherapy group, and a personal group experience over an extended period of time.

The group's purpose is to examine and explore the behavior of the group members as it occurs with a view toward permanent change.[11] One of the ways in which clients are helped to behave in their most basic "real" or "irrational" way is to create a situation that provokes some slight anxiety. If clients are allowed to remain comfortable or relatively unanxious in a group, their defenses will continue to operate in an optimum way and they will not change. If they are anxious, however, their defenses will be so sharply exaggerated that all will notice them and begin to explore them to the clients' benefit. This stirring up of anxiety which the therapist continues to do may be thought of as "stirring up the dust to see how it settles." The group leader, therefore, is constantly alert to group process and offers comments from time to time. For example, one member mentioned that she has had extensive group experience and was interested in seeing how the leader would operate. The leader asked her later, "Am I doing all right so far?" This comment by the leader had the effect of stimulating the group to notice the process, but it was not a heavy-handed and pedantic remark like "I notice that you want to compete with me." This comment would only tend to bring on a fierce denial, while the first one would tend to bring a laugh and then a quiet consideration of what has just happened.

There are certain expectations which the leader has of the group members.[12] Table 10-4 lists these expectations, possible client behavior, and appropriate leader intervention.

When a new group is being formed, the leader should keep in mind that the first session sets the stage for all that is to follow. It is extremely important that the leader be as accepting yet nondirective as possible. If the leader can manage to sit back and let the group start itself, members will realize from the outset that the group is their responsibility. On the other hand, if the leader adopts an "I am the expert" attitude, the group members will sit back and wait for therapy to be "done to" them. This is antithetical to the principles of group psychotherapy. A rule of thumb for leaders to bear in mind is that they should never do for the group what the group can do for itself.

The leader's most important task is to watch the evolving group process and to stimulate the members to act within the context of this evolution. This often involves making overt that which is covert. The leader must be constantly alert to the covert or latent process and stimulate its emergence in relation to members' intrapsychic lives. Table 10-5 outlines growth-inhibiting behaviors to be avoided and some growth-promoting alternatives which may be used by leaders.

Problems of Beginning Group Leaders

Beginning group leaders need to be aware of the fact that they will experience a level of anxiety which is based on their need to maintain a good self-image and their need to gain control of the group. Table 10-6 lists some of the common irrational and nonproductive needs of beginning group psychotherapists. Fearful fantasies are expressed by inexperienced leaders in a variety of ways. This can be problematic for both clients and leaders. Supervision is essential in assisting new leaders to understand what is occurring within themselves and how it affects the group process.

Phases of Group Development

The phases of group development can be divided into four categories. These are—sequentially—uncertainty, overaggressiveness, regression, and adaptation. While new groups do move through these stages sequentially, there is often overlapping of behaviors from one phase into another.

Table 10-4 Leader's Expectations of Clients, Possible Client Behavior, Leader Intervention

Expectation	Possible client behavior	Appropriate leader intervention
Members will attend every session or tell leader beforehand if they must miss one. (Voiced by leader.)	Leave message with another client, secretary, or answering service.	Tells members they must speak to leader directly. Explores need to avoid leader in in this case.
	Miss sessions without notice.	Asks members about absence. Explores meaning if appropriate.
	Call to cancel with vague excuse. ("I'm not feeling up to it.")	Strongly encourages members to come anyway, pointing out that not feeling well may be related to feelings about the group.
Members will be as open as possible. (Not voiced by leader.)	Conscious deception. Members feel one way (e.g., angry) but act another (e.g., sweet).	Point out inconsistency: "You look angry, but you're acting sweet."
	Unconscious deception. Member seems to feel one way but does not seem aware of it and acts another.	Point out inconsistency or question in a gentle way: "Are you sure you're not angry?"
No physical violence will occur. (Not voiced by leader.)	Members threaten violence.	State that physical violence is not allowed, but encourage verbal exploration of reason for violent feelings.
Members will not discuss group matters outside the group with those who are concerned in these matters. (Not voiced by leader.)	Members break group confidentiality.	Explore this in the group.
Members will not meet outside the group, or if they do, they will discuss their meetings in the group. (Voiced by the leader.)	Two members form a sexual relationship.	Intensive exploration in the group of the meaning of the relationship vis-à-vis the group itself, the leader, and past relationships with significant others.
	Two members of the group appear to be attracted to one another.	Intensive exploration of the relationship in the group, as above, in order to "nip it in the bud" and deal with the motivation rather than have it acted out.

New members coming into a group which is on-going will also move through these stages.

Uncertainty Phase

The uncertainty phase lasts up to twenty sessions. It is the time in the life of the group when many demands are made on the leader. Table 10-7 outlines the dynamics often present in the uncertainty phase. In this phase, members often feel that comment or interpretation by the leader means that they should not continue to do what the leader has observed. Therefore, the leader must often say,

"Not that you shouldn't" in an attempt to point out that only an observation and *not* a criticism has been made.

Overaggressiveness Phase

When a group or a new member in a group has gotten over the feeling of uncertainty and grasped how the group might operate, there follows a phase of overaggressiveness. This occurs as a defense against what is to follow, that is, regression and adaptation. In this phase of group development hostility is often displayed toward other

Table 10-5 Growth-Inhibiting Behaviors (to Be Avoided by Leaders) and Growth-Promoting Alternatives

Growth-inhibiting behaviors	Growth-promoting behaviors
Starting sessions by introducing members or explaining the purpose of group therapy.	Waiting for members to begin on their own. Avoiding lengthy explanations of anything.
Bringing food or drink for group members.	Exploring dependency needs in the context of the group and the members' lives outside the group.
Calling on specific members to talk.	Allowing silences to continue until a group member breaks them, or after a few minutes commenting on the silence. Allowing other members to deal with consistently silent members.
"Going around" the group, requiring that each member talk in turn.	Allowing members to talk at random as they please.
Pushing for closure on a topic or summing up sessions at the end.	Realizing that there is no "final solution." Allowing issues to be discussed, explored, examined by anyone in the group, with interest and respect shown to all. Allowing sessions to end "up in the air," with some members feeling anxious.

members and toward the leader. Frequently that which the other members receive is actually felt toward the leader. In addition, an attraction is beginning to take place between members, and this is frightening to them. Such attraction may be the seed of a mutually intimate relationship, which is anathema to most group therapy clients. Table 10-8 lists the dynamics experienced in the group during the overaggressiveness phase.

Regression Phase

The third phase of group development comes about when clients are no longer afraid to regress. The earlier defenses are put aside and the member experiences pure anxiety, anger at more primitive sources, dependency, fear, longing, envy, jealousy, and other forms of pain. There is no longer a felt need to pretend to be in control. Regression does not arise from a desire to manipulate others

Table 10-6 Common Irrational and Nonproductive Needs of Beginning Group Psychotherapists

Need to maintain a "good" self-image

    Need to be liked

    Need to avoid exposing self as "human"

    Need to impress group with knowledge and authority

Need to maintain control of the group

    Need to prevent group disintegration

    Need to prevent regressive behavior

    Need to prevent resistance

    Need to prevent expression of hostility

    Need to prevent acting out

    Need to avoid "taboo" topics

    Need to prevent intensive, multiple transference reactions

    Need to prevent the examination of individual or subgroup problems

    Need to restrict process that does not "go through" the therapist

Table 10-7 Behavior, Examples, and Leader Intervention in the Uncertainty Phase

Behavior	Example	Leader intervention
Initial anxiety	Pacing the floor. Leaving and returning. Hallucinations and delusions. Excessive intellectualization. Organization of a "group plan."	Comment about the anxiety. Question what members fear happening in the group.
Demands on leader to explain purpose or provide structure	"Do we begin now?" What is supposed to happen here?" "How does this work?"	Communicate to members that it is their group. ("Let's see how things go.")
Competition	Comparison among members of past group experience, past number of years of psychotherapy, knowledge of the leader, etc.	Point out that competition is taking place, being careful to communicate that it is not wrong and should not necessarily stop just because it is noted.
Excessive politeness	Members feel anxious and angry about the lack of structure from the leader, but they are afraid to show this. Instead, they react with inappropriate kindness. To a monopolizer: "You certainly are talkative today."	Note the covert feeling and ask if it is present. ("Are you a little irritated by all that talking?") Encourage openness rather than politeness.
Silence	All members sit for 5 minutes staring at the floor or occasionally glancing at each other.	Comment on the silence. ("I guess everyone is afraid to start.") Comment on some nonverbal behavior. ("Mary, I notice you're staring at John. Do you wish he'd speak?")
Questions about the leader's personal life, qualifications, and competence	Member asks: "Are you a mother?" Member asks: "Are you an MD?"	"No. Are you afraid I won't know how to care for you because I'm not?" "No, I'm a psychiatric nurse. Are you afraid I won't know enough to do things right?"
Avoidance of involvement in the group	Schizophrenic member talks to voices instead of other group members. Members intellectualize about their problems. Members adopt roles which were used in their families to reduce anxiety but which are not appropriate in the current group (e.g., the buffoon, the boss, the incompetent person, the ingenue).	Comment that these are methods to avoid reacting emotionally to the current group. Explore why this is feared and avoided.
Strong, irrational reactions to the leader	The leader is seen as a "savior" with all the answers. The leader is seen as using power to manipulate or humiliate members and as having a secret reason for every comment or move.	Explore why a "savior" is necessary. Explore the meaning of these ideas in the context of the members' lives.

Table 10-8 Behavior, Examples, and Leader Intervention in the Overaggressiveness Phase

Behavior	Example	Leader intervention
Criticism of one another	One member who is very lonely but leads the life of the happy, sophisticated swinger is critical of another member whose isolation and loneliness are all too stark and evident.	Ask whether the "swinger" is reminded of herself by the isolated member. Explore their similarities and the resultant anxiety.
	One member becomes enraged when another acts stubborn and impenetrable.	Ask whether there was someone else in the member's life that he could not "get through" to.
Anger at one another for using their own defenses in a clumsy way	One obsessional member begins sentences with "Please don't think I'm trying to be controlling but. . . ." Another obsessional says "Don't warn us so obviously. It only calls our attention to the fact that you are!"	Point out the dynamic that people feel their own defenses should be used only in their own unique way and are spoiled or "exposed" if used "incorrectly."
Ganging up	One member who is secretly anxious about almost everything arrives late to group each week, giving various weak excuses. He refuses to acknowledge that he might have wanted to miss part of a session or that he may have wanted to stir everyone up.	Examine and explore both sides of the process, why the member is so provocative as well as why members cannot resist being provoked.
Hostility toward the leader	Clients distort the leader's behavior. ("You do nothing to help us.") Clients point out real eccentricities of the leader. ("You are too compulsive!")	Accept their hostility in a nondefensive way. Avoid a win-lose approach. Weaknesses and eccentricities may be acknowledged freely. It is often a great relief to members to see that the leader is human and does not mind if this shows.

but occurs spontaneously. At first, other members may feel anxious and may even begin to cry themselves or want to leave or stop the member who is regressing. It is important at this time for the leader to move in and question the regressed member about what is being experienced, what led to this feeling, and so on. Actually, this is an extremely important period in psychotherapy, for it is in these regressed states that heretofore repressed or dissociated material can come into awareness. An example will illustrate: A client, Mary, who has never felt love or acceptance from her parents but rather has felt like the "ugly duckling" in the family, perceived her brothers and sisters as more attractive and "successful." During a session, she began to feel that all the other members were more "loved" by the therapist and that she was the "reject." She began to cry and to express the pain she was experiencing. Clients are often surprised at the feeling of support they receive from other members, having believed previously that to lose control would lead to disaster. The others, by the same token, often like the regressed member better after such an episode has occurred, feeling that they share a common bond of humanness.

During this period, the leader often takes on a new image and is seen as an expert resource person, not as an "idol" or "enemy" as before. Just as the other members' humanness has begun to be tolerated, so is the leader's.

Adaptation Phase
This is the fourth stage of group development. In this stage, members accept one another in spite of

their weaknesses and faults. While their behavior to one another is fairly nonthreatening, it is nonetheless explored in depth and in a relatively nondefensive way. This does not mean that members in this phase do not ever respond to one another irrationally, for if this were to happen the therapeutic effectiveness of the group would be sharply decreased. Therefore the leader must continue in this phase to "stir up the dust" and poke away at unresolved conflicts and wishes.

The relative stability and comfort of this phase can be a disadvantage. This is one reason why open-ended groups are preferable to those in which all members start together and remain together. In open-ended groups, where the membership varies every so often as one member leaves and another joins, there are more new stimuli to react to, more exposure of more aspects of the personality, and hence more exploration. For example, a very narcissistic client will evoke rage and indignation at first. Then, eventually, the others will react with acceptance and toleration. This toleration may decrease the amount of "work" done in relation to the client's narcissism. However, a new client in the group will be astonished by the first member's narcissism and by the group's tolerance of it. This client will shake things up a bit and lead the group members to further exploration of both their own and the narcissist's experiences.

Central Concepts of Group Psychotherapy

There are four central concepts which combine to form the essence of intensive group psychotherapy. They are *transference* (and its reverse, *countertransference*), *resistance, acting out,* and *insight.* Each of these will be considered separately.

Transference

Transference occurs when the client transfers onto the therapist feelings, wishes, conflicts, and so forth which were originally felt in relation to the parents or significant others. Usually this is an unconscious process at first. The client begins to experience feelings about the therapist which are distortions of reality. For example, a young woman might say to the therapist, "You prefer all the others to me." In reality this has never entered the therapist's mind, and on reflection the therapist does not feel this way. With exploration, it is learned that the client had a "Cinderella" role in her family and therefore tends to distort the mildest slight as a reenactment of her early disappointments. Thus she "transfers" onto the therapist her mother's rejecting behavior. These distortions are very important to examine, and the group setting provides an excellent opportunity. When a client begins to react irrationally to the therapist, other clients will notice and talk about this. The client who is doing the transferring or distorting will, at first, defend this perception of reality; but when confronted by a group of surprised faces, he or she will frequently begin to question it. It is then that the client may recall earlier treatment by a parent or significant other which was similar to that which is being experienced in the present. Often other clients will remember something helpful about the client who is making the transferral. Through this process, the client is enabled to see the distortion and to begin to experience reality.

Countertransference

Countertransference occurs when the therapist transfers onto the client feelings, wishes, conflicts, and so forth which originated with the therapist's own parents or significant others. In other words, the therapist begins to experience feelings about the client which are distortions of reality. This usually begins first with the therapist noting a feeling of anxiety or anger in regard to a particular client. For example, there may be a feeling that the client is a "jerk" or, the converse, that the client is "special." In both cases, the therapist is experiencing some kind of distortion which can be either helpful or destructive to the client.

Group leaders can be helpful in the following way: If the client does indeed act like a jerk in an attempt to avoid growing up or to anger others, then it is helpful to point this behavior out in a tactful way. Countertransference becomes destructure only if (1) the therapist is not aware of the powerful reaction to the client and just reacts automatically or (2) the therapist is aware of the countertransference but cannot stop reacting. In the latter case, the situation should be discussed carefully with a supervisor, or another knowledgeable, disengaged person. Countertransference is most frequently present in the beginning therapist but generally decreases in amount and intensity as the therapist matures. Its existence, however, is one good reason why group psychotherapists should receive personal psychoanalysis as well as supervision over time.

Resistance

Resistance occurs when powerful *unconscious* forces prevent the client from giving up distortions and from experiencing reality. Clients may feel unable to understand what others are saying about them and may instead feel "blank" or even angry. More subtle forms of resistance are operating when the client is habitually late or absent or feels reluctant to come to sessions. This resistance usually increases when the client is either (1) under pressure from the others to experience reality or (2) under pressure from "inside" to experience reality. For example, as the client begins to improve and feel more open to life, there is a kind of internal pressure to experience more and more of life. As others observe this about the client, they move more toward relating in a realistic way with the client.

An example of resistance occurred with a kind of tough, flippant young woman who kept people at a distance with wit and sarcasm. She began after some time to miss sessions and to hate coming when she did appear. This coincided with the group's first glimpses of her toughness as a mask, a time when they began reacting to her in an unintimidated manner. Unconsciously fearing this closer, more intimate way of relating, she did not want to continue.

It is not uncommon for clients to resist just when they are growing closer to others or are improving in other ways. At these times, the therapist must help clients to notice what it is that is

frightening them so that the resistance can be overcome and they can progress to more rewarding levels of experience.

Acting Out

Acting out occurs when the client relives or reproduces—through actions rather than words—the feelings, wishes, or conflicts which are operating unconsciously. Instead of talking about buried conflicts, feelings, and wishes, the client dramatizes them in a disguised form. For example, the client may secretly wish for a close, special relationship with the therapist. Instead of talking about this, the client enters into a sexual relationship with a member of the group who is most like the therapist. In the case of acting out, the therapist must try to understand the symbolic meaning of the behavior and explore it in depth with the clients involved. The symbolism may be very evident if the client is schizophrenic. One client, for example, vomited during the session. The therapist might then have asked, "What is it here you can't stomach?" The purpose of analyzing the acting out is to help the person experience directly the wishes and conflicts that are disguised. If they are simply acted out and not interpreted, they can never come into conscious awareness and will prevent the client from growing.

Insight

Insight occurs when the client is able to see the connection between unconscious feelings, wishes, and conflicts and conscious behavior. In order to make this connection, the client must first fully experience these unconscious feelings, wishes, and conflicts in conscious awareness. This then produces *emotional* insight, which is distinctly different from *intellectual* insight. In the latter case, the client "knows" intellectually why certain behaviors occur but is powerless to stop them. When true emotional insight occurs, the problem behavior vanishes. Pat, a client, may know intellectually that she is resisting group interaction because of her fear of closeness. One evening she attends the group and feels a kind of shakiness and fear accompanied by a desire to be close to the others. This marks the beginning of emotional insight. Intellectual insight almost always precedes emotional insight. Clients often say, "Now I *know* why I do this, but I can't stop, so what good does it do?" Of course there is no simple answer, but the therapist can encourage clients by saying, "The rest will come" or "It does take time."

Termination

Therapists vary in their opinions about when termination of intensive group therapy should properly occur. It is generally agreed that both the client and the therapist should feel ready at the time of termination. Freud once stated that termination occurred when one was *"able to love and work."*[14] In general, it is hoped that the client will be able to relate to others in a basically nondefensive way and that there will be other signs of healthy self-esteem. At termination, the client should feel satisfied with life on the whole and able to recognize the unsatisfying parts that cannot be changed. The client should find contentment in self-directed pleasures as well as happiness in relationships with others. All these criteria can be observed in the group. Other members can be helpful to clients who wish to terminate by pointing out resolved as well as unresolved areas.

References

1 Helen Durkin: *The Group in Depth,* International Universities Press, New York, 1964, pp. 12–14.

2 Sigmund Freud: *Group Psychology and the Analysis of the Ego,* Bantam, New York, 1960.

3 George Homans: *The Human Group.* Harcourt, Brace & World, New York, 1950.

4 Peter Blau: "A Theory of Social Integration," *The American Journal of Sociology,* vol. 45, pp. 545–556, May 1960.

5 Dorwin Cartwright: "The Nature of Group Cohesiveness," in D. Cartwright and A. Zander (eds.), *Group Dynamics,* Harper & Row, New York, 1960, p. 91.

6 Georg Simmel: *Conflict and the Web of Group Affiliations,* Free Press, New York, 1969.

7 Albert Pepitone and George Reichling: "Group Cohesiveness and the Expression of Hostility," in D. Cartwright and A. Zander (eds.), *Group Dynamics,* Harper & Row, New York, 1960.

8 Jerome Frank: "Some Determinants, Manifestations, and Effects of Cohesion in Therapy Groups," *International Journal of Group Psychotherapy,* vol. 7, pp. 53–62, 1957.

*9 Shirley Armstrong and Sheila Rouslin: *Group Psychotherapy in Nursing Practice,* Macmillan, New York, 1963, pp. 48–49.

10 Joseph J. Geller: "Group Psychotherapy in the Treatment of the Schizophrenic Syndromes," *Psychiatric Quarterly,* vol. 63, pp. 1–13, 1963.

*11 Suzanne Lego: "Five Functions of the Group Therapist—Twenty Sessions Later," *American Journal of Nursing,* vol. 66, pp. 795–797, 1966.

12 Milton Wilner: "Group Therapy in a Day Hospital Setting," unpublished paper.

13 Irving Yalom: *The Theory and Practice of Group Psychotherapy,* Basic Books, New York, 1970, p. 277.

*Recommended reference by a nurse author.

11

Family Theory and Application

Patricia Winstead-Fry

Learning Objectives

After studying this chapter, the student should be able to:

1 Introduce the systems concept as applied to families
2 Define the functions of the family
3 Introduce the primary concepts in family dynamics
4 Present a definition of a dysfunctional family
5 Present a brief method of assessing a family's level of differentiation
6 Present the goals and techniques of family therapy

Historical Perspective

Prior to World War II, Ackerman, known as the grandfather of family theory, published his ideas on extending psychoanalytic concepts to include the family. After the Second World War, six forces contributed to the rapid growth of family therapy practice:

1 World War II created the need to modify the classic psychoanalytic approach so that a larger number of clients could be reached.

2 Psychiatric practitioners, due to their wartime experiences, were willing to experiment with novel treatment approaches.

3 Returning members of the Armed Forces, trying to reintegrate themselves into their families, often created upheaval, leading some people to seek psychotherapy for family-related problems.

4 As childhood hospitalization became more common, the separation anxiety associated with it highlighted the need for a mothering one and focused attention on families.

5 Some psychiatric practitioners became concerned about the familial consequences of individual psychotherapy—for example, the situation in which a wife becomes dysfunctional as her husband improves.

6 A rapidly accelerating divorce rate led to questions about how families function and why 'some marriages succeed.

Definition of Family Theory

A family may be defined as a group united by marriage, kinship, or adoption. Currently, families are commonly regarded as systems. The field of family theory is most accurately called relationship theory, as it can contribute to the understanding any relationship. Historically, theorists "borrowed" from communication theorists like Watzlawich to study families. Phenomenologists like R. D. Laing made significant contributions to family theory by defining "mystification," "rules," "metarules," etc. (see Chap. 4).

Functions of a Family

There is no such thing as an absolutely healthy family. Every family, by virtue of its existence over time, will experience some dysfunction periodically. Fluctuations in jobs, amount of money available, births and deaths, developmental needs of children, and the many other facts of everyday life would rule out an absolutely harmonious family life over 40 or 50 years.

Ackerman notes that the family has two basic functions, the first of which is to ensure the physical survival of the young. Physical well-being, sufficient food and clothes, and safety are characteristic of a successful family. The second function of families is to provide the framework in which a person's humanness can grow. The affectional bonds among family members are the matrix within which personal identity, sexual identity, social responsibility, and learning develop.[1] A healthy family may be defined as one that fulfills these two functions adequately.

Systems Framework

Family theory is based on systems theory. A *system* is a totality, or more than the sum of its parts. The family is a totality, a system. *Subsystems* are units which interact within a system. Individuals in families are subsystems interacting to form a system, the family.[2] The idea of a system is illustrated diagrammatically in Fig. 11-1.

Peter, Tom, Mary, and Sue each have individual identities, as indicated by the lines around the names. The space between them (dotted in the diagram) is the relationship area. According to systems theory, one could not understand Peter unless one understood Peter in relationship to Sue, Mary, and Tom as well as the totality of the relationship. The line drawn around Peter indicates a self-boundary, but the self can only be defined in relationship to others. It would be absurd to define Peter as an 18-year-old black male college freshman if there were no other persons to give these designations meaning. Being 18 years old has meaning because there are 4-year-olds and 20-year-olds. Peter's age makes a difference

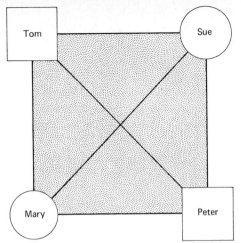

Figure 11-1 A relational system.

in relation to the age of others. The same is true for maleness, blackness, and being a freshman. These designations would be useless if there were no females, nonblacks, or nonfreshmen.

Characteristics of Systems

Physics and cybernetics have contributed a great deal to the refining and exploring of systems concepts. On the basis of this work, those concerned with human systems also concern themselves with matter, energy, information, meaning, and feedback. In modern physics and in family systems theory, matter and energy are interchangeable. The primary manifestation of these systems properties which interests the family therapist is their *expression in action*. One cannot act in a vacuum. The very concept implies actions against another or the environment and, by extension, it also implies some relationship.

Communication

The second characteristic of a system is *communication*. There are three components of the communication process: information, meaning, and feedback. By *information* the systems theorist means the feelings or ideas that a system or subsystem may convey by means of symbols, messages, or signals.[3] These behaviors are partly culture-bound. The physical distance one person keeps from another may convey information. For instance, in exchanging endearments, people usually move very close together. When discussing the weather, people stand farther apart. The ability to express a wide range of emotions and ideas is part of the information process.

The various nonverbal cues (e.g., an index finger to the lips saying "be silent") are other components of the information process.

The information is conveyed to another person, who assigns it a *meaning*. People often find that a piece of information they have sent has been given the wrong meaning by the recipient. Messages can be confused or misinterpreted in several ways: if we use unusual words, if the emotional tone of the message is different from what one would expect from the words ("I love you" said sarcastically), or if the nonverbal message is different from the verbal one. The recipient of contradictory messages usually feels confused or disconfirmed if the various components of the information do not match.

The third phase of the communication process is *feedback,* or what the receiver of the information conveys back to the sender. There are two types of feedback: *negative,* which causes no change in the sender of the message, and *positive,* which does cause change in the sender of the message.[4] With feedback, the communication component of the system meshes with the action component. Feedback may result in an action or may call for more information.

If the sender acts in response to feedback by the recipient, the action is simultaneously a piece of information for the recipient and the communication process continues. The action and communication process is shown diagrammatically in Fig. 11-2.

Theory of Family Dynamics

Family therapy requires an understanding of the dynamics of family systems. An understanding of the family as a system in relationship to the large system, society, is essential for the nurse who

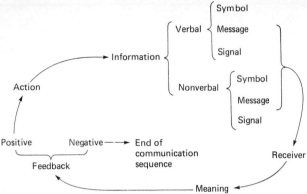

Figure 11-2 Communication process.

practices total care. Knowledge of the levels of differentiation within families, of triangling patterns, and of the multigenerational transmission process is theory which provides the framework for the nurse to both understand pathology and to practice family therapy.

The family is viewed as the system which is the interface and major source of feedback between its individual members and society. The family receives actions and information from society in the form of values, norms, economic status, and so forth. It applies meaning to these, and it gives feedback to the society and to its individual members. The family system is simultaneously maintained by the action and information exchange of its individual members.

The family as a system in relationship to a large system, society, is represented diagrammatically in Fig. 11-3.

The broken lines convey the hundreds of bits of information and action that a society produces. Some penetrate through the family system and touch one or two members; some stop at the outer shell of the family. Not all families are equally influenced by the messages of their society. Of those messages that impinge on the family, some are more meaningful to one member than to another. The solid lines (from the family) convey the feedback the family as a whole gives to its individual members and to society. The curved lines (from individual family members) convey the feedback the individual gives to the family system and

to society. There are limitless possibilities for actions and interactions within families.

Using a systems framework to assess families, four basic issues are explored: (1) individual boundaries, (2) levels of differentiation, (3) triangles, and (4) the multigenerational transmission process.

Individual Boundaries

A boundary for the individual, a sense of "I," must exist for each family member. This "I" must be unique and different from others. Simultaneously, a person must be able to cooperate collectively with others. Family life, with its forced closeness, is the primary place where this individual-collective tension is enacted. It is not uncommon to find families that have attempted to resolve this tension by going to either of two extremes. At one end is the extreme of *the family* focus. Here there is little individuality and members seem lost in the family system. At the other end of this imaginary scale is *the individual* focus. Here there is little sense of cohesion or family identity. As opposed to the obviously fused family, this family is outstanding for the emotional distance members keep from one another. They may be emotionally detached or geographically distant. Family members may look "mature" and "independent" on the surface, but they experience interpersonal discomfort because they have difficulties with closeness. At both extremes, there is an undifferentiated family ego

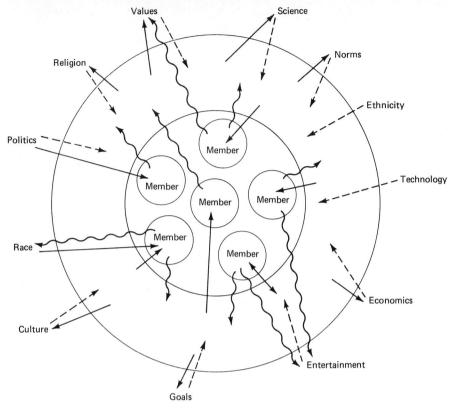

Figure 11-3 Relationship of family system to societal system. Broken line: information offered by society to family; solid line: feedback of family to society and individual members; Wavy line: feedback of individual to family and society.

mass, a family "stickiness" that prevents the members from developing a sense of separate identity.[5] In the first case, the fusion is obvious; in the second, the lack of differentiation is disguised by distance.

Whether the lack of differentiation is handled by fusion or distance, a family that is less differentiated is prone to dysfunction in one or several of the members. Dysfunction of a family system may take the form of physical or mental illness and/or social disorganization. The family with a delinquent or an alcoholic member, for example may be labeled dysfunctional.

Levels of Differentiation

Determining levels of differentiation is another tool used in the assessment of families. Following the classic concept, a family begins when two persons, a man and a woman, marry. The individuals come from family systems, and they bring their families' generational processes and levels of differentiation to their new relationship. Generally, people are attracted to others who are like themselves in terms of their sense of "I," or differentiation. Differentiation is similar to self-concept, self-esteem, or self-actualization.[6] (See Chap. 19.) They all refer to the individual's sense of worth and separateness as a unique person. This level of differentiation is a basic aspect of the person and is not related to such accomplishments as education, economic success, social status, or physical abilities.

Bowen conceptualizes a range of differentiation from the lowest level, characterized by little sense of self, to the highest level, characterized by a real sense of self.[5] Persons lowest in differentiation are *pseudoselves*. They have tenuous identities built on facts, beliefs, and feelings borrowed from others. Pseudoselves may act assertive and outgoing, but inside they feel afraid and sure that no one will love them. People in this lowest range are most prone to physical and mental illnesses or social disorganization. Parents at this level will have more trouble providing for the physical needs of their children and will experience overwhelming difficulties with the second function of the family (developing humanness) because they have such tenuous identities themselves. These people live in a feeling-dominated world; the action-information component of the system is dysharmonic. Decisions are based on what feels right or what decreases anxiety. The intellectual use of communication barely exists for these people, while the search for good feelings and comfort leaves them little energy for anything else.[5] If such a person meets someone who is similarly concerned, a marriage that "feels good" may result. This marriage may go along well enough for some time, but it is highly vulnerable to stress caused by social crisis, the needs of a dependent infant, or some other upsetting event.

Spouses in this group are more prone to overadequate-inadequate reciprocity.[5] In this phenomenon, one spouse benefits from the fusion and actually functions better; the other may be dysfunctional to the point of symptom formation. Schizophrenic families fall within this very undifferentiated range. A little further up the scale are persons with some ability to allow the intellect to influence their emotions. The self in a member of this group may attach itself to a cause or belief and become lost in it, in effect using the cause as an identity. (The cause is usually one that fits with the person's emotional needs.) Persons on this level, like those further down, are predominantly motivated by feelings. They are tremendously sensitive to the feelings of those about them and react to these feelings. Their goal is emotional comfort.[5]

Further differentiated are those who have some sense of self. These persons have differentiated sets of beliefs and values on important issues; under stress, however, emotions will dictate their decisions. Very often such a person will avoid antagonizing others by remaining silent.[5]

At the highest level of functioning is the differentiated person, a rare example of one who is goal-directed and has a firm set of principles. Such people are flexible and can discard beliefs if the evidence does not support them. In their interpersonal relationships, they do not need to use others to satisfy unmet ego needs. Both persons in such a relationship have a sense of commitment and of freedom. Neither needs to remake the other to conform to an idealized image. Both can relax their self-boundaries during sex relations or other intensely emotional periods, but they can reinstate the self at will.[5]

In view of these descriptions of the levels of differentiation, it becomes clearer why persons marry others at their own level. Ways of thinking and feeling are too different among the levels to allow a person from one place to be comfortable with someone from another.

Triangles

Using triangles to assess families is an additional tool nurses may use. This concept helps one to assess the specific relationships among family members. Looking at a family in terms of triangles helps to distinguish areas of fusion from areas of differentiation. A *triangle* is a predictable pattern of interaction among three persons, two being fused and the third in a distant position.[5] All of us are in many triangles. The more differentiated we are, the less the triangle will result in automatic, predictable behavior.

A triangle occurs when a person in a dyad, already fused, begins to experience stress. To handle this, the person pulls in someone else (the triangled one), often telling the partner a story about this person. This reduces the tension in the dyad.

In the family today, a common pattern is for the wife to handle fusion with her husband by triangling in a child or children, making the husband an outsider. The husband may respond to this by triangling in his job.

Triangles always have two positive positions

and one negative one.[5] The people on the positive lines have warm, close feelings for one another. The one on the negative side feels distant and tense around the others. The intensity of these feelings varies with the importance of the relationship and the degree of undifferentiation. The concept of triangling sheds light on many common family concerns. A frequent event in divorce is fighting over custody of the child or children. Figure 11-4 illustrates the negative relationship created by wife–mother—husband–father—when triangling occurs with the children. If the parents are less differentiated, they are going to react with emotionality rather than rationality to the divorce. The child (children) is positive to both parents, each of them wants the child, and the parents are negative to each other. Fighting is the expected outcome. The fact that the child (children) is in the positive position is not meant to imply that the parent wants custody of the child for "good" reasons, that is, reasons that will lead to happiness and humanness for the child. The child of undifferentiated parents may be so fused in the parents' minds with themselves that both need the child for all sorts of reasons that will interfere with the child's emotional growth.

Triangles are fluid, changing parts of a family system. It is when a triangle gets stuck that problems occur. Figure 11-5 diagrams the expected crisis of the birth of the first child. Both parents are happy to have the baby. If the mother is the primary caretaker, it is expected that she will be very

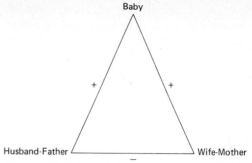

Figure 11-5 Normal triangular stress of first baby. Expected crisis at the birth of the first child.

involved in the baby and "ignore" her husband for a while. In the usual flow of family life, the mother will gain confidence in her abilities as caretaker; then she will want to get back to wearing stylish clothes and to be sexual again. She will want to show the baby off to family and friends. The husband, simultaneously, will want to have his sex partner back and to show off his new family to others. The father-mother-baby triangle will integrate with the husband-wife-baby triangle, as illustrated in Fig. 11-6.

This diagram shows the tension most adults feel with a young baby. The husband-wife dyad want time by themselves to be adults together; the baby sometimes interferes with this. The mother and father concern themselves with the baby. The more differentiated couples have a greater ability to integrate the contradictory demands of these roles, reducing the degree of negativeness in the

Figure 11-4 Negative-positive triangle over divorce. Illustrates the negative relationship created by wife–mother—husband–father when triangling occurs with the children.

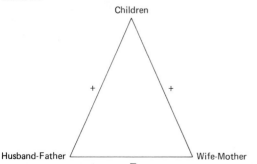

Figure 11-6 Integrated triangle. The father—mother—baby triangle integrates with the husband—wife—baby triangle.

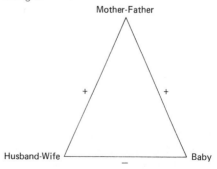

triangle. Less differentiated couples may not be able to begin integrating the roles; then the family will remain triangled, with the mother and/or father overinvolved with the baby and distant from the other parent.

Triangles do not exist in a clear, neat way. If the wife triangles in the child to decrease fusion with her husband, he may triangle in someone or something else to decrease his loneliness (Fig. 11-7).

Since husbands and wives are also the children of families (the extended family), the triangling process begins to look like Fig. 11-8.

Each person is involved in many triangles throughout life. It is not the presence of triangles that causes pathology but rather the strength of the undifferentiated bonds in important relationships.

Multigenerational Transmission Process

The final theoretical concept pertinent to understanding family systems is the *multigenerational transmission process.* Each person brings to marriage a piece of the undifferentiated ego mass he or she grew up in. If one of the spouses was the scapegoat in his or her family, this experience will be brought to the new marriage and will influence what goes on there. A child who grew up outside the projection process may be more differentiated than anyone else in the family. This accounts for families that produce a functional child and a nonfunctional one. The generational transmission

process is diagnosed through the genogram, a drawing of the generations (see Fig. 11-9).

The genogram in the diagram presents the basic facts of family existence. It is a guide for following the action of the family over three generations. Using the genogram, one finds out about each member: who is close or distant (triangles), what the people are doing at present, how marriages are working out, what illnesses there have been, who gets into trouble, and so forth. Row 1 in Fig. 11-9 represents the grandparent generation. Row 2 illustrates the parental generation. The line with 1965 on it shows that Mr. Smith married Ms. Jones in 1965. Row 3 presents the children of the marriage between Mr. Smith and Ms. Jones.

Genograms often give professionals working with families valuable clues. Triangles can be noted, as well as the degrees of fusion which exist among members of the extended family. A simple genogram often provides information which would take months to obtain through interviewing.

In summary, the basic ingredients of the family system are the degree of fusion or undifferentiated ego mass, the generational transmission process of unresolved conflicts and issues, and triangles. The relative health of the family depends on the degree to which the system and its individual members are differentiated from generational problems. The "healthier" family is characterized by a sense of system integrity; there is enough positive feedback to maintain an identifiable family and, simultaneously, enough negative feedback to give individuals a sense of separate identity and the family a sense of changing over time. The triangles in a healthier family are not so rigid that the action and communication components of the system are dichotomized. Actions directed toward society, others, and self are based on a communication process wherein information is clearly sent and appropriate meanings are assigned to messages.

The Dysfunctional Family

The term "dysfunctional family" is relativistic. Increasingly, family therapists are seeing families

Figure 11-7 More complex triangle around birth of first child. If the wife triangles to the child, the husband may triangle to someone or something else.

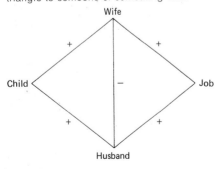

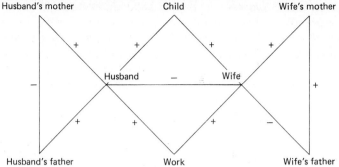

Figure 11-8 Extended family triangles illustrate that husbands and wives are also children from other families.

who are upset by generational conflicts, families who are concerned over areas of dissatisfaction (although the marriage is basically satisfactory), and couples who are weighing the advisability of divorce. If one used this portion of the population as a criterion for the dysfunctional family, then any family dissatisfied with some aspect of its functioning would qualify. More specifically, however, a *dysfunctional family* is defined as a family fused to such a degree that marital conflict is unresolvable by the spouses, that a child shows symptoms of disturbance, or that a spouse is incapacitated by mental, physical, or social illness.[5]

Assessing the Dysfunctional Family

Professionals involved in family care are often those who diagnose a family as being dysfunction-al. Questions that may be asked in assessing a family's level of differentiation are the following:

1 What actions does the family engage in?
2 What is the predominant "mood" of the family?
3 How satisfied do the family members say they are?
4 Are there indications of fusion? What are they?
5 Where are the triangles in the family?
6 What important issues does the genogram suggest for this family?

The family therapist's exploration of the area encompassing the action-information component of the family system (questions 1 through 3), shows how the family organizes itself around meeting goals. To what degree are decisions based upon

Figure 11-9 Genogram of three generations. □ = male, ○ = female. x = dead. Row 1 = grandparent generation. Dates indicate year of deaths of grandparents. Row 2 = parent generation. Row 3 = children of marriage in 1965 between Mr. Smith and Ms. Jones.

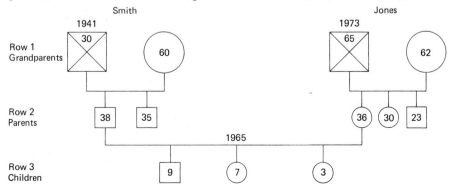

intellect informed by feelings—as opposed to doing what "feels right" or intellectual attitudes uninformed by feelings? If the system is malfunctioning around this issue, action and information will be dichotomized instead of being in harmony. This enhances marital discord and is a direct reflection of the amount of fusion in the family system.

Next, the family worker looks for the degree of fusion or enmeshment among family members[5,7] and for the degree to which a sense of "I" is lacking or present in family members (questions 4 through 6). The fusion between the spouses may show itself in three ways: as marital discord, as overadequate-inadequate reciprocity, or in the form of projection onto a child or children.[5]

If a couple is fused, neither has much sense of "I." Each partner is very needy and is tuned in to any real or threatened rejection by the other. Each is on the offensive and watches the other very carefully for the anticipated rejection; each is ready to do battle to fend off "assaults." These are the families that will be characterized by marital conflict. This is not to suggest that fights are bad for marriages, but there are different types of fights. The fusion fight referred to here is one wherein the anger is out of proportion to the offense; the issue that starts the fight gets lost in the shouting and is never resolved. A nonfusion fight—where one spouse is angry at another for a reason, shares the anger, and then moves toward resolution—adds spice and growth to a marriage.

The second way a couple may handle fusion is through overadequate-inadequate reciprocity; this is the most common method for handling fusion.[8] In this instance, the fusion leads one spouse to draw strength from the undifferentiated ego mass and the other to be weakened by it. One of the two will actually function better. There are marriages that go on for years with one spouse functioning well and the other being sick, either physically or mentally.

The final way fusion may be handled between spouses is through projection onto a child or children.[5] If spouses are unable to deal with angry feelings, it is not unusual for one child to be seen as angry or sullen, and indeed the child will act this way. If one child gets more of the parental projection, that child becomes the family scapegoat. The child selected for this process is usually one who was born at a time of stress, is unwanted, resembles some other family member in some way, or is physically or mentally defective.[9] Once the scapegoat role is learned, this child causes the family much pain and worry, thus further keeping the parents from focusing on their problems. Sibling position is an important concept in determining whether there is parental projection. Toman has documented very clear differences between siblings occupying different positions in a family.[10] If children do not behave as one would expect them to from their position and especially if they are more infantile than their chronological age would suggest, there may well be parental projection.

Children may also react to family fusion by distancing themselves. A distancer may flee the family, moving away or breaking all ties. This person is still stuck in the fusion, however, because it takes so much energy to stay away. People may talk about how much they hate their family, saying that they never see them. This is done with such vehemence that an observer can sense that there are still strong emotional ties. Other children may stay near home or maintain a connection by telephone, thus remaining overtly fused with the family system.

Most families, as they attempt to keep fusion from becoming intolerable, will use a combination of these three processes. There will be some fights, some dysfunction in a spouse, and some projection onto children. Each family, based upon its unique history, will evolve a pattern that "works" for it.

The Schizophrenic Family
An example of a dysfunctional family is the schizophrenic family. Such a family is very undifferentiated. it is so fused that one member may actually know what others are thinking; sometimes they even dream the same dreams.[11] A common pattern

is the distant father and an enmeshed mother-son dyad (the triangle of the "schizophrenogenic mother").[12] The action-information subsystem in these families may be so undifferentiated that feelings and thoughts seem the same and thinking something, to these people, is the same as doing it. This is the action-information level of the young child.[13] The information system is generally characterized by the *double bind*. The double bind is a communication wherein the verbal message is contradictory to the nonverbal one, but the child *must* obey both. Since children cannot question either message, they are "damned" no matter what they do. It is like being told to turn left and right simultaneously—it cannot be done! However, developing schizophrenics do not know this because this form of communication is so common in their lives. They have no other option but to move into a world of hallucinations.

Family Therapy

Just as, theoretically, there is no such thing as the absolutely healthy family, so also there is no such thing as the absolutely sick family. Changing life circumstances cause stress in all families. Frequently families seek help around stressful issues, such as limit setting for adolescents, the "empty-nest syndrome" when the last child leaves home, and the spouses' adoption of conflicting goals. Family therapy should be considered the treatment

of choice in dysfunctional families characterized by marital conflict, projection onto a child or children, and overadequate-inadequate reciprocity.

Dysfunctional families are often symptomatic in a way that is upsetting to them or to society. When the basic issue is child projection and the child has been delinquent, the family is often referred to the therapist by a judge. The teacher or guidance counselor may refer the family because of a child's academic failure, misbehavior in school, isolation, and/or lack of friends. Generally, the family has little insight into its own problems: They generally want the therapist to "shape up" the child, whom they see as ruining the family. In overadequate-inadequate reciprocity, the inadequate member usually has a diagnosis from some other health professional. The overadequate member generally comes along to therapy to "help" the therapist with the sick person. In a situation of marital conflict, the partners come to therapy to convince the therapist how unassailable their respective arguments are. Each sees the other as bad, unreasonable, or uncaring.

Goals

Family therapists usually have four general goals in treating their clients. These are charted in Table 11-1.

The first goal—to rephrase the problem as a family one—is very important both to establish a

Table 11-1 Goals of Family Therapy

Goal	Intervention
1 Rephrase the problem as a family one.	Explore what the problem does to everyone. Find out who feels lonely, angry, attacked.
2 Create a family client, not an individual one.	Highlight the family members' involvement in the symptom. Explore how each benefits from the symptom.
3 Help the family understand the operation of family triangles.	Show how a member of the dyad signals to a third party. Explore the needs that prompt the third party to respond to these signals. Assign tasks that realign the triangle.
4 Help each member to differentiate a sense of "I."	Encourage separate activities. Insist that people speak for themselves, not for each other. Assign tasks that bring different people together in novel ways.

contract and in order to diagnose the degree of fusion in the family. The more resistant the family is to dealing with the family issues, the greater the degree of fusion. The therapist can also begin to get a sense of the interlocking triangles that keep the symptoms going during this negotiation phase. For example, Johnny, age 8, is truant and failing in spite of an IQ of 140, a good record for attendance, and high grades in earlier years. The therapist, in exploring what happened this year to change things, may find that Johnny's father began a job that requires much traveling. If the fusion is very strong, the family will argue that this was not upsetting the family *even if* Johnny says it was. A less fused family may quickly realize that everyone feels bad since the father left home, but that only Johnny is expressing the family's sadness. Even though the basic triangle is the same in this case, there is less fusion, so it will be easier to "unstick" Johnny. Negotiating with the family for a contract that defines the problem as a family one is the first goal of family therapy.

The second goal is to create a *family* client instead of an *individual* client. The overadequate husband is going to have to begin to look at how his wife's headaches help him. The inadequate wife will have to look at her fears of being powerful. The scapegoated child will begin to see how he stabilizes the family by his "evil," and the family will have to begin to deal with whatever multigenerational issues the child's behavior is masking.

Helping the family understand how their triangles operate is the third goal of family therapy. They need to understand that triangling is operating when Mom and Dad are angry at one another, cannot express their anger, and signal one of the children to do something to focus attention away from their anger. Each person must be aware of how he or she fits into the overall system and how each reacts emotionally to that system. The therapist helps family members separate the I-we dimensions so that their action-information subsystems can operate on clearer messages. Ultimately, each member of the system, so far as his or her developmental level allows, should be an expert on the family system so that each can self-correct it

and prevent future problems.[8] The final goal is to help each member to differentiate a sense of "I," thereby decreasing the fusion and the probability of dysfunction.

Initial Interview

In keeping with the therapist's first goal, the initial interview begins only when the whole family has arrived.[14] It is not uncommon to see people trailing in one at a time or for one parent to show up with the child who is the "problem." No matter how they arrive, the therapist waits for the whole family when the contract is for family therapy.

Sometimes one family member does not come at all. In this case, the therapist may begin the session but should not "buy" the family's excuses for the absent member. In one case, a depressed looking young mother of three arrived without her husband. She proceeded to tell the therapist that her husband did not care for her or the children and that he was inconsiderate. The more she went on in this vein, the more the therapist was "clued in" that the woman had somehow signaled her husband not to come. The therapist recognized that the woman was utilizing a triangling technique by talking about her husband. To avoid being triangled in on one side, the therapist can use one or more of the following techniques:

1 Leave a vacant chair in the conversation space to hold a place for the spouse.
2 Make it clear that there will be no secrets; that the therapist will not withhold information from the partner.
3 Explain to the spouse who is present that the absent partner will be expected to attend the next session.
4 Do not call the absent person, because that would convey to the one present that the therapist may be "helping to handle the inconsiderate spouse."
5 Show interest in how the present partner gets the spouse to come to sessions.

The family therapist remains outside the system—sometimes as a participant observer. The initial task of the systems theorist will be a family assessment and history. Those doing therapy will construct a genogram with the help of the family (see Fig. 11-9). This begins in the first session. The depth to which it is pursued depends on what else is going on in the family.

A therapist would not do a detailed genogram if a family is in crisis. The genogram may be begun to initiate the idea of multigenerational issues, but the crisis must be handled first.

Based on the information given in row 1 of the genogram illustrated in Fig. 11-9, the following questions may be asked by nurses when doing a family assessment:

1 What happened to Grandfather Smith, who died at 30 years of age?
2 What did this do to the family?
3 How did Grandmother Smith manage?
4 What do the sons remember of their father?
5 How did the family mourn his death?
6 What are the implications for this family that each of the parents was an oldest child? (See row 2.)

Following Toman, one wonders what happened to the issue of responsibility in this marriage, as oldest children are usually very responsible.[10]

Suppose the Smiths came to see the family therapist because Melissa, the 7-year-old, has chronic headaches. Looking at the genogram, the therapist already has a clue. Barring a physiological cause, headaches can be the results of worry. The therapist has already wondered how responsibility (of which worry is a part) is handled between the parents. Now the therapist goes a step further and wonders if there is fusion between the parents around responsibility and if, because of projection, Melissa is the family worrier. With this hypothesis, the therapist would begin to explore the function Melissa's worrying serves for the family.

The genogram serves the therapist's purpose of creating a systems attitude; at the same time, it helps the family. Children may never have known, or may have forgotten, that their parents were once happy. Parents themselves may have forgotten! A therapist can usually count on a "good story" around how the parents met and ultimately married. Even in the most depressed families, this story engenders a sense of happiness and hope. A genogram also helps to decrease guilt in individual family members. It shows that the issues which occupy them and cause them distress have a history in the family. It is not that the individuals are uncaring or unlovable but rather that the family, over generations, has been characterized by emotionally distant men or women. Acknowledgement of past health and happiness serves to spur well-intentioned parents to work at therapy so that their children will not have to suffer similar painful experiences.

Techniques

The goals of family therapy are to decrease fusion among members, to increase the family's ability to handle stress, and to help them avoid falling into triangular communication patterns. Techniques used by the therapist are directed to these aims. Because family therapists have all the members of the family to work with, they are not limited by the perceptions of one member talking about the rest of the family. The therapist has enough "material" to be able to move quickly toward a problem. Work toward developing transference with the therapist is not necessary because the major transference objects are present (mother-child and husband-wife dyads). The trust relationship is with the family, not with individuals. There are no secrets between the therapist and individual members. The therapist can help individuals to share any secrets they may have and relieve the family of the burden of a taboo area. Table 11-2 lists the various techniques utilized by nurses and family therapists.

Family Theory in Nursing Practice

Nurses are concerned with people and their environments in health and illness, from before birth

Table 11-2 Techniques Used in Family Therapy

Technique and definition	Principles
Cotherapy—more than one therapist.	Advantage: two therapists can more easily accumulate data, make observations, and keep track of interactions.
	Cotherapists must work out their own relationship.
	If male and female, cotherapists can be role models for parents.[6,15,16]
Multiple family therapy—more than one family seen simultaneously by one or more therapists.	Families can help one another see problems and possible solutions.
	Competition between families is engendered, leading to faster progress in therapy.
	This approach is more economical.[17,18]
Network therapy—the extended family and all social systems that interact with the family are seen together.	All the healing forces of society are brought to therapy: teachers, coworkers, and so forth.[19]
Operational mourning—highlights loss of significant members and how insufficient mourning for them has caused current problems.	Loss of significant people through death, marriage, and so forth is explored and mourning reinitiated with sufficient support to complete it.
	Decreases need to project characteristics of the lost person onto children.[20,21,22]
Sculpting—family member arranges others as he or she perceives them relationally.	Highlights, through physical activity, the triangles affecting the family.
	Valuable with young children who cannot verbalize feelings well.
	Family can physically try to realign themselves in ways that would make relationships more satisfying.[23]
Freezing—a family member pantomimes a situation that is problematic, then freezes at that point.	Allows person who is freezing to discuss how it feels to be stuck, to look at triangles that are maintaining the problem, and to explore alternative behaviors.[24,25]
Role playing—family members act parts of other members.	Allows people a chance to see how they look to others.
	Increases understanding of feelings people are unable to express.
	Participants can perceive how triangles are maintained.[26]
Paradoxical injunction (prescribing the symptom or reversal) — therapist instructs family members to do consciously what they are doing unconsciously.	Behavior changes because consciously controlled behavior cannot serve unconscious purposes.
	Should be used only by skilled therapists who are sure of the forces acting within the family; otherwise the family will perceive it as sarcasm.[27]
Making assignments—therapist assigns family members a task.	Rearranges triangles.
	Opens up feelings between distant persons that are blocked.[7]
Home visit—therapist visits a client's home and conducts one or more therapy sessions there.	Homes express the feeling of the people who live in them.
	Family is on its own "turf" and less likely to be overly polite, etc.[8,28]

until death. The nurse is constantly seeking, through research and clinical expertise, correlates of health and illness. Family theory offers a perspective on a major source of health in individuals, families, and communities. No matter what the area of practice, nursing diagnosis and treatment can be enhanced by a family orientation.

Primary Prevention

In primary care (e.g., in prenatal work and in maternity units), where the goal is promotion of health, nurses can utilize this framework to aid the young family. The birth of the first child is especially pivotal. It is at this point that the adult, parental dyad moves to a triangle. All the other triangles that the parents are involved in undergo change. The parents move from a relatively adult relationship to a relationship that incorporates a dependent, needy infant. Exploring with expectant parents the meaning of the baby, their plans for its care, and how this will change their relationship to each other and to their extended families can give the nurse valuable information on triangles and plans for intervention. Families that are relatively differentiated can benefit from education about the developmental process and about the fact that the baby is going to change their current life. Parents need to know that although babies are "bundles of joy," they are also separate people who have needs and personalities different from those of the parents. (See Chap. 32 for a detailed discussion of these issues.)

Another major area of primary care is that involving the dying. Paul's work, referred to earlier, makes it clear that death is a significant family event that may reverberate in the system for generations. Many nurse practitioners, using family theory and Kübler-Ross's work on dying, have done excellent work in helping clients and their families move through the crisis to a higher level of differentiation.[29,30]

Secondary Prevention

The major focus in secondary care is early case finding and, even more desirable, prevention. The nurse in pediatrics is in a unique position in regard to secondary care. It is obvious from the theoretical presentation that children, especially sick children, are very vulnerable to family fusion. The pediatric nurse can be of great assistance in clarifying to the child and the family the meaning of a diagnosis. Many families who have experienced a great deal of illness will react with guilt and blame when a child is sick. It is almost as if they believed in a genetic cause for every illness. The nurse, through teaching and counseling, can help the family understand the true nature of the illness and take steps to stop the projection process or minimize its strength. The nurse needs to be aware that many of the current medical practices push the mother to be the caretaker of the sick child and make it difficult to include the father. This could result in distancing the father. The pediatric nurse should try to include the father in classes and discussions.

The nurse who works in medical or surgical nursing can utilize family theory in understanding why, for example, Mrs. Smith becomes ill at the same time every year. It may be a response to familial stress or to an unresolved death. This may lead the nurse to consider family therapy as a useful adjunct to the medical and nursing regimens.

Tertiary Prevention

Since it is unusual to find whole families hospitalized, the nurse who works in the psychiatric unit of a hospital may find few examples of family therapy. However, family therapy concepts can be very helpful to these nurses also, helping them to understand some of the reactions of clients and families during visiting hours. Knowledge of the double bind can be useful in understanding why hospitalized schizophrenics often seem more disturbed after visiting hours. The sensitive nurse can spend time helping the disturbed client put the visit in perspective.

Nurses in a community mental health setting may find whole families in treatment and may be therapists for these families. Such nurses would need to pursue their understanding of families further through reading, attendance at conferences, and perhaps advanced study in family therapy.

Regardless of the settings, nurses' responsibility for giving comprehensive care to their clients can be carried out better with the help of an understanding of family theory. Whether the illness is an acute, brief one or whether it is chronic, the client's family will be strongly affected by the situation and therefore in need of the nurse who is knowledgeable in family theory.

References

1 Nathan Ackerman: *Psychodynamics of Family Life*, Basic Books, New York, 1958.

2 Ludwig von Bertalanffy: *General Systems Theory,* Braziller, New York, 1968, p. 83.

3 James G. Miller: "Living Systems: Basic Concepts," *Behavioral Science,* vol. 10, pp. 393–411, July 1965.

4 Paul Watzlawick, Janet Beavin, and Don Jackson: *Pragmatics of Human Communication,* Norton, New York, 1967.

5 Murray Bowen: "Use of Family Theory in Clinical Practice," in Jay Haley (ed.), *Changing Families,* Grune & Stratton, New York, 1971, pp. 172–192.

6 Gene Abrams, Carl Fellner, and Carl Whitaker: "The Family Enters the Hospital," *American Journal of Psychotherapy,* vol. 127, pp. 99–106, April 1971.

7 Salvador Minuchin: *Families and Family Therapy,* Harvard University Press, Cambridge, Mass., 1974, pp. 54–56.

8 Donald Bloch: "Clinical Home Visit," in D. Bloch (ed.), *Techniques of Family Psychotherapy,* Grune & Stratton, New York, 1973, pp. 39–45.

9 R. S. Postner et al.: "Process and Outcome in Conjoint Family Therapy," *Family Process,* vol. 10, pp. 451–474, 1971.

10 Walter Toman: *Family Constellation,* Springer, New York, 1969.

11 Murray Bowen: "A Family Concept of Schizophrenia," in Don Jackson (ed.), *The Etiology of Schizophrenia,* Basic Books, New York, 1960, pp. 346–372.

12 C. L. Winder: "Some Psychological Studies of Schizophrenia," in Don Jackson (ed.), *The Etiology of Schizophrenia,* Basic Books, New York, 1960, pp. 191–247.

13 Jean Piaget: *The Language and Thought of The Child,* Meredian Books, New York, 1955.

14 Paul Franklin and Phoebe Prosky: "A Standard Initial Interview," in D. Block (ed.), *Techniques of Family Psychotherapy,* Grune & Stratton, New York, 1973, pp. 29–38.

15 Carl Whitaker, Thomas Malone, and John Warkentin: "Multiple Therapy and Psychotherapy," in J. L. Moreno and F. Fromm-Reichmann (eds.), *Progress in Psychotherapy,* Grune & Stratton, New York, 1956.

16 August Napier and Carl Whitaker: "A Conversation About Co-Therapy," in Andrew Ferber, M. Mendelsohn, and A. Napier (eds.), *The Book of Family Therapy,* Science House, New York, 1972, pp. 480–506.

17 H. Peter Laquer: "Mechanisms of Change in Multiple Family Therapy," in C. J. Sager and H. S. Kaplan (eds.), *Progress in Group and Family Therapy,* Brunner/Mazel, New York, 1972, pp. 400–415.

18 Peggy Papp: "Multiple Ways of Multiple Family Therapists," *The Family,* vol. 2, pp. 20–25, Spring 1975.

19 Ross V. Speck and Carolyn L. Attneave: *Family Networks,* Pantheon, New York, 1973.

20 Norman Paul: "Effects of Playback on Family Members of Their Own Previously Recorded Conjoint Family Material," *Psychiatric Research Reports,* vol. 20, pp. 175–187, 1966.

21 Norman Paul: "The Role of Mourning and Empathy in Conjoint Marital Therapy," in G. Zuk and Ivan Boszormenyi-Nagy (eds.), *Family Therapy and Disturbed Families,* Science and Behavior Books, Palo Alto, Calif., 1967.

22 Norman Paul and G. Grosser: "Operational Mourning and Its Role in Conjoint Family Therapy," *Community Mental Health Journal,* vol. 1, pp. 339–345, 1965.

23 Frederick Duhl, David Kantor and Bunny Duhl: "Learning Space and Action in Family Therapy: A Primer of Sculpture," in Don Bloch (ed.), *Techniques of Family Psychotherapy,* Grune & Stratton, New York, 1973, pp. 47–64.

*24 Helen Pazdur Monea: "Family in Trouble," *Perspectives in Psychiatric Care,* vol. 12, pp. 165–170, 1974.

25 Paul Watzlawick, John Weakland, and Richard Fisch: *Change,* Norton, New York, 1974, pp. 67–73, 113–114.

26 Murray Bowen: "Principles and Techniques of Multiple Family Therapy," in J. O. Bradt and C. J. Moynihan (eds.), *Systems Therapy: Selected Papers,* Groome Child Guidance Center, Washington, D.C., 1971, pp. 187–206.

27 R. Fisch et al.: "On Unbecoming Family Therapists," in Andrew Ferber et al. (eds.), *The Book of Family Therapy,* Science House, New York, 1972, p. 613.

28 A. S. Friedman: "Family Therapy as Conducted in the Home," *Family Process,* vol. 1, pp. 132–140, March 1962.

*29 S. B. Goldberg: "Family Tasks and Reactions in the Crisis of Death," *Nursing Digest,* vol. 2, pp. 21–26, May 1974.

*30 E. E. Reniar: "Helping the Survivors of Expected Death," *Nursing 1975,* vol. 5, pp. 60–65, March 1975.

*Recommended reference by a nurse author.

12

Sex Theory and Application

Anita M. Leach

Learning Objectives

After studying this chapter, the student should be able to:

1 Be aware of sexuality as an integral part of the total person
2 Describe the value-formation process
3 Understand the relationship between love and sex
4 Define the four basic components of the sexual system: biological sexuality, sexual identity, gender identity, and sex-role behavior
5 Describe the anatomy and physiology of the male and female
6 Name the characteristics of each stage of psychosexual development
7 Define "coitus," the functions of coitus, and coital approaches
8 Describe the phases of orgasm and the physiological reactions which occur during each
9 Name and define the disorders of sexual functioning

10 Understand sex therapy and the nurse's role in the treatment of disorders of sexual functioning

11 Describe the problematic variations of sexual aim and sexual object

12 Understand the rapist and the rape victim and be able to describe the rape trauma syndrome

13 Be familiar with the nursing intervention necessary for the rape victim

14 Describe homosexuality

15 List the theoretical causes of homosexuality

16 Define "homosexual panic"

17 Define and describe other alternative sexual behavior

18 List appropriate nursing interventions for relating to clients about their sexuality.

Sexual behavior has always been with us. During the last 10 years, however—which have been called the age of sexual enlightenment—a total reevaluation and redefinition of sex and sexuality has been in progress. Sexual values, which were once based on ignorance, superstition, and restriction, have now evolved to the point where sexual pleasure is considered a normal part of human existence, important to all people and their development.

Nurses need an understanding of their own sexuality if they are to enter meaningful relationships with others. When nurses interact with clients of either sex, they must acknowledge the feelings generated by the client's gender and sexual identity. An in-depth understanding of human sexuality is part of the total body of knowledge in the practice of the therapeutic use of self.*

Values

Those who, across the ages, have researched and written about sexuality have brought their personal

*The intent of this chapter is to emphasize sexuality as an integral part of the total person. Students are referred to one of the many available textbooks on human sexuality to expand their knowledge of the concepts presented here.

sexual attitudes to their work. In the process of acknowledging their sexuality, individuals must also confront the cultural and social influences that have been part of their environment. Adult values are *individualized* rules by which people live their lives. They govern and influence the way people behave. The process of forming one's own values involves looking *objectively* at parental and cultural influences and at the value base or philosophy which influences the formation of values. This process generally begins in adolescence and ends when individuals accept, reject, or modify the values of the influential others in their lives. Value formation implies making a *choice*. Before people can form adult values, they must be exposed to and learn about the object of the value (sex and sexual activity) either by real experience (intercourse or other sexual activity) or through intellectual pursuits (sex education). A young girl, for example, who has been sheltered and never exposed to heterosexual relationships educationally or actually, will not experience a need to form an adult value which governs her sexual behavior with males. Inherited parental and cultural values will suffice. Exposure to sexual knowledge or *experience* creates a need for a personal value and is the first step in adult value formation.

Individuals must then look at such exposure in

the light of a *chosen value base* (religious doctrines, philosophy, scripture, the golden rule, etc.). Thoughtful comparison and sometimes new learning takes place before a decision is made. Values are decisions which, when adhered to, result in behavior that is satisfying to an individual's self-esteem. Adult values and behavior must jibe if an individual is to be free of guilt. Individuals must, therefore, confront the sexuality of their parents and culture and form sexual values for themselves.[1]

The process summarized here involves *exposure* or *experience* which create a need for the value. Thoughtful *consideration* and *comparison* follows. The key in value formation is the *choice* or *decision*. *Behavior* or *action* results from the choice and is a public affirmation of one's value.

Nurses possess a variety of unique values. In their work with clients, however, they must be careful not to impose this value system on others. They must also assess the client's value system in order to plan change and intervention consistent with it.

Love

The English word "love" has many meanings. Love as it relates to sex is referred to as *erotic* love. Sullivan states that when the satisfaction or security of another person becomes as significant as one's own satisfaction or security, love exists.[2] Rado has defined "love" as a sustained emotional response to a known source of pleasure. He states that in a love relationship three major components—the *sexual*, the *magical*, and the *sensual*—are in balance and constantly interweaving.

The *sexual* component of love is the desire for shared orgasmic release. The *magical* is the belief that the love object is powerful and wise enough to provide care and security, much as one's parents did in childhood. Finally, the *sensual* component is an appreciation of the physical attractions of a loved one and an idealization of him or her on a highly subjective level.[3]

Some believe that a condition more realistic than love in meaningful human relationships is *intimacy.* It is seen as fundamental to love. Time and privacy are basic requirements for the evaluation of the five components of intimacy: choice, mutuality, reciprocity, trust, and delight. Each of these components develops from the previous one. In intimacy, two people delight in each other as whole persons and express this delight in various ways. One of the most meaningful of these—because it is one of the most delightful—is sexual expression.[4]

Sexual fulfillment and love satisfy human needs of significant importance in the formation of the self (see Chap. 19). The complex relationship between these needs is often controversial. Some say that sex is empty and animalistic without love, while others argue that sex can be fun and enjoyable without love. Some say that those who insist upon imposing love on a sexual relationship are guilty about sex and are trying to convince themselves that the act can somehow be made acceptable.[5] It is possible to love without having sex and to have sex without love. Both will satisfy needs. The difficulty arises when partners do not agree on the meaning of their sexual relationship or when self-awareness is minimal. For some, the sexual relationship may be a way of expressing love. For others, it may be a way of discharging physical energy or tension. For still others it is a *search* for intimacy and feelings of closeness. Nurses need to be aware of the meanings that the love-sex relationship has for them personally. The nurse must also be nonjudgmental in exploring with clients their views of love and sex in their relationships with others.

Sexual Systems—Sexuality

There are four basic components of the sexual system: biological sexuality, sexual identity, gender identity, and sex-role behavior. Patterns of sexual behavior vary among individuals. Sexual functioning, therefore, cannot be too rigidly or restrictively defined. Sexual fulfillment is a basic need that is highly individualistic despite existing legal, moral, and cultural norms.[6]

Biological Sexuality

Biological sexuality refers to the chromosomes, hormones, and primary and secondary sex characteristics which distinguish male from female. For purposes of discussion, biological characteristics will be considered separately. It should be remembered, however, that the human person is a totality and cannot be artificially compartmentalized. Anatomical structures as well as social, cultural, and psychological factors influence sexuality. Likewise, mood and environment influence biology and function. In-depth information of biological sexual characteristics is the realm of sexual researchers and practitioners.

The sex of a human being is determined at the time of fertilization. Chromosome combination determines whether fetal gonads develop into testes or ovaries. In the genetically normal male, the chromosome combination determining sex is XY; and in the female, it is XX. The presence or absence from the normal pattern of chromosomes of any type will likely produce abnormalities.[7] Male and female gonadal structures are recognizable in the embryo by the fourth week of development. By the seventh week, male and female morphological characteristics can be distinguished.[6] A large number of the anatomical characteristics typical of one sex are also present in the other, but in modified form.

Many hormones are involved in the sexual maturation process. They are produced in sex glands or gonads (ovaries and testes) and are controlled by the secretions of the pituitary or master gland. Hormones influence the development of secondary sex characteristics during puberty and also control the reproductive functions of sperm and ovum formation as well as the menstrual cycle. Knowledge of the workings of the sex hormones has led to medical contraception through use of "the pill," utilization of hormones for the maintenance of pregnancy, and the hormonal treatment of sex-related disease. A list of the sex hormones and the function of each follows:

Follicle Stimulating Hormone (FSH) Stimulates ovaries to manufacture female sex hormones.

Luteinizing Hormone (LH) Stimulates the production of estrogen and progesterone in the female.

Interstitial-Cell-Stimulating Hormone (ICSH) Stimulates manufacture of testosterone in the male.

Progesterone Female hormone, influential in maintaining pregnancy and the menstrual cycle.

Estrogen Female hormone, stimulates development of secondary sex characteristics during puberty, influences menstruation, stimulates growth of the glandular surface of the endometrium.

Testosterone Male hormone, responsible for the development of secondary sex characteristics during puberty.[8]

Male Biological Characteristics

Male anatomical structures are complementary in function and design to those of the female. The male genitalia produce sex hormones and sperm. They provide the means for conveying sperm from the male gonads to the female vagina. The male organs consist of two gonads or testes, located in the scrotum; a series of ducts that drain the sperm from the testes to the exterior of the body; the penis; and numerous glands which aid in the manufacture of sperm. Figure 12-1 illustrates the male pelvis, genitalia, and adjacent parts. Table 12-1 lists some male anatomical structures and their functions.[7]

The male reproductive role is dependent on the manufacture of semen and its deposition, via erection and ejaculation, in the female vagina. In addition to *sperm*, semen contains *water*, the vehicle for the transport of sperm; *mucus* to lubricate the male ducts and tubes; certain *bases*, which neutralize the acidity of the male urethra and female vagina, making these environments more hospitable to sperm; *fructose sugar*, the energy source for sperm; *salts* and *minerals*; temporary coagulators, which cause clotting of semen in the vagina and prevent leakage of sperm out of the woman's body; and *prostaglandins*, the chemicals

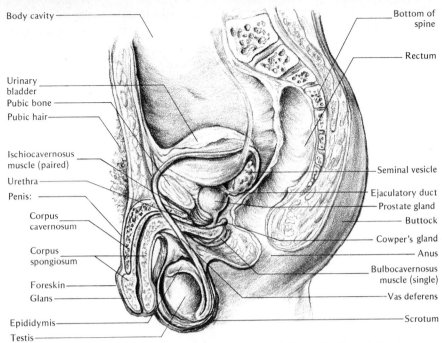

Body cavity
Urinary bladder
Pubic bone
Pubic hair
Ischiocavernosus muscle (paired)
Urethra
Penis:
Corpus cavernosum
Corpus spongiosum
Foreskin
Glans
Epididymis
Testis

Bottom of spine
Rectum
Seminal vesicle
Ejaculatory duct
Prostate gland
Buttock
Cowper's gland
Anus
Bulbocavernosus muscle (single)
Vas deferens
Scrotum

Figure 12-1 Male pelvic structures showing testis, genitalia, and adjacent structures. (Adapted from Bernard Goldstein, *Human Sexuality*, McGraw-Hill, New York, 1976.)

that cause the uterus and fallopian tubes to contract. It is suspected that these contractions of the uterus and fallopian tubes facilitate the movement of the sperm to the egg.[7]

An *erection* occurs when the penis widens, lengthens, and hardens as it becomes congested with blood. This process, referred to as *tumescence*, is necessary for ejaculation. *Ejaculation* is

Table 12-1 Male Anatomy

Anatomical part	Description	Function
Scrotum	Highly wrinkled, dark, hairless skin making up a sac which hangs behind penis and holds testes.	Protection of the testes.
Testes	Two oval-shaped gonads or reproductive glands contained within scrotum.	Production of sperm (male germ cells or semen); production of sex hormones (testosterone, estrogen, and androgens).
Epididymis	Highly coiled duct interposed between tubules of the testes and vas deferens.	Sperm maturation, accumulation, and selection.
Vas deferens	Long tube or sperm duct (cut in vasectomy).	Holding area for mature sperm; during ejaculation, serves as conduit for sperm to exterior of body.
Penis	Erectile organ made up of shaft, glans (tip), corona (crown), and foreskin (hood); contains urethra.	Copulation, urination, delivery of sperm.
Urethra	Canal within penis conducting urine and semen.	Conduction of urine and sperm through penis.

the transport of semen out of the body. The force of the ejaculation or of semen leaving the penis is influenced by factors such as age, length of time between ejaculations, consistency of sexual activity, and degree of sexual arousal. Whether or not ejaculation occurs, the erect penis gradually returns to a state of flaccidity. This process is called *detumescence.*

Female Biological Characteristics

Male and female anatomical structures are complementary. The female role in reproduction requires reception of the semen (sperm) and nurturance of the fertilized ovum after its eventual union with the sperm. Female anatomical structures parallel those of the male. They include the external genitalia (vulva) and internal structures, namely, the vagina, uterus, two ovaries, fallopian tubes, and a number of glands. Figure 12-2 illustrates the female pelvis, genitalia, and adjacent structures. The functions and appearance of female internal and external reproductive organs are outlined in Table 12-2 and 12-3.

Female genitalia have been the subject of art and pornography throughout history. The *hymen,* in its intact state, is a delicate pinkish membrane at the orifice of the vagina; it has no known physiological function but does have psychological and cultural significance. Most hymens will permit the passage of a finger or sanitary tampon but usually cannot accommodate an erect penis without tearing. The hymen can also be torn accidentally. The condition of the hymen, despite cultural beliefs to the contrary, is unreliable as evidence for or against virginity.

Breasts

Breasts are mammary glands that serve to suckle the young. Although they are not classified as sex organs, breasts do have great erotic significance. The nipple is highly sensitive and plays an important part in sexual arousal. The sensitivity and function of the breast, despite the myths, is unrelated to its size and shape.[10] Women may experience body-image insecurities, however, because of breast size. Such concerns, usually the result of

Figure 12-2 Female pelvis showing ovary, genitalia, and adjacent structures. (Adapted from Bernard Goldstein, *Human Sexuality,* McGraw-Hill, New York, 1976.)

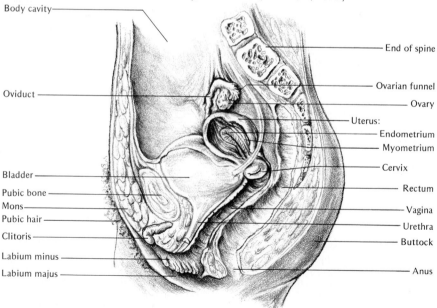

Body cavity
End of spine
Oviduct
Ovarian funnel
Ovary
Uterus:
Endometrium
Myometrium
Bladder
Cervix
Pubic bone
Rectum
Mons
Pubic hair
Vagina
Clitoris
Urethra
Buttock
Labium minus
Labium majus
Anus

Table 12-2 Female External Genitalia

Organs	Description
Vulva	Collective term to describe the external female genitalia. Includes the mons pubis, major and minor labia or lips, clitoris, vaginal opening, and urethral opening. Also called the cunnus.
Mons pubis	Soft, rounded elevation of fatty tissue over the pubic symphysis. Most visible part of genitalia. Becomes covered with hair during puberty.
Labia majora	Major lips. Two elongated folds of skin that run down and back from the mons pubis.
Labia minora	Minor lips. Two folds of skin located between the major lips.
Vaginal vestibule	Enclosed by labia minora. Includes vaginal and urethral orifices and the duct openings of glands.
Clitoris	Resembles a miniature penis. Located in upper portion of labia minora and contiguous with it. Organ of sexual stimulation and arousal in female (see writings of Masters and Johnson).[9]

societal pressure, resolve into insignificance as women realize that the appeal of the breast varies widely from culture to culture and era to era and that anatomy is only one part of the total person. Nurses encounter these concerns when they care for the woman faced with a mastectomy or when they themselves are confronted with body-image problems.

Menstrual Cycle

Reproduction begins when the female produces an ovum (egg) that unites with the male's sperm. As a rule, only one egg is released by the woman each month during ovulation. Multiple sperm, however, are ejaculated by the male with each copulation. If the egg is not fertilized by sperm during its journey through the fallopian tube, it disintegrates and a so-called menstrual cycle begins again. *Menstruation,* or periodic uterine bleeding, has a complete cycle of approximately 28 days and occurs in most females from the onset of puberty until menopause. The duration of actual bleeding varies from 3 to 7 days in most women.

The phases of the menstrual cycle are under the control of hormones. There are four phases in the normal cycle:

1 *Proliferative or preovulatory* Reconstruction of endometrium takes place. Lasts from day 1 to day 14 in a 28-day cycle.

2 *Ovulatory* Occurs 14 days before menstruation, when the ovum or mature egg is released into the fallopian tube. Time of greatest fertility.

3 *Secretory or postovulatory* Occurs after

Table 12-3 Internal Female Reproductive Organs

Organs	Description	Functions in reproduction
Ovaries	A pair of almond-shaped female gonads or sex organs; they lie vertically flanking the uterus.	Production of ova (egg). Secretion of estrogen, progesterone, and androgens.
Fallopian tubes (oviducts)	Paired tubes extending between the ovaries and the uterus.	Conduits for transport and maintenance of sperm, oocytes, and zygotes.
Uterus (womb)	Pear-shaped organ connecting the vagina with the fallopian tubes.	Site of implantation of a fertilized egg. Houses and nourishes embryo from conception to birth.
Vagina (sheath)	A collapsed muscular tube or canal extending from vulva to the uterus.	Passage of discharge during menstruation, recipient of semen and of penis during coitus, passage of baby during birth.

ovulation and—when egg has not been fertilized—lasts until menstruation takes place.

4 *Menstrual* Endometrium is shed through the cervix and vagina.

The fall of hormonal levels (estrogen) causes the secretion of FSH, and thus the proliferative phase of the next cycle occurs again.[8] If the egg has been fertilized, a *zygote* is formed. The fertilized ovum travels down the fallopian tubes and is implanted in the unshed endometrial lining of the uterus. This takes approximately 14 days and is the initial phase of pregnancy (see Chap. 32).

Sexual Identity

Sexual identity is based on a person's inner feelings of and about maleness or femaleness. It includes both gender and sex-role identity. It is an acknowledgement of how well a person's traits correspond to the concept he or she has of an ideal male or female. The biological component of a person's identity is assigned at birth, but in the maturation process individuals must actively choose maleness or femaleness in order to be comfortable with their sexuality in adulthood. The choice of male or female is closely interwoven with a self-identity (see Chap. 19). This decision significantly influences behavior in later heterosexual and homosexual relationships.[8]

Gender Identity

"Gender identity" refers to a person's sense of masculinity or femininity. The product of biological, environmental, and intrapsychic forces, it is a highly individualistic adult choice influenced by cultural traditions, education, and environmental factors.[7] Each man and woman must make a personal choice regarding the unique role that is *masculine* or *feminine* for him or her. The expression "tomboy," for example, implies a female who does not conform to the cultural traditions of femininity. A woman, however, may feel very feminine in this role. Another example is that of nursing, which has traditionally been identified as a profession for women. But a male nurse does not feel less masculine because he has chosen a career in nursing.

The ideal woman has been portrayed as passive, submissive, and obedient, while the male is traditionally seen as superior in all things sexual, social, and individual. "Feminine" has been equated with housewife and mother while "masculine" has meant father and breadwinner. While these traditional roles are adhered to by some, the advent of the "women's movement" and the stepped up efforts in male consciousness raising have begun to revolutionize traditional roles. One has only to notice the unisex trend in clothing and hairstyles to realize that traditional roles are no longer valid for many individuals.

Sex-Role Behavior

Sex-role behavior includes components of both sexual identity and gender identity. Sexual behavior is motivated by a desire for sexual fulfillment (ultimately orgasm). It is directed at the fulfillment of basic biological needs and may include masturbation as well as heterosexual and homosexual experiences. "Gender behavior" refers to what is masculine or feminine for an individual. The interplay between a person's value system and his or her gender, sexual identity, and biological identity leads to the sex-role behavior selected. Sex-role behavior may be described as the acting out of a person's sexual desires in the highly unique way that provides pleasure for that individual.

Stages of Psychosexual Development

Psychosexual development is the maturation and development of the psychic phase of sexuality from birth to adult life (see Chaps. 4 and 5). Sexual behavior throughout the life cycle is a unique experience for each individual. Although social, cultural, and ethnic differences exist in sexual development, there are commonalities shared by the majority of people. Normal or average sexual behavior is described as what is most typical for the majority at a given point in time.[6] It is these commonalities which will be noted here as they occur across the life span.

During the *oral* stage of development, or a child's first 18 months, the major source of satisfaction is the mouth. Pleasure is derived from touch and oral exploration.

The *anal* stage follows and lasts from 18 months to 3 years. Children receive pleasure from the acts of urination and defecation until parents interfere and teach *control.* They develop a sense of privacy and make the association between sexual feelings and the genitals during this period.[6] Masturbation begins, but fantasy and recognition of eroticism is absent.

The *phallic* stage lasts approximately from 3 to 6 years. The child works through the beginning relationship with the parent of the opposite sex and lays the foundation for future healthy heterosexual relationships. (Resolution of the Oedipus and Electra complexes is discussed in Chaps. 4 and 5.) Masturbation continues intermittently and curiosity about the genitals of the opposite sex characterizes this age. The ages between 6 and 11 have been referred to by Erikson as the *latency* stage of development (see Chap. 5). Peer relationships with members of the same sex develop and sex play begins during this period. Morality and attitudes toward sex are subtly taught and learned. It is an age of relative sexual tranquility.

Adolescence or puberty begins at about age 12. There is slow biological development of secondary sex characteristics in both the male and female. Girls begin menstruating and boys gain the capacity to ejaculate. Masturbation occurs frequently and, because of its private nature, leads to an independent commitment to genitality and either heterosexual or homosexual behavior during the remainder of adolescence. However, when masturbation or other sexual behavior occurs (necking, petting, and especially intercourse), the adolescent sometimes feels intense anxiety and guilt.[6]

A sense of autonomy begins to develop in the adolescent between the ages of 16 and 18. There is no great peer pressure to pursue dating, although attempts are made to assert masculinity or femininity through the language of sexual activity ("scoring," "getting laid," etc.). By the age of 18, most male adolescents have engaged in heavy *petting* (genital involvement without coitus). The older male adolescent generally has greater opportunity to become involved in coitus than does his female counterpart. Females generally have more restrictions placed on them by their parents than do males. When coitus does occur at this age, it is generally part of a nonserious relationship of short duration. This may be reflective of the inability of adolescents to manage the emotional requirements of the intimate relationship.[11]

Early adulthood has its onset around age 18 and lasts until age 23. It is a time of preparation for marriage as well as of maximum interpersonal and intrapsychic sexual self-consciousness (see Chap. 4). The issue of premarital intercourse is confronted, and sexual freedom becomes the norm for most men and a majority of women during this period.[10] Anxieties about sexual competence, impotence, and penis size commonly occur among men. Women's anxieties tend to focus on fears of unwanted pregnancy or rejection by the male because of reluctance to engage in intercourse.

Between the ages of 23 and 30, sexual access tends to be less of a problem and attention is focused on the activity itself. Marriage and parenthood, with their accompanying anxieties, occur for many (see Chap. 32). Masturbation continues as a sexual outlet and is often performed mutually by sexual partners.[11] Extramarital activity is relatively rare during these early adult years, but its incidence tends to vary from class to class and culture to culture.

The point of maximum involvement in careers, family, child rearing, and the social life of a community occurs in *middle adulthood* (31 to 46 years). Sexuality is then at its peak, giving rise to new sexual experiences. The occurrence of conflict about extramarital relations increases.[6] Kinsey reported that about half of all men and a quarter of all women reported at least one instance of extramarital activity.[10] For men, the extramarital activity serves to validate masculinity; for women, it justifies and confirms a romantic self-image.[6]

In the *later adult years* (46 to 60), differences between the sexual activity of men and women become evident. It takes men longer to reach orgasm, and the pleasure associated with it declines. For women, on the other hand, there appears to be stabilization or an increase in the pleasure derived from coitus, perhaps because fears of pregnancy are lessened. During this time it is important that both partners continue sexual activity. Long sexual abstinence makes it harder for either partner to continue to function even at a reduced level.[9] Mutual masturbation, because it involves less physical strain, is often chosen as a means of sexual fulfillment by those in the later adult years. Menopause occurs for women during this stage (the average age is 50).[6] For some, the empty-nest phenomenon occurs simultaneously, compelling husband and wife to confront their mutual conflicts and one another directly (see Chap. 32).

Old age in American society begins at about age 60. Sexual activity at this period of a person's life often depends on his or her earlier attitudes toward sexuality. Masters and Johnson point out that couples in their seventies and beyond can have an active and enjoyable sex life.[9] American society and older adults themselves, however, do not always believe this, and consequently many older people suffer guilt and shame when they engage in sexual activity. Nurses who work in settings with older adults can reduce the anxiety of couples about their sexual activity through sex reeducation and by recognizing the clients' need for privacy. The older adults of today are much healthier physically and younger in spirit, consequently they have continuing sexual needs which can be fulfilled through masturbation or through heterosexual or homosexual activity.

The Sex Act

"Coitus," "copulation," and "intercourse" all refer to the sex act. The word "coitus" is derived from the Latin *coitio,* meaning "a coming together." It refers to the penetration of the penis into the vagina. "Fornication," "adultery," and "sodomy" are legal terms associated with the coital act. *Fornication* is voluntary coitus between adults of the opposite sex who are not married. *Adultery* refers to voluntary coitus performed by a married person with someone other than his or her spouse. *Sodomy* refers to any sex act other than face-to-face coitus between a man and a woman. It has multiple legal meanings from state to state.[7]

Functions of Coitus

Sexual intercourse is essential to reproduction in Homo sapiens and many other species. It is also biologically one of the most important but not always accepted ways in which humans play. It implies a kind of acceptance by another human being and successful establishment of sex-role identity. A primary function of coitus is the development and expression of a reciprocal love relationship. Because coitus is positive and pleasurable, it has also been used to exploit and manipulate the behavior of others.

Factors Influencing the Sex Act

Healthy sexual functioning occurs when emotions such as fear, apathy, anger, mistrust, and concerns about pain and disease are absent from the relationship. The sex act is enhanced by such feelings as pride, joy, and love. Studies have shown that love for the partner is the single most significant factor in a healthy sexual relationship. Overall *health,* because it contributes to the well-being of individuals, likewise influences the coital act. A *mood* which is a mix of seriousness and lightheartedness is often most effective. There are no absolute standards, however, since different occasions require different attitudes. Healthy sex requires honesty and mutual concern as well as the realization that there will, from time to time, be environmental situations, techniques, and positions which do not particularly please one partner but provide tremendous pleasure to the other.[8]

Techniques of Arousal

Masturbation

One of the many techniques for achieving sexual fulfillment, either alone or with a partner, is masturbation. *Masturbation* is the sexual arousal of oneself or another through manual, oral, or mechanical stimulation of the sex organs. It is part of the normal process of sexual development in both sexes, beginning early in childhood and increasing in frequency during adolescence.

In the psychoanalytic literature, *autoeroticism* or solitary masturbation for the sake of erotic pleasure is looked upon as the primitive phase in the development of object relationships, the phase preceding the narcissistic state. Recent literature, however, contends that masturbation is healthy at all stages of development and retards ego development only when it is compulsive and *the exclusive* sexual activity.[10] Masturbation then becomes a symptom not because it is sexual but because it is compulsive.

Fantasy plays a major role in masturbation. Since it is readily accessible, it serves as a source of pleasure. For the ill or tired, it substitutes for physical action. Fantasies can compensate for unattainable goals (wish fulfillment) or those that an individual may not want to attain, or they may replay infantile or oedipal wishes. The fantasy which accompanies early autoeroticism serves as a sort of rehearsal for future object relationships.[8]

Kinsey reported that the incidence of masturbation is high for Americans of both sexes: 85 to 96 percent of males and 50 to 80 percent of females have experienced masturbation to orgasm at least once in their lives. Frequency ranges widely, from zero to several times daily.[10] Myths contend that masturbation can be harmful both physically and mentally; in fact, however, no form of injury has been directly attributed to masturbation. Guilt about masturbating does exist, however, primarily because of religious and cultural outlooks. The current belief is that masturbation is part of the normal developmental process of both sexes and it serves the adult as a method of releasing tension when coitus is not available. Mutual masturbation is a frequently used method of foreplay and is sometimes a technique advocated by the sex therapist to help in the treatment of sexual dysfunction.

Nurses need to be aware of their attitudes toward masturbation in order to deal with clients objectively. A nurse who scolds an adolescent or older adult for masturbating will mobilize the client's guilt and will accomplish nothing in the way of eliminating or modifying the behavior. Nurses must recognize that masturbation is part of the normal developmental process and a means of fulfilling sexual needs. They should discuss its occurrence in a nonjudgmental, objective way with the client. The nurse may suggest that clients confine masturbation to the privacy of their rooms. Acceptance and objectivity about the behavior will contribute to the total well-being of clients who engage in masturbatory activity.

Other Techniques of Sexual Arousal

A variety of other activities precede sexual intercourse and serve to increase sexual arousal. The stimuli are received via the senses of sight, hearing, smell, and touch. Previous conditioning must occur for a person to interpret a particular stimulus as an erotic one. The physical contact or touching which purposely increases sexual arousal prior to intercourse is called *foreplay* or *petting*. The Kinsey report described the following methods, arranged in the order of frequency, of foreplay utilized in the United States:[10]

General body contact—hugging, body caresses

Simple kissing

Tongue kissing

Manipulation of female breasts

Manipulation of female genitalia

Oral stimulation of female breasts

Manual stimulation of female breasts

Oral stimulation of male genitalia (fellatio)

Oral stimulation of female genitalia (cunnilingus)

Oral stimulation of anal area (anilingus)

Painful stimulation (scratching, punching, and biting)

Besides tactile stimulation, persons are also capable of being aroused by things they see, smell, hear, or think. Social factors also enhance sexual arousal. Diversity and variation in the sex act; uninhibited expression of affection between partners; the capacity to perceive, listen, and communicate desires; patience, tenderness, honesty, truth, integrity, and the elimination of exploitation all enhance the sex act.[7]

Coital Positions

Human beings are known to employ hundreds of coital positions. Variations maintain the novelty of the sex act, although most people tend to settle on a few preferred techniques. The most important consideration is that the flow of sexual activity be mutually acceptable and that the couple feel free to speak openly with one another about their thoughts and feelings regarding coitus. Table 12-4 lists the various approaches and their advantages and disadvantages.[7,8] Each of the approaches described, along with variations, is illustrated in Figs. 12-3 to 12-9. The purpose of these positions

Table 12-4 Coital Approaches

Approach	Advantages and disadvantages
Face to face (man on top), Figs. 12-3, 12-4, and 12-6.	Opportunity for direct interaction (kissing). Numerous alternatives for woman's legs. Maximum friction. Little likelihood that penis will slip out of vagina. Most acceptable to many people because woman is accommodated effortlessly. Most likely to lead to pregnancy. Man's weight may be a problem. Man's hands not free for stimulation of partner. Restriction of woman's movements. Expresses male psychological supremacy. (Stout or pregnant variation — woman across bed — Fig. 12-7.)
Face to face (woman on top), Fig. 12-5.	Opportunity for direct interaction. Many variations possible. Weight of woman less a problem. Man less immobilized. Woman has opportunity to express herself fully. Some men feel threatened. Mutual stimulation possible.
Side by side, Fig. 12-8.	Penetration difficult—woman must lift upper leg. Maximum play possible. Eliminates weight on both partners. Prolonged and leisurely.
Rear entry, Fig. 12-9.	Great variety (sitting, standing, kneeling). Easy for man to fondle woman's breasts and stimulate genitals manually. Isolates partners, who cannot conveniently see each other. Penetration not deep. May be impossible for obese people.

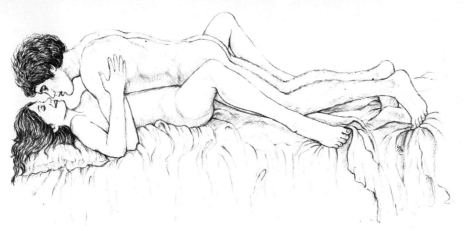

Figure 12-3 Man-above, woman-below, face-to-face coital position. High male overriding may be achieved in this position. (From Bernard Goldstein, *Human Sexuality,* McGraw-Hill, New York, 1976.)

Figure 12-4 Woman's legs are fully elevated; axis of approach is varied. (From Bernard Goldstein, *Human Sexuality,* McGraw-Hill, New York, 1976.)

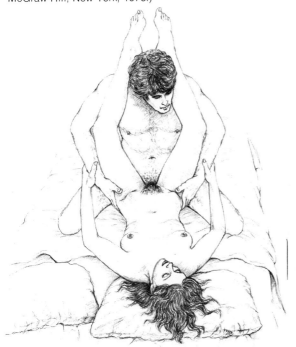

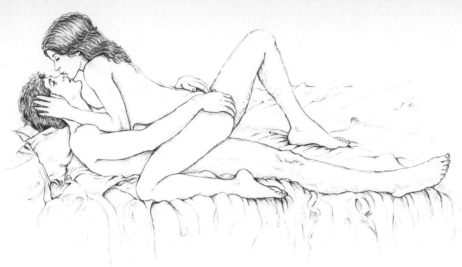

Figure 12-5 Woman-above, man-below, face-to-face coital position. (From Bernard Goldstein, *Human Sexuality,* McGraw-Hill, New York, 1976.)

Figure 12-6 Face-to-face standing allows maximum freedom of movement for both partners. (From Bernard Goldstein, *Human Sexuality,* McGraw-Hill, New York, 1976.)

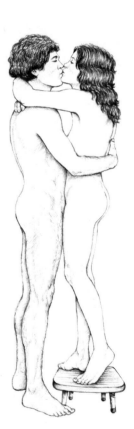

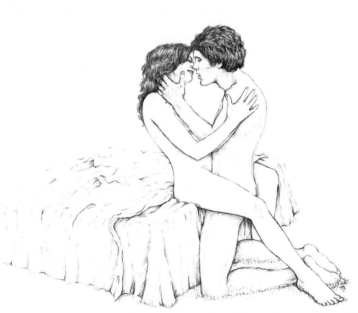

Figure 12-7 Woman across bed. A variation of face-to-face position. (From Bernard Goldstein, *Human Sexuality,* McGraw-Hill, New York, 1976.)

190 < Entry into psychiatric treatment

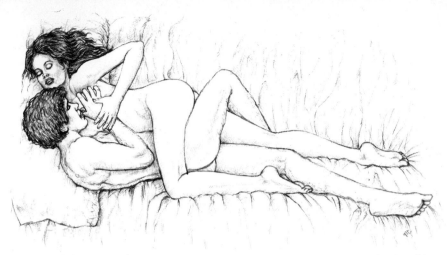

Figure 12-8 Side-by-side, face-to-face position. Masters and Johnson claim that this position and the woman-on-top position allow maximum stimulation of the female. (From Bernard Goldstein, *Human Sexuality,* McGraw-Hill, New York, 1976.)

is to provide variety and pleasure for the partners. During sexual intercourse, genital organs cease to be the exclusive possessions of the male and female but are instead shared.

Orgasm

Orgasm is an extremely pleasurable response involving the feeling of physiological and psychological release from maximum levels of sexual excitement. In heterosexual coitus, females are multiorgasmic as long as male partners sustain their erections. Ejaculation is the mark of male orgasm; it usually occurs once in each union.

Sexual Response Cycle

Masters and Johnson characterized the sexual response cycle as having four successive phases: excitement, plateau, orgasm, and resolution. The

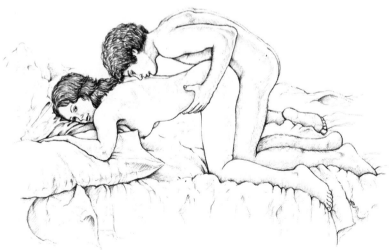

Figure 12-9 One of several rear-entry postures. (From Bernard Goldstein, *Human Sexuality,* McGraw-Hill, New York, 1976.)

excitement phase involves a gradual increase in an individual's level of sexual arousal. If there is adequate erotic stimulation, the *plateau* phase occurs; here sexual excitement is intensified to levels approaching orgasm.[9] *Orgasm* is a highly pleasurable generalized peak response of sexual excitement. It is of short duration and is physiologically a response of the entire body. The *resolution* phase is a physiological and psychological return to a state in which there is no sexual arousal. The male experiences a refractory period and loss of erection while the female can readily return to orgasm or experience loss of pelvic vasocongestion. Responses of the body are not restricted to the sex organs. Table 12-5 outlines body reactions during the sexual response cycle.

Disorders of Sexual Functioning

More than half the married couples in the United States have some sexual problem. About 20 percent of clients seeking treatment for relief of sexual dysfunction are found to have a biological or physical cause for their difficulty such as early diabetes, alcoholism, narcotics use, local pathology of the genitals, neurological disease, or severe depression (see Chap. 21). Depression, stress, and fatigue can damage sexuality and are frequently the cause of sexual dysfunction.[12]

Kaplan states that the immediate cause of sexual dysfunction is often an antierotic environment created by the couple which is destructive to the sexuality of one or both. Openness and trust, on the other hand, allow the partners to abandon themselves to the erotic experience. Among the specific causes of sexual dysfunction are failure or avoidance of sexual behavior that is exciting and effectively stimulating, fear of failure or an over-anxiety to "please" or perform, perceptual and intellectual defenses against erotic pleasure, and failure of communication about feelings, wishes, and responses.[12]

In contrast to the client who enjoys sex, the dysfunctional client suffers from inadequate sexual response and does not enjoy sexual intercourse.

A *sexual dysfunction* is a psychosomatic disorder which makes it impossible for individuals to have and/or enjoy coitus. The male who experiences sexual dysfunction may suffer from impotence, retarded ejaculation, or premature ejaculation. The female may suffer from vaginismus, frigidity, or orgasmic dysfunction.[12]

Impotence and Frigidity

Impotence is the inability to achieve or maintain an erection. It is referred to as *erectile dysfunction.* It is analogous to frigidity or general sexual dysfunction in women. Both conditions are characterized by the inhibition of the local vasocongestive phase of sexual response. In the man the penis remains flaccid, while in frigid women the vagina remains tight and dry. Fear of failure or "performance anxiety" is the most common causative factor. Biological factors are also frequent causes of impotence and frigidity (see Chap. 21).

Premature Ejaculation

Premature ejaculation is best defined as the inability of a man to exert voluntary control over his ejaculatory reflex. Once he is aroused, orgasm is reached very quickly. The reasons why voluntary control of ejaculation is not possible for some men are not clear. However, it has been speculated that clients fail to acquire ejaculatory control because they have not received or allowed themselves to receive the sensory feedback which is necessary to bring any reflex under control. The object of therapy becomes to teach the client voluntary control over the ejaculatory reflex.[12]

Retarded Ejaculation

Retarded ejaculation is a condition in which clients are able to respond to sexual stimuli with erotic feelings and a firm erection but, despite desire, are unable to ejaculate. Masters and Johnson have labeled this condition *ejaculatory incompetence.*[9] It is analogous to orgasmic dysfunction in the female and is thought to be a specific inhibition of the ejaculatory reflex. Strict upbring-

Table 12-5 Reactions during Sexual Response Cycle

Male	Female
Excitement phase	
Penile erection (within 3–8 seconds)	Vaginal lubrication (within 10–30 seconds)
Thickening, flattening, and elevation of scrotal sac	Thickening of vaginal walls and labia
Partial testicular elevation and size increase	Expansion of inner 2/3 of vagina and elevation of cervix and corpus
Nipple erection (25%)	Tumescence of clitoris
	Nipple erection (consistent)
	Sex-tension flush
Plateau phase	
Increase in penile circumference and testicular tumescence (50–100% enlarged)	Orgasmic platform in outer 1/3 of vagina
Full testicular elevation and rotation (orgasm inevitable)	Full expansion of 2/3 of vagina, uterine and cervical elevation
Purple hue on corona of penis (inconsistent, even if orgasm is to ensue)	"Sex skin" or discoloration of minor labia (constant if orgasm is to ensue)
Mucoid secretion from Cowper's gland	Mucoid secretion from Bartholin's gland
Sex-tension flush (25%)	Withdrawal of clitoris
Generalized skeletal muscle tension	Sex-tension flush (75%)
Hyperventilation	Hyperventilation
Tachycardia (110–170 beats per minute)	Tachycardia (100–160 beats per minute)
Orgasmic phase	
Ejaculation	Pelvic response (vasocongestion)
Contractions of accessory organs of reproduction (vas deferens, seminal vesicles, ejaculatory duct, prostate)	Contractions of uterus from fundus toward lower uterine segment
Relaxation of external bladder sphincter	Minimal relaxation of external cervical opening
Contractions of penile urethra	Contractions of orgasmic platform
Anal sphincter contractions	External rectal sphincter contractions
Specific skeletal muscle contractions	Specific skeletal muscle contractions
Hyperventilation, tachycardia (100–180 beats per minute)	Hyperventilation, tachycardia (100–180 beats per minute)
Resolution phase	
Refractory period with rapid loss of pelvic vasocongestion	Ready return to orgasm with retarded loss of pelvic vasocongestion
Loss of penile erection in primary (rapid) and secondary (slow) stages	Loss of "sex skin" color and orgasmic platform in primary (rapid) stage
Sweating reaction (30%–40%)	Remainder of pelvic vasocongestion as secondary (slow) stage
Hyperventilation, tachycardia (150–80 beats per minute)	Loss of clitoral tumescence and return to position
	Sweating reaction (30%–40%)
	Hyperventilation, tachycardia (150–80 beats per minute)

Source: Adapted from Herant Katchadourian and Donald T. Lunde, *Fundamentals of Human Sexuality,* Holt, New York, 1972; After Frank A. Beach (ed.), *Sex and Behavior*, Krieger, Huntington, New York, 1974; and William H. Masters and Virginia E. Johnson, *Human Sexual Response*, Little, Brown, Boston, 1966.

ing which engenders sexual guilt, intrapsychic conflict deriving from an unresolved Oedipus complex, suppressed anger, ambivalence toward a partner, fear of abandonment, or specific sexual distress are all proposed causes. The goal of therapy is to eliminate the inhibitory process which has become uncontrollable for the client.[12]

Orgasmic Dysfunction

Orgasmic dysfunction is the specific inhibition of the orgasmic component of the female sexual response. A woman who suffers from *primary* orgasmic dysfunction is one who has never experienced orgasm. A woman who has *situational orgasmic dysfunction* has previously experienced orgasm through masturbation or coitus but is currently nonorgasmic. If the disorder develops after a period of having been able to reach orgasm, it is considered *secondary* orgasmic dysfunction.

The essential pathology in orgasmic dysfunction is the involuntary inhibition of the orgasmic reflex. Orgasmic dysfunction may occur because orgasm has acquired symbolic meaning, because its intensity frightens the woman, or because unconscious conflicts are evoked by erotic feelings. Ambivalence about the relationship, fears of abandonment or of asserting independence, guilt about sexuality, or hostility toward a partner all contribute to overcontrol of the orgasmic reflex and the resulting orgasmic dysfunction. The objective in the treatment of orgasmic dysfunction is to diminish or eliminate the involuntary overcontrol of the orgasmic reflex.[12]

Vaginismus

Vaginismus is defined as the irregular and involuntary contraction of the muscles surrounding the outer third of the vagina whenever there is an attempt at coitus. It results in the closing of the vaginal opening before penetration by the penis. Even the thought of coitus can produce vaginismus in some women. Clients with vaginismus are usually phobic about coitus and vaginal penetration due to sexual inhibitions associated with strong religious family life, traumatic sexual experiences, or painful intercourse. Treatment aims at

modifying the immediate cause of the disorder through behavioral conditioning. Masters and Johnson have reported a cure rate for vaginismus of 100 percent through the use of conditioning techniques.[9]

Sex Therapy

Sex therapy is the active treatment of sexual dysfunctions. The increased understanding of human sexuality that has resulted from the pioneering work of Kinsey and Masters and Johnson has led to innovative new approaches in the treatment of sexual dysfunctions. Treatment is of *a couple,* on an outpatient basis. It focuses on relief of the sexual problem and the attainment of improved sexual functioning. Clients usually require from six to fifteen visits during which learning-theory techniques, behavioral modification, and psychoanalytic methods are employed by the therapist.[12]

Nursing Intervention

Nurses are involved in referring clients to reputable sex therapists. They should be aware of the credentials and training of local therapists. All nurses need knowledge and awareness of sexual dysfunctions, although only those with advanced educational preparation should practice sex therapy. Clients see nurses as informed authorities and are receptive to their attitudes about sexual functioning. Nurses are often the recipients of confidences which provide them with an opening to discuss the usefulness of sex therapy with a troubled client. Likewise, they are aware of the biological/physical factors which are causative of sexual dysfunction. Nurses should be frank, warm, and objective when approaching clients to discuss sexual dysfunction. An open, direct, and nonjudgmental approach is most appropriate. Respect for the client's feelings, empathy, and reassurance will help allay the anxiety the client may feel.

Problematic Sexual Behavior

To define what is normal sexual behavior is difficult. Goldstein states that any sexual act between adults that is consensual, lacks force, and is performed in private away from unwilling observers should be considered normal. The key words are *adult, privacy, consent,* and *lack of force.*[7] For some, sexual gratification falls into the realm of the problematic, primarily because of legal or cultural sanctions which prohibit the preferred behavior. As a general rule, problematic sexual behavior is that which excludes the possibility of an adult sexual *relationship* or is harmful to the sexual partner or victim.

Deviations can be considered variations in sexual behavior. Freud assumed that any form of sexual behavior that took precedence over heterosexual intercourse represented a defect in psychosexual development. He felt that in the healthy, mature adult, an adult of the opposite sex would be the *sexual object* and the wish for coitus the *sexual aim.*[13] Incest, pedophilia, zoophilia, fetishism, and transvestism are variations of the sexual object. Rape, voyeurism, frottage, exhibitionism, sadism, and masochism are variations of the sexual aim.

Variations of Sexual Object

The term *incest* refers to sexual relations between parents and offspring. The definition has been extended to include sexual relations between close relatives such as siblings, cousins, uncles, etc. The incest "taboo" is age old and is believed to have evolved as an attempt to safeguard the integrity of the family unit. Incestuous relationships often continue for some time before they are suddenly discovered by a spouse or reported by the victim because of anger for some unrelated reason.[8]

Pedophilia is the act of obtaining sexual pleasure by molesting a child. Child molesters are often male and in their late thirties or early forties. They lack feelings of emotional security and self-confidence and have often been recently rejected by an adult sex partner. A child represents a less threatening sex object. The offender is often familiar to the child and may be a relative, friend, or acquaintance (see Chap. 36). *Gerontophilia,* or sexual assault of an elderly person, and *necrophilia,* or sexual contact with a corpse, are behaviors

which result from dynamics similar to those found in a person who commits pedophilia.[7] *Zoophilia* or *bestiality* is sexual contact with animals. Kinsey reported that about 8 percent of adult males and 3 percent of females reported such contacts.[7]

Another variation of behavior involving sexual aim is *transvestism.* A transvestite is a person who derives sexual pleasure from wearing the clothing of the opposite sex. This variation is closely linked to fetishism. Some transvestites are transsexuals. Others are homosexuals using female clothing to attract other homosexuals.[8] *Fetishism* is the act of deriving sexual pleasure from an inanimate object. It is a focus on paraphernalia or a body part to the exclusion of everything else. Generally, the fetishist eroticizes certain nonsexual objects because of frequent associations with actual sexual parts and functions or because previous chance associations occurred under emotionally charged conditions.[8]

Variations of Sexual Aim

Among behaviors which vary sexual aim is *voyeurism.* Voyeurism involves sexual arousal through the *viewing* of sex organs or sex acts. The voyeurist is one who receives full sexual satisfaction primarily by viewing the behavior of victims. The family history of a voyeur often involves an incident of viewing parents engaged in sexual intercourse, and the adult behavior is thought to be a pursuit of this scene in hopes of coping with it.[8] A person who becomes sexually aroused by rubbing up against someone, usually without specific genital contact, is a *frotteur.* Frottage usually occurs wherever people congregate, generally in crowded buses and trains. Victims are often oblivious to the contact.[7] *Exhibitionists* derive erotic pleasure from briefly exposing their genitals to a surprised victim, generally in a public place. Their pleasure stems from seeing the shocked reaction of the viewer. The exhibitionist, generally a male, will often masturbate to orgasm following the incident. Dynamically, it is thought that the exhibitionist has a weak sex-role identity and constantly needs to confirm his masculinity by showing that he indeed has a penis.

Sadism is a term used to describe sexual pleasure and erotic gratification which is derived from the infliction of pain. A sadist achieves orgasm via sadistic acts even when other sexual outlets are available. The desire to dominate, rather than physical violence, seems to be the primary requirement for the sadist. *Masochism* is defined as sexual pleasure and gratification obtained by experiencing physical or mental pain and humiliation. The masochist wants to be dominated in the sexual relationship and is excited by the idea of being the recipient of pain. The sadist and masochist are often paired, one deriving pleasure from inflicting pain and the other from receiving it. This relationship is part of the psychodynamic pattern of alcoholics and their spouses (see Chap. 15).

Hypersexuality

Nymphomania (in women) and *satyriasis* (in men) are conditions characterized by an excessive and constant preoccupation with the desire for coitus. Both are usually associated with compulsive masturbation. The search for intimacy and love, the need to prove masculinity or femininity, and unresolved oedipal conflicts in which individuals are unconsciously searching for their parents of the opposite sex are among the underlying dynamics leading to hypersexuality.

Rape

Perhaps the most problematic type of sexual behavior involving sexual aim is rape. The act—a crime—generally lacks the elements of privacy, consent, and lack of force which are components of "normal" sexual behavior. *Rape* is rather an act of intercourse or penile-vaginal contact that is forced upon an unwilling victim.

The Rapist

Most rapists are younger men, between 24 and 25 years of age on the average. They are often the victims of broken homes, intellectually dull, amor-

al, aggressive, and in need of immediate gratification. Their previous relationships with adult women have generally been poor and they have probably relied on prostitutes for sexual pleasure. An excessive intake of alcohol figures in many rape situations.

Burgess has cited four clinical classifications of rape in terms of the motivation of the rapist:[14]

Aggressive Aim The rapist displaces anger felt toward a significant woman onto the victim. Rape occurs when irritation and anger have built up and control is weak. Something in the victim, a stranger, prompts the rapist to commit the rape.

Sexual Aim The rapist is motivated by an image or sexual behavior. This type of rapist is less violent and is acting with sexual gratification in mind and as a defense against strong homosexual wishes.

Sex-Aggression Defusion This type of rapist is rare but the most dangerous. Motivation is sexual combined with deep-seated hatred and aggressive feelings toward women in general. This type of rapist is aroused by the aggressiveness of the sexual act rather than the act itself.

Impulsive This type of rape does not involve interpersonal issues. Rather the rapist, in executing another crime, exploits any opportunity which may present itself, such as a potential rape victim.[14]

Nurses encounter the rapist in jails, hospitals, or rehabilitation settings. They must remember that the rapist is as much a client as the rape victim herself. Female nurses must confront fears, prejudices, and anxieties within themselves before they are able to be therapeutic with the client. The identified rapist is often sociopathic and manipulative. Nurses must be aware of their own anger in response to this behavior and be able to respond appropriately (see Chap. 17). The nurse needs to adopt a nonjudgmental attitude which conveys to the client that it is his *behavior,* rather than he as a person, that is unacceptable and the reason why professional help is being offered.

The Rape Victim

The average age of the rape victim is 14, although the age ranges from 1 to 88. The majority of victims are single and alone rather than married. In about one-third of reported rape cases, the victim knew the rapist, although the victim is most frequently assaulted by a stranger.[14] One possible (but controversial) cause of rape is seductiveness on the part of the victim. In one study, Schiff found that 16 percent of the rape victims studied had been behaviorally seductive at a party or bar prior to the rape.[15] Therefore, because other victims had engaged in such seductive behavior, the victim may have to cope with a negative attitude on the part of police and caretakers.

The most common emotional response to rape is fear of injury, mutilation, and death. Other feelings include humiliation, degradation, shame and guilt, embarrassment, self-blame, anger, and revenge. Most of these emotions arise immediately after the rape. Burgess talks of a *rape trauma syndrome* which she states occurs in two stages, the *immediate* and *acute* phase. Initially, the victim's life is completely disrupted by the crisis. This is followed by a long-term process during which the victim reorganizes a disrupted life-style. Physical, emotional, and behavioral stress reactions resulting from the life-threatening rape occur in both stages. During the period of time immediately following reported rapes, the police are involved. They need to collect evidence that will prove or disprove three elements of the crime: that sexual intercourse (penetration) did occur, that it was committed by force, and that it was committed without the consent of the victim.[14]

Nursing Intervention

The nurse meets the rape victim in a variety of settings and sometimes at various times in the rape counseling process. Crisis-intervention clinics and hospital emergency rooms are two of the settings in which the nurse meets the rape victim in the initial phase of crisis. Short-term, issue-oriented intervention must begin immediately to help the victim recover from the physical, emotional, social, and sexual disruption which has occurred. Focus is on the rape crisis situation and not on previous problems. It is assumed that the victims are "normal" and have been managing their lives adequately prior to the crisis (see Chap. 5). At this time, the nurse should take great care in preparing the medical record, since this will be used later to help in a criminal court case.

The record should include notation of a complete physical assessment. Notes should include the presence and location of abrasions, bruises, swellings, lacerations, or teeth marks. The gynecological examination should be carefully noted, indicating whether penetration took place. Photographs should be taken with the permission of the victim. Clothing should be carefully removed from the victim and given to the police. A brief, concise, and complete account of the incident should be entered in the record. The signs of emotional trauma should also be noted. Tears, trembling, sobbing, hyperventilation, or withdrawal should be recorded. In a court trial, it is assumed that the record is correct. It is helpful if it contains as many of the victim's own words as possible.

Nurses may also become involved with rape victims in the follow-up phase of intervention. Follow-up intervention with the rape victim is counselor-initiated. A telephone call or a home visit is utilized by the nurse-counselor rather than an office appointment. During this follow-up contact, the nurse needs to be alert to the "silent reactions to rape."[14] Long periods of silence during the interview, blocking of associations, minor stuttering, and physical distress are manifestations of anxiety and emotional discomfort. Reports by the client of sudden marked irritability, avoidance of relationships with men, or a marked change in sexual behavior are signs of unresolved emotional reactions to the rape. The sudden onset of phobic reactions to being alone, going outside, or being inside are all indications to the nurse that further intervention is necessary. Some rape victims have also experienced a loss of self-confidence and self-esteem, have developed an attitude of self-blame, find themselves feeling paranoid, or experience nightmarish, violent dreams.

All such reactions are cause to refer the rape victim for continued counseling.[14] Nurses in settings such as schools, industry, and colleges can provide primary preventive counseling by teaching clients how to avoid rape.[7]

Alternate Sexual Behavior
Homosexuality and Lesbianism

The term *homosexual* has been applied to sexual relations between individuals of the same sex. The homosexual is an adult who seeks out and prefers members of the same sex for sexual contact. A *lesbian* is a female homosexual. A *bisexual* is a person who enjoys sexual contacts with individuals of both sexes. In 1953, Kinsey reported that 3 to 16 percent of males between the ages of 20 and 35 were homosexual and 1 to 3 percent of females in the same age range were exclusively lesbian. About 60 percent of preadolescent boys engage in homosexual activities.[10] More recent research indicates a higher incidence of homosexuality, probably because of its current acceptability as a legitimate means of sexual fulfillment.

Causes of Homosexuality

There are a multitude of theories regarding the dynamics of homosexuality. It should be remembered that those who go for treatment provide the information which forms the basis of these theories. Many of these persons are dysfunctional in a general way and not specifically because of their sexual orientation. The possible theories seem to fall into three broad categories involving hereditary tendencies, environmental influences, and/or imbalance of the sex hormones. That multiple causes have been suggested should not be surprising, since homosexuals, like heterosexuals, have widely varying character traits, personalities, and family histories.

According to all recent research, genetic or hereditary theories should be rejected.[7] Hormonal theories, like those based on genetics, are also generally rejected by most psychologists. It is the

learning and psychodynamic theories that describe the psychological basis of homosexual behavior. Environmental pressures and other conditioning factors are the more likely causes of homosexuality. A pleasurable homosexual incident in childhood or the experience of being segregated with others of the same sex for long periods of time sometimes lies at the root of homosexual behavior.

Classic environmental explanations include the theory that the male homosexual's family life patterns include a mother who is unhappy with her marriage and turns to her son in a seductive, intimate way. Although this seductiveness stops short of physical contact, it is thought that the relationship engenders guilt in the son because of his desires toward his mother. This guilt causes him, eventually, to avoid all women. Generally the father of a homosexual boy discourages masculine growth in a subtle way by favoring his daughters. The father resents his wife's attention to his son and may also be a weak, aloof, and ineffectual force in his son's life. Thus the boy comes to develop an excessive attachment to the mother, which he never outgrows.[5]

Some homosexuals have fathers who are harsh, overly aggressive, and too much the tough guy to allow their sons to enter into close relationships with them. In such a situation the boy is unable to identify with his father and therefore does not learn a masculine role. The son becomes frightened of the masculine role epitomized by his father and is unable to accept it. Instead, he assumes a feminine role, with its implications of warmth and understanding. This is a defense against the unsatisfying relationship he has had with his father.[5] Converse dynamics can cause a young girl to choose a lesbian life-style. She may be excluded by a rejecting mother and may seek from another older woman the maternal love that she was denied as a youngster.

The desire of parents to have a child of a specific sex may be another cause of homosexuality when they convey to their child that they reject its sex. Or a child's sex education may be faulty and loaded with guilt. Finally, there are cases where the relationship between parents is so bad that the child chooses homosexuality to escape from the feared and contemptible example of the heterosexuality that is witnessed at home.

Sociologically, another causative factor may be unsatisfactory and threatening early relationships with members of the opposite sex. A sensitive girl may be rejected by a boy she loves and therefore decide not to run the risk of another rejection. Labeling is another determinate. A parent or teacher may call a child "queer" as the result of some experimentation that is quite common and normal. Guilt and the belief that they are truly homosexual can cause such children to act out this sexual orientation. Strong castration fears and sexual (oedipal) attachment to the mother is the classical psychoanalytic explanation for homosexuality.[5]

Homosexuality—A Life-Style

The terms "gay," "homogenic love," "contrasexuality," and "homoeroticism" all apply to homosexuality. The gay culture has received increasing attention in the media during the past few years. Current psychiatric thinking is that homosexuality is a preferred sexual orientation or life-style, and many homosexuals and lesbians have long-term, loving relationships. However, the attitudes of Americans in general have a long way to go in allowing homosexuals to come out of their "closets." It is postulated that the homosexual confronts the latent tendencies of those whose sexual orientation is "straight" or heterosexual.

Male homosexuality is a greater threat to men than female homosexuality is to women. Men have an underlying fear of their own homosexual tendencies and are frequently abusive in their attacks on homosexuality. Those who have dealt with their own homosexual feelings are most understanding and relaxed in their relationships with people of homosexual orientation. Recent thinking has definitely refuted the concept that homosexuality is an illness. Recently the term *homodysphilia* has been applied by the APA to describe homosexuals and lesbians who are unhappy with their sexual orientation and desirous of hospitalization or psychiatric intervention to change it.

Homosexual Panic

When confronted by a situation where denied homosexual longings can no longer be repressed or when open exposure of this psychosexual orientation is threatened, *men* whose homosexual desires are latent may react violently with behavior described as *homosexual panic*. This panic takes on the proportions of a true psychosis but is usually of short duration. It is not known to occur in women. When such a panic becomes apparent, the client should be separated from others and be provided with a single-room setting. Generally, such behavior is indicative of dependency. Sulking, demanding special attention, protective behavior, sarcasm, and hostility often follow an episode of homosexual panic and are signs of this dependency.

Differentness—Homosexual Defense

The special defense of the homosexual is *differentness*. Homosexual clients in treatment take great pains to cultivate the illusion that they are indeed different. They cling to the chauvinism of the gay culture. If homosexuals wish to reorient their sexual preference, they must revise patterns which have become established and ingrained. This is a long and often painful psychoanalytic process. If, on the other hand, psychotherapy is aimed at other goals, the defense of differentness must first be challenged and replaced.[16]

Transsexualism, Transvestism, and Triolism

Transsexualism and transvestism are often confused with homosexuality. *Transsexualism* is a relatively rare phenomenon associated with gender identity. It refers to a person who is psychologically identified with one sex but belongs to the other sex physically. A *transvestite* is a person who derives pleasure or increased sexual arousal from wearing the clothing of the opposite sex. Another term sometimes associated with homosexuality is *triolism*. This is defined as a sexual variance in which three people—two men and a woman or two women and a man—participate in a series of sexual practices including homosexual contact. *Group sex* is a growing alternative to sexual intercourse between two persons of the opposite sex.

Nursing Intervention

Nurses encounter clients with sexual dysfunctions in many settings. Nurses working in inpatient and outpatient mental health settings meet clients with defined problematic behavior. Nurses are also asked to work with clients who adhere to sexual orientations different from their own. There are several facts the nurse should keep in mind when intervening with clients who have sexual concerns or problems. Nurses need insight into their values and beliefs regarding sexuality. They must therefore be tolerant of values and behaviors that differ from their own, avoiding any judgment about the behavior or orientation of the client. They need to watch their nonverbal communication in order to avoid conveying personal values or a sense of discomfort to the client.

Nurses must be aware of what they consider sexually normal and abnormal for themselves and others. They must think about and examine their values about premarital and extramarital coitus, premarital pregnancy, homosexuality, masturbation, abortion, conception, divorce, and the effect these values have on their interaction with clients. They must allow clients to arrive at their own answers when exploring sexual issues. Clients need to discover for themselves what their personal values are regarding sexuality. Hence nurses should avoid projecting their own problems onto the client.

Counseling and interviewing techniques are important when discussing sexuality; both privacy and confidentiality should be ensured during such discussions. Listen. Avoid note taking. Allow enough time to discuss and explore needs, attitudes, feelings, values, expectations, practices, anxieties, fears, and problems.

Be frank, warm, objective, respectful, comfortable, open, unevasive, unmoralistic, reassuring, empathetic. When possible, interview the husband and wife as a marital unit when sexual dysfunction is the problem. Clarify vocabulary. Words have different emotional connotations for each individual. Help clients to describe their sexual concerns accurately. Note the client's choice of words. Do not overgeneralize or oversimplify. Avoid labeling clients. Assume that the client is anxious. Decide how much detail to obtain based on the client's physical and emotional actions and reactions. Assume by the form of the question used that the client has had the sexual experience under discussion. Do not ask questions just out of curiosity but only to obtain information that will be useful in helping the client. Be aware of anxiety, which may take the form of silence, jokes, covert complaints, testing, distortions, or trying to please when both partners are present. Do not take sides with either partner, as this may reinforce a client's defenses and lead to misinterpretations.

References

1 Carlfred B. Broderick and Jessie Bernard: *The Individual, Sex and Society,* Johns Hopkins, Baltimore, 1969.

2 Harry Stack Sullivan: *Conceptions of Modern Psychiatry,* Norton, New York, 1953.

3 Alfred M. Friedman, Harold Kaplan, and Benjamin J. Sadock (eds.): *Comprehensive Textbook of Psychiatry,* Williams & Wilkins, Baltimore, 1972.

4 Mary S. Calderone: *Sex, Love and Intimacy—Whose Life Styles?* SIECUS, New York, 1971.

5 James Leslie McCary: *Human Sexuality,* Van Nostrand-Reinhold, New York, 1973.

6 Benjamin J. Sadock, Howard I. Kaplan, and Alfred M. Freedman (eds.): *The Sexual Experience,* Williams & Wilkins, Baltimore, 1976.

7 Bernard Goldstein: *Human Sexuality,* McGraw-Hill, New York, 1976.

8 Herant Katchadourian and Donald T. Lunde: *Fundamentals of Human Sexuality,* Holt, New York, 1972.

9 William H. Masters and Virginia E. Johnson: *Human Sexual Response,* Little, Brown, Boston, 1966.

10 Alfred C. Kinsey, Wardell B. Pomeroy, and Clyde E.

Martin: *Sexual Behavior in the Human Female,* Saunders, Philadelphia, 1953.

11   Warren J. Gadpaille: *The Cycles of Sex,* Scribner, New York, 1975.

12   Helen Singer Kaplan: *The New Sex Therapy,* Brunner-Mazel, New York, 1974.

13   Sigmund Freud: *Three Contributions to the Theory of Sex,* Dutton, New York, 1962.

*14 Ann Wolbert Burgess and Lynda Lytle Holmstrom: *Rape, Victims of Crisis,* Robert J. Brady, Maryland, 1974.

15   A. F. Schiff: "Rape," *Medical Aspects of Human Sexuality,* vol. 6, no. 5, pp. 76–84, 1972.

16   Lee Birk: "Group Psychotherapy for Men Who Are Homosexual," *Journal of Sex and Marital Therapy,* vol. 1, no. 1, pp. 29–52, Fall 1974.

*Recommended reference by a nurse author.

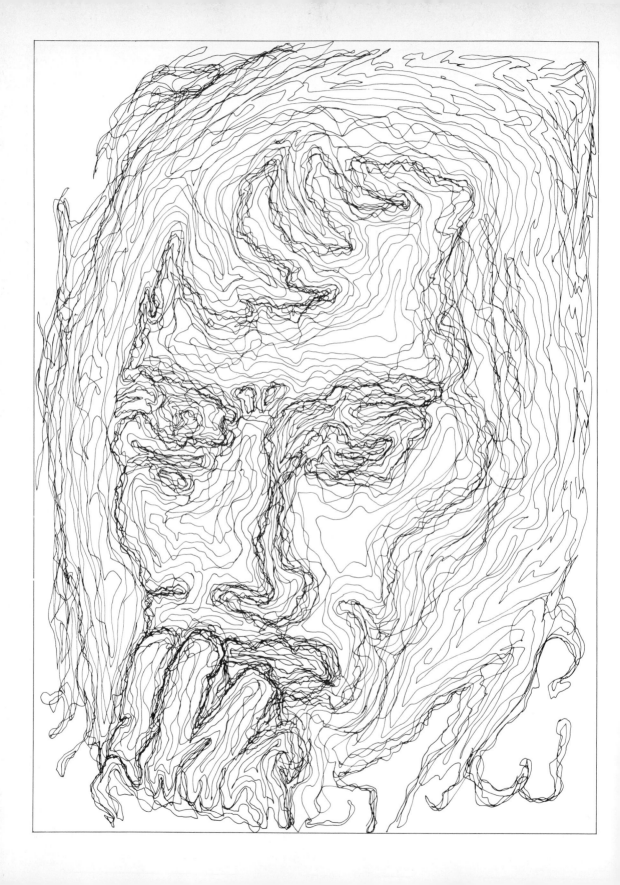

Three

Nursing Management of Clients

Chapter

13

Self - Awareness

Judith Haber

Anita M. Leach

Sylvia M. Schudy

Barbara Flynn Sideleau

Learning Objectives

After studying this chapter, the student should be able to:

1 Identify the relational aspects of the nurse-client relationship
2 Define the components of the self
3 Identify the steps leading to self-awareness
4 Describe the application of self-awareness to the nurse-client relationship
5 Analyze interactions in order to identify therapeutic blocks which occur as a result of low levels of self-awareness
6 Assess his or her own level of self-awareness
7 Assess client levels of self-awareness
8 Identify the steps by which the nurse assists the client to achieve higher levels of self-awareness

Nursing takes place in an interpersonal setting and deals with relationships and interactions concerning the self, the self and others, and the environment. Feelings, thoughts, and behaviors continually emerge and change as a result of the dynamic, reciprocal interaction between nurses and clients.

Traditionally, the nurse has been identified as one who cares for, nurtures, and gives to clients. The nurse has been the giver and the client the receiver. The feelings and needs of the client have been of paramount importance. More recently, caring has been viewed as a relational experience. Within such a relationship, the nurse and the client *both* have feelings and needs which affect their interaction and are communicated verbally or nonverbally from one to the other. This is a mutually interactive process which plays a major role in the development of empathy and identification.

The Self

The basic therapeutic tool used by the nurse is the self.[1] Therapeutic use of self requires that nurses be aware of and confront their thoughts, feelings, and actions. This is a prerequisite to developing insight about how these factors are affecting the nurse-client relationship. One's own feelings are a key to understanding how the client may be feeling. Insight into their own feelings increases the ability of nurses to empathize with clients and to intervene effectively on the basis of realistic client needs.[2]

An individual, whether nurse or client, comes to each interaction with a *unique* pattern of values, attitudes, feelings, and needs.[3] This pattern results from a biological hereditary endowment, attitudes developed within the family, culturally accepted values, formal learning experiences, and need-fulfilling interpersonal relationships. Together, these factors contribute to the formation of the self: the individual personality (see Chap. 23).

The self is never constant. It is forever changing and responding to interactions with people and the environment. The self has four distinct components: (1) the public self, the self that is

presented to and observed by others; (2) the semipublic self, the self as others perceive it and of which one may not be aware; (3) the private self, the self that is known but not revealed to others; and (4) the inner self, the self that is unconscious and unknown even to the individual because its content is too anxiety-provoking to be consciously acknowledged.[4-6] Table 13-1 gives a diagrammatic outline of the components of the self.

Self-awareness allows an individual to get in touch with the various components of the self as they exist at any point in time and space. There are three steps to developing self-awareness: listening to yourself; listening to others; telling others about yourself, and letting others listen to you.

First, listening to oneself involves becoming aware of a feeling at a given moment, identifying the feeling, and searching for the cause of the feeling. A nurse engaged in this process might ask the following questions:

1 How do I feel now?	Good, bad, relaxed, tense.
2 What is the feeling I am experiencing?	Fear, anger, guilt, joy, sadness.
3 Why am I feeling this way? What happened to make this feeling arise?	Client told me I'm a lousy therapist. Client remains aloof and bizarre despite the nurse's efforts.

Second, by listening to others, people learn a lot about *themselves*. The feedback mechanism of communication opens up area II of the self—the semipublic self (see Fig. 13-1)—and leads people to develop a greater awareness of themselves as others see them. When listening to others, people also learn a lot about *the other person* in the interaction. *Listeners* tend to picture themselves in a situation similar to the one described by the speaker and usually compare their own feelings and responses with those of the other person. This inner activity stimulates greater insight into the self and an empathetic understanding of the other person's uniqueness.

Table 13-1 The Self

	Known to self	Not known to self
Known to others	I Public self	II Semipublic self (blind area)
Not known to others	III Private self	IV Inner self (area of unknown)

Source: Joseph Luft, **Group Processes: An Introduction to Group Dynamics**, National Press Books, Palo Alto, Calif., 1970. Reprinted with permission.

Third, telling others about oneself and letting others listen involves self-disclosure. Self-disclosure is a prerequisite to developing greater awareness of oneself. It is only as we reveal ourselves that we become more aware of our feelings, strengths, weaknesses, and areas for growth. This step involves risk taking because what is being disclosed usually belongs to area III on Fig. 13-1, the private self, that which a person avoids or hides from others. A high level of honesty about self and trust in others must be present for such sharing to occur, and it ultimately creates a feeling of greater closeness to people.[3, 7]

As a person becomes more knowledgeable about and comfortable with areas I, II, and III on Fig. 13-1, there is less need to be highly defended against area IV, the inner self. This allows the person to get in touch with and work through that which is anxiety provoking, a process which leads to greater self-acceptance.

Once people acknowledge, accept, and deal with their own feelings, they are freer to acknowledge, accept, and deal with the feelings, thoughts, and behavior of others.

The Relationship

In a therapeutic nurse-client relationship, the nurse's cognitive and affective spheres need to be balanced if the nurse is to intervene effectively on the basis of realistic client needs. When the cognitive is overwhelmed by the affective, the nurse is unable to operate objectively, in a rational manner, because feelings supplant thinking. When feelings predominate, decision making and problem solving are impaired because the data base is distorted by the decreased perceptual field and erroneous conclusions result. An example of this occurred with a young nurse named Cindy who was working on an inpatient unit of a psychiatric hospital.

Jerry, aged 19, was a client on the unit. Overtly, he was a handsome, well-dressed, charming, intelligent, witty adolescent. He was "into" Zen and other mystical religions. In fact, he had spent some time in India studying with a guru. Cindy liked him and said to the rest of the staff, "He's not crazy, he's a free spirit; and he reminds me of my younger brother." At the same time, Jerry's impulsivity and destructiveness were driving the rest of the staff to distraction. Cindy was unaware of this behavior because of her affective distortion and overidentification with the client. The treatment plan consisted of limit setting and consistency. Cindy did not agree with the rest of the staff nor did she see the need for this approach. Thus, she sabotaged the treatment plan by not enforcing the limits agreed upon by the team.

Nurses spend most of their time trying to help clients who are operating on an affective plane to learn how to make greater use of their cognitive skills. Before nurses can do this with their clients, they must be able to do it for themselves. A myriad of feelings are generated in the nurse-client relationship because it is a reciprocal process. The process of self-awareness is utilized to examine the feelings at hand and to restore a sense of objectivity and empathy. Some of the questions the nurse may ask in such a situation are:

Who is this client?

What does the client mean to me?

What is the behavior being exhibited?

What does the behavior mean to me?

How do my perceptions compare with those of other team members?

It is only when the cognitive and affective spheres

are rebalanced through self-awareness that the nurse is able to perceive how self and feelings are influencing client behavior and care. The acknowledged feelings may be unpleasant, but once understood, they pose less of a threat to the self. When nurses have developed skill in listening to themselves and are ready to acknowledge and accept that which they feel, they are ready to begin listening to clients and to hear what they are saying. They will then be better able to understand the psychodynamics of client behavior and focus more on the *process* of interactions rather than the *content*.

In the therapeutic setting, nurses help clients to become aware of and to disclose feelings, desires, and thoughts. If these feelings are validated by another as being acceptable, then clients feel that they are "OK," and this leads to greater self-acceptance. Self-acceptance leads to the ability to sort out feelings and thoughts and discover how they mutually interact as well as to take risks in developing alternative behaviors that may be more satisfying.

Therapeutic blocks occur in the nurse-client relationship, when expectations are not met and feelings are experienced which may or may not be consciously acknowledged (see Chap. 6). Feelings that are not acknowledged cannot be analyzed and worked through in a therapeutic manner; hence they lead to a vague sense of threat which gives rise to anxiety. Rising levels of anxiety further undermine awareness and control while also leading to stereotyping and judgmental behavior. When this occurs, both nurse and client must return to the self-awareness process to identify feelings and determine what is causing the block. It is only when the issues and feelings are resolved that therapeutic progress can resume.

Nurses valuing self-disclosure in a society which says "Mind your own business" and "Don't ask personal questions" face a difficult challenge. However, awareness of the breadth and depth of their own selves puts them in a much better position to empathize with clients and encourage self-disclosure. The student and beginning practitioner needs to learn when and how to use selective self-disclosure as it relates to the process and content of the nurse-client interaction. Clients move toward wellness as they are helped to become aware and accepting of their real selves.[8]

The nurse-client interaction pivots around the six core dimensions of empathic understanding, concreteness, respect, genuineness, confrontation, and immediacy—all of which require self-awareness on the part of the nurse in order to be implemented within the nurse-client relationship (see Chap. 6). The nurse's understanding of the client is in large part a result of an awareness of the feelings generated in self by the client. The cognitive and affective components of the nurse's awareness facilitate the helping process, which moves the client toward health. Thus, the nurse is better able to assess the client situation, understand the dynamics of the client's behavior, formulate nursing diagnoses, plan goals, and carry out nursing interventions in a more accurate comprehensive way. The nurse is then not bound up in hiding from feelings and thoughts but is free to delve into the self and explore the impact and purpose of client behavior; thus it becomes possible for the nurse to formulate interventions which will effectively deal with the issues at hand.

Nurses can be assisted with the self-awareness process through team meetings, supervisory conferences, use of process recordings, and personal introspection. Nurses need to trust the environment so that they feel that the risk of venturing into the process of achieving self-awareness will be rewarding and stimulating.

The subsequent chapters of this section reflect a commitment to the philosophy of self-awareness. Within the framework of the nursing process, selected client behaviors and psychodynamics will be explored; the nurse's response to client behavior will be discussed; assessment factors will be identified; and interventions will be formulated on the bases of the nursing diagnosis and goal formulation.

References

1 Madeleine Clemence, Sr.: "Existentialism: A Philosophy of Commitment," *American Journal of Nursing,* vol. 66, no. 3, pp. 500–505, March 1966.

2 Hildegard Peplau: *Interpersonal Relationships in Nursing,* Putnam, New York, 1952.

3 Gertrude Ujhely: *Determinants of the Nurse-Patient Relationship,* Springer, New York, 1968.

4 Leda Saulnier and Teresa Simard: *Personal Growth and Interpersonal Relations,* Prentice-Hall, Englewood Cliffs, N.J., 1973.

5 Joseph Luft: *Group Processes: An Introduction to Group Dynamics,* National Press Books, Palo Alto, Calif., 1970.

6 Marilyn Bates and Clarence D. Johnson: *Group Leadership: A Manual for Group Counseling,* Love Publishing Company, Denver, 1972.

7 Sidney Jourard: *The Transparent Self,* Van Nostrand-Reinhold, New York, 1971.

8 Martin Buber: *I and Thou,* Scribner, New York, 1970.

14

The Client Who Generates Anxiety

Sylvia Theresa Schwartzman

Learning Objectives

After studying this chapter, the student should be able to:

1 Identify the stages of anxiety
2 Relate these stages to normal behavioral manifestations of anxiety as seen in healthy clients
3 Relate these stages to the pathological behavioral manifestations of anxiety as seen in psychotic clients
4 Recognize the underlying needs met by various client behaviors
5 Assist clients to identify healthier ways of meeting their needs, thus enabling them to achieve a higher level of interpersonal functioning
6 Define the general guidelines for nursing interventions in working with clients experiencing anxiety reactions
7 Define the general guidelines for nursing interventions used in working with clients manifesting psychotic behaviors

The Anxious Client

Anxiety is a universal condition of humankind. Everyone experiences it to a greater or lesser degree at some time in life. Anxiety strikes people in all walks of life, not singling out any special age group, sex group, socioeconomic level, religious affiliation, or vocational group.

People experience anxiety to varying degrees and it becomes manifest in different ways. It covers the gamut from birth trauma to old age and impending death. Anxiety is a sense of uneasiness, apprehension, or tension caused by a vague, nonspecific danger or threat.[1]

Selected Client Behaviors

Anxiety, the underlying component of neurotic and psychotic behavior, is a global condition. Many people arrive at their doctor's office presenting a myriad of somatic complaints such as fatigue, anorexia, irritability, headache, and chest tightness. They are quite unaware that the source of their problem is anxiety. It is also exhibited in a wide variety of other maladaptive patterns such as eating disorders, ritualistic behavior, assaultive behavior, hallucinations, delusions, withdrawal, and suicidal preoccupation. Anxiety is a major mental health problem and one on which a great deal of attention is being focused in terms of primary, secondary, and tertiary prevention. Anxiety, like stress, is a paradoxical phenomenon. It serves as a warning; it is a physiological and psychological way of preparing to deal with danger. Anxiety does not always imply something malignant but often signals a struggle within the personality, indicating that something is amiss. The anxiety experienced when one is in a high place or preparing for an exam can mobilize one's coping behavior. If looked at within this context, anxiety can serve as a motivating force and warn the individual to avoid or correct threatening situations.

Psychodynamics

Several theorists have varying points of view on the psychodynamics of anxiety.

Freud states that anxiety is a response to danger which has its roots in the separation that occurs with the birth trauma.[2] This has a varied effect in intensity and severity. If, during infancy, the baby experiences frequent and heightened tension from nongratification of needs, feelings of helplessness and powerlessness predominate. The degree of anxiety experienced by the infant and the infant's ability to cope are factors determining how well the person will be able to control anxiety in threatening situations in the future. The diffuse anxiety experienced in infancy becomes the prototype of affective responses in later life.

Later, in defense of a real danger and the anxiety generated thereby, the individual calls into play a variety of coping mechanisms (see Chap. 4) and engages in either a fight or flight pattern (see Chap. 25). These mechanisms are ways the ego uses to minimize anxiety and protect itself from further assault; they are unconscious, and the person using them is not aware of doing so. These operations are not in themselves pathological but are ways of keeping anxiety at manageable levels so that the individual can cope effectively on a daily basis.

If the effort to remove the self or the threatening object from the dangerous situation has been unsuccessful, then feelings of ambivalence, helplessness, and powerlessness are elicited. The ego experiences the trauma passively and the response pattern to danger of ambivalence, anxiety, and helplessness is initiated. If the pattern is reinforced, it will be elicited automatically in future situations.

Anxiety also occurs when feelings and impulses unacceptable to the ego come into consciousness. In order to cope with the anxiety, repression of unacceptable impulses and feelings occurs. If the defenses against the danger and impulses are inadequate or tax the individual's coping capacity, there is symptom formation to avoid anxiety. In this instance the source of danger from without is dealt with by measures taken from within. For example, fear of castration by the father, accompanied by eroticized feelings and impulses toward the mother, is the primary theme of the

Oedipus complex. These feelings toward the mother are unacceptable. The young boy, fearing his powerful father's retaliation, experiences fear and hostility while at the same time feeling warmth toward the father and desiring his love. Developmentally, the use of the coping mechanisms of ambivalence and repression at this point and in latency to deal with the admonishments of the superego is appropriate. These mechanisms are effective and allow for comfortable growth and development unless additional stresses weaken them. In that case, a growing awareness of discomfort occurs because of the unacceptable feelings and impulses and the anxiety associated with them; hence symptoms are formed as an expression of anxiety.

The young man whose unresolved fears of his father are rooted in this developmental stage may, as an adult, be in conflict and feel ambivalence about pursuing a career which would enhance his own power. Inadequate defenses allow the symptom *fear of success* to develop. This symptom reduces the anxiety generated by the conflict between the desire for personal success and the fear of paternal retaliation. The young man inhibits his ambition, and the needs which would be satisfied by its fulfillment are superseded by the need for security.[2]

Sullivan saw anxiety as the experience of tension that results from real or imaginary threats to one's security (see Chap. 4). The threat is transmitted to the infant by the "mothering one," who expresses anxiety in her looks, tone of voice, touch, and general demeanor.[3] Threat without relief becomes an expectation, and relationships continue to be perceived in similar ways throughout the life span. Loss of physical well being, prestige and status as well as affronts to self-esteem also generate anxiety.

Threats may be physical, as when one is confronted with actual bodily assault or lack of food, or psychological, as, for example, when a person who has been working as a supervisor is faced with unemployment after 35 years of loyal service. Social threat may arise when a family moves to a distant place and is faced with isola-tion, loss of friends, and loss of position in the community. Loss or threat of loss of a significant, valued possession such as identity, role, home, or status has the potential for causing anxiety (see Chap. 23). How these threats are perceived and how intense the reaction is is unique to each individual. One person suffering a job loss may be anxious, upset, and immobilized for days or weeks after the loss. Another individual may shrug, say "So what," and proceed to check out want ads and employment agencies as soon as possible in order to gain another position.

Sullivan states that anxiety is a symptom of all forms of mental illness. It tells people that something is amiss in their interpersonal relationships, and it is often felt as powerlessness or extreme discomfort. Individuals utilize automatic defensive operations (coping mechanisms) to obtain a feeling of restored control and power. In this way relief is derived.

Hays has operationally defined anxiety in the following way:

1 Expectations of self are incorporated into the self system.

2 In a stressful situation, these expectations are activated.

3 These expectations are not met, and there is a fear they will not be met.

4 Because of this, anxiety is felt as a threat to the self system.[4]

She has identified four stages of anxiety: mild, moderate, severe, and panic. Each stage reflects a level of awareness which affects the individual's ability to perceive and evaluate the environment (see Table 14-1, columns 1, 2, and 3). *Alertness* is the first level of awareness and corresponds to *mild levels of anxiety*. The individual is able to perceive events and relationships accurately and minimal distortion is present.

Reduced ability to perceive and communicate is the second level of awareness and is referred to as *selective inattention*. It corresponds with *moderate to severe levels of anxiety*. The individual fails to notice what is occurring in situations out-

Table 14-1 Stages of Anxiety

Stage of anxiety	Operations	Variations in the form of operation	Learning tasks of the anxious person
Mild anxiety	Alertness.	Noises seem louder. Restlessness. Irritability.	Recognition of anxiety as a warning sign that something is not going as expected. This can be done by: 1 Observing what goes on 2 Describing what was observed 3 Analyzing what was expected 4 Analyzing how expectations and what went on in the event differed 5 Formulating what can be done about the situation in terms of changing the situation or changing expectations 6 Validating with others
Moderate anxiety	Reduced ability to perceive and communicate. Increased tension.	Concentration on a problem. Someone talking may not be heard. Part of the room may not be noticed. Muscular tension, pounding heart, perspiration, gastric discomfort.	Recognition that in moderate and severe anxiety, the focus is reduced and connections between details may not be seen; also that anxiety provides energy which can be reduced to mild anxiety and then used to find out what went wrong.
Severe anxiety	Only details are perceived. Physical discomfort. Emotional discomfort.	Connections between details are not seen. Headaches, nausea, trembling, dizziness. Awe, dread, loathing, horror.	Moderate to severe anxiety may be reduced by: 1 Working at a simple, concrete task 2 Talking to someone who can listen 3 Playing a simple game 4 Walking 5 Crying
Panic	A perceived detail is elaborated and blown up.	Inability to communicate or function.	The person experiencing panic needs help in getting more comfortable. (In this stage learning cannot be expected to take place.)

Source: Dorothea R. Hays, "Teaching a Concept of Anxiety to Patients," **Nursing Research**, vol. 10, pp. 108–113, Spring 1961.

side of immediate focus but *can* notice them if attention is pointed there by another observer.[5] For example, Bob's attention was focused on the solution of a math problem for a test tomorrow. He was unaware of his father calling him to the telephone until he was tapped on the shoulder by his mother who said, "Your father's calling you."

An increasing inability to perceive what is going on in a situation is the third level of awareness and corresponds to *severe and panic levels of anxiety.* Dissociating tendencies operate to prevent panic. There is an inability to notice what is going on, especially in reference to communication about the self, even when attention is pointed in this direction by another observer.[5]

During the mild to moderate stages of anxiety, learning can take place. During moderate to severe stages of anxiety, learning is impaired because the focus is reduced and connections between details are not seen. If the anxiety is reduced, the extra energy can be utilized to find out what went wrong and corrections can be made. During severe to panic levels of anxiety, learning does not occur. Instead, behavior is directed toward obtaining immediate relief from intense discomfort through automatic use of coping mechanisms (see Table 14-1, column 4), and the person is immobilized in terms of effective action (see Chap 4).

Physiological Manifestations of Anxiety

Accompanying the psychological responses to anxiety are various physiological symptoms that are regulated by the autonomic nervous system. These are palpitations, tachycardia, sweating, urinary frequency, vertigo, chest pains, headaches, dryness of the mouth, diarrhea, anorexia or excessive eating, and increased rate and depth of respirations; they may occur alone or with other psychological symptoms. The physiological symptoms of anxiety indicate that the ego is in distress and is seeking to reestablish stability, release tension, and find relief from intolerable anxiety (see Chap. 25).

When ego integrity is *severely* compromised, anxiety precipitates psychotic behavior. In this instance the client regresses to an earlier stage of development, hallucinates, is delusional, and displays general behavioral disorganization.

Total decompensation is the alternate way in which anxiety is manifested. This most malignant type of anxiety often results in psychogenic death from the uninterrupted and unrelenting state of anxiety. One sees this "finale" to anxiety in the individual who commits suicide (see Chap. 20). This state of anxiety represents for Menninger a fifth order of dyscontrol, wherein the individual experiences total collapse. The ego is pushed to the extreme, all prior defenses fail, and the only appropriate behavior seems to be self-extermination.[6]

Nurses' Response to Client Behavior

Clients experiencing intolerable anxiety may display excessive physical activity to relieve tension. These behaviors may include wringing the hands, rubbing the body, wiping the brow, and trying to catch the breath. Such clients engage in repetitive foot swinging, finger tapping, cuticle picking, and nail biting. They simply exude tension. These behaviors are communicable. Being with a very anxious client tends to increase one's own anxiety. Thus nurses also experience increasing inner tension. They often feel unsure about what they can do to relieve the clients' distress. This generates a sense of inadequacy and a feeling of helplessness. Consequently, the nurses' own anxiety increases, and this creates a reciprocal pattern of escalating tension. When that happens, nurses may experience a need to withdraw from the client and engage in other activities to reduce their anxiety.

When nurses identify with the client's anxiety because of previous life experience, their empathy is distorted, and this leads them to entertain the idea that they may be able to rescue the client from this intolerable dilemma. Anxious clients often attempt to seduce the nurse into the role of problem solver or healer. Clients who demand that the nurse alleviate their pain and supply answers to their problems create a heavy burden for the nurse and an impossible expectation. Nurses who fall victim to this seduction impair the clients' ability to assume responsibility for their difficulties and inhibit them from learning problem-solving behavior. If nurses assume the role of problem-solvers, the solutions they identify are usually rejected or not implemented by the client. Clients who do attempt to implement suggestions often do not succeed. This may be due to their own pathological dynamic or to intervening variables and stress which are beyond their problem-solving abilities. The ability to integrate learning is missing when the client is experiencing more than mild levels of anxiety (see Table 14-1). This may lead nurses to become frustrated and angry at their inability to help the client progress.

During an acute state of anxiety, other clients may lash out physically or verbally at the staff. This generates fear and feelings of rejection in the caretakers. When conflict is perceived and threat to the self is present, individuals tend to withdraw from the situation to protect their self-esteem and physical integrity (see Chap. 15). In the clinical setting, this is demonstrated when the nurse physically and interpersonally leaves the nurse-client relationship. The perception of the underlying dynamic of anxiety is masked by the hostility of the conflict. The focus shifts from the issue of amelioration of anxiety to the imposition of control measures to deal with the overt hostility.

Nurses working with anxious clients who withdraw from others or who continue to say, "Nobody can help, its all my fault," may feel inadequate, helpless, frustrated, and fearful of rejection. The nurse's self-image is that of one who gives help, but these clients may frustrate the attainment of this professional goal (see Chaps. 16 and 18).

Agitated clients may ignore verbal requests. Using selective inattention, they may continue in an activity they are pursuing or violate unit rules. These clients require repeated reinforcement and reminders, but to give these is time consuming, repetitive, and frustrating. Another frustrating dynamic is the clients' repeated harassment, pleading, or requests for attention. The tendency may be to withdraw, reply with platitudes, or promptly reassure these clients.

Self-awareness and being tuned in to one's own feeling state is of paramount importance if nurses are to be sensitive to clients' needs, changes in mood, behavior, and thought processes.

Nursing Assessment

People experiencing anxiety with which they cannot cope seek relief in a variety of places. Some appear in emergency rooms or psychiatric agencies in acute distress. Others seek medical care from family physicians or clinics for relief from their somatic and psychiatric symptoms.

Nursing assessment must encompass the physiological and behavioral manifestations of anxiety, the family, and the environment. The most sensitive tools the nurse can bring to the situation are skillful observation and effective listening. Analysis of a broad data base contributes to the differentiation of symptoms with a physical base from those of psychological origin and can help to determine whether elements of both are present.

Information regarding clients' previous ability to cope with stressful events and their use of resources is useful in predicting how they will progress in therapy. The clients' perception of their problems and of the role of professionals influence the way in which they will enter and participate in treatment. If the client views hospitalization as simply an opportunity to rest and be medicated, then efforts to explore the problem and the feelings associated with it—as well as all other problem-solving activities—will be resisted.

Nurses must determine how realistically clients perceive past and present events contributing to their anxiety. Thus the broad data base which includes previous records, family and client perceptions, and observations collected from all caretakers involved with the client is necessary to making an accurate diagnosis.

Coping Patterns

Assessment of an individual's coping patterns will identify strengths and weaknesses in confronting and dealing with anxiety. Coping patterns are those anxiety-reducing devices that people employ when they have a specific problem or crisis. What specific coping pattern or skill will be utilized generally depends on which methods have successfully relieved anxiety in similar past situations. Such commonly employed defense mechanisms as displacement, denial, projection, rationalization, and others are described in Chap. 4. People also attempt to relieve anxiety by talking with friends, yelling, cursing, slamming the door, going for a walk, or taking a nap. These behaviors help to relieve the tension and assist the person to reexamine the problem with a fresh perspective. They can therefore be identified as strengths. It is also important to identify how the client has coped with anxiety previously. When coping mechanisms are used excessively and contribute to an individual's distorted perception of the problem, the coping pattern can be defined as a weakness. For example, Sarah G. took twenty-five sleeping pills. Her husband found her unconscious when he came home from work and rushed her to the hospital. When she regained consciousness and was questioned regarding the overdose, she proceeded to minimize her actions and deny the seriousness of her depression. She said, "I was feeling a little blue and I thought I'd get a little rest." This remark shows lack of congruence between feeling and action.

Perception of the Problem

If the perception of the precipitating event is distorted by the client, there may be no recognition of the relationship between the event and the stress being experienced. The client is unable to connect the anxiety with a cause. Identification of a cause should suggest a solution, which would alleviate the anxiety. But without a cause or solution, the client is left feeling more anxious, insecure, and inadequate.

During initial interviews, changes in client behavior which serve to avoid a topic or which indicate increasing anxiety suggest that the interviewer is dealing with an emotionally charged area. When anxiety is increasing, clients may become distracted, lose their train of thought, look out of windows, wipe their lips, and demonstrate increased body tension (as evidenced by rhythmic tightening of the jaw muscles and other body musculature), perspire excessively, or fail to respond verbally to the nurse. When a client exhibits extreme agitation on the admission interview, the sensitive areas are not exposed or explored, the interview is postponed, and the client may be brought directly to the unit (see Chap. 7). However, at a later point during treatment, these behaviors would be utilized in the therapeutic relationship to help the client recognize and label this anxiety and connect it with the stress-producing event.

Determinations must be made of the level of anxiety being experienced by the client (see Table 14-1). This will enable the nurse to formulate a nursing diagnosis and an appropriate treatment plan.

During the nurse-client interaction, the client may experience *encounter anxiety* (resistence), which is the fear of exposing inner thoughts and feelings in a new situation or relationship. Fearing censure and rejection, the client experiences vulnerability and accompanying anxiety. To deal with the anxiety, the client avoids any recognition of its existence. For example, following the client's return to the unit after a weekend pass, the nurse asked Mr. Jones how things went with his wife. Mr. Jones responded by saying, "Oh, everything was just fine. I have to bring my things to my room. See you later." Then he abruptly walked away. Later explorations regarding the weekend revealed that the client found it painful and that his expectations of self and family were not met.

During the later stages of the nurse-client relationship, the client is better able to recognize and deal with the encounter anxiety and utilize it as a learning experience. For example, Mrs. Smith had been meeting with her nurse-therapist for 6 months. During the sessions, she had repeatedly blamed others for her continual failures in life. She stated that her husband divorced her; her parents could not afford to send her to college, and therefore she has no job skill; nobody appreciates her, so that it is difficult for her to retain friends. As the relationship developed, the therapist focused on Mrs. Smith's projection and anxiety, stating, "I hear you telling me that others are responsible for your problems, but you look uncomfortable saying this. Your eyes are averted, you're shifting in your seat. I sense that you're not so sure that others are to blame. It's difficult for you to tell me how you're really feeling." The therapist used the anxiety exhibited by the client to confront the discrepancy between content and affect.

Gradually, Mrs. Smith was able to recognize that she was the one who had manipulated these failures, perhaps unconsciously, and that she had caused her life to take the form it did. This revelation about self is often painful, but it is a healthy sign that the client is learning to become aware of and make connections about feelings and behavior. It is important for the nurse to understand this therapy-related anxiety and allow it to occur without attempting to allay it. (There is a further discussion of resistence under "Nursing Intervention" in the second half of this chapter.)

Clients may exhibit anxiety as an "anniversary reaction." Traumatic events in the past such as divorce, suicide of a significant other, or death of a parent may cause feelings to recur on or about the date of the incident in succeeding years. During the assessment process, the nurse seeks to identify past situations which have potential for causing such a reaction. This anxiety is most apt to arise when the client has unresolved ambivalent feelings toward the lost person or traumatic event. For example, Mrs. Jackson exhibited shortness of breath and chest pains on the anniversary of her husband's death. In this situation, the client identified with the deceased and took on the symptom complex of the acute myocardial infarction which had caused his death.

External Support System

People within the client's environment provide situational and emotional support and serve as resources for the client. Such supports include family members and close friends. The client's relationship with these significant others must be assessed. Determinations must be made as to whether these people are rallying around the client, abandoning the client, projecting hostility, or sabotaging treatment.

Two points on a continuum of family relationships can be identified, ranging from abandonment to smothering. Family visiting behavior, contact with the treatment team, and participation in the treatment program serve as criteria for determining where the client falls on the continuum. Families characterized by an undifferentiated ego mass resist the client's efforts to differentiate, causing the client to feel guilty or trapped. In some instances, hospitalization represents rejection of the family by the client. Their anger is manifested by infrequent visiting behavior and depreciation of the treatment team and program. They abandon the client when he or she is most in need of them.

Environmental supports are those material objects in the environment that the client depends on in time of stress.

Clients who have a supportive family, educa-tional skills, and a job to return to after hospitalization are far better off prognostically speaking than those who are without family supports, permanent housing, employment, or visible outside means of financial support. Thus, if overall supports are favorable and available, these would tend to protect the client from feelings of insecurity and reinforce feelings of ego strength and control.

This assessment process is analogous to putting together a puzzle. Initially the pieces seem unrelated when looked at separately. However, when these pieces are assembled, a picture emerges which reveals the roots of the problems, immediate intrafamily and intrapsychic dynamics, resources, and alternatives for resolution.

Nursing Diagnosis

The analysis of the data previously collected is used to formulate a nursing diagnosis. In making a nursing diagnosis, the extent to which the anxiety has disrupted the client's life and factors influencing the situation are identified.

The following are examples of nursing diagnoses applicable to the anxious client:

1 Feels inadequate as a wife and mother
2 Exhibits helplessness in interpersonal relationships
3 Is unable to perceive situations clearly and therefore distorts reality
4 Shows selective inattention
5 Communication with others is disruptive
6 Manifests anniversary reaction to death of spouse
7 Not recently employed; skills obsolete

The process of formulating such diagnoses is illustrated by the case of Mrs. J, a woman who had been functioning well until the birth of her child. She gradually found housework, adjusting to the child, maintaining a full-time job, and being a "good wife" just too overwhelming. She began to experience palpitations, headaches, nausea, restlessness, insomnia, feelings of helplessness, loss of appetite, and unprovoked episodes of crying. Her husband finally noticed that Mrs. J was not coping well as she was neglecting the infant's care and had missed many days at work. She cried over seemingly insignificant issues. A visit to her family physician resulted in a referral to a psychiatric agency. Based on this information, the following nursing diagnoses might be formulated:

1 Physiological and behavioral manifestations of severe anxiety
2 Inability to perform activities of daily living
3 Excessively demanding life-style
4 Husband lacking awareness of and sensitivity to wife's inability to cope effectively

Planning and Implementation

Goals

Goals are established to give direction to both the client and the professional. They provide a framework for identifying priorities and suggest the interventions appropriate to the solution of problems. Goals can be further subdivided into the short-term and the long-term. The former are those attainable within a short period of time, while the latter represent the outcomes for the treatment program.

In the case of Mrs. J, the following goals might be established. For the short-term:

1 To help the client assess her current situation
2 To help client examine her roles and responsibilities in the family
3 To help client and husband become aware of needs and determine how these needs can and must be met
4 To help husband and wife in negotiating a division of labor
5 To initiate learning experiences that facilitate effective problem-solving

For the long-term:

1 To facilitate effective family communication
2 To help the family establish a healthier life-style

3 To help the family develop a sound knowledge base and skill in parenting

Nursing Intervention

The problem-solving learning approach is the primary form of interpersonal nursing intervention utilized with the anxious client. The steps of this process as defined by Peplau include the following: observation, description, analysis, formulation, validation, testing, and integration.[7] The client is helped to deal with anxiety and to develop more effective coping patterns (see Chap. 6).

Observation

It is vital for clients to verbalize their anxiety. Initially, they may not be able to do this. The nurse, acting as a role model, may have to perform this task for them. Verbal acknowledgement of a client's feelings and symptoms is supportive and assists clients to recognize and label what they are experiencing.

For example, Mr. Z's family had just left the unit after visiting hours and he was pacing the lounge. Operationally, the nurse might say to him, "I notice you seem restless. Are you feeling anxious or uncomfortable now that your family has gone home?" By verbalizing their observations of the client's anxiety, nurses can obtain consensual validation.

This message is also intended to help the client to:

1 Acknowledge distress
2 Label the restless feelings as anxiety
3 Make a connection between the anxious feelings and the departure of the family

If the client does not affirm the presence of anxiety, the nurse should turn the client's attention to another subject since the client obviously is not able to deal directly with the anxiety at this time. Further exploration will only increase the anxiety. In time, once the client has some relief from medication (see Chap. 9) and the relationship with the nurse has developed a workable level of trust, the nurse can, if necessary, "press" the client toward recognizing the anxiety and exploring the dynamic in order to pursue healthier ways of dealing with it.

When clients do acknowledge the presence of anxiety, this gives nurses a clue that they can engage in further exploration of the feelings generated and the dynamics of the situation. The recognition of anxiety often proceeds from denial, to ambivalent feelings, to awareness, and finally to direct confrontation.[8]

Description

Working with the anxious client, the nurse focuses on the feelings the client may be experiencing rather than on the symptoms. It becomes unproductive and tedious to allow the client to give a recital of symptoms which blocks dealing with the anxiety. This avoidance pattern is a relief behavior and a signal to the nurse that the client is not ready to confront feelings. It is exemplified by the client who changes the subject when the focus becomes too threatening. Repeated use of this avoidance maneuver causes the relationship and the therapeutic process to get bogged down. Identification of the level of anxiety is necessary to determine the appropriate intervention task.

To facilitate description the nurse should use terminology that is consistent with the client's understanding and level of awareness. If the client defines anxiety as feeling "uncomfortable," then this is the word the nurse should use when interacting with the client, thus avoiding further confusion and heightening of anxiety. For example, the nurse may say, "Tell me, Mr. Jones, what are some of the things you have done in the past to deal with this uncomfortable feeling?" Mr. Jones might report that he yells, screams, goes for a walk, or goes to sleep in order to avoid the situation. The client's response will reveal the coping behavior that was used to decrease anxiety. The nurse can then make a judgment as to whether coping patterns have been healthy or pathological and can work with the client to strengthen positive strategies and devise alternative strategies to replace those that are not effective in decreasing anxiety.

Analysis

The third step in the learning process is to help the client make the connection between the anxiety-producing event and everyday-life situations. In the example of Mrs. J, the nurse can help her to realize that she becomes restless, has palpitations, and feels like crying when she must prepare to leave for work and get the infant ready to go to a baby-sitter. In this way the nurse is helping her to make the very important connection between felt anxiety and the events contributing to it. After exploring family relationships, clients must be helped to understand why some dimensions of the event are disturbing. To formulate connections, clients must be able to verbalize the relationship between the feeling and the precipitating event. This serves as an anticipatory planning approach. If Mrs. J can understand that she feels pressured, inadequate, and helpless in dealing with all her responsibilities, then she can begin looking at alternative ways of structuring her life-style. The client utilizes the nurse-client relationship to check out the validity of perceptions and connections.

Formulation, Validation, Testing, and Integration

Next, the client must be helped to identify alternative behaviors and their consequences. The nurse helps the client to set up realistic methods for handling anxiety-producing situations and provides opportunities for testing new behaviors. This must be done so as to assess realistically the extent to which the support system can be utilized. If a strong support system exists, then clients should be taught how to enlist the support and assistance of significant others in working through their anxiety. This is particularly important when the client resides outside the protection and support of the hospital setting. Some clients cannot ask for help, so that this kind of assistance can be meaningful to them.

The client must be helped to implement plans and cope with subsequent problems of everyday living in the home environment. The new behavior learned in the therapeutic process is tested, validated, and then used, in an anticipatory problem-solving manner, independent of the guidance and support of the professional. The problem-solving process and the feedback in the therapeutic relationship has the potential for expanding awareness and promoting growth. Such learning can only occur in the presence of mild to moderate anxiety and is not as useful or workable when the client is experiencing overwhelming anxiety in severe or panic proportions. In such instances, the anxiety level must be reduced before learning can take place. Table 14-1 shows that the problem-solving approach enables clients to understand what goals, values, and expectations are threatened and to see how conflicts develop and precipitate anxiety. This learning seeks to develop a degree of self-awareness by dealing constructively with the anxiety and confronting the problems directly. It is imperative that nurses engage in ongoing self-assessment so that self-awareness may guide the selection of nursing intervention.

Evaluation

The effectiveness of the therapeutic intervention can be determined by the following self-assessment guide:

1 Did the client recognize and verbalize the anxiety?
2 Did the client devise healthier ways of dealing with the anxiety?
3 Did the client experience a decrease in the anxiety as a result of the above?
4 Did the nurse alleviate the client's increased anxiety? How?
5 How did the nurse feel in this interaction with the client? For example, were there feelings of insecurity and inadequacy?
6 Has the nurse acted as the client's advocate and enlisted the aid of significant others to assist the client to cope with anxiety?

Answers to the above questions will enable nurses to enhance their self-awareness and growth as practitioners, to learn from their interactions with clients, and to improve the quality of care provided.

The Psychotic Client or the Client Who Has Difficulty Evaluating Reality

This section of the chapter discusses the client whose coping devices fail and whose anxiety continues to mount to severe or panic proportions because there is no control over these overwhelming and overpowering feelings. To understand how the individual can move from a relatively healthy to a psychotic state such as schizophrenia, one must have an understanding of the self-system.

According to Sullivan, the self-system evolves from early childhood. The child first becomes aware of self through the appraisals of the significant others in the environment. The child internalizes these appraisals into a formulation of the self: a self-system. This development involves the evolution of "me" as the "good-me," the "bad-me," and sometimes the "not-me."[9]

The good-me develops from gratifying, satisfying, and rewarding experiences with a tender, nurturing significant other, usually the mother or the mother substitute, through whose ministrations the child comes to see the self in a positive light. The bad-me, on the other hand, evolves from increasing anxiety transmitted to the child by the mothering figure. This interpersonal transaction is often fraught with tension and forbidding, distancing behavior on the part of the mother. The child does not get good "vibes" from the mother about its behavior and consequently does not feel good about the self. The not-me, which also develops out of experiences with significant others, is usually one laden with intense anxiety that results from parental inconsistency and subtle rejection. Such children never get a clear message as to who they are and what is expected of them.

about the self. The not-me, which also develops out of experiences with significant others, is usually one laden with intense anxiety that results from parental inconsistency and subtle rejection. Such children never get a clear message as to who they are and what is expected of them.

When repeated perceptual distortions occur as a result of the severe levels of anxiety, logical connections between events and relationships cannot be made. Consequently, the child is prevented from grasping or understanding the particular circumstances which dictated the experience of intense anxiety (see Table 14-1). The not-me part of the child feels unwanted, unloved, unlovable, inadequate, rejected, isolated, and inferior. The not-me becomes the psychotic-me when threats to the self-system become overwhelming, anxiety rises to panic levels, and the person is no longer able to cope.

Individuals who become psychotic often have severe problems in evaluating reality. They are in a great deal of psychic anguish and feel vulnerable to people or forces outside themselves. This is particularly true of *schizophrenic* clients, who attempt to protect or insulate themselves from these feelings by communicating in distorted fashion so as to keep others at a "safe" distance. By doing so they are also preventing their own involvement in meaningful relationships and hence denying their own and others' identities. All this is done in an attempt to feel less anxious, less vulnerable and ward off further assaults on a fragile self-system.

Cameron cites five general situations that make a prepsychotic person especially vulnerable to a schizophrenic psychosis:

1 Loss or threatened loss of a major source of gratification
2 Loss or threatened loss of basic security
3 Upsurge of erotic or hostile impulses
4 Sudden increase in guilt
5 Reduced general effectiveness of ego adaptation or defense[10]

The above often occur as the adolescent or young adult moves out of the safety of the home into an independent life-style such as a college career, marriage, and parenthood. The coping patterns which were adequate for living in a "secure" home environment become ineffective. This age group is concerned with issues of intimacy and sexuality. The person may be faced with a situation calling for close interaction with another, and the resulting interpersonal demands may overwhelm the one whose ego, self-esteem, and identity are weak. These demands may create an upsurge of erotic and hostile impulses which generate guilt in the person and render coping mechanisms ineffective. Thus a psychotic episode may be precipitated.

Etiology of Schizophrenia

In addition to the interpersonal theory of schizophrenia outlined above, there is a plethora of other theories based on genetic, biochemical, social, familial, and psychological foundations. One thing all the researchers and theorists agree on to date is that the etiology of schizophrenia remains a clouded debate.

The following theories provide a broader perspective in understanding some of the hypotheses that have been formulated.

Genetic Theory

Many studies have been conducted to clarify the role of heredity in schizophrenia. There has been a strong impression that children of schizophrenic parents develop schizophrenia more frequently than do children of parents in the general population. The application of statistical methods suggests that hereditary factors may be involved. Investigators have studied groups of individuals in whom the diagnosis of schizophrenia has been established and have then attempted to accurately determine the incidence of the syndrome in relatives of these clients. Investigators are attempting to find a statistically significant level of correlation between the closeness of kin relationship and the incidence of the disease. To do this, relatives are ranked in decreasingly similar pairs in terms of genetic makeup. If a hereditary factor is present, the incidence rate for closer members of the series should be greater than for those who are further removed.

Other studies, using identical twins reared from birth in different environments, attempt to eliminate environmental biases. If an increased incidence of schizophrenia were found in this group as compared to the general population, this would constitute strong support of a hereditary factor as a contributory cause of schizophrenia. The studies that have been made *do* in fact provide such support: they suggest that there is a *hereditary predisposition* but no direct cause-and-effect relationship has been identified in the development of schizophrenia.

Biochemical Theories

Amine Theory

The drug amphetamine has been used for many years by persons trying to control their weight and by others to gain "pep" or stamina. It has, however, been found to produce a clinical syndrome called *amphetamine psychosis* that is often indistinguishable from schizophrenia. This amphetamine psychosis may indeed be a model for some forms of schizophrenia by producing a hyperactive dopaminergic system. The phenothiazine drugs—major tranquilizers used in the treatment of schizophrenia—seem to act mainly by blocking dopaminergic receptors; in a study by Wise and Stein, there was found to be decreased dopamine β-hydroxylase in schizophrenia.[11] Therefore, an imbalance in the amine regulatory system may be found to be responsible for the syndrome known as schizophrenia.

Schizophrenic Cognitive Mode Theory

This theory states that the schizophrenic person is open and very vulnerable to incoming and outgoing stimuli of all kinds. Because of an ineffective stimulus filter, these persons are so acutely bombarded by the environmental input that they often do not know how and to which stimuli they should respond. The schizophrenic is unlike other people who can respond selectively and discriminately to stimuli in the perceptual field, thus focusing on the more relevant task at hand.[12]

Family Systems Theory

The dysfunctional family has low levels of *differentiation.* The family ego mass is *fused;* there is little sense of separation between members. The concept of "I" as a separate, worthwhile person is absent in varying degrees. Family members become lost in the family system. They rely on the family myths and rules to validate their identities. Children remain enmeshed with the family because they do not develop a separate sense of self. An example of the dysfunctional family is the schizophrenic family. Fusion is so great that one family member may know what another thinks, and they may even dream the same dreams. A common pattern is the enmeshed mother-child dyad and the distant father. The mother and child remain overtly fused and the father handles the fusion by distancing himself from their relationship. The child never individuates but remains a fused part of mother. (See Chap. 11 for a discussion of scapegoating and other family dynamics.)

Another way of handling fusion is through *overadequate-inadequate reciprocity.* In a marital relationship, one spouse draws strength from the undifferentiated ego mass and the other is weakened by it. One partner will function productively and the other will develop symptoms such as those of schizophrenia (see Chap. 11).

Role reversal within the family plays an important part in the development of the child's sexual identity. A domineering, aggressive mother and a passive, dependent father will present confusing sex-role models for the child to identify with; that is, the child will not learn what behavior is generally expected of men and women as they participate in interpersonal situations, Thus, the child is deprived of appropriate sex-role modeling. This can result in withdrawal from interpersonal situations due to feelings of inadequacy and confusion. Arieti states that these children also experience feelings of rejection from both parents and consequently have difficulty identifying with either sex or gender. This leads to incomplete identity formation and repeated sexual uncertainty throughout life.

Pathological Communication Theory

Bateson and his associates theorize that there is considerable ambivalence toward the child on the part of significant others. The double-bind message is one way of communicating this ambivalence. The child receives a message with two opposing, conflicting meanings, both of which must be obeyed. However, because acting on both messages at the same time is impossible, the child is in a dilemma as to which one to respond to first. An example of this is the mother who tells her child she loves him, but when he runs over to embrace her, she holds him at a distance. The child may resolve the dilemma by:

1 Trying to figure out which message is really intended

2 Responding to one communication and ignoring the other

3 Dealing with this ambiguous situation by not responding to either message and withdrawing into a world of fantasy

The child does not confront the inconsistency because of accompanying high levels of anxiety, frustration, and the need to maintain positive parental images and love. Consequently, the child develops a sense of insecurity and confusion which inhibits the ability to relate trustingly to other people. Such children come to feel mistrustful about incoming messages and fear that they will be rejected or that their well-being will be threatened.[13]

Some double-bind communication is a normal part of the communication process and most children learn to deal with it adequately. But the person who becomes schizophrenic seems unable to deal with the multiple aspects of communication at the same time. Consequently many repeated experiences with double-bind communication lead to a generalized anticipation of disapproval or punishment. If these people have enough double-bind experiences, they may feel that they are "damned if they do and damned if they don't." They tend to perceive everyone in their environment as capable of putting them in a double bind. They may eventually choose to pull further and further away from people and retreat into their own made-up world of unreality, where they feel "safe" and free from the anxiety that others seem to inflict on them (see Chap. 11).

The preceding section represents many of the theories that explain the etiology of schizophrenia. A combination of theories known as the multicausational theory has been advanced. This identifies schizophrenia as resulting from coexisting genetic, biochemical, and environmental factors. Researchers and clinicians still find that schizophrenia is a puzzle in terms of etiology—a puzzle that calls on them to expend long hours and boundless energies in piecing together the parts.

Definition of Psychosis

The client labeled psychotic is one who experiences difficulty in evaluating reality. This individual often has problems in ego functioning characterized by mood changes, perceptual disturbances, disordered thinking, and a general impoverishment in interpersonal relationships resulting in social isolation and withdrawal from the world.

High levels of anxiety contribute to this development in that the individual cannot obtain any relief from anxiety, intense awe, and feelings of threat to the self-system. In this state, the coping devices are not functioning effectively, so that the person experiences a loss of ability to focus on contents of awareness (selective attention). The person attends to everything yet misses relationships between ideas. There is continual physical discomfort without amelioration and a general reduction in the ability to adapt to the environment and relate meaningfully to others. One can see how the schizophrenias belong under the heading of psychotic conditions from this brief description of psychosis.

Selected Client Behaviors

There are many diagnostic labels for the different schizophrenic psychoses depending on the behaviors associated with them. These are listed in the appendix at the end of this book.

Simple schizophrenia may begin early in life, generally in late adolescence or young adulthood. It may or may not be precipitated by an external event. Symptoms may appear abruptly or the onset be characterized by a slow and insidious reduction of interpersonal interests, by apathy, and by indifference leading to impoverishment of interpersonal relationships, mental deterioration, and adjustment on a lower level of functioning. These behaviors are less dramatically psychotic than those classified as hebephrenic, catatonic, and paranoid.

Hebephrenic schizophrenia is characterized by disorganized thinking, superficial and inappropriate affect, unpredictable laughter, silly and regressive behavior and mannerisms, and frequent hypochondriacal complaints. Delusions and hallucinations, if present, are transient and not well organized.

There are two types of *catatonia*. One is characterized by excitation and the other by withdrawal. The excited form is marked by excessive, sometimes violent motor activity and agitation, whereas the withdrawn type is characterized by generalized inhibition manifested by stupor, mutism, negativity, and waxy flexibility. In time, some clients may deteriorate to a vegetative state. Abrupt onset is seen with these types of disordered behavior.

The onset of *paranoid* behavior usually occurs later in life. This type schizophrenia is characterized by grandiose delusions, suspicion, and a mistrust of others which takes the form of persecutory delusions, hostility, and hallucinations. Excessive religiosity is sometimes seen as well. The coping mechanism most frequently utilized by the paranoid client is that of *projection,* which ascribes to others characteristics the individual cannot accept within the self.

Acute schizophrenic episodes occur precipitously. Behavioral symptoms are associated with confusion, perplexity, turmoil, ideas of reference, excitement, depression, dreamlike dissociation, and fear. Characteristic of the acute psychotic episode is reconstitution. Frequent remissions may be followed by recurrence. Over time, these cycles may lead to gradual deterioration of cognitive and affective functioning.

Some types of schizophrenia are characterized by an affective disturbance as the primary symptom and are called *schizoaffective* type. These disturbances may be either of two subtypes, elated or depressed, depending on which affect or mood seems predominant. (See Chaps. 18 and 19 for a discussion of the affective psychoses.)

Another type of schizophrenia involves a mixture of symptoms characterized by thought, mood, and behavioral disorganization which is not classifiable under the more clearly definable affective and cognitive labels. This is referred to as *undifferentiated* schizophrenia.[14]

Psychodynamics

Retreat from Reality

Schizophrenics retreat from the real world because they cannot face or deal with the exigencies of life around them. The retreat from reality is manifested in their regressive behavior. They withdraw their energy from the environment and focus it instead on the self (thoughts, the body, and the self-concept). *Regression* is the basis for cognitive changes such as autistic thinking and loss of the ability to test reality. It is also associated with feelings of unreality, estrangement, and bodily change.

Autistic Thinking

Retreat from reality is manifested by disordered thought processes. In the absence of consensual validation, psychotics engage in an autistic thinking process. The ideas, beliefs, and perceptions they process are based on their distorted view of the world and on imaginary creations.[17]

Autistic thinking is a normal part of each child's development. But if for some reason the child is stifled or repeatedly experiences high levels of anxiety, consensually validated thinking will suffer. The normal process in the development of thought are (1) free association, (2) autistic thinking, (3) creative imagination, and (4) reasoning.[15]

When people are not permitted to "check out" their interpretations of actions, words, and gestures, they resort to autistic invention to explain what is going on around them. As individuals develop, they see, hear, and attempt to make some sense of stimuli they are receiving from within and without the self. This is an important part of developing the ego function of cognition or thinking. However, if they are given either no corroboration or disputation to validate or invalidate information which they are attempting to assimilate, they will use themselves as the focal point of reference in their thinking. Thus, an intrapersonal, autistic communication system develops. This form of thinking is not reality-based and consequently consists of distortions. Lacking satisfaction from the outer world—the environment around them—these individuals resort to their inner world for reward. This self-centered thinking fosters fantasy and daydreaming, which substitute for reality. Individuals apply their own personal and private meanings to situations and words rather than those that are consensually validated. One can see autistic thinking in progress with the use of several different cognitive mechanisms.

First, return of *primitive thinking* involves a loss of abstract, connotative thinking. It is replaced by *concrete, denotative* thought processes. There is an absence of conceptual meaning for thoughts and words. The client attends to the discrete details of a thought rather than to the main idea of a subject.[16] For example, when such a client is asked how a pear and a banana are alike, he or she may say, "They are yellow," responding to the concrete, denotive color of each. When asked to say more on how they are similar, the client cannot respond. A more *abstract connotative* response might be "They are both fruits," or "They are picked from trees to be eaten by people."

Second, the disordered thinking in the psychotic client leads to *disordered communication,* which serves the specific purpose of destroying the message and its meaning for others. By doing this, the client negates communication and hence also any relationship with another person. Such behavior may indicate to others that the individual is "crazy" and not responsible for what is being said or done.

Examples of distorted communication are *neologisms,* words or groups of words that have meaning only for the speaker and are not understood by others. When the client says, "Today is a good day to *peshwar* in the *beavoir* with *sigrum*," he is using *neologisms.* The italicized words have meaning for no one but the client.

Other examples of distorted communication are *echolalia,* which is the pathological repetition of phrases and words, and *word salad,* a form of speech in which words and phrases have no apparent meaning or logical connection.

A third form of disordered thought process is *looseness of associations.* This occurs in the schizophrenic client who is suffering from disordered communication ability and thinking and therefore expresses successive ideas which appear to be unrelated or only slightly related to one another. These persons do not indicate any intention to change the subject, nor do they explain sudden transitions. There is an obvious interruption of the train of thought by the expression of irrelevant ideas. Consequently, they are prevented from pursuing a single concept to its logical conclusion. As a result, communication is confusing, bizarre, difficult to follow, and incorrect. For example, the client might be asked, "How old are you?" to which she replies, "Blonds have more fun," or a client's stream of thought might run "Going, going, blue, green, house, sky, dirt, in, out, bones, more, more, cover it up."

Magical thinking is a fourth type of primitive thought process normal to the preschool child but seen as a regressive behavior in schizophrenic clients. The individual attaches personal meaning or power (omnipotence) to objective events or neutral situations. For example, through watching a television program in which someone is taking a trip, the client may become convinced that the protagonist is sending a magic message telling the client how and where to join him on vacation and where to find the necessary money. This form of thinking seems to stem from a desire to be wanted, loved, and needed. The thought fulfills these needs in ways that are not based on reality. For example, a female client claimed she possessed radar capabilities that gave her the power to keep track of her eight dead children.

Dysfunction of Reality Testing
Regression is also displayed as a dysfunction or impairment of reality testing as characterized by illusions, hallucinations, and delusions.

Illusions are misinterpretations of *real,* external sensory experiences. For example, a cloud is seen as a flying saucer or a linen sheet on a clothesline is perceived as a ghost. However, in both these examples, the cloud and the linen sheet are indeed actually real and present in the outside world. They are not parts of an internalized system. The illusion is a healthier sensory misperception than the hallucination. One sees varying degrees of such misperception among people who range from the "normal" to the psychotic.

An *hallucination*". . . is an inner sensory experience expressed as though it were an outer event. It arises out of the dissociated motivations of the self-system and is an uncanny, yet real, experience for the person."[17] The hallucination is the experience of a sensory perception in the *absence* of actual environmental stimuli. It is brought about by emotional and/or other factors such as drugs, alcohol intoxication, or incipient brain tumor (see Chaps. 15 and 17). With an *olfactory hallucination,* clients may smell odors that seem to be emanating from their bodies. With *auditory hallucinations,* clients hear voices that are not audible to others. One client, who was experiencing guilt and anxiety about an abortion, heard the voice of God berating her for her sexual transgressions. *Gustatory hallucinations* are those affecting the sense of taste. A client who has a bad taste in the mouth which is not relieved by mouthwash or spicy food may be experiencing gustatory hallucinations. When *visual hallucinations* occur, psychotic cli-

ents may see figures which are grotesque and frightening or companionable and pleasant. With *tactile hallucinations,* clients may feel creepy, crawling bugs, spiders, or animals all over their bodies.

Hallucinations often meet needs that the client feels cannot be met in the real world, such as the need for relatedness, communication, and control. The hallucination often has dynamic significance for the client.)For example, a female client who was hallucinating was being told by the "voices" to "urinate in people's mouths." This auditory hallucination seemed to fulfill an unconscious aggressive wish. During a therapy session, she reported to the nurse that the voices had told her to "pee in people's mouths" immediately after the nurse attempted to structure the client's activity away from the hallucinations. This was not in accord with the client's wishes at the moment. She communicated her anger to the nurse by using this veiled language. She could not relate her anger directly for fear of possible rejection or retaliation from the nurse, so the forbidden feeling was expressed via the hallucination, which the client did not perceive as coming from within herself. In this instance, the hallucination served the purpose of expressing a forbidden aggressive wish.[18]

There are four phases in the development of hallucinations that help to explain how anxiety, when out of control, can become translated into the hallucinatory phenomena.[19]

During the first phase, the client experiences increased anxiety, feelings of loneliness, and increased stress. The client focuses on comforting thoughts so as to relieve the tension of this anxiety; but the anxiety continues to mount and the person recognizes these thoughts as part of the self even though their perceptual quality is heightened. The client still has control over focal awareness.

During the second phase, the anxiety increases and the client puts the self into a "listening state" for the hallucination; inner thoughts become more accentuated and the client begins to be fearful that others will hear, steal, and repeat them. The client is ineffective in controlling these thoughts and may experience terror as a form of rising anxiety over them; anxiety continues to mount and the client attempts to put distance between self and the hallucination by projecting experience outward as if the hallucination were coming from another person or place.

During the third phase, the hallucination becomes seductive and controlling; the client gets used to it and submits to it; often the hallucination affords the client temporary security in this phase.

During the fourth phase, the client feels helpless to free the self from the hallucination and so feels unable to form meaningful relationships with real people. The anxiety continues to rise, and the hallucination is continually elaborated on in an endless but unsuccessful effort to satisfy the needs it is partially serving. The client loses all control over focal awareness, withdraws from others, and is almost constantly in terror. This process may become chronic if intervention is not forthcoming.)

The *delusion* is another phenomenon that may result from impairment of reality testing. A delusion is a false belief that is held without appropriate external stimulation and is firmly maintained in the face of contradicting data. There are several types of delusions: The *persecutory delusion* is a false belief that one is being harassed or persecuted by others. The *delusion of reference* is a false belief that the behavior of others refers to oneself. An example of this is the client who sees two people talking and believes they are speaking about him. The *delusion of control/influence* is a false belief that one is being controlled by others. This is exemplified by the person who believes the radio announcer is controlling him through radio waves. The *delusion of infidelity* is the false belief, derived from a pathological jealousy, that one's lover or spouse is unfaithful. The *somatic delusion* is a false belief about one's body. An example of this is the client who believes her heart has stopped pumping. Finally, there is the *delusion of grandeur,* in which the client harbors an exaggerated belief of self-importance. An example of this is the female client who believes she is the Blessed Virgin about to give birth to the Christ Child.

A delusion develops by way of the following steps:

1 The client may feel anxious, threatened, perhaps harassed, leading to feelings of being locked in and powerless. The client is aware that something ominous is happening.

2 The client attempts to deny a part of the objective reality—that which is happening—by making desperate attempts to regain control through elaborate schemes of body and character building.

3 The client *projects* inner thoughts and feelings onto the environment so that they seem to be coming from outside rather than from within the self. The element of the delusion that has been projected outward is the key tipoff to understanding the client's need to distort reality.

4 The client then attempts to justify or rationalize personal interpretations of reality to self and others. This is the step in which the firm entrenchment of the delusion may occur in that the client's belief in the delusion may become unshakable—that is, it becomes a fixed delusion.[20]

The underlying need satisfied by the delusion can be met by healthier, nonpathological means, and the delusion may then be relinquished. Delusions meet needs for self-esteem, control, expression of hostility, sexuality, and dependency in inappropriate ways. The female client who believed she was the Blessed Virgin about to give birth to the infant Jesus may have been having a delusion of world salvation to compensate for feelings of inadequacy and powerlessness.

Body Changes: Hypocondriasis and Depersonalization

Regression and the inability to test reality result in a withdrawal of interest from the environment. This is accompanied by a failure to find gratifying relationships with significant others. Attention becomes focused on the client's own body and self-concept. Clients may feel intensely anxious about their impending doom and complain about a myriad of physical symptoms. This symptom cluster is called *hypochondriasis*. Such clients are narcissistically preoccupied with self.[21] One client complained that he could not eat because his intestines had shriveled up.

Depersonalization is an affective disturbance in which there is a feeling of unreality concerning the self or the environment.[22] The person may experience a sense of estrangement or bodily change. This results from a lack of ego boundaries which makes it difficult to separate the self from the not-self. Clients may feel as though they were living in a dream. Activity may also have a dream-like quality. For example, a male client said, "I feel like a shell. I don't know who I am or where I belong. I am apart from life." A female client awakened in the middle of the night and screamed for the nurse. She stated that upon opening her eyes she lifted her arm and it looked as though it had turned to stone. Another male client persistently complained that the furniture in his room looked different and that he could not recognize it from day to day.

Retreat from Emotion

Behind all mental disorders rests an element of anxiety and loneliness. Loneliness is usually not a chosen condition; and what is experienced by the client is not so much loneliness as estrangement, unexpected dread, desperation, or extreme restlessness (heightened anxiety). Often, these feelings are so intense that automatic responses (coping mechanisms) are activated.[23]

These feelings stem from early life experiences in which remoteness, indifference, or emptiness were the principal themes that characterized the child's relationships with others. These early experiences contribute to the child's feelings of isolation from the world and sense of failure in terms of establishing meaningful relationships. They carry into adult life and nourish the development of loneliness.

To insulate themselves from loneliness, clients:

1 Resort to fantasy by daydreaming and contriving imaginary situations in their minds.
2 Worship others from afar.

3 Engage in somatic symptom formation in an attempt to gain attention from others as secondary gains.
4 Resort to a world of knowledge and intellectual pursuits which substitute for relationships with people. An example of this is the person who reads extensively and seems on the surface to be the "intellectual" but who has difficulty in social relationships.
5 Engage in frankly psychotic behaviors (for example, autistic thinking, hallucinations, and delusions).
6 Exhibit psychogenic death, whereby the individual removes the self completely from intense feelings of anxiety and loneliness.

Schizophrenic clients may and often do experience feelings of emotional emptiness—manifesting flat affect, inappropriate affect, and ambivalence—because they have withdrawn from any affective display of feeling.

Flat affect is a form of mood change in the schizophrenic in which there is a loss of feeling tone. The client feels "blah," inert, and incapable of any emotional display. There is also an absence of emotion in the tone of voice (verbal communication) and kinesthetic movements (nonverbal communication). Although we all experience dull periods from time to time, these periods are exaggerated in duration and intensity in the psychotic. For example, during the psychiatric admission interview, Carol described her 3-year-old son's sudden death under the wheels of the family car in the driveway in a monotone voice and with no facial expression or verbal evidence of distress.

Inappropriate affect is affect which is incongruous to the situation, content of thought, and ideas expressed. Bob, in discussing the recent death of his mother, described her funeral as if it had been a party, laughing and smiling throughout the narrative.

Ambivalence refers to conflicting feelings experienced within the self. Ambivalent feelings are normally present in all relationships. However, the schizophrenic person experiences excessive ambivalence. It has an unrealistic quality in terms of objects, people, and situations. For example, Susan would often make obvious opposing statements about her mother such as "I love you. I hate you." Or "I want to live on my own, I need my parents so much."

Relationships become dominated and stifled by ambivalence. This results from early communication experiences with double-bind messages, high levels of anxiety, and lack of consensually validated experiences. The client has never learned how to synthesize feelings and identify a dominant emotional state. This does protect the client from feeling positively or negatively about others, thus dampening feelings of love, anger, and rejection. However, the constant indecisiveness that results creates an internal, self-contained, double-bind feeling state which actually increases anxiety and discomfort. A young male client was so ambivalent about forming a therapeutic relationship with a nurse that he would frequently tell her "I want to be here, but I have to go. I want to be like other people, but I'm afraid." Ultimately, clients may be so immobilized by their conflicting feelings that they withdraw from relationships with others and society. The behavior is characterized by disorganization, social isolation, and dependency.

Retreat from Society

Behavioral disorganization is the result of disordered thinking. For example, individuals may change their clothes several times a day in attempting to find their identity. Their ego boundaries are so fluid that they often feel a fusion of self with others and/or the environment. One client needed to go barefoot in order to feel "where I stop and the floor begins." To deliberately try to make this client wear shoes for the sake of cleanliness, for instance, would demand that the client maintain body boundaries which do not exist and cause the client to panic. Identity confusion can also be seen in the client who approaches the nurse, touches her, and states, "I am you." This client feels that he has been incorporated into the nurse (see Chap. 23). Such confusion about one's identity makes it impossible to reach out to others.

Consequently the client may retreat to the extreme degree of mutism, catatonia, or a stuporous state. In such an instance the client becomes merged with the environment, like an object.

Social isolation is another way in which the psychotic person withdraws from society. Burnham and his coworkers have spoken of the "need-fear dilemma" of schizophrenia in which the schizophrenic is poorly differentiated and integrated, lacking reliable internal structure and autonomy. They comment further that the client needs others to provide organization and regulation of drives but, on the other hand, fears others, perceiving them as dangerous and fearsome, since the client can be destroyed through abandonment. So the schizophrenic needs yet fears and distrusts others, thus being in a need-fear dilemma which often results in social withdrawal and isolation. The client may attempt to deal with this anxiety by denying the need for others or the fear of separation from them. Or schizophrenics may make insatiable pleas or demands on others, as proof of their endurance and sincerity, in an attempt to alleviate the threat of loss due to their own instability.[24] For example, a male schizophrenic client who has been working closely with a nurse-therapist over a period of approximately 3 months, and who is developing an interpersonal relationship with the nurse, may suddenly stop seeing her. The client may do this because he feels threatened by this new relationship and is not able to trust his newly developing ability to form a trusting relationship with another human being. Or the client may abruptly terminate therapy because he feels fearful of an impending loss. He may imagine that the nurse-therapist will have to leave to change jobs or go on vacation. Thus, the client wards off possible feelings of abandonment by anticipating abandonment and doing the abandoning himself, thus trying to prevent further damage to an already fragile ego. The client, although needing the nurse-therapist, is fearful of separation, so he resorts to withdrawal in order to "resolve" this dilemma. In fact, the client is his own worst enemy and actually takes refuge in his isolation.

Dependency is part of the need-fear dilemma.

The schizophrenic client wants desperately to be dependent but fears possible rejection or retaliation. Yet despite experience with rejection and disapproval, such a client remains dependent and continues to make impossible demands on others. These behaviors stem from the fact that the schizophrenic's ego strength is very tenuous, largely because this client has never differentiated from the family ego mass and developed a separate identity, sense of autonomy, or self-esteem. The nurse must be wary in working with such a client so as not to encourage too much dependence, because the client will never feel that enough has been given. Such clients simply seek more and more and may sap the unwary therapist's own ego strength.

Nurses' Response to Client Behavior

Schizophrenic clients generate diverse feelings in caretakers. Their aloofness from interpersonal situations tends to arouse anxiety in others. Nurses feel that the client is unapproachable and are often uncertain as to how best to intervene. The client's behavior is also chaotic and confusing to self and others, including nurses, doctors, family, and friends. For example, when the nurse approached, a client stated, "I am dead" and then began to scream loudly in the corridor saying, "I'm crazy. What do you want to do with me? Crucify me for the world's injustices? I'll never get well. It's all your fault. Leave me alone!" Such communication tends to make the caretakers feel anxious and helpless. They may label the client a hopeless case and blame his failure to respond on him rather than themselves. When this happens, the staff may begin to avoid the client. This pattern of client pushing staff away and nursing staff ignoring the client has been termed *mutual withdrawal*.[25] According to Will, the interpersonal context consists of failure with regard to the client. Caretakers "feel indifference and apathy toward these clients, guilt about avoiding them and may label them as hopeless to avoid this guilt, and rationalize the avoid-

ance by saying that they could not tolerate closeness."[25] The bizarre behavior of schizophrenic clients generates chaotic and confusing feelings in those who attempt to help them unravel anxious feelings and their behavioral manifestations.

In addition to feelings of anxiety, hopelessness, frustration, and anger, the nurse may experience exasperation and sadness. Psychotic clients who retreat from others require patience and perseverance. It is often very difficult to establish rapport and a level of trust with them which permits exploration of significant issues. Often the nurse feels frustrated, incompetent, angry, and exasperated when efforts to "make contact" are repeatedly thwarted by the client. The temptation is to throw one's hands up and say, "I give up, let someone else work with this client!" Yet perseverance is more necessary in working with the schizophrenic than with any other type of client in order to overcome, *with* the client, the testing, trying, and manipulative ways of communicating. These clients have to find out for themselves whether they can trust others in meaningful ways, and they must test the therapist in order to establish this.

Therefore, supervision is very helpful to those who work with psychotics. In the supervisory relationship, nurse-therapists examine their relationships with clients. The content and process of meetings with the client are explored. The supervisor assists the nurse-therapist involved by sharing perceptions of the therapeutic process. The nurse-therapist is thus enabled to examine and work through feelings generated by the client so that they will not interfere with the nurse-client relationship and the therapeutic process.

Nurses may also experience amusement as they work with psychotic clients. Often, a sense of humor helps nurses deal with feelings of anxiety and discomfort. Laughter serves as an escape valve for anxiety, and once this is released, nurses are once again able to work effectively with their clients. Laughter and giggling are common in a situation involving stress or embarrassment, not so much because the incident was funny as because people did not know what to say or how to act. To find amusement in such a dilemma helps to relieve tension. Another instance in which humor serves the nurse's relationship with the client is when they both share their appreciation of a humorous episode. Humor can be therapeutically useful when it is exercised judiciously in the sense of "laughing with" rather than "laughing at" the client.

Anxious clients often have difficulty interpreting communications from others. Their own faulty communication system distorts messages. This misinterpretation can block communication, impair the therapeutic relationship, and distort any humor the nurse is displaying. Nurses who laugh and talk within the view of paranoid clients may be seen as talking about *them*. It is mandatory that nurses be aware of their feelings and actions. They should share with the client, when appropriate, feelings relevant to their interaction.

Nursing Assessment

The nurse must observe client and family behavior objectively in order to formulate a valid data base. Initially, the team tries to validate the etiology of the behavioral constellation. The psychotic behavior can be due to:

1 A functional psychosis such as schizophrenia
2 A toxic problem such as an acute drug reaction
3 An organic problem such as a brain tumor or anoxia
4 A religious inner experience

It is important to obtain information from the client as well as significant others. Perceptions of the situation may vary, and it is important to attain a complete picture (see Chap. 7).

Case Study
Howard L is a 21-year-old male who has been hospitalized, for the first time, for emotional problems. Howard was the first of three children of a middle-class family. He has two sisters aged 16 and 18. Howard's mastery of developmental tasks

was normal. He was obedient and did well in school but had few friends. He was not very athletic and did not join any team sports. Mr. and Mrs. L state that they have had a fairly happy marriage. However, Mr. L travels a great deal on business and has always been very wrapped up in his work. Mrs. L was the major caretaker during Howard's childhood. Mrs. L states she was often lonely and perhaps gave too much attention and affection to Howard, who often tried to be the "little man" of the house when his father was away.

Howard graduated at the top of his high school class and went to college in a distant part of the state on a scholarship. Mrs L stated, "It broke my heart when he left, I was so alone." Howard replied, "But that's what you wanted me to do. She never tells you what she really wants. It's always a mystery. She's always treating me like a little boy but telling me to be a man." Howard made dean's list for 1½ years of college. During the last semester of his second year, he wanted to join a fraternity. During initiation week, he stopped going to classes and complained about the senior fraternity members "hazing" him. He complained that they were playing tricks on him, hurting him in some way, and that he was a social flop. He left school and returned home, remaining in his room and emerging only to eat. He stated, "I was so frightened, I couldn't concentrate." This behavior diminished after a week. He got a job at a printing firm and learned typesetting. He did his job but made no friends. His only socializing was an occasional beer at the local tavern.

Howard had become more withdrawn in the past 2 months, following attempts to date a girl at work that failed to work out. His boss wanted to promote him to supervisor, but Howard declined. His mother told him, "You'll never amount to anything, no friends, no ambition, no education; you don't even help me." Howard quit his job and has spent the past 2 weeks curled up in the fetal position in bed, talking to himself. He has eaten little; this morning he hid under the covers, mute, refusing to get up. His younger sister tried to mobilize him but was told, "You're part of the conspiracy. Get them all out of here, debug the place! The electricity will kill us all!" The family dressed Howard and brought him to the emergen-cy room of the general hospital. He is to be interviewed by the team and admitted to the psychiatric unit. Table 14-2 illustrates an assessment

Table 14-2 Assessment of Client and Family

Assessment questions	Response of the client and family	
Behavioral assessment		
What does client perceive as the problem?	Client:	I don't have any problems. They brought me here, it's a plot, the FBI are behind this.
What does the family perceive as the problem?[3,4]	Family:	He sleeps all day curled up under the blankets, has quit work, won't eat, is scared there is a plot against him.
What particular circumstances precipitated the behavior?	Client:	They don't like me—don't appreciate me. They're sending people after me now to make me pay for quitting.
	Family:	It seemed to happen all of a sudden. Within 2 weeks, he had stopped seeing friends, stating they're no good; quit work, saying "They're always criticizing me—it's a lousy job anyway." Began spending time in his room, stopped eating. Stayed in bed, couldn't get him out for anything. Would hear him walking about his room in the middle of the night.
What purpose does the behavior serve for the client?	Client:	I'm scared, I feel safe in bed.
Affective assessment		
What is the client's affect? Are thought and affect congruent?	Client's face remains blank when relating "scary" experiences of past 2 weeks. Client giggles suddenly when talking about the plot against him.	
What objective data is client presenting? Gestures, posture, gait, tone of voice, mannerisms.	Client is seated on a chair curled up with face turned away from family and nurse. Arms are wrapped tightly around his sides, and he does not maintain eye contact when speaking.	
	Family:	He's stayed in that position for days, no matter where he is. When he walks, he runs as if to get away from people as far as possible.
Cognitive assessment		
Does client present evidence of thought disorder? (Loss of abstract thinking, hypochondriasis, depersonalization, magical thinking, autistic communication.)	Client:	I feel empty sometimes, like all my insides have been eaten away. Other times I feel electrical power pumping through my body. It feels like I'm going to electrocute anybody who is near me.
Does client present evidence of impaired reality testing? (Hallucinations, delusions.)	Client appears to look off into space, lips moving, talking to people who are not there.	
	Client:	The FBI are after me, it's a plot to find out all the secrets I know. When all is known, the truth about who I am will be revealed. I'm traveling incognito right now. If you really want to know, I'm the right arm of God.

guide that highlights key areas to be considered in assembling a comprehensive data base for the client and family.

The nurse needs to assess other areas of behavior once the client is in treatment, either in the hospital or in the outpatient setting. Other

Table 14-2 Assessment of Client and Family (continued)

Assessment questions	Response of the client and family	
Environmental assessment		
Who are the client's significant others?	Client:	I have nobody that I care about, nobody cares about me.
What is the composition of the family?	Family:	He lives at home with father, mother, 18- and 16-year-old sisters.
What is the relationship between client and parents.	Client:	I have no relationship. They're always on my back telling me what to do, who to have as friends.
	Family:	He's always been a good boy, obedient, shy, and not too talkative with us, but never any trouble till now.
What is client's sibling position in the family?	Client:	I'm the oldest with two bratty sisters.
	Family:	He is the oldest, 21 now. Sometimes you'd never know it. We've always had to look out for him.
Who were the primary caretakers?	Client:	I take care of myself.
	Mother states she has always been at home caring for children, looking out for all their needs. Father travels, is away a great deal. Relatives live in a distant state.	
What is the family communication pattern and network?	Client:	Things are never said straight. She tells me to go out and have a good time with friends. When I do, she tells me they're no good, I'm not going to the right places and am staying out too late. That's how its always been. They never really listen to me either.
	Mother attempts to speak for whole family and explain the situation. Father sits quietly beside her, saying, "Yes dear," when she asks for validation. Communication from mother contradicts son's perceptions.	
What are the relationships within the family? What role models has the client had to identify with?	Client:	Mom's the boss, Dad says, "Yes, dear." He's never around anyway, even when he's there.
	Family:	My husband's away a great deal, so I've had to take hold of things. The girls have always helped.
Social, economic, and educational assessment		
Does the client have friends? Does the client make friends easily and/or have any sustained relationships?	Client:	I've never made friends easily. I had a buddy in high school, but we drifted apart when I went to college. Now no one's good enough that I bring home. Girls were never much interested in me.
	Family:	He's always been a loner.
What is the client's level of education?	Client:	Two years of college.
	Family:	He dropped out, the pressure was too much.

Table 14-2 Assessment of Client and Family (continued)

Assessment questions	Response of the client and family
What is the client's employment history? (Type of job, length held, job satisfaction, relationships at work.)	Client: I've been working since I left school. Work in a printing firm. I do typesetting. It's OK; everybody leaves me alone . . . until they hatched this plot. Family: He's too bright for this job . . . they don't appreciate him. But he won't go after anything that would challenge him or where he'd meet people.

questions to be answered in an ongoing assessment are:

1 What purpose does the behavior serve for the client? What need is it fulfilling? The client's auditory hallucinations may be fulfilling a need for interpersonal intimacy in the presence of intense loneliness.
2 What is the impact of the client's behavior on staff and other clients on the unit?
3 What is the probability of effecting change in the client's interpersonal relationships, feelings about self and life-style?
4 What is the client's response to the treatment program?

Nursing Diagnosis

Nurses will be able to make initial nursing diagnoses about the client and family system by utilizing observations and communication skills. Table 14-3 illustrates an initial problem list.

As the nurse develops a relationship with the client, other problems will become evident. In order to make a comprehensive nursing diagnosis, the process must be ongoing. Resolution of current problems leads to the identification of new problems on a different level of client integration.

Nursing Intervention

The client usually arrives at the treatment setting feeling frightened, isolated from others, and experiencing reality from a different perceptual stance.

The client and/or the family may be upset about separation at this time.

The client needs skilled nursing attention, good judgment, and respect. The most valuable tool the nurse has is the therapeutic use of self to intervene with the schizophrenic client in group and individual interactions. The nurse must be able to adjust the nursing care to the current needs of the client. This may include assisting the client to develop trust in others, decrease anxiety, define reality, and increase self-esteem. The nurse is also involved in meeting the physical and safety needs of the client.

The environment of the schizophrenic client needs to be managed in a flexible manner. Because of the client's retreat from reality and consequent thought disorder, the client communicates and experiences reality on many different levels. Control also varies from time to time.

Management of the Environment

The environment should be simple, predictable, and consistent. Upon admission, the client is often experiencing an overload of sensory stimuli. Therefore, immediate involvement in a variety of complex, stimulating activities such as ward government meetings, group therapy, and dances may be contraindicated. If the clients are not able to participate effectively, their anxiety level will rise further and they will feel incompetent and bewildered. Client involvement in an activity program is modified according to the individual's capacity for involvement (see Chap. 8).[26,27]

Table 14-3 Problem List and Goals

Behavior	Problem	Goal
Fetal position. Pulls away when touched. Verbally noncommunicative, no eye contact.	Mistrust, withdrawal.	Develop trust. Decrease withdrawal in presence of others. Increase eye contact. Increase client-initiated verbal communication. Increase client response to communication initiated by others.
Has not eaten solid food in 2 days.	Resistance to eating.	Increase nutritional intake.
Refuses to change clothes or wash.	Poor body hygiene.	Improve self-care patterns, hygiene and grooming.
Mother sends mixed messages.	Double-bind communication patterns.	Increase direct, open communication between family members.
Mother negates son's plan to move out of the house.	Fusion relationship between mother and son.	Differentiation of client from family ego mass. Increase independent decision making and life-style.
Son acts bizarre when marital conflict is focused on.	Scapegoating of son.	Increase acceptance of client's feelings.
Mother acts as spokesperson for the family.	Overadequate-inadequate reciprocity, lack of role complementarity.	Increase role complementarity.
"The FBI is after me. I can't eat. They've poisoned my food."	Impairment of reality testing; delusion of persecution.	Increase reality orientation. Decrease threat of relatedness. Increase relatedness to others.
"The voices are telling me it's not safe. I have to believe them."	Auditory hallucinations. Repression of anger, powerlessness, loneliness.	Increase successful decision making. Increase task mastery. Increase verbal expression of anger through body language (i.e., movement therapy).
No friends	Low self-esteem.	Increase self-esteem.
"I'm scared; I can't concentrate."	Severe anxiety.	Decrease anxiety.
Quit his job.	Unemployed	Return to economic self-support.

The nurse's initial goal is to establish an accepting environment in which the client is comfortable. The nurse strives to begin communication with the client so that a relationship is initiated. It is important for them to spend time together so that the nurse may talk with the client, become comfortable with him or her, and listen to the client. When communication is established, the nurse is better able to pursue an understanding of client behavior. The client, feeling that attempts at understanding are being made, feels more secure and confident in the nurse.[26]

The nurse listens to the client to determine client goals, that is, what the client hopes to achieve from treatment. Listening skills enable the nurse to hear and analyze what the client is saying and respond in an accepting, nonjudgmental way. The underlying meaning or theme of the client's communication is utilized by the team members in formulating effective intervention. Specific areas of intervention will be discussed in terms of behavioral themes.

Mistrust

The schizophrenic client exhibits profound mistrust of others and the environment. Mistrust is derived from interpersonal experiences which have been perceived as threatening, anxiety-laden, and disappointing. As a result of these experiences, the client utilizes defensive maneuvers such as avoidance, resistance, testing, and manipulation to protect the self from further harm.

Intervention is directed toward developing a sense of trust. *Trust* is a feeling of dependability, safety, and confidence in others. In establishing a nurse-client relationship, efforts must be made to be consistent and reliable as to scheduled appointments. Nurses must be sensitive to the importance of reliability for clients, whose apparent indifference to the nurse's presence or absence is often a facade, thus it usually takes a good deal of time to recover therapeutic ground after an unexplained absence. Clients are sensitive to the genuineness of others.[28] They have discarded the masks of sanity and are very perceptive about inauthentic behavior in others. They may or may not indicate this awareness at the beginning of a relationship. For example, a nurse asked many questions of a client who was always busy talking with her hallucinatory voices. The client finally turned to the nurse and said, "Stop those questions, stop acting like a 'shrink'. Let's see you! You're all right!"

The nurse must meet the client at the current level of behavior and be honest and undemanding. Many clients have persistently experienced conditional love; caring attached to a demand or expectation. They have difficulty believing that others may like them just for themselves. They mistrust caring because they are waiting for the "catch"; the demand. Nurses who expect recognition or social courtesies are often disappointed. They must often work with clients for months without a hello, thank you, eye contact, smile, or verbal response. To demand such appropriate behavior may cause clients to reject further contacts, for they may feel that the expectations of the nurse are unrealistic and not respectful of their needs.

Another barrier to trust is the need-fear dilemma. The client both needs and fears others. The need of others is caused by dependency and the fear of others is caused by the threat of abandonment. Therefore these clients may engage in approach-avoidance behavior. For example, Timmy, a young client, would stand at the door each Monday morning waiting for his nurse-therapist to arrive. The minute she came through the door Timmy would say hello and either pace the floor of the dayroom for the hour or retreat to the bathroom and sleep. As the end of the hour approached, he would come out, see her sitting in their meeting place, and say, "It's 10:30 now and time for you to go." But at the door he would ask her if she was coming back the following week.

The client attempts to deal with the anxiety surrounding relationships by denying the need for others and the fear of separation from them. Lucy, a female client, had been working with a nurse for 3 months and they were developing a close relationship. Lucy suddenly began missing appointments. When the nurse asked her about the absences, Lucy replied, "Oh, it's nothing, I just forgot. I'll be there next time." She continued to miss appointments until she was transferred to another unit. The client was threatened by the closeness of the relationship. She was afraid to trust her ability to form a significant relationship with another human being and feared another disappointment.

The nurse must understand the purpose served by such behavior. Reliability, patience, and perseverance will usually demonstrate to the client that the nurse is sincere and trustworthy. Additionally, the nurse should state her observations about the client behavior so that the issue can be confronted and dealt with in an open way. The content of communication—"Go away leave me alone"—and the behavior that accompanies it are often misleading. The nurse must respond to and comment on *thematic* material that more accurately represents the client's underlying feelings of anxiety and discontent—the feelings which give rise to the distorted communication and behavior. Then, the nurse tries to identify environmental or interpersonal cues that stimulate these feelings, such as having gotten too close to the client. Timmy's nurse-therapist would often say to him, "You've spent the hour in the bathroom today and now you're pacing the floor. I sense that you're feeling uncomfortable about something."

Changes in schedule and anticipated absences should be mentioned in advance so that opportunities for fantasy about abandonment are minimized. Very often, the client will react to anticipated abandonment by initiating the process before it is begun by others. For example, a female client abruptly terminated meetings with her therapist. When asked about her decision, the client said, "My therapists are changed every year, so I figured why wait?"

Testing and manipulation are also components of mistrust. Clients may, for instance, engage in socially unacceptable behavior. One such client in the early stages of the nurse-client relationship would sit and pick his nose. When that didn't ruffle the nurse, he would say, "Go away girl, you do me no good; go away girl." The nurse might have intervened by recognizing the purpose of the message and identifying its theme: "You're wondering if I'm going to stay with you, if I'm really sincere about wanting to spend time with you." Clients need to see that nurses will not be thrown by attempts to drive them away. Then, as trust develops, testing behavior diminishes. The client needs to hear that the nurse will not be destroyed or scared away by clients who fear the effect of their secret hostility and violence on others. For example, Mary, a client, became very aggressive toward others on the unit one morning. She threw chairs around the dayroom and hit and bit everyone in sight, including her nurse. Later, after she had been sedated and was spending time in a quiet room, her nurse appeared for their regular hour. Mary looked up at the nurse as she entered the room and said, "You realize I could have knocked you out?"

The nurse replied, "Yes, Mary, I realize that.

Next time, please come and tell us that you are feeling anxious and out of control. We can help to protect you."

"You still want to be my nurse?"

"Yes, Mary, I want to spend time with you."

Nonverbal clients may manipulate the nurse into an unwitting acceptance of their nonverbal communication. They may exploit the nurse's sympathy by giving the impression that they are too sick to speak. Nurses who work with catatonic clients often find themselves responding to them in similar nonverbal ways. Susan, one such client, usually sat silently curled up in a chair in the corner of the lounge. On approaching the client to spend their daily hour together, the nurse waved hello, motioned for Susan to move her chair aside, and sat down. She did not greet the client verbally or ask her to move over. The rest of the hour was spent in silence.

The nursing intervention is initially directed toward recognition of the process that is occurring between client and nurse and making observations to the client about what has been happening. "Susan, I'm finding myself responding to your gestures with my own nonverbal gestures rather than with words." Then, by verbalizing for the client, the nurse can help the client learn to speak for herself. Fromm-Reichmann describes this process as observing the client's nonverbal behavior and then verbalizing aloud what the client appears to be experiencing.[28] For example, the nurse observes Susan seated in a corner chair, curled up with her knees against her chest. The nurse sits down next to her and tells Susan that she is here for their daily half-hour together. The nurse notices Susan peeking out at her from between her fingers. As soon as Susan makes eye contact with the nurse, she quickly hides her eyes. The nurse observes this behavior and tries to verbalize Susan's thoughts. "You seem to be wondering whether it's safe to be with me, and I guess you haven't quite decided yet." This remark calls for affirmation or denial from the client, which may be given in words and is frequently accompanied by a display of affect. In this instance, the nurse saw a small smile pull at the corners of Susan's mouth while her eyes lifted to meet the nurse's gaze. She said, "Sometimes I never decide." The nurse had (1) acknowledged the manipulation and (2) encouraged the client and herself to utilize more appropriate verbal behavior. In this way the nurse acted as a role model and a bridge for communication, setting kind but firm limits on the continuous nonverbal behavior.

Anxiety

Resistance is the behavioral mode the client uses either consciously or unconsciously to avoid anxiety that is provoked when security operations are challenged. Psychotic clients have elaborate security systems to avoid the disapproval they expect from others, as well as the accompanying anxiety. In the nurse-client relationship, any attempt the nurse makes to help the client clarify problems, explore feelings, or examine relationships with others may be viewed by the client as threatening. Therefore defensive maneuvers will be utilized to ensure self-protection. Low self-esteem, shame, and guilt regarding previous thoughts, feelings, and actions relating to hostility and aggression are a few of the myriad of reasons a client may have for avoiding a discussion of issues with the nurse.[29] Pat, a female client, was initially quite verbal in her sessions with the nurse. She gave, in great detail, information about herself and her family, However, as the relationship progressed and the nurse began focusing on the feelings Pat was experiencing, Pat would not respond, lose eye contact with the nurse, look across the room, or say, "I'm finding it hard to get into this today. I have nothing to say. Let's talk about the barbecue next week." At such times the nurse must help the client to notice what is happening and identify what it is that is frightening, so that resistance can be overcome and they can progress to more authentic levels of experience (see Chap. 6).

Resistance may also be manifested by regression. Some clients who have begun to progress may suddenly again become highly delusional, withdrawn, incontinent, symbolic in their language, and inappropriate in their responses. Other clients will only regress in one area. The client is usually responding to inner or outer pressure to experience reality more completely and is communicating that the therapeutic pace is proceeding too rapidly or that a letup is needed. Maladaptive behavior patterns that have persisted over long periods of time are difficult to dislodge. Clients often need to regress temporarily to a lower but better-integrated level of adjustment in order to reach a firmer basis for improvement.[28] They need to retreat to the safety of their psychosis to consider new feelings, perspectives, and behaviors. This often occurs as clients approach discharge from the treatment setting, but the regression is usually only temporary. *Anxiety* rises regarding the newly planned independence and responsibility. Clients need assistance in identifying what is frightening them, and it is important to convey understanding—through support, flexibility, and acceptance—to them. The clients then feel safe and not abandoned. These periods may require intensive nursing interventions and additional supportive measures such as medication, a special environment, and specific activities.

Low Self-esteem

The nurse may have to spend a great deal of time with a schizophrenic client before realizing the full extent of the client's low self-esteem. The client feels totally unlovable, different from others, and incapable of accomplishment. Intervention must be directed toward creating a climate of acceptance. The nurse may spend time with the client in an undemanding way, listening to the client's communication and responding in a nonjudgmental manner. The nurse needs to indicate that the client's ideas and feeling are not shocking or very different from those of other people. Opportunities should be provided for the client to experience success in interpersonal and task areas. An initial success might consist of no more than 30 minutes during which the client and nurse sit together comfortably in silence. This may not sound like a milestone, but it may be just that for one who has always experienced intense anxiety with other people. The client should gradually be introduced to the company of others, and the nurse can serve as facilitator and role model when engaging the client in such interaction. Respect, attentiveness, and sharing of experience will allow the client to incorporate positive feelings and take a more positive attitude toward the self. Additionally, the nurse must clarify any communication that is not understood. When clients feel misunderstood, their self-esteem declines. The client feels that "If they cared, they'd ask me what I meant and not just say umhmm." (See Chapter 6.)

Opportunities for task mastery should be provided. Movement therapy allows the client to experience the body in positive and negative ways. It provides a vehicle for the expression of feelings without censure. Occupational therapy, recreational therapy, and on-the-ward activities also present opportunities for individualized, graded accomplishment. Positive reinforcement for interpersonal or task accomplishments should be given in a realistic way. Too much praise is often regarded as insincere by the wary client and is incompatible with the client's negative self-concept.

Social Withdrawal

The schizophrenic client has difficulty relating to people, is often lonely, and feels unlovable. Additionally, negative interpersonal experiences from the past are transferred to present situations and thus current relationships are distorted (see Chap. 6). The role of the nurse is to help clients to look at their feelings and perceptions. Dialogue between client and nurse can assist the client in gaining a more objective, reality-oriented view of current relationships. For example:

Nurse: What are your plans after you are discharged?

Pat: There you go again, asking me for specifics, telling me to shape up.

Nurse: I wonder if you've heard this message before from other people in your life.

Pat: You sound just like my father, always on my back, always wanting me to have a plan for what I'm going to do.

Nurse: My asking you about what you were going to do after you leave the hospital reminded you of your father doing the same thing?

Pat: Yes, only he'd never really let *me* make the decision. He'd do it for me before I had a chance.

Nurse: You feel that I'm directing your life in the same way.

Pat: Your saying it reminded me of it so clearly. I can hear his nagging voice. I know, though, that you're not doing that. I know I have to decide what I'm going to do. This time I'll decide what I want to do and what's best for me.

Through this exchange, the nurse helped the client to remove distortions from past relationships that were affecting the current interaction. Pat went on to discuss how past experiences cloud her ability to evaluate people in her current life, and that this was something she would have to watch out for in future situations.

The nurse can also assist the client to gradually enlarge social relationships. This may consist of providing social situations in which the client is comfortable. Relatedness must proceed at a pace which meets client needs. A group walk, a concert, or a play allows for relatedness but does not demand communication. When such clients enter verbal groups, they may initially need permission to participate on a nonverbal level. As anxiety decreases, participation may increase and become more appropriate. The nurse must assess the client's anxiety level and either assist the group in helping the client handle the discomfort or help the client to withdraw from the group without losing face.[30] The nurse acts as a role model for appropriate communication and encourages the client to participate. The client may never enjoy relatedness even after discharge; therefore the client's life may have to be structured to permit minimal interaction. The client may pursue a career and attend parties and meetings but still remain essentially alone, without sustained relationships.

Defining Reality

Because the client has thought disorders and places much autistic meaning and distortion into verbal symbols, it is often difficult for nurses to know how to respond. They should speak clearly and concretely and make meanings as commonplace as possible. This will minimize ambiguities and distortions in communication. For example, let us suppose that the doctor has come onto the unit. He has entered his office, closed the door, and begun to plan his morning interviews with the clients. Mary knocks on the door asking to see the doctor. As the nurse says, "He's busy right now," Mary hears him talking to another nurse about another client saying, "She's getting worse." Mary thinks he was talking about her, turns, and runs from the office crying. The nurse follows her, sits down with her, and attempts to clarify the reality aspects of the situation by saying, "You heard the doctor talking to the nurse. You heard the doctor say something; it got you upset. This happened today outside the nurses office."

The schizophrenic client also has difficulty differentiating between thought, feeling, and action. For example, a client with intensely hostile, murderous feelings toward his wife may believe that he has actually killed her. The nurse must help the client see the reality of the situation: having murderous feelings does not mean that they have been put into action.

Nurse: I know that you have been feeling angry with your wife and believe that she is dead.

Client: She's gone, she's dead.

Nurse: Sometimes people feel angry with others and think about hurting them.

Client: I can see it in my head.

Nurse: Thinking of hurting someone doesn't mean you have actually done it.

(Client looks at nurse silently.)

Nurse: Feeling angry toward another person is not so unusual and it's OK.

The nurse in this situation acknowledges and verbalizes the client's feeling tone and presents the reality of the situation. The nurse indicates the healthy aspects of expressing anger and lets the client know that there is a difference between thought and action; that feelings such as anger do not destroy others. The distorted feelings of omnipotence are thus placed in better perspective and the magical thinking is clarified. The nurse must try to understand the client's private world, what it means, and why the client has retreated into it. When clients see the nurse trying to understand their dilemma, fright, and pain, they become more trusting and confident in the nurse and feel freer to share their perceptions and feelings. The nurse can then act as a bridge for the client in defining reality.

Hallucinations and delusions are very real and usually more vivid than reality-based experiences to the schizophrenic client. During the early or acute stages of schizophrenia, such experiences can be very frightening and may be accompanied by a great deal of anxiety. Many authorities feel that hallucinations and delusions may disappear in the course of therapy as overall anxiety decreases. To directly confront the unreality of psychotic thoughts and feelings is to increase the client's already severe estrangement.

Many chronic schizophrenic clients retain their delusional or hallucinatory thoughts and perceptions and live quite comfortably with them.

Hallucinations

The attitude of the nurse who is interacting with a hallucinating client is very important. It must be accepting and nonjudgmental. Reasoning, arguing, or attempting to prove the client wrong only serve to entrench the hallucinatory perception. However, the nurse should clearly indicate that the client's sensory perceptions are not shared by others; the nurse does not see or hear what the client does and does not evaluate the facts (information) in the same way. The following exchange illustrates the correct approach in responding to such a client:

Nurse: Mr. Jones, you say that you are hearing voices telling you to kick your wife? I understand that this is very real to you, but I do not hear that voice.

(Client looks distressed; frown creases face.)

Nurse: You appear distressed by what you say you hear.

It is important for the nurse not to enter the psychotic world of the client by "going along with the hallucination"; in fact, the nurse should cast doubt on the reality of the hallucination. For example, one client believed that every time she heard an airplane fly overhead, the airplane was telling her to smash windows. The response of a nearby attendant was, "Wait a minute. I'll call the airport and tell the control tower to tone down the planes so you won't have to listen to them telling you this." This response was *nontherapeutic* because it did not help the client to correct her perceptual distortions. It reinforced the client's belief that the plane could "talk" to her. In fact, it would lead the client to believe that the attendant shared this information, so that it has been consensually validated for the client. A more *therapeutic* response would have been to remark, "You say you're hearing noises that make you feel like smashing windows."

Staff must beware of becoming involved in the client's psychotic world. The nurse's nonjudgmental attitude coupled with a different set of data permit the client to look at two sets of information objectively and facilitate the possibility of choice for the client. This provides a safe climate for validating the reality or unreality of the client experience. The nurse should also observe the client's nonverbal behavior. When a client moves his lips or cocks his head to the side in a listening stance, the nurse can tell that the client is hallucinating. The nurse can utilize this observation to elicit a description of the experience and the events that preceded it. The nurse helps the client to make connections between anxiety-producing events and the hallucinations. The following example of a client who had been hospitalized for the third time in a year for an acute schizophrenic reaction will clarify this process:

Mary: Gee, Ms. F, I sure look fine today; I think I'll see the doctor today about going home. I'm ready to take on the world. (States this with a frown on her face and voice trembling.)

Ms. F (Nurse): You're all dressed up today, Mary; you're looking fine . . . you're going out to show everybody. But I see you're frowning. Are you really as ready inside as you look on the outside?

(Client looks off to the other side of the room. Her lips begin moving; she giggles and puts her hand over her mouth.)

Ms. F: Mary, we were talking about your readiness to go home. You suddenly looked away from me and began moving your lips.

Mary: It was Satan again. Whenever I start thinking about feeling good, going, and doing, he's there reminding me that I don't have wings. Maybe I'll just rest awhile longer before I try to fly.

[The client's shaky self-esteem and her underlying anxiety regarding her ability to be independent had clearly risen and called into play the hallucination, which confirmed her basic negative self-appraisal.) The thematic material of low self-esteem needs to be connected to independence, success, and the anxiety surrounding these. The nurse might respond to Mary's last statement by stating, "The voices you say you hear seem to appear when you and I talk about your getting better and living successfully on your own. I'm wondering if you are concerned about being able to do this." Thus, the nurse helps the client focus on the feelings, situations, and/or people in the environment which evoke anxiety and trigger hallucinatory experiences.

Clients who are experiencing hallucinations often feel out of control. The nurse must supply external controls for such clients at certain times. The development of trust is facilitated in clients who feel that the nurse understands and cares enough to prevent them from harming themselves when they are out of control. A client who is hearing voices telling him to jump out the window needs the nurse to say, "We don't want you to do what the voices tell you to do. We won't let them control you. You come to one of us when the voices bother you." Such a client feels more secure knowing that others are supplying the needed controls. Limit setting needs to continue as long as the client is exhibiting out-of-control behavior. Monitored restraints, continuous supervision, a quiet environment, and medication may be adjuncts to verbally stated limits. As anxiety decreases, the client becomes more self-directing and capable of greater self-control.

In dealing with hallucinations, the nurse should also respond verbally to anything real and appropriate in the client's conversation. This will reinforce reality and redirect the client's attention from the hallucination.[31] The nurse can also utilize reality-oriented tasks such as sewing, art work, or folding laundry as a means of involving the schizophrenic client in the real world as readiness is indicated. Nonverbal responses should be avoided, such as shaking one's head or gesturing with one's hands, since these behaviors are ambiguous and may be misinterpreted by the client involved in a hallucination.[18]

Delusions

There are many similarities in working with delusional and hallucinating clients. Although a delusion is a false belief or thought that has no basis in reality, the nurse must initially listen to a description of the client's thoughts to determine the validity of the information before making a nursing diagnosis of delusional thought pattern. Culturally related beliefs are sometimes interpreted by staff as delusional information. Such seemingly farfetched beliefs must be validated with the client and family for accuracy.

The nurse should not attempt to convince the client that the delusion is false and "argue the client out of it." Rational explanations on the part of staff will only make the client adhere more firmly to the belief, and the client often ends up trying to convince the nurse of its legitimacy. Nurses must affirm reality by stating that they do not share the client's belief. For example, a client who believes that the FBI is after him should not be told that he is wrong or that nobody is chasing him. Rather, the nurse should respond to the theme of the message by stating, "Mr. Jones, you say the FBI is after you. I don't have any evidence of that, but this must be a frightening feeling for *you.*"

Delusions usually have symbolic meaning for the client which may exist on an unconscious level. Feelings relating to powerlessness, loss of control, and low self-esteem are converted into delusions via projective coping mechanisms. Consequently, the nurse is most effective when responding to the *feeling tone* or *theme* of the delusion rather than the verbal content. For example, a client who had been hospitalized for 10 years had lost six children in childbirth. Her husband had died and her home was demolished during highway construction. Her delusional thoughts revolved around the removal of her vital organs by bad people. A poor response to this client would be, "Your body looks complete to me." This reply challenges the client's belief. Instead, the nurse could respond, "You're feeling empty inside; lots of what you had or wanted is gone now." This response also shifts the focus of the interaction to a more reality-oriented direction.

The nurse must be aware of (1) the purpose the delusion serves for the client and (2) the underlying need met by the delusion (power, control, self-esteem), so that the nurse can work toward meeting the client's needs in more satisfying, socially acceptable, reality-oriented ways.

The nurse should also focus the client on unambiguous reality-oriented activities that provide opportunities for mastery and positive appraisal which will increase ego strength. If engaged in concrete tasks, the client will have less time to dwell on delusional thoughts. Grandiose clients will want to engage in activities or tasks that may be beyond their current capacity. For them, graduated task accomplishment is more appropriate. Suspicious clients should be involved in activities which provide minimum levels of competition and which prevent them from dominating others. Such clients are always trying to be "one up" on others and cannot tolerate losing. Activities must be provided which will allow them to gain satisfaction without losing face.

Physical Needs

Clients with acute psychosis experience high levels of anxiety, and their reality orientation is poor. Antipsychotic drugs such as the phenothiazines are usually administered to decrease the anxiety and are often effective in reducing psychotic behaviors such as hostility, withdrawal, hallucinations, and delusions. Nursing intervention is directed toward monitoring the effectiveness of the medication regimen, assessing the incidence of side and toxic effects (such as parkinsonian symptoms, skin rashes, photosensitivity), and coordinating periodic laboratory tests. Clients must know what drugs they are receiving and be knowledgeable about the side effects so that they can report them. Providing client education about medications is an ongoing responsibility for the nurse in both inpatient and outpatient settings. (See Chap. 8 for an extensive discussion of psychotropic drugs.)

Because the reality orientation of these clients is generally poor, they often fail to attend adequately to their own grooming, nutrition, and safety. Nursing intervention involves assessing the level of self-care, providing the equipment for self-care, and assisting the client to meet these needs. Direct care such as bathing and dressing is sometimes necessary when the client is in a catatonic stupor. When delusional thoughts make the client suspect that food has been poisoned, the nurse must be prepared to make special adjustments so that adequate nutritional intake is maintained. Such situations provide a good opportunity to meet the clients' most basic needs and provide the positive nurturing experiences that have been absent in their lives. However, dependency should not be fostered. The client is assisted to move gradually toward increased reality orientation and independence in the activities of daily living.

Poor reality orientation, poor judgment, and impulsivity make it necessary to monitor these clients' safety needs closely. Harmful objects should be removed from their environment. Firm limits must be set to protect them from their own impulsiveness. A client who is standing at a window touching the glass should be removed to another area at once, since powerful hallucinatory voices may be telling this client to jump. Touching the glass may be a move toward putting a hand or the body through the glass. Behavior that is out of control represents an increased level of anxiety. Allowing it to continue perpetuates the anxiety cycle. The client becomes terrified and frightened. Therefore, such behavior must be arrested at the earliest possible moment.

The Community

Discharge planning is begun when the client enters the treatment setting. The family is involved in the therapeutic process through family therapy and mutually negotiated treatment goals, and they remain involved throughout the treatment program. Community services need to be identified as potential resources that the client and family can turn to after the client has been discharged.

The Family

The client is an integral part of the family system. Nurturing patterns, communication, roles, and self-concept are developed within the family milieu. The family cooperates in the development and maintenance of psychopathology in one or more members. Removal of one member for treatment and growth disrupts the family's homeodynamic balance. If the identified client is to maintain change and successfully return to the family or negotiate an alternate life-style, all family members must be involved in the therapeutic process. Communication patterns, role designations, family rules, and family myths must be explored, clarified, and changed so that a more effective family interaction pattern can emerge. It is only then that the family system can begin to discard pathological modes of interaction and achieve a healthier level of integration. (See Chap. 11 for an extensive discussion of family therapy.)

Community Resources

Clients come to an outpatient treatment setting for weekly or monthly supportive group therapy sessions. The goal of such groups is to increase and maintain appropriate social functioning and participation. Group therapy gives clients an opportunity to discuss the problems they have encountered in their transition to social responsibilities. The group provides a milieu for receiving feedback regarding the clients' experiences, testing of alternative approaches, and progress in achieving acceptance and social interaction with peers.

The halfway house is a transitional facility for clients who have been hospitalized, who are homeless, or who are best advised not to return to their families. Halfway houses provide the sort of group living that facilitates a graded return to the community. Each resident has a room for which each is personally responsible. In addition, each client has certain responsibilities toward general maintenance of the house. From the halfway house, the client goes to an aftercare center, work, or school. The house provides supervision from a resident counselor as well as a social milieu in which clients can interact.

Clients who have been hospitalized for many years are often unequipped to return to the community without supervision. Apartments which are supervised by a landlord-supervisor are being successfully utilized. The landlord supervises the client in activities of daily living, and gradually the client is encouraged to assume increasing responsibility for the daily routine. The cooperative apartment becomes the person's home, for often these clients are homeless after many years of hospitalization. The cost of such living facilities is far lower than that of hospitalization or life in a halfway house.

People within the community are trained as paraprofessionals to assist clients in dealing with activities of daily living following discharge. This is most appropriate intervention for those clients who are not returning to a structured setting such as a halfway house or cooperative apartment. Living alone or within the family, the client can turn to a resource person for help on an as-needed basis. This facilitates the movement of the client away from the hospital and back to the community.[32]

Primary Prevention

A great deal of research is being conducted relating to the identification of "high risk" children, that is, children either or both of whose parents have had a schizophrenic episode. Outreach programs designed to find such families are very important. Following identification, such families are candidates for a variety of mental health programs:

1 Parent education classes to enhance parental knowledge and effective nurturing patterns.
2 Community health programs which work with schools, teachers, and other social agencies to effectively anticipate and deal with problems as they arise.
3 Programs that work with children in meaningful ways within the family when exacerbations in parental coping patterns occur. Children can be helped to understand the parents' absence so that fantasy, magical thinking, and guilt are minimized.

Identification of social conditions and problems within the community that contribute to the incidence of mental illness is another area of primary prevention. Crowding, inadequate housing, poverty, unemployment, poor nutrition, substance abuse, and delinquent behavior are among issues that need to be priority items for social intervention. Delineating "pockets" of illness within a community can lead to a reorganization of mental health workers to act as a first line of defense for education, case finding, and treatment.

Evaluation

The effectiveness of nursing intervention can be determined by changes in client thoughts, affect, and behavior. The nursing staff must compare the behavioral outcomes to the goals formulated in the care plan. The behaviors exhibited by the client should reflect the achievement of the goals. For example, social isolation should become less intense, although it may never disappear. The client who has experienced intense loneliness during a psychotic episode may feel less estrangement from others and may show this in a willingness to reach out and initiate social interaction. Although a gap between self and others may still be felt, it is not experienced as an insurmountable chasm.

References

1 Basic Systems Inc.: "Anxiety: Recognition and Intervention: Programmed Instruction," *American Journal of Nursing*, vol. 15, pp. 129–152, September 1965.

2 Sigmund Freud: *The Problem of Anxiety*, Norton, New York, 1936.

3 Harry Stack Sullivan: "The Meaning of Anxiety in Psychiatry and in Life," *Psychiatry*, vol. 11, pp. 1–13, 1948.

*4 Dorothea R. Hays: "Teaching a Concept of Anxiety to Patients," *Nursing Research*, vol. 10, pp. 108–113, Spring 1961.

*5 Hildegard E. Peplau: "A Working Definition of Anxiety," in Shirley F. Burd and Margaret A. Marshall (eds.), *Some Clinical Approaches to Psychiatric Nursing*, Macmillan, New York, 1963, pp. 323–327.

6 Karl Menninger: *The Vital Balance*, Viking, New York, 1964.

7 Hildegard E. Peplau: "Process and Concept of Learning," in Shirley F. Burd and Margaret A. Marshall (eds.), *Some Clinical Approaches to Psychiatric Nursing*, Macmillan, New York, 1963, pp. 333–336.

*Recommended reference by a nurse author.

*8 Shirley F. Burd: "Effects of Nursing Intervention in Anxiety of Patients," in Shirley F. Burd and Margaret A. Marshall (eds.), *Some Clinical Approaches to Psychiatric Nursing*, Macmillan, New York, 1963, pp. 307–322.

9 Harry Stack Sullivan: *The Interpersonal Theory of Psychiatry*, Norton, New York, 1953.

10 Norman Cameron: *Personality Development and Psychopathology*, Houghton Mifflin, Boston, 1963.

11 C. D. Wise and L. Stein: "Dopamine β-hydroxylase Deficits in the Brains of Schizophrenic Patients," *Science*, vol. 181, pp. 344, 1973.

12 J. Chapman: "Early Symptoms of Schizophrenia," *British Journal of Psychiatry*, vol. 112, pp. 225–251, 1966.

13 Gregory Bateson et al.: "Toward a Theory of Schizophrenia," *Behavioral Science*, vol. 1, October 1956, pp. 251–264.

14 *Diagnostic and Statistical Manual of Mental Disorders*, 2d ed., American Psychiatric Association, Washington, D.C., 1968.

15 Gloria Oden: "An Outline of the Normal Thought Process," in Shirley F. Burd and Margaret A. Marshall (eds.), *Some Clinical Approaches to Psychiatric Nursing*, Macmillan, New York, 1963, pp. 3–10.

16 Silvano Arieti: *Interpretation of Schizophrenia*, Bruner, New York, 1955.

17 Katherine H. Gravenkemper: "Hallucinations," in Shirley F. Burd and Margaret A. Marshall (eds.), *Some Clinical Approaches to Psychiatric Nursing*, Macmillan, New York, 1963, pp. 184–188.

*18 Sylvia T. Schwartzman: "The Hallucinating Patient and Nursing Intervention," *Journal of Psychiatric Nursing and Mental Health Services*, vol. 13, November–December 1975, pp. 23–36.

*19 Janice Clack: "An Interpersonal Technique for Handling Hallucinations," in *Nursing Care of the Disoriented Patient*, Monograph 13, The American Nurses' Association, New York, pp. 16–26.

20 Barbara K. Dixson: "Intervening When the Patient Is Delusional," *Journal of Psychiatric Nursing and Mental Health Services*, vol. 7, pp. 25–34, January–February 1969.

21 Harry Stack Sullivan: *Clinical Studies in Psychiatry*, Norton, New York, 1956.

22 Alfred M. Freedman, M.D., Harold I. Kaplan, M.D., and Benjamin J. Sadock (eds.), *Comprehensive Textbook of Psychiatry*, 2d ed., Williams & Wilkins, Baltimore, 1975.

23 Hildegard E. Peplau: "Loneliness," *American Journal of Nursing,* vol. 55, pp. 1476–1481, December 1955.

24 Donald L. Burnham, Arthur I. Gladstone, and Robert W. Gibson: *Schizophrenia and the Need-Fear Dilemma,* International Universities Press, New York, 1969.

*25 Gwen E. Tudor Will: "A Sociopsychiatric Nursing Approach to Intervention in a Problem of Mutual Withdrawal on a Mental Hospital Ward," *Perspectives in Psychiatric Care,* vol. 8, pp. 11–35, 1970.

26 David Raskin: "Problems in the Therapeutic Community," *American Journal of Psychiatry,* vol. 128, no. 4, pp. 124–125, October 1971.

27 Theodore Van Putten: "Milieu Therapy: Contraindications?" *Archives of General Psychiatry,* vol. 29, November 1973, pp. 640–643.

28 Frieda Fromm-Reichman: *Principles of Intensive Psychotherapy,* University of Chicago Press, Chicago, 19

*29 Alice Stueks: "Resistance" in Shirley F. Burd and Margaret A. Marshall (eds.), *Some Clinical Approaches to Psychiatric Nursing,* Macmillan, New York, 1963, pp. 96–104.

30 Jurgens Ruesch and Gregory Bateson: *Communication—The Social Matrix of Society,* Norton, New York, 1968.

31 Jeanette P. Grosicki and Marguerite Harmonson: "Nursing Action Guide: Hallucinations," *Journal of Psychiatric Nursing and Mental Health Services,* vol. 7, May–June 1969, pp. 133–135.

32 Ann Wolbert Burgess and Aaron Lazare: *Psychiatric Nursing in the Hospital and the Community,* 2d ed., Prentice-Hall, Englewood Cliffs, N.J., 1976.

15
The Client Who Generates Fear

Eugenia McAuliffe Kelly

Learning Objectives

After studying this chapter, the student should be able to:

1 List four precursive signals to violent and assaultive behavior
2 List five environmental factors that perpetuate violence in our society
3 Describe how assaultive and/or homicidal behavior can result from
    a a psychotic state
    b an organic condition
    c a depressive state
4 Design a plan of intervention to control a client's assaultive behavior with attention to
    a use of medication
    b use of restraints
    c role of the police
    d need for hospitalization
5 Design a plan of care for a day-hospital client who "acts out" in an assaultive manner, with attention to issues for discussion in psychotherapy, setting limits, activity program, and alternate ways to express aggressive energies

To understand the client who generates fear in others, it is necessary to know something about fear. Human beings are afraid of many things, depending on their perception of external reality and their sensitivity, based on prior experience, to this reality. For example, most people are afraid of explosives, but not everyone is afraid of mice. Thus, fear can be a very personal experience for nurses as they care for clients; its extent depends on what fears they have as people and what they perceive as "fearful" in the client. In this chapter, we will deal with the fear that is common to all human beings: the fear of death or bodily harm from violence or threatened loss of control.

The threat of death or bodily harm is felt with clients who are assaultive or homicidal or who "act out" in a violent fashion. The violence may be deliberate, as in premeditated homicide, or it may occur because the client loses control over aggressive impulses. Fear is also felt with clients who act out impulsively and aggressively to get their needs met without considering the consequences of their behavior for others.

It is important to distinguish between aggression and violence. Aggression is a natural drive in human beings. Under the direction of the ego, the aggressive drive can be channeled into higher-level productive activity (sublimation) which helps us to master other animal species, control the environment, and achieve goals in industry, commerce, and science. In times of threat, aggressive instincts directed by the ego enable us to protect ourselves even to the point of killing others. The aggressive drive is both a motivating force and an enabling power. When aggressive instincts are not sublimated, molded, and controlled in the service of life and growth, they can very easily be used to do harm and wreak destruction. The aggressive drive can be used deliberately in the service of violence. For example, it can be used to kill, injure,

plunder, rape, assault, and abuse other human beings. All people are born with a natural instinct for aggression; it is through learning and socialization that this instinct is turned toward constructive or destructive goals. *There is no instinctual-survival need for men to act violently towards men. . . .* All acts of violence are learned. It is not only the when and how to kill in a homicide which are learned, *the act itself is socially conditioned, rationally defined.*"[1]

Aggression is a natural drive for human beings, but how one uses the drive is learned. Violence is the expression of the aggressive drive in the service of destruction. This destructive expression is something one learns, just as the constructive use of aggression is learned. Violence can be learned directly through exposure and imitation or indirectly when one is not taught to channel aggressive impulses constructively. Some people who learn violent ways of acting feel guilty about their behavior. Others do not. Since humanity has generally been more violent in the past, working against the violent use of aggression continues to be a personal and evolutionary struggle—one which is thought to be pivotal in striving for mental health. "In our present evolutionary state man is struggling to control the aggressive impulses that are still within him. This struggle . . . is one of the greatest causes of tension,"[2] and it can be the most powerful catalyst for growth. There remains some pessimism as to whether humanity will ever conquer the violent expression of aggression. But Sherwood and Harding[3] point out that language is not the only thing people learn easily. "We have a biology that allows us to control rage and the degree to which humans are able to control this emotion is remarkable when we look at nonhuman primates."

The author acknowledges the assistance of Dr. Lewis Glickman, Chief of Psychiatry Consultation Service at Kings County Hospital, Brooklyn, New York, in the preparation of the sections of this chapter entitled "Psychophysiology of Client Behavior" and "Nursing Intervention."

Selected Client Behaviors

Clients can generate fear in others by being assaultive or homicidal. They can arouse fear through violent behavior or threats of violence.

Clients can generate fear whether the assaultive or homicidal behavior is deliberate and calculated or when it results from the loss of control. As far as health professionals are concerned, assaultive behavior is primarily the result of (1) a psychotic state, (2) an organic condition, or (3) some depressive state. But assaultive behavior can also be (4) a way of acting out. The term "acting out" refers to a life-style in which actions tend to be impulsive and not adapted to reality. Actions are aimed at relieving unconscious tensions without consideration of the effect on others and without an attendant sense of guilt over the consequences.[4]

The violence of the client classified as assaultive or homicidal is deliberate and destructive in intent; it stems from the client's perception of real or imagined threats. Clients in the acting-out group use violence as a way of getting their needs met immediately. The assault or killing is merely the most expedient way of achieving this, and the "conscience" or superego is not strong enough to restrain the violent behavior. Many members of this group are also considered criminals by society because their behavior runs counter to the law. Thus caretakers in correctional facilities may see more of these people than do the nurses in health-care settings. Clients who act out in an assaultive manner in psychiatric settings represent only 2 percent of psychiatric clients. However, caretakers spend much more than 2 percent of their time in coping with the threat of danger that these clients present.

Psychophysiology of Client Behaviors

People use assaultive behavior primarily to protect the self against a real or imagined danger. Where the threat is objectively real, we do not have much difficulty in understanding assaultiveness. An example of this would be the violent behavior that is seen during natural disasters such as fires, floods, and hurricanes. However, the thought processes of psychotics are so disordered that thought, feeling, and behavior are not connected in a logical fashion. Those interacting with the psychotic client cannot validate the client's subjective reality or predict the associated behavior. The client's need to protect the self is based on a personal or autistic perception of danger which is often difficult to understand (see Chap. 14).

Acute attacks of paranoia are psychotic episodes which can result from a functional mental disorder or from an organic brain syndrome. These clients represent the greatest danger to others. The pattern of thought is projective and leads to the development of delusions which are usually persecutory in nature (see Chap. 14). In this disorder, reality testing is impaired. If it remains uncorrected, the delusions persist, causing the client to perceive the environment as hostile and destructive. The client then becomes assaultive in an effort to protect the self. In episodes of acute paranoia, there are often unfamiliar visual and auditory hallucinations; these are confusing and frightening to the client, who is unable to test the external reality. Hallucinations that are bizarre, cruel, or commanding cause the client to see reality as dangerous; thus he or she is forced to use assaultive acts to protect the self.

Since the client is often unable to communicate his or her uniquely personal perceptions of danger, health personnel may have only vague hints of the impending violent behavior. The most reliable are (1) increase in psychomotor activity and rapidly expanding body space which communicates the need for distance; (2) intensity of affect; (3) verbalization of delusional thinking, especially that which is threatening; (4) hallucinations that are threatening, new, commanding in nature, or in any way upsetting; (5) prior history of violent behavior when under stress.

Clients may also suffer from defective thinking and impaired reality testing due to organic or toxic physical states. Such a mental condition is called an organic brain syndrome. These clients may resort to violent behavior in an effort to protect themselves, as in the psychotic group. In this group, there is the added problem of disorientation of time, place, and/or person, and there is a much higher incidence of visual hallucinations. Organic states are particularly dangerous because they may come on without warning. Often there is no prior history available of either organicity or assaultive behavior. Intervention must be immediate. In the organic group, in particular, the client may not be able to communicate either the fear of being harmed or the impending loss of control. Therefore, health personnel must be especially on guard for assaultive behavior in the groups discussed in the following paragraphs. (See Chap. 35.)

Epileptics may suddenly become violent at the beginning of a seizure. However, these attacks tend to be less dangerous than those suffered by clients who are not diagnosed as epileptic but who have "seizure equivalents" that is, disorganized discharges of energy leading to unprovoked fights.

Clients with metabolic or endocrine imbalances, including high fevers, will be toxic to the point where the physiology required for logical thinking is impaired. Some of these may indeed become assaultive, especially if they have been violent under stress in the past.

Client with space-occupying lesions, including brain tumors, may have violent episodes. These episodes may be difficult to understand, especially if the brain tumor's growth has been insidious. If such a client has had a lifelong tendency to be explosive as well as a prior history of unexplained violence, the current, organically based explosive behavior may be misunderstood. Keep in mind that any organic brain syndrome causes, among other things, an extension or magnification of preexisting behavior trends.

The person in either impending or full-blown delirium tremens (alcohol withdrawal syndrome) is always assaultive and belligerent. Clients in drug withdrawal or those who are coming out of a drug overdose (especially barbiturates) are also violent and assaultive due to the irritability of the central nervous system.

Clients prone to depressive states may become violent and assaultive or even, on occasion, homicidal in an attempt to release some of their pent-up rage and thus relieve their depression. Such situations are more unpredictable and hence dangerous if the depression is associated with psychosis. Depressed individuals are often abusers of alcohol and addictive drugs. Their defenses against rage are often lifted temporarily by these substances, especially alcohol, leading them to become belligerent, assaultive, homicidal, and/or suicidal (see Chap. 17). In 1975, it was estimated that in more than 50 percent of all murders committed, either the victim or the perpetrator had been drinking. Depressed mothers may inflict physical abuse on their children while drinking and may be irritable with them when "hung over." (See Chap. 34.)

Other clients who may elicit fear through their violent and assaultive behavior are those who act out in a violent fashion. These people often manifest dysfunctional behavior patterns called *character disorders*. (See Chap. 17.) This term refers to lifelong syndromes of behavior which require long-term, consistent therapeutic intervention to be changed.

Fenichel[4] defines *acting-out characters* as "those in whom transference . . . is extrordinarily strong; the patients repeatedly perform acts or undergo experiences, identical or very similar ones, that represent unconscious attempts to get rid of old instinctual conflicts (such as rage at the parent), to find a belated gratification of repressed impulses, or at least to find relief from some inner tension." For these persons the environment is only an arena in which to stage their internal conflicts. Common to all acting-out characters is their impulsive haste to get their needs met and their lack of any guilt feelings for the consequences of their behavior.

Among people with character disorders, those that can evoke fear in others are the paranoid personality, the antisocial personality (criminals, addicts), and the explosive personality. All these people have strong security and dependency needs along with an inadequately developed conscience or superego. They often go out and aggressively take what they want or discharge rage and frustration in assaultive and murderous ways.

Fenichel[4] points out that acting-out characters are not happy "narcissistic psychopaths" who can get all their demands gratified. They are people who have not had lasting object relationships in early childhood or whose relationships were so traumatic that their development was arrested, making the complete and definite establishment of the superego or conscience impossible. For example, the parental figures may have changed in such rapid succession that there was no time or opportunity to develop lasting relationships and identifications or to internalize ideas of right and wrong. Or the parenting ones may have been so abusive that all experiences were frustrating and the child developed rage reactions. Such children would come to accept the parents' behavior—internalize the parents' rage and destructive aggression as "normal." The resulting ambivalent attitudes of love and hate toward the parents would then, later on, be acted out violently in relation to others. "The superego is not lacking but is incomplete or pathological, and the reactions of the ego to the pathological superego reflect the ambivalences and contradictions which these persons felt toward their first objects."[4] Some people do feel a degree of remorse after violent behavior, but others have never internalized the wrongness of the destructive use of aggression and hence either do not experience guilt or displace the guilt onto something other than the self.

Worthy of special mention are violence-prone children,[5] usually from our big cities, some of whom have already committed homicide. These young people of grammar- and junior-high-school age are categorized as "juveniles" but are capable of killing and inflicting severe physical harm. The psychoanalysis of juvenile delinquents gives examples of distorted relations toward the superego. These are comprehensible in terms of childhood history characterized by (1) a frequent change of milieu, (2) a loveless or inconsistent environment, and (3) a resolution of the Oedipus complex which was disorganized, weak, and inconsistent.[4] Some of these youths simply have never learned to develop object relationships. They need to be considered separately owing to

their unfinished, incomplete psychological development (see Chap. 5).

Nurse (and Staff) Response to Client and/or Family Behavior

The nurse's response to client behavior is based on the nurse's perceptions, thoughts, and feelings in response to given stimuli. The client who is violent or about to become violent is a given stimulus. The nurse perceives the threat of violence via the senses: eyes, ears, skin, and "gut reactions." When a client has suddenly begun to pace and to mumble angrily, the nurse senses that the client is behaving strangely, that people nearby may be in danger, or that the client may be self-destructive. Nurses will assess this potential for danger not only on the basis of the perceived external reality but also in terms of their prior experience. Thus, nurses who have seen these warning signs before will sense danger more quickly.

After the perception and thought have been formed, there is an attendant feeling. The first and universal feeling the nurse or anyone will experience is *fear*. As discussed, the threat of death or bodily harm elicits fear in all human beings. There is nothing weak or shameful in this. This natural feeling state of fear, once recognized and accepted, can be used as an effective danger signal when violence may be impending. Since an individual cannot remain in a state of fear, the feeling will be converted into another state that permits action. The degree to which nurses can feel fear and understand what it is signaling will affect their ability to take action.

Fear gives way to *anger* or to continued fear, which leads to *flight* or to *vigilance*. Anger will be a response in many situations of threatened violence, depending on the degree of danger. Persistent fear is often the response where the threat is strong and immediate and the nurse does not feel adequate to meet the threat and effect some controls. In such cases, there is a decided impulse to run away in an attempt at self-protection. Vigilance is the response that would be expected from health professionals, since this response allows for better definition of the threatening situation and formulation of a plan of intervention—either by the nurse or with the assistance of others under the nurse's direction.

Of special significance is the fear that is transformed into anger or rage. Such a reaction is common and is seen when caretakers use provocative behavior that generates assaultiveness in patients. This sets up some common countertransference problems (see Chap. 6), especially where the nurse and staff have to manage the violent client over a longer period of time (e.g., inpatient psychiatric wards, day hospitals, chronic-care facilities, residential treatment settings, prisons). King[1] points out that countertransference responses are an integral part of staff reactions to a client and are inevitable. However, they need to be as limited as possible and should be used to understand and work with the patient's emotional problems. The following are three common countertransference problems:

Rejection This is different from running away. It refers to a rage-helpless reaction which pushes nurses to rid themselves of the violent client.

Wish to Punish This reaction in the staff is prompted by the defiant, remorseless, threatening attitude of the client. The staff wish to punish the client by taking away privileges or conveniences, by locking the client up, or even by sending the client away (banishment).

Appeasement and Identification This happens when there is periodic, temporary integration of the violent person, who attempts to conform and cooperate. This leads the staff to take on an appeasing stance lest the client again become violent. Concessions that are blatantly out of keeping with the client's adjustment goals are made. There is also a problem when staff members regard their clients' aggression as a form of healthy machismo.

The ability to intervene in violent or assaultive behavior depends on a sensitive awareness of one's own perceptions and of one's usual response pattern. Until nurses understand their feelings and responses and use them as helpful cues in life-threatening situations, they will never be effective in designing and implementing plans for intervention. Because their fear will persist, their actions will be aimed at fleeing from the client. The client's behavior will not be dealt with, and there is nothing so dangerous as a potentially violent client to whom no one is paying attention.

Not everyone has the makeup or experience needed to work with violent clients, and nurses should know whether they can handle these situations or not. "Those believed to be potentially dangerous should be dealt with by mental health professionals who have had considerable exposure to the behavior of patients and particular training in handling highly disturbed people."[6] Thus medical and nursing staff in emergency rooms or on the wards of general hospitals should not hesitate to call the psychiatrist and psychiatric nurse-clinician for assistance with assaultive patients. All health professionals, including psychiatric staff, should feel comfortable in calling for police assistance and supervising the police in the plan of care.

Assessment of Present Environmental Factors

Nurses are continuously involved in the job of keeping clients from becoming assaultive or intervening when there is violent behavior. Nurses are also concerned with helping parents to socialize small children in nonviolent ways. Nurses are concerned about the safety of society at the hands of violent and potentially violent criminals. Nurses work in correctional facilities and residential treatment settings to teach clients new ways of coping to replace impulsive, violent, and homicidal acting out. However, the client, the child, the citizen, and the prisoner live in a community or must return to a community. This community must be considered because it so often condones, supports, and creates breeding grounds for continued rage and violence. Certain factors and situations exist in our environment which contribute to the perpetuation of violence and violent behavior. These factors cause frustration to build up, and many people either lack outlets whereby to discharge their aggressive energy or have never learned how to channel it in constructive ways. Moreover, there certainly exist in our society models for the destructive channeling of aggression. This combination—the buildup of frustration with either no outlets or unacceptable outlets for the constructive expression of aggression—serves to perpetuate violent behavior.

Marriages are breaking up and youngsters becoming the products of divorce and broken homes[8] more often than ever before, while children from broken homes or even some that are "intact" are often victims of child abuse or neglect. Frustrated parents with "poorly modified sadistic impulses" use the child for their own "aggressive gratification."[9] Often, these children in turn become abusive adults. The extent to which the violence that is shown on television affects the behavior of children is a question that is still being studied by the Surgeon General's Office. Already we see an increase in violent behavior in "aggression-prone children," i.e., those from broken homes and high-crime areas and those with abusive parents. Moreover, children aged 3 to 12 often watch as much as six hours of TV a day.[10]

During the last decade, many young people rebelled against the prevailing culture, tried to change it, and finally suffered disillusion. These events will have their effect on society, but the long-range adaptations of those who attempted to free themselves from the "confused ideologies" of the 1960s by becoming part of a "counterculture" of new myths or adopting the "passive entertainment of drugs" are still unclear.[11] Economic inequities which followed the boom of the sixties have tightened the job market and negatively affected the health and welfare agencies. There has been a corresponding increase in crime. Violence means survival. Shooting, stealing, fighting, and over-powering buy time from being killed, robbed, assaulted, or starved. Frustration leads to aggression. Exploitation leads to fruitless rage. The total social context gives a specific frustration its devastating power.[7]

Nursing Diagnosis

It is important for the nurse to know how to intervene in a client's violent behavior when it is already in progress. It is equally important to be able to predict that a client is about to act violently and to take steps to interrupt this. It is not difficult to make a nursing diagnosis of violent and assaultive behavior that is already going on. The skill comes in assessing those clients who are about to lose control and in intervening before they do. With regard to those clients who have a history of violent outbursts, the skill lies in knowing at what point and under what conditions they will lose control.

In order to make a nursing diagnosis of impending dangerous behavior, the nurse needs to have an array of tools. Some of these tools will be derived from a variety of theories and some will come from experience. But an invaluable tool and one not to be underestimated is the nurse's perception of signals of impending violence, many of which come from what are called gut feelings or intuitions. The personnel with the greatest success in dealing with asaultive clients are those with highly developed perceptual antennae for picking up signs of impending danger. There are various observations that may impinge on one's gut feelings before they are integrated by the brain, and these should be given the utmost attention by the nurse. An example is the feeling that a client seems to have or actually does have a hair-trigger temper or a chip on the shoulder. Again, where the nurse has a sense of having to "walk on eggs" around a client or where a client has to be "handled with kid gloves," the nurse should take this as a signal for danger.

Besides the help a nurse will get from personal intuition, there are other guidelines to assist in diagnosing possible loss of control in a client. For example, it is held that the incidence of violent behavior is greater in some places than in others. Such areas include emergency rooms of general hospitals, intensive-care units, scenes of accidents or natural disaster including war, scenes of crimes, barrooms and taverns, jails and prisons, and acute inpatient psychiatric units. Here there is a greater risk of violence because of the higher incidence of stress, disordered thinking, abnormal organic states, and opportunities for acting out. The possibility of violence should be kept in mind and anticipated in these areas because, as West[12] points out, there are four immediate causes of violent behavior:

1 Alcohol or drug intoxication
2 Criminal activity related to the desire to obtain addictive drugs
3 Acute episodes of functional mental disorders such as paranoia or agitated depression
4 Acute physical illness or brain injury, including delirium tremens

When any of these factors arises in one of the previously listed areas, the possibility that assaultive or homicidal behavior will occur is greatly increased. It is not enough for the nurse to know the locations and circumstances most commonly associated with violence. The nurse must also be able to assess the degree of potential violence in a particular person at a given moment for the purpose of preventing the outburst and/or restoring control. Table 15-1 identifies six criteria or cues which can help nurses to predict when assaultive behavior may occur in a particular client.

Where any of these six criteria applies, the nurse can diagnose a potentially assaultive client. The next step is to determine just how dangerous the client is or will become. The more sudden the change in behavior and the more signs present, the more out of control the client is or will become. It goes without saying that once there is a violent or potentially violent situation, health personnel must take steps to return the client to control and/or to prevent further loss of control. To ensure safety, they must be one step ahead of the client. The following case is an example of a client's loss of control. A 42-year-old woman became belligerent on a medical ward, heard doctors "plotting" outside the door "to get rid of me," and refused to eat because "the food was poisoned." Her daughter denied any previous similar behavior. Soon after, laboratory studies revealed a BUN (blood urea nitrogen) of 54, which would account for the increasing confusion and belligerence.

Planning Nursing Care and Intervention

In the interests of prevention, nurses must think about the kinds of clients for whom they will be caring. They must be aware of child abuse, through which children learn violence at first hand from parents and guardians. (In studies of assaultive criminals, a very great percentage were found to be victims of child abuse; see Chap. 36). Less significant but worthy of note is the connection between criminal violence and deformities, scars, and other physical defects. The dynamics vary, but in general there is a higher incidence of violent acting out among the deformed and scarred. Finally, children in our society are generally not taught to respect nonviolence. The popular concept of *machismo* and the approval of warfare show where the society's values lie.

The immediate goals of nursing intervention in relation to assaultive or homicidal clients are (1) to prevent further loss of control and (2) to restore control in clients already behaving in a violent and/or assaultive manner. The long-range goal of nursing care is to remedy early manifestations of violent behavior, especially in children, and to try to correct longstanding habits of violence in clients of any age. Once the nurse has determined that the client is potentially violent, the following recommendations for intervention apply:[12]

1 Be aware of precursive signs—especially agitation, threatening verbalizations and gestures, sudden signs of organicity, the presence of drugs and/or alcohol—and use them as an index to monitor whether the patient is regaining or further losing control.

Table 15-1 Criteria for Assessing Assaultive Behavior

Criterion	Behavior	Comment
1 Increase in motor agitation	1 Pacing 2 Inability to sit still 3 Sudden cessation of motor activity	1-2 These are attempts to discharge aggression via large muscle activity. 3 The stillness is uncomfortable, like the "calm before a storm."
2 Threatening verbalizations or gestures toward real or imagined objects	1 Retaliation toward actual persons who are seen as threats 2 Aggressiveness in response to threatening visual or auditory hallucinations 3 Aggressiveness in response to expansion of delusional thinking	 2 Such hallucinations are bizarre, threatening, unfamiliar, or confusing. Many psychotics do live comfortably with an entourage of *familiar* "voices." 3 The degree of violence is related to how desperately client perceives the need to protect the self.
2 Intensification of affect	1 Very tense expression 2 Jumpiness 3 Elated expression	1-3 Such intensification indicates loss of control, especially if accompanied by laughing.
4 Prior history of assaultive behavior	1 Has acted assaultively in the past 2 Has been violent under stress in the past 3 Has never been assaultive in the past	1-2 One who has used violence in the past is likely to do so again. 3 One who has never been violent and suddenly becomes so may be suffering from organic illness.
5 Use of alcohol or addictive drugs	1 Intoxication with drugs or alcohol 2 Withdrawal from drugs or alcohol	1 Client can act out rage with inhibitions dissolved. 2 Violence is due to irritability of the central nervous system.
6 Presence of acute organic brain syndrome	1 Sudden rise or fall in level of consciousness 2 Disorientation as to time, place, person 3 Impairment of recent memory 4 Auditory hallucinations within the psychic horizon (i.e., within earshot) 5 Visual hallucinations without drug involvement 6 Abnormal muscle movements such as tics, jerks, tremors, asterixis	1 Sense of time is lost first. 2 Especially significant where no memory impairment existed before. 3 Such are heard coming from under the bed or outside the door. "Voices" out of earshot, as the voice of God or sounds from another planet, indicate functional mental disorder. 4 These are rarely functional in our culture except in religious people. 5 These are significant only where none existed before.

For example, a client on the medical ward may at first express general suspicion of all hospital personnel and gradually, with treatment, complain only about those who are not wearing white. There is still a potential for violence, but it has been diluted.

2 Reduce stimuli by withdrawing from the environment any object or person which appears to frighten the patient. Get the client into an area where there are fewer people and less noise, light, activity, etc.

3 Allow distance between the client and the examiner. Examiners should explain who they are by giving a name and position; the client should be called by his or her full name (Mr. Smith, Mrs. Jones), though the first name may

be used if the client appears frightened. Nicknames are to be avoided. It is most helpful for the health professional to be further identified by a uniform or at least a name tag. It is not uncommon for a nurse in uniform to be able to get closer to a violent client than a doctor in street clothes would be able to do. In addition, clients who tend to use paranoid coping mechanisms relate better to staff of the opposite sex, especially where physical contact must be made. This is because people suffering from paranoia fear attack or intrusion from outside, often in the form of homosexual attack. Physical contact by a staff member of the same sex can be interpreted by the client as a homosexual overture, and this heightens the potential for homosexual panic. Such panic, in turn, increases the risk of violent acting out. If a female nurse must give an injection to a paranoid female client, a male staff member should be in attendance to communicate protection.

4 Give assurance to clients by explaining what is happening, telling them that they will be safe and asking them whether they have any questions. Express an attitude of helpfulness and calm. Under no circumstances allow a power struggle to develop between the client and the staff. If such a conflict has developed, make every effort to acquiesce to the client provided that it is safe to do so. For example, give the client a choice of sitting in a chair or lying in bed, provided that the client stays in a certain room. If the client's demands pose risks, explain these to the client.

5 Like those who threaten suicide, those who threaten violence must be taken seriously. If a client expresses a fear of committing a violent act, estimate the seriousness of the danger and initiate steps to avert it; e.g., remove weapons or objects that could be used in a destructive fashion. It is important to note here that client confidentiality does not extend to situations where the client may be dangerous to others. If the nurse learns that a client has a gun at home and has been having impulses to kill someone, it is the nurse's responsibility to notify the psychiatrist. They will then decide together whether to hospitalize the client and/or ask the police to arrest the client.

6 Whenever a client shows signs of impending assaultive behavior, every effort should be made to find the cause and correct it. However, while this search is taking place, the potentially violent client should be prevented from becoming overtly violent. In addition to the steps already recommended, sedation should be considered. For example, a 72-year-old woman had become suspicious of staff on a medical floor and was about to assault anyone who came near her. It was discovered that she was experiencing cerebral anoxia due to a hemoglobin of 6 g. In order to correct the low hemoglobin with a blood transfusion, she had to be sedated with chlorpromazine until she would permit the staff to come close enough to begin the transfusion.

When the nurse has a client who is overtly violent, more immediate and stringent intervention is recommended in the following five steps:[12] First, as pointed out before, health personnel should never attempt contact with a violent client alone. Get immediate emergency help, preferably from people trained in the techniques of restraint, such as trained psychiatric attendants or police. Professional staff not trained in the use of restraint should keep away from the client and supervise the emergency help from the sidelines. No one should approach an overtly violent client alone, not even the psychiatric attendants or the police. If professionals want to make an impact on the client prior to the arrival of the police, they can enter in numbers of three or more by way of a "show of force."

It is important to note that the nurse should never hesitate to call on the police to restrain a violent client. Since the need to act assaultively comes from a real or imagined loss of inner control on the client's part, the client often calms down just at the sight of a number of blue uniforms representing external control. In fact, to a confused client, a blue uniform is often more understandable and reassuring than a white one. "At their best, policemen appear to respond well when confronted with persons they can clearly identify as sick and in need of help."[6] However, mental health personnel should never leave the restraint of a violent client up to the police entirely. "Whenever the authority of the police is required in dealing with an aggressive patient, a mental health professional should also take part in the procedure. There should be a close and friendly relationship between the emergency service and the police through which the information and experience of each can become known to and appreciated by the other."[6] Police use various techniques in restraining a violent person, from "talking the person down" to body contact, cloth restraints, and handcuffs. They use what they feel is necessary for safety until the client calms down naturally or with the help of medication. Nurses should collaborate with the police on the methods they select.

Second, if clients do not quickly calm down by their own efforts, medication will probably be necessary. The nurse must make this assessment and call the physician to further evaluate the client and to order sedation. The mental hygiene law in most states is quite specific about how long a patient may legally be restrained. (See Table 15-2.) Most laws stipulate that restraints may be applied if the client is a danger to self or others, but this "danger" must be reevaluated every few hours, and restraint should be continued only until "more humane methods" (i.e., medication) become effective. This becomes a problem in the treatment of violent clients who are intoxicated or overdosed on drugs. It is usually not possible to give any sedation until the alcohol or drug is metabolized; in such instances, therefore, restraints with continued observation are necessary. Seclusion, like restraint, is discontinued as soon as possible. Either the patient becomes somnolent from medication or the patient communicates that control has been regained.

Overtly violent clients respond quickly to intramuscular doses of major tranquilizers like chlor-promazine and haloperidol. Some clients have been given slow-acting barbiturates (amobarbital, Benital) or diazepam intravenously if they need to be sedated quickly. This route carries a risk of respiratory depression; therefore the nurse should be sure to have the equipment for intubation available. The IM route for barbiturates and diazepam is slower but less risky.

When a violent client must be kept sedated, especially over a period of time to permit workup and treatment of an organic condition, the major tranquilizers have been most effective. Chlorpromazine should be given intramuscularly in 25-mg increments every hour until the client is somnolent but arousable to eat and speak. With geriatric clients, the chlorpromazine should be given in 10-mg increments. The blood pressure should be checked before and one half hour after each dose and the medication should be held only if the systolic pressure is below 90 mm Hg. When the maintenance dose has been reached, the amount should be doubled and given in oral liquid concentrate form every 4 hours. The often-publicized problem side effects of Thorazine are not likely to develop in the average client, and certainly not during the time of the emergency. In fact, clients with violent outbursts from hepatic encephalopathy have been satisfactorily sedated with chlorpromazine with no further compromising of the liver condition. In any case, the risk of side effects must be weighed against the risk of harm to self or others.

Third, the nurse who is dealing with an overtly violent patient should attempt to get the client's history from anyone who accompanied the client, such as relatives or police, or anyone who was a witness to the client's difficulties. The nurse may have to telephone other agencies that know the client, the client's landlord, or the client's building superintendent. The following questions should be asked: Has the client taken a hallucinogenic drug? Is he or she on any other type of medication? Is the client physically ill? Has the client ever been treated for mental illness? Been in a psychiatric hospital? Is the present behavior like or unlike the client's problem behavior in the past? A chronic

Table 15-2 Nursing Care Checklist for the Client in Restraint

	Record	Time	Record	Time	Record	Time	Record	Time
☑ Physician's order for restraints								
Camisole								
Wrist								
Ankle								
☑ Airway patent Vital signs (record q 30 min.)								
P								
R								
BP								
☑ Circulation intact								
L Ankle								
R Ankle								
L Wrist								
R Wrist								
☑ Elimination								
Bowel								
Bladder								
☑ Hydration (record amount)								
PO liquids								
IV liquids								
☑ Medication (record type and route; e.g., chlorpromazine 24 IM)								
☑ Physician's order to continue or release restraints q 2 h								

schizophrenic who is suddenly agitated and paranoid may be going into kidney failure (uremia) and not having an acute psychotic episode. This information should be recorded and shared with other concerned professionals.

Fourth, the nurse must continue to monitor the client for further violent outbursts using the six criteria discussed under "Nursing Diagnosis." Any hint of another violent episode should cue the nurses to reactivate their plan of intervention.

Fifth, a decision may have to be made regarding hospitalization. If clients remain dangerous to others by virtue of a functional mental illness, they must be hospitalized and treated in an inpatient psychiatric setting. If clients are violent due to an organic illness, they may have to be hospitalized in a general hospital and followed psychiatrically until the physical illness is corrected. Such patients *must* be followed psychiatrically because they induce fear in other patients on the ward. In the general hospital, the nurse should use the plan of intervention discussed in the first four steps. If a client who is mentally ill has an injury because of a violent episode (e.g., putting a hand through a glass door and thus severing tendons), the physical condition takes precedence. The client would be hospitalized in a surgical unit and followed, with the psychiatric plan of intervention as discussed, until the surgical problem was corrected. Then a plan for psychiatric treatment could be instituted.

Intervention with Clients Who Act Impulsively
Clients who are potentially or overly violent because of psychotic states or organic conditions are not the only ones with whom nurses will have contact. Nurses have many opportunities to work with clients who act out their rage or their urge to kill in an impulsive manner. These can be clients of any age, and their impulsive assaultivness is part of their repertoire of coping behavior. The behavior is used when frustration builds and superego controls are poor. These are the clients who are not psychotic, nor are they suffering from an organic illness. Rather, they have *character*

disorders; they are people who use impulsive acting out in order to get their needs met on an ongoing basis. (See App. A.)

Nurses may have contact with these clients anywhere: schools, hospitals, prisons, day hospitals, clinics. These clients are often known to the police because criminal charges have been brought against them for assaultive or homicidal behavior. Many clients of this group are put on probation or parole on the condition that they pursue psychiatric treatment. Their potential for improvement under the conditions imposed—i.e., when they have not freely chosen to accept treatment—is a topic of much debate among both law enforcement and mental hygiene professionals. In the care of adults who are in treatment due to difficulties in controlling their hostile, violent impulses, there are specific steps that the nurse and treatment team can take to teach their clients to (1) recognize the problems they create through their violent behavior and (2) cope with hostile feelings in ways that will not inflict trauma on self and others.[13,14,15]

Nurses must first feel comfortable with their own feelings of violence and aggression and be aware of how they were conditioned as children to respond to angry outbursts. Only when nurses are aware of their own aggressive feelings and their reactions to violence in others, and when they endeavor to bring these feelings under rational scrutiny, will they be effective members of the treatment team. This is extremely important because, before violent clients can be treated, they must feel assured that they will not be allowed to be destructive. "The first inroad into violent behavior is the patient's perception and eventual belief that the therapist can control the client's rage and impulse to destroy."[1] Nurses must, of course, work on their own personal awareness, but the treatment team must have constant cooperation, review, and supervision from consultants and each other in the management of the violent client.

The team approach is recommended because it is a constant "show of force" and sign of external control for the client. Also, a team approach helps to dilute both the transference and countertransference problems. The goal of the team is to bring into disciplined play the understanding of feelings. In general, this is done by assisting the client to (1) control or set limits on impulsive aggressive behavior, (2) examine the immediate situation which promoted the impulsive reaction, and (3) learn alternate methods of reacting in similar situations or other ways to discharge aggressive energies on an ongoing basis.

Some of the most rewarding results in working with violent clients over an extended time period have been seen in inpatient psychiatric services, or in day hospitals where the client comes in contact with the home environment every day. Until they are able to respond to the "protective" limits set by another human being or to a set of rules, clients need to be in an area where physical protection is built in. Thus, violent clients may first need to be in seclusion or in a locked inpatient unit with barred windows; but when they are ready for a day hospital, the area may simply be one where heavy or dangerous equipment has been removed. Next, clients feel external control by limit setting, which is conveyed by (1) short, direct commands like "Don't hit her!" or "Hold your arms still!" or (2) a set of rules and regulations that the whole group follows, such as "No alcohol or drugs allowed," or "No physical contact except in sports or games." Finally, the client further feels external controls when outlets for aggression are part of the program. These can be heavy cleaning, competitive games, walks, calisthenics, and sports. Special mention should be made of the particular benefit of sports through which aggressiveness can be channeled. In addition, sports afford a reward system of activity, support from others, emotional involvement, and social position.[3] For the violent client, motor activity involving the large muscles is of great value as a means of discharging rage and aggression. Thus, sports and strenuous walks should be encouraged regularly.

A 23-year-old man was admitted to the inpatient psychiatric unit after he had become violent at home, had broken furniture, and had finally put his fist through the television screen. This behavior had followed an argument between the mother and the father. The client was kept in the unit as a way of protecting him until he regained inner control. This was done both by removal from the home environment and by some medication. After 3 weeks, the client was discharged from the inpatient unit to attend the day hospital. Coming to the hospital every day and returning home at night enabled the client to examine in a supervised way the situation that had led up to his violent behavior prior to admission and in the past, i.e., the parental arguments.

After the client feels external controls, intervention for developing internal controls may be instituted. The ability to control violent impulses by oneself implies a strengthening of ego functions plus basic mental health learning. As with any dysfunctional coping behavior, resorting to assaultive and/or violent coping behavior is related to an increase in anxiety. When anxiety levels get dangerously high, the risk of violence increases. This happens when the anxiety builds up above the frustration-tolerance level and is too much for the already tenuous and fragile ego to monitor. The weak ego is incapable of channeling the aggressive energy constructively and the client reverts to the more primitive discharge of aggression in a chaotic and destructive fashion. This behavior resembles the temper tantrum or rage reaction of a frustrated child, whose ego is not yet fully developed.

Even though medication can alleviate anxiety, it is of paramount importance that the violent client first learn to recognize high tension levels within the self and to associate them with the possibility of violent acting out. Association is a built-in step which blocks action and enables the ego to *decide* to channel the violence in a way that is not harmful to self and others. So many assaultive clients react to an impulse without thinking. A "stop and think" step prevents the impulsive action, dilutes some of the aggression, and gives the client an opportunity to express aggression in an alternate way.

After the "trigger signs" are recognized and the impulsive action is stopped, the client should gradually be encouraged to talk about the feeling and any connection it may have to the surrounding environment. Concomitant circumstances, particularly interaction with other human beings, should be recognized. When the nurse who is assigned to the patient follows this procedure, the groundwork for learning can be laid. The client will gradually come to trust the nurse, who is seen as the *significant other*. With sufficient trust, the client will begin to come to the nurse to verbalize a feeling of rage and to report the action taken. As trust grows, the client will want to discuss not only the action taken but also—in an attempt to understand—whatever led up to the rage or near-violent state. This is a step toward internalizing reality.[14] For example, the client gradually comes to associate the urge to hit someone with an immediately preceding argument with his wife. In treatment, the argument can serve as a signal for the client to take a long walk or play a game of paddle ball. Then the argument with the wife can be discussed.

In addition to helping the client to internalize reality, the nurse and staff also serve as models with whom the client may identify. A nurse who handles reality in nonviolent ways can effect great change in the client who sees the nurse as a role model. Approaches which would *prevent* the team from successfully intervening in violent behavior are:[13]

- Reacting inconsistently
- Reacting with hostility
- Conveying the idea that it is wrong to feel hostile
- Focusing attention primarily when the client is acting counter to the goal
- Subtly reinforcing behavior that meets staff needs (e.g., for a scapegoat, for excitement)
- Showing fear of being the object of verbal or physical abuse
- Avoiding the client
- Defending yourself
- Reacting with icy courtesy

It must also be remembered that probing which is too deep or premature precipitates confusion, panic, and antagonism in the client, and these damage rapport (see Chap. 6).

Evaluation

Hard work at developing rapport at a pace the client sets can assure the goals of (1) controlling impulsive, violent behavior; (2) examining the immediate situation which promoted the impulsive reaction; and (3) learning alternate methods of reacting in similar situations. When previously violent clients can consistently suspend impulsive action and choose nonviolent ways of discharging aggression, they are on the way to being rehabilitated.

References

1 Charles H. King: "Counter-Transference and Counter-Experience in the Treatment of Violence Prone Youth," *American Journal of Orthopsychiatry* vol. 46, pp. 43–52, January 1976.

2 Ainslee Meares: *Relief Without Drug,* Doubleday, Garden City, N.Y., 1967, pp. 43–44

3 Sherwood L. Washburn and Robert S. O. Harding: "Evolution and Human Nature," in Silvano Arieti (ed.), *American Handbook of Psychiatry,* Basic Books, New York, 1975, vol. 6, pp. 3–13.

4 Otto Fenichel: *The Psychoanalytic Theory of Neurosis,* Norton, New York, 1945, pp. 375ff., 506–507.

5 Charles H. King: "The Ego and the Integration of Violence in Homicidal Youth," *American Journal of Orthopsychiatry,* vol. 45, pp. 134–145, October 1975.

6 Raymond M. Glasscote, Elaine Cumming, Donald W. Hammersley, Lucy D. Ozarin, and Lauren H. Smith: *The Psychiatric Emergency: A Study of Patterns of Service,* The Joint Information Service, Washington, D.C., 1966, pp. 29–33.

7 Erik H. Erikson: *Childhood and Society,* Norton, New York, 1963, pp. 418–419.

*8 Kay Tooley: "Antisocial Behavior and Social Alienation Post Divorce: The 'Man of the House' and His Mother," *American Journal of Orthopsychiatry,* vol. 45, pp. 33–42, January 1976.

*Recommended reference by nurse author.

9 Albert J. Solenti and Melvin Lewis: "Promising Directions in Psychoanalysis," in Silvano Arieti (ed.), *American Handbook of Psychiatry,* Basic Books, New York, 1975, vol. 6, pp. 692–706.

10 Beatrix A. Hamburg: "Social Change and the Problem of Youth," in Silvano Arieti (ed.), *Handbook of Psychiatry,* Basic Books, New York, 1975, vol. 6, pp. 385–410.

11 J. Shick, E. Fred, and Daniel X. Freedman: "Research on Nonnarcotic Drug Abuse," in Silvano Arieti (ed.), *American Handbook of Psychiatry,* Basic Books, New York, 1975, vol. 6, pp. 552–622.

12 Louis Jolyon West: "The Violent Patient—Causes and Management," *Practical Psychiatry,* vol. 2, pp. 1–4, April–May 1974.

*13 Ethel M. Rosenfeld: "Intervening in Hostile Behavior Through Dyadic and/or Group Intervention," *Journal of Psychiatric Nursing,* vol. 7, pp. 251–254, November–December 1969.

*14 Rita Sue Henschen: "Learning Impulse Control Through Day Care," *Perspectives in Psychiatric Care,* vol. 9, pp. 218–224, May 1971.

*15 Maxine E. Loomis: "Nursing Management of Acting-Out Behavior," *Perspectives in Psychiatric Care,* vol. 8, pp. 168–175, April 1970.

*16 Judith Ann Coffman: "Anger: Its Significance for Nurses Who Work with Emotionally Disturbed Children," *Perspectives in Psychiatric Care,* vol. 7, pp. 104–111 May–June, 1969.

*17 Gertrude E. Flynn: "Nursing Intervention in Hostile Behavior," *Perspectives in Psychiatric Care,* vol. 7, pp. 177–189, July–August 1969.

*18 Kathleen Jurgensen: "Limit Setting for Hospitalized Adolescent Psychiatric Patients," *Perspectives in Psychiatric Care,* vol. 9, pp. 173–183, April 1971.

19 J. Lion: *Evaluation and Management of the Violent Patient,* Charles C Thomas, Springfield, Ill., 1972.

*20 Meg Penalver: "Helping the Child Handle His Aggression," *American Journal of Nursing,* vol. 73, pp. 1554–1555, September 1973.

21 *Mental Hygiene Law of the State of New York, State Department of Mental Hygiene,* July 1972.

22 *One Step Ahead,* 16-mm film produced for Motorola Teleprograms, Inc., by American Image Films, Ltd., 1975.

Chapter

16

The Client Who Generates Frustration

Hope Fox

Learning Objectives

After studying this chapter, the student should be able to:

1 Identify experiences which commonly give rise to frustration in nurses
2 Identify two common human experiences which result from feelings of frustration
3 Differentiate personal needs from clients' needs when establishing nursing goals
4 Identify the etiology of hysteria, obsessive-compulsive neurosis, and phobic neurosis
5 Identify the mental mechanisms employed in hysteria, obsessive-compulsive neurosis, and phobic neurosis
6 Identify common client behaviors associated with hysteria, obsessive-compulsive neurosis, and phobic neurosis

7 Differentiate nursing interventions appropriate to hysteria, obsessive-compulsive neurosis, and phobic neurosis

8 Construct a nursing-care plan for a client with hysteria, obsessive-compulsive neurosis, or phobic neurosis

9 Distinguish between normal personality traits and the symptoms of hysteria, obsessive-compulsive neurosis, and phobic neurosis

Frustration is the feeling experienced when one's expectations in a situation are not met.[1] The frustrated person experiences a generalized uneasiness and irritability which blossom into anger if unchecked or unresolved. An important criterion for maturity is the ability to tolerate frustration and traumatic events and to utilize them in forming better adaptive modes of behavior.

The feeling of frustration is uncomfortable. The individual feels unworthy, futile, and defeated as well as blocked from being able to accomplish the desired goals. This is detrimental when experienced within the nurse-client relationship.[2]

Selected Client Behaviors

Psychoneurosis is characterized by particular ways of thinking and perceiving: ways of experiencing emotions and modes of subjective experience and activity. These particular ways of behaving in response to intolerable anxiety are manifested in syndromes such as *hysteria, obsessive-compulsive neurosis,* and *phobias* (see appendix for APA diagnostic classification).

Development of these neurotic patterns in individuals seems to be influenced by the underlying personality structure, and the symptoms seem to fit the person's life-style.[3] For example, the hysterical neurotic who frequently exhibits inauthentic emotional outbursts may earn a living as a performing artist in the theater. The meticulous accountant is more apt, under intolerable stress, to

exaggerate already ingrained behavioral patterns and exhibit compulsive behavior rather than hysteria. The phobic housekeeper may be a woman who tells others that she really wants to get out of the house and do things in the community but is unable to do so because of a fear of being outdoors.

Neurotic people generally experience chronic low self-esteem. They feel that their efforts are unappreciated by others. In addition, they have a low level of self-acceptance and therefore feel of little value to others.

Psychoneurotic clients exhibit their distress in ways which tend to frustrate the helper. In attempting to control intolerable anxiety, the client exhibits a variety of behaviors such as physical symptoms which have no organic basis, inauthentic emotion, repetitive and ritualistic actions, and excessive fears. Some of these behaviors can be disconcerting to others, especially if a knowledge of the underlying dynamics is lacking.

Client Behavior in Hysteria

"Hysteria" is a term applied to various sensory, motor, or psychic disturbances.[4] The behavior of clients with such symptoms may be not only bizarre but mind-boggling. Manifestations of hysteria include somnambulism (sleepwalking), amnesia ("fugue states"), multiple personalities (dissociative experiences), apparent paralysis of a limb, deafness, and the inability—unaccompanied by an organic problem—to walk or speak (conversion reactions).

The primary mode of cognition in hysteria is *repression.* This adaptive process results in a tendency toward forgetfulness. The memory function is impressionistic and global, lacking sharpness.[3] As a result, the hysteric lives in a fairly nonfactual world and is often remarkably deficient in knowledge. This is often seen by others as naiveté. In addition, the hysteric is incapable of persistent, intense intellectual concentration and is easily distracted.

Along with the symptoms, the client exhibits a noticeable lack of affect, in proportion to the apparent severity of the symptoms. This is so characteristic of hysterical manifestations that Janet[5] gave it the name *la belle indifférence,* describing the patient's marked complacency in the presence of gross objective disability. For example, a middle-aged woman experienced total blindness and all organic causes were ruled out. When the nurse spoke with the client, she did not deny the blindness but rather seemed calm and unconcerned about her loss of sight. She asked no questions and expressed no anxiety about her condition, nor did she ask about the medical team's estimate of her prognosis. This is typical of the behavior of someone experiencing hysterical blindness. The nurse's expectation that the client would be frightened, anxious, or depressed about the sensory loss is not met. The nurse is disconcerted and unprepared to care for a client who *should* be engaged in mourning a loss but seems instead to be unconcerned at the physical deficit and change in life-style. Attempts to help the client confront her loss are thwarted by inappropriate affect.

Hysteria occurs in many forms. The example given, of hysterical blindness, falls into the category of *conversion reaction.* This means that the underlying psychological conflict is literally *converted* into a physical manifestation.[4] The complacency seen in the client occurs because anxiety is not manifest but rather has been completely invested in the symptom, bringing psychological relief to the individual. It does, of course, accomplish other things as well. It usually places the client in a "sick role," which calls forth the expect-

ed nurturing responses from significant others in the environment (see Chap. 25). This extra attention satisfies dependency needs, which usually are also repressed. The results are *secondary gains,* which are those "fringe benefits" a person derives from the environment during illness. Thus there is a real danger of an acute episode becoming chronic. This is a significant factor to be taken into account when planning nursing care.

In conversion reaction, the mental functioning of the individual remains intact in spite of the often profound psychic symptom, such as muscular paralysis. This form of hysteria is quite common and may take on other forms such as tremor of limbs, convulsions, contractures, astasia or abasia (inability to stand or walk), or speech disorders such as aphasia.

Another form of conversion hysteria which is commonly seen is *convulsive hysteria.* In this condition the presenting symptom is a convulsive seizure closely resembling epilepsy. The convulsion serves as a symbolic rage reaction or temper tantrum for the client and has its origin in frustration or fear of sexual wishes of a genital nature. It is often difficult for the professional person to differentiate between idiopathic epilepsy and the hysterical form. Convulsive hysteria may be suspected when the following characteristics are in evidence during seizure:

1 No full loss of consciousness
2 The episode occurs only in the presence of others
3 No dangerous falls occur
4 Pupillary and deep reflexes are present
5 No biting of tongue
6 No loss of bladder or bowel control
7 Facial flushing present, but no cyanosis or pallor
8 Attempts to open eyes are resisted
9 Pressure on the supraorbital notch causes withdrawal of the head[4]

Dissociative reaction is still another form of hysteria. This type is characterized by *amnesia, fugue, somnambulism,* or the *multiple personality* syndrome. Janet[5] defined hysteria as a malady of the personal synthesis. The dissociative states most typify that definition. In this emotional disorder there are episodic disturbances in the stream of consciousness when a group of ideas or emotions which are *ego-alien* occupy the field of consciousness. These thoughts or feelings may be excluded from the individual's normal stream of consciousness.[4]

Although there is no primary thought disorder, the individual who is experiencing a dissociative reaction does not act in a normal fashion yet is not considered irrational. The best example is the sleepwalker who, of course, is not acting normally yet upon awakening is perfectly rational.

A *fugue state* may precede amnesia. The fugue state is a restriction in the field of consciousness. People suffering from this disturbance may leave their homes and usual way of life and engage in activities which have no connection with their usual habits.[4] This phenomenon may occur with the appearance of one or multiple personalities that arise from different ego-alien components of the self-system. There are well-known fiction and nonfiction stories that deal with this phenomenon, such as *Dr. Jekyll and Mr. Hyde,*[6] *The Three Faces of Eve,*[7] and, more recently, *Sybil.*[8] The wanderings of clients in a fugue state are symbolic of the underlying conflicts affecting them. Often their condition represents an exchange of the present for the past.

Client Behaviors in Obsessive-Compulsive Neurosis

Obsessive-compulsive neurosis is one of the less common forms of psychoneurosis, representing only 5 percent of all psychoneurotics. No significant difference exists in the incidence with regard to sex. It is interesting to note that a large number of persons in this classification remain unmarried: 50 percent in some surveys.[9] This neurosis is more frequently seen in the upper middle class and in individuals with higher intellectual functioning. The symptoms tend to appear in the mid-twenties, though it is not uncommon to see them in people

under the age of 10 (see Chap. 34). Some theorists indicate that a first onset rarely appears as late as the fortieth year of life. An acute attack is often precipitated by a stressful environmental incident.

Obsessive-compulsive neurosis is characterized by a number of symptoms that often occur together. An *obsession* is a repetitive thought which the individual is unable to control. Anyone who has ever had the experience of having some ridiculous little tune (usually a commercial jingle) repeating in their head for a portion of the day will understand, to a mild degree, what an obsession is. A *compulsion* is an urge to act that cannot be resisted without extreme difficulty. The compulsion is often an irrational impulse and the person to whom it happens has insight and recognizes the absurdity of the compulsion. A great deal of psychic effort goes into controlling the impulse so that it does not become an irrational act.[9]

There is a need on the part of these clients to maintain rigid and purposive activity with continuous self-imposed pressure. They feel that they act in response to some objective necessity, particularly a moral necessity. The "shoulds" in their life-style are issued by the self. This eternally driven activity makes relaxation impossible. They are so overcontrolled from within that they feel nonpurposive, nondirected activity to be unsafe and bad. Pleasurable activities bring them discomfort.

The thinking processes of obsessive-compulsive clients are characterized by rigidity, intellectuality, and sharply focused task orientation. Although they focus and concentrate on detail, they are often unproductive in work situations because they are limited in both mobility and range of ideas. This hampers creative thought and recognition of alternative solutions to problems. In interpersonal relationships, there is no meeting of minds. There is neither agreement nor disagreement when issues arise. One gets a feeling of not having been heard or of being given perfunctory attention.[3]

Characteristic rituals in which the obsessive-compulsive client may indulge are dressing and undressing a number of times, placing of articles in a specific way, hand-washing, and intensive cleanliness. If the ritual is inadvertently thwarted, often by some "well-meaning" family or staff member, the client feels compelled to start the ritual all over again. If the ritual is consistently thwarted, a panic state may occur due to the buildup of intolerable anxiety.

Ritualistic speech is another client behavior commonly seen in obsessive-compulsive neurosis. One such patient, Mrs. W, was being seen in family therapy sessions. Each time the nurse asked Mrs. W a question, she would launch into a lengthy narrative, stating *repeatedly* "I never should have sold my house. I never would have had these problems with my son if we hadn't moved."

Clients who fall into this diagnostic category may present the greatest challenge to the mental health worker. Their behavior markedly frustrates the environmental routines within both the family and hospital settings.

Client Behavior in Phobia

A *phobia* is an irrational fear.[9] It is a fairly common phenomenon not unfamiliar to most of us and often quite compatible with normal functioning. However, when the phobia takes on such monumental proportions that it immoblizes the individual to the extent that normal, routine functioning ceases, then a phobic neurosis is present. Some more common phobias are fear of heights, open spaces, closed spaces, crowds, animals, darkness, trains, planes, cars, boats, and water. Table 16-1 is a brief list of the scientific names for some of the more common phobias.

Although a phobia is specific and object-oriented and therefore quite circumscribed, such fears may present profound problems to the clients who suffer them. The limitations to the client's life-style can be extreme, depending upon the nature and extent of the phobia. Fear of the outdoors, for instance, can be far more immobilizing to a city dweller's daily activities than fear of rabbits.

Usually, the phobic client has had a specific fear since childhood and as an adult is fairly well adjusted and free of other neurotic symptoms. Referral usually occurs as a result of the intensification of fear and a recent change in the environment which transforms a simple phobia into a more paralyzing phobic neurosis. Phobias are also found to be common in conjunction with other psychiatric syndromes such as depression and obsessive-compulsive neurosis.

It is important to differentiate between normal fear and phobia. *Normal fear* has an object; it is adaptive and is therefore a healthy response to danger or threat. The feeling of fear, with its attendant "fight or flight" reaction, serves to help the individual take quick protective action to avoid an object or situation which can be potentially harmful. Phobia has an object, but it is maladaptive. One teen-ager was unable to enjoy bathing in

Table 16-1 Common Phobias[10]

Object feared	Scientific term
Height	Acrophobia
Outdoors	Agoraphobia
Closed spaces	Claustrophobia
Animals	Zoophobia
Night and darkness	Nyctophobia
Thunder/lightning	Astraphobia
Blood	Hematophobia
Water	Hydrophobia
Speaking	Glossophobia
Dirt	Mycophobia
Eating	Sitophobia

the ocean with her peers because of a fear (which *she* labeled ridiculous) that her body would suddenly fold in two, like some inflated object cleaved in the middle, if she were to float on the water. In all other respects she appeared to be a normal adolescent. The phobia, rather than being adaptive like normal fear, was inhibitory to normal development and peer relationships.

There are three major components to phobic reactions: (1) subjective experience of fear and anxiety accompanying contact with a specific object or situation, (2) physiological changes associated with such contact, (3) behavioral steps to avoid or escape it.[11]

The three main types of phobic neuroses are (1) agoraphobia, (2) social phobias, and (3) specific phobias.

The most common phobia is *agoraphobia.* This is the fear of going out, especially alone. People who are severely affected are unable to leave home alone or travel at all. It is obvious that this malady becomes extremely disabling for the client and burdensome to family and friends. Milder forms may be restricted to specific activities like shopping or travel by bus or train. The symptoms may be relieved when the client is accompanied by a companion. One young woman was unable to go out alone but had an infant with a blood disorder which required weekly trips to the pediatrician. Friends and neighbors had to mobilize to provide transportation and companionship in connection with these medical visits. The young woman also feared traveling on buses. This example illustrates how the phobic neurotic manipulates the environment and compounds dependency needs.

In *social phobia* there is a fear of eating, drinking, speaking, writing, blushing, or vomiting in the presence of others. General anxiety and depression may occur as well. The client in this instance is more likely to come for help voluntarily as daily functioning becomes more restricted. The sexes are equally affected.

These social phobias may present management problems for the family of the phobic person as well as the staff of residential settings. Some-times the phobia makes it necessary for the clients to have meals in their rooms away from the rest of the community. This special arrangement can be misconstrued by siblings, other clients, or staff as preferential treatment, causing further interpersonal stresses to the environment in which the client lives.

Specific phobia, as the name implies has a foundation in the fear of one special object (see Table 16-1). In all phobias of this type, factors such as size, movement, distance, and color may play important parts in generating the fear. A moving insect may elicit more fear than a stationary one. Large dogs may activate the phobic reaction, while small ones may not.

Psychodynamics
Psychoneurosis

Freud's earliest manuscripts revolved around the study of neurosis generally and hysteria specifically, as well as his attempts to cure these emotional disorders. Out of these studies rose the whole science of psychoanalysis with its many present-day offshoots, which took form as new investigators devised newer theories.

Freud concluded that neurotics were people who experienced opposing wishes called *mental conflicts.* These conflicts exist as a result of id urges relating to *sexuality* and *aggression* and the ego's attempts to repress them. Freud believed there would be no neurosis without psychological conflict between the id, ego, and superego. The symptoms which neurotics present are substitutions for satisfaction of the id impulses.[12] They afford a temporary and partial solution to the conflict situation.

Hysteria

Hysteria arises from a fixation in early psychosexual development at the Oedipal level,[13] when the individual fails to give up the incestuous tie to the loved parent. This leads to anxiety and a conflict regarding sexual drives in adult life. The incestuous wishes and attendant anxiety are *repressed.* (*Repression* is the primary coping mechanism utilized in hysteria.) The tension which arises from the forbidden sexual drive is converted into the hysterical symptom. The manifestation of the symptom provides both a symbolic expression of the drive and protection from conscious awareness.[12] This phenomenon is most clearly recognized in conversion hysteria. It is especially important to be aware that the symptom has symbolic meaning. For example, Jane D, during her childhood, had deep unconscious guilt feelings due to early masturbatory experiences. Later in adult life, after her first sexual experience, she developed paralysis of the right arm. It was subsequently discovered, during treatment, that this right arm was actively used both in the early and later sexual experiences. The hysterical paralysis served to express her deep sexual guilt.

Obsessive-Compulsive Neurosis

Freud[12] placed the origin of obsessive and compulsive characteristics in the anal stage of development, when holding back (of feces) and learning to let go is a significant developmental task. The child gains pleasure from controlling its own body and, indirectly, the actions of significant others.

Erikson[14] defines the second stage of development as autonomy versus shame and doubt. Children at this level have the option of giving up excretions as required by the parent or holding onto them if perversity prevails. To be neat and tidy brings parental rewards of approval. To be messy, which the child longs for, brings criticism and rejection. In other words, to be *good* is to be neat and controlled. To be *bad* is to capitulate to impulses to be dirty and aggressive.

The obsessional character develops out of the need to obtain approval by being excessively tidy and controlled. At this time of development, the child is reacting to standards set by the parents. It is not uncommon to find that some of these standards are sometimes excessively high and conflict with normal developmental tasks necessary for healthy personality growth. In such cases, frustra-tion continually exists between the child's normal developmental tendencies and the parental taboos. This type of experience often contributes to the incidence of obsessive-compulsive neurosis.

Obsessive-compulsive behaviors are an unconscious attempt by the client to reduce an intolerable level of anxiety: the more anxiety there is present, the more attention the client will devote to the elaboration and maintenance of a rigid routine. Symptom formation occurs on the basis of several coping mechanisms. First, the client's handling of feelings and thoughts through ritualistic behavior represents a return to earlier, *regressive* methods of dealing with anxiety. Second, obsessive thoughts as they present themselves to clients are either devoid of feeling or attached only to anxiety. When ideas become detached from emotions, *isolation* is being used. Third, the client's overt attitude toward others is usually the opposite of unconscious feelings. Thus *reaction formation* is exhibited. Fourth, compulsive rituals are a symbolic way of *undoing* or resolving underlying conflict. In the presence of critical life events, the symptoms, as defensive attempts to deal with anxiety, may become worse. For example, a client who feels responsibility and guilt about the death of a spouse may engage in excessive hand-washing to deal with feelings of guilt and responsibility.

It is important to differentiate between obsessional or compulsive *character traits* and obsessive-compulsive *neurosis.* All too often, students of psychology, medicine, and nursing judge themselves and their acquaintances too harshly in that they tend to see gross pathology in what is, in fact, normal behavior. Actually, some of the characteristics which typify obsessional traits can be helpful to have if they are present in moderation. Some of these traits are tidiness, orderliness, preciseness, punctuality, concern for detail, perseverance, and a sound sense of caution. These are most helpful in professions requiring neatness and precision and are associated with intelligence. Such traits differ quite radically from the crippling slavery to certain rituals which typify the neurotic person. Neurotic behaviors are protective ways of acting that occupy the whole day and result in a totally destructive and nonproductive pattern of behavior.[3]

Thus we see that, within normal limits, a few compulsive *traits* are helpful in getting the work of the world done. The crucial difference between mental health and illness lies in the ability to function and to control these traits rather than being controlled by them.

Phobias

Present knowledge of phobias is based primarily on principles formulated by Freud.[12] The chief experience of the client is intolerable anxiety characterized by feelings of apprehension, uncertainty, and helplessness. The roots of these feelings go back to anxiety experienced during the oral phase of development, due to the loss of love and support from the nurturing figure. These dynamics place the foundation of this disorder in the area of dependency, with the symptom generating increased dependency requirements for the client. The primary coping mechanism used is *displacement*.[3] The person combats the diffuse anxiety by displacing it onto a particular object or situation. The specificity of the fear makes it manageable. Thus, we see that normal anxiety present in one situation is heightened and then displaced onto another situation in the environment. Binding of fear to the external object occurs. This can be a learned response as a result of early conditioning experiences, when the parent or caretaker communicated their own inappropriate fear and displaced it onto something in the environment.

For example, Mrs. R has had extremely poor eyesight from a very early age. Now, in late middle age, she has developed agoraphobia. She never ventures out of her home unaccompanied, and even going out in company results in moderate to severe anxiety. The nurse-therapist sees Mrs. R in the client's home because of her reluctance to go out. In the course of therapy, it becomes obvious that the agoraphobia is a displacement of anxiety related to the near blindness which Mrs. R experiences but has never dealt with realistically.[15]

The true meaning of any symbol can be determined by listening to the associations of the client. Recall of childhood experiences closely associated with the present fear often can lead to clarification of the phobia.[16]

For example, a 9-year-old girl, small for her age, was frequently left in the care of her 14-year-old brother, who was instructed by the working parent to take his sister wherever he went. This led to the young girl's participation in activities which were often beyond the physical ability of a person her age. She found this frightening. One of these activities involved sneaking into the local movie house by climbing to the third-story top of the fire escape and entering a fire-exit door which led to the balcony. In adult life, while on a camping trip with her family, this woman attempted to climb a fire tower which was a popular tourist attraction in a state forest. She experienced no discomfort initially, but upon reaching the third landing, she was seized by a sudden, profound, and paralyzing fear and was unable to continue.

This is a good example of a phobia occurring many years after the initial feared experience. The relationship to the earlier childhood situation was subsequently brought out in therapy.

Within the environment, "phobic partners" may emerge. These are convenient "helpers" who stand by and protect the person from acute panic or anxiety. These partners usually serve to further the unconscious wish of the phobic to be taken care of. In this way, secondary gains become evident.

Nurses' Responses to Client Behaviors

Nurses' role perceptions of themselves affect their interaction with clients. Likewise, clients' perceptions of the nurse as mother, counselor, doctor's assistant, or administrator influence how they interact in the relationship. Thus, when nurse and client perceptions and expectations are incongruous, conflict arises. If, for example, the nurse's self-perception is one of helper and counselor but the client does not allow this role assumption, then frustrated feelings are engendered in the nurse.[2] When the professional person moves towards lofty, self-imposed goals but encounters barriers in the form of client behaviors which challenge these goals, frustration results. If the nurse has a reasonable and realistic expectation of self and client, then, when feelings of frustration are encountered, they are not intensified. Instead, new directions for problem solving are sought.

However, when the satisfying feelings of direction and striving are thwarted, they are frequently converted into their opposites: unsatisfying feelings of *anger* as well as *hopelessness* and *helplessness*.[2] Skills are felt to be useless and, in defense of their own egos, nurses attempt to coerce the client to conform, withdraw, or strike out in anger.

Exploration of Anger

As defined in Chap. 17, anger is a means of avoiding the anxiety which arises in response to interpersonal threat. Nurses are threatened by frustrating client behaviors which generate feelings of incompetence and helplessness. The client's behavior produces a barrier to the help which the nurse wants to provide. Consequently, the nurse focuses attention on the objectionable *barrier behavior* in an attempt to eliminate it. However, these barrier behaviors are the client's best way of coping. When nurses are not aware of their frustration and anger, they become less effective and displace their anger with the client on to the environment, or else they turn it inward. This displacement reduces the intensity of their own feelings of anger, tension, or anxiety. Meanwhile the needs of the client go unmet and escalate.

With experience and more specialized knowledge, the nurse can, in time, learn to share how the behavior barriers generate frustration and anger, which block the client's need gratification. This feedback from the nurse helps the client develop a more realistic image of the nurse as a *feeling* human being and, in turn, enhances the nurse's image as a role model of healthy behavior.

People who are psychoneurotic are keenly aware of the strangeness of their own behavior. They often have a certain detachment about their own actions and act "as if it were all happening to someone else." In addition, there is an absence of primary thought disorder in these clients. They are oriented to time and place, can converse normally with others, usually speak rationally and intelligently, and are cooperative in many other respects. Because of their rational behavior, nurses often lose sight of the clients' illness. When the client does exhibit symptoms, nurses may feel impatient and think that the client is "acting up" or "looking for attention," because the nurse acts on the erroneous assumption that the client's symptoms are within conscious control.

Nurses' Responses to Client Behavior in Hysteria

There are many characteristics of hysteria which cause frustration in the helper. Hysterical clients tend to romanticize reality through a repressive mode of cognition and have an affinity for distorting reality to fit their subjective view of life and events. This behavior causes confusion and eventual distrust among family and staff. For example, a young woman diagnosed as a hysterical personality convinced herself that a male psychiatric aide was madly in love with her because he had "gone out of his way to do special favors for me." In actuality, he was fulfilling his usual role according to his job description. The client embellished his actions with her own interpretations. When the client's interpretations of the aide's actions were revealed in team conference, he was embarrassed and angry.

Nurses' Responses to Client Behavior in Obsessive-Compulsive Neurosis

Nurses often feel frustrated when interacting with compulsive individuals because they make the professional feel helpless. Mrs. S, an obsessive-compulsive woman with ritualistic behavior who was residing in the psychiatric unit of a general hospital, fell while showering, requiring immediate x-ray to determine the extent of her injuries. This unanticipated event so interfered with all her usual rituals that it took the ultimate in patience and creative nursing measures to succeed in moving her off the unit, completely exhausting the entire staff.

Another source of discomfort to the nurse dealing with obsessive-compulsive behavior is the identification of certain elements of the client's behavior with one's own. It becomes obvious to the nurses that like the client, they too pay careful attention to routine and ritual. In preparing medications and carrying out nursing procedures, the nurse goes through carefully defined rituals. Therefore the client's behavior may seem like a caricature or mockery of nursing activities.

Nurses' Responses to Client Behavior in Phobic Neurosis

In caring for phobic clients, nurses encounter symptoms with which they identify. Nurses may also suffer from phobic symptioms, as do many individuals in the general population. However, the nurse, functioning successfully in the work-a-day world in spite of this benign symptom, may have difficulty accepting the client's disability. There may be a tendency on the part of the nurse to urge the client to "shape up"; especially if the feared object or situation appears ridiculously ignominious to others. Fear of spiders or snakes we can all understand and sympathize with, but *feathers?*

Some phobias are so specific that the professional person is doubtful of the validity of the fear and tries to "trap" the client, through a series of planned encounters, into a confrontation. For instance, the person may fear a moving insect but not a stationary one. In the presence of a nonaccepting and judgmental nurse, the client may not react to a stationary insect. This may lead the nurse to conclude that the client's insect phobia is not genuine.

Assessment

Nurses may come into contact with clients who generate frustration in many ways. They may be already diagnosed and receiving treatment in a community health facility on an inpatient or outpatient basis, or they may be undergoing treatment at home, where they are periodically seen by the community health nurse. In situations such as these, the nurse is part of an established health team and the nursing-care plan encompasses the range of services being offered to the client and family by all members of the team. The nurse may also be an independent practitioner in the community, in which case the client may seek help on a one-to-one, group, or family basis. In this instance, the nurse may make an assessment alone or in consultation with others.

Nurses play a major role in case finding, recognizing behavioral deviations and assisting the client to obtain help in an appropriate treatment setting. Some of these deviations may be observed as behavioral cues which signal the presence of one of the neuroses and should be considered as assessment factors (see Table 16-2).

Nursing Diagnosis

A *nursing diagnosis* is a statement of conclusions about the areas in which the person assessed needs nursing intervention.[17] The judgment of these areas is based on a comparison of norms to data collected. Bear in mind that a nursing problem is a client's problem in coping with daily life in relation to the deviation from health. Some people deviate from health but still cope well on an ongoing basis.

The behavioral nursing diagnosis should allow for as open-ended a system as possible, since clients vary so widely in their behavioral dynamics. It is important to express the nursing diagnosis in terms of client experience. For example, a nursing diagnosis for a client with obsessive-compulsive neurosis would be "inability to concentrate due to severe anxiety level." Based on the more common symptoms identified in the disorders that generate frustration in others, additional examples of nursing diagnoses are outlined in Table 16-3.

Table 16-2 General Assessment Factors

1 Identify precipitating event and its symbolic meaning to the client.

   a Evaluate stress factors, both internal and external.

2 Evaluate how the client deals with actions, feelings, and thoughts.

   a Hysteria: Global response, use of superlatives, extremes of behavioral responses. For example,

       Interviewer: "How was your vacation?"

       Client: "Great!" or "Like wow!" or "Oh, it was just awful!"

   b Obsessive-compulsive: Gives much detail, but never states affective reality. For example,

       Interviewer: "How was your vacation?"

       Client: "I did Paris in 48 hours. I got to see all the museums, cafes, and nightclubs. Saturday morning I awoke at 7 A.M. to get an early start . . ." etc.

   c Phobic: Describes experiences in terms of personal fearfulness. For example,

       Interviewer: "How was your vacation?"

       Client: "I couldn't go to the observation tower because I'm afraid of heights. There were so many people . . . mobs of them. I couldn't catch my breath. I had to stay in my room and the rest of the group went on the tour without me."

3 Evaluate the client's style of dress.

   a Showy and extreme

   b Rigidly neat, nothing whatsoever out of place

4 Evaluate the client's level of anxiety (see Chap. 14).

   a Mild

   b Moderate

   c Severe

   d Panic

5 Evaluate defensive patterns or security operations utilized to reduce anxiety.

   a Repression

   b Conversion

   c Intellectualization

   d Regression

   e Displacement

   f Isolation

   g Undoing

   h Reaction formation

6 Evaluate interaction patterns within family.

   a Do family patterns tend to reinforce deviation?

   b Do family patterns tend to lessen deviation?

7 Does client engage in manipulative behavior?

8 Does client engage in acting-out behavior?

9 What is the client's decision-making ability?

10 What is the client's problem-solving ability?

11 What is the client's life-style like? How does it reinforce maladaptive behavior?

Table 16-3 Nursing Diagnoses

Hysteric
1 Secondary gains from assumption of sick role through functional paralysis of sensory or motor ability.
2 Affective overreaction to interpersonal encounters with staff members of opposite sex.
3 Sudden outburst of dramatic emotionality such as crying or temper tantrums without apparent provocation.
4 Selective forgetfulness (amnesia); inability to recall recent educational, employment, and family history.
5 Client assumes alternate identities and disappears from family periodically as a way of avoiding responsibility or open resolution of family conflict.

Obsessive-Compulsive
1 Inability to concentrate due to severe levels of anxiety.
2 Inability to carry out activities of daily living due to ritualistic behavior such as hand-washing (or any other behavior).
3 Anxiety produces recurring thoughts which are not dispelled by logic.
4 Rigid inflexibility in the face of change leads to repetitive verbalizations about inability to participate in new activity programs.
5 Hostile reaction to unscheduled change leads to outburst of verbal hostility directed at staff and other clients.
6 Difficulty following directions which interfere with ritualistic activities.
7 Panic levels of anxiety when limits are set on ritualistic behavior.

Phobic
1 Unfounded, morbid fear of a seemingly harmless object.
2 Increased dependency on others due to agoraphobia.
3 Constriction of life-style and limitations on range of social activities due to fears.
4 Interference with assumption of personal responsibility and freedom to function effectively in activities of daily living.
5 Depressed affect.
6 Severe levels of anxiety when confronted with a phobic object or situation.

Goals

The ongoing evaluations of nursing actions are measured against the nursing goals established for the individual client. In general, the nursing goals involve helping the client cope with the experience of illness. In the disorders discussed herein, some of the nursing goals include assisting the client to:

1 Decrease anxiety
2 Recognize authentic feelings
3 Express feelings openly and directly
4 Decrease manipulative behavior
5 Increase constructive social interaction
6 Decrease ritualistic behavior
7 Decrease dependency needs
8 Become desensitized to fears

Primary Prevention

Most theorists agree that early child-rearing patterns, along with stressful events in a person's life, are the significant etiological factors in the development of neuroses. The nurse's role in *primary prevention*, therefore, is the organization and implementation of programs that will help people become more effective parents by assisting them in exploring, understanding, and accepting their feelings; enhancing their ability to communicate; and developing a sound understanding of normal growth and development. School nurses, community health nurses, and psychiatric liaison nurses are found in a variety of settings within the community. Opportunities for them to plan preventive programs such as parent education classes and community workshops are numerous.

Nursing Intervention

Neurotic behavior patterns develop over extended periods of time; therefore their treatment may also be long and slow. Most clients come for help only after they have unsuccessfully tried remedies suggested by well-meaning family and friends. Clients who have neurotic symptoms have usually developed them as defenses against anxiety. Therefore, if clients are urged to approach that which they fear or are forced to relinquish their symptoms, their anxiety levels will rise. If the client does comply and the particular symptoms do disappear, others equally if not more frustrating and debilitating may appear in their place. Simply extinguishing the problematic behavior, then, prevents the client from seeking the underlying reason for the symptom's development.

Intervention with clients who generate frustration begins with the caretaker. The attitude of the nurse affects the client immediately. Self-awareness of the feelings generated by the client is a prerequisite for understanding client behavior. Nurses who do not understand the clients' need to behave as they do may directly or indirectly indicate to them that their behavior is unacceptable and must be modified. This attitude arises from the nurses' discomfort with client behavior and an inability to examine its meaning and purpose for the client.[19]

The nurse needs to have the capacity to empathize with clients—the ability to understand client motives and the willingness to listen to clients' expressions of what they are thinking and feeling.[18] An attitude of calm reassurance coupled with warmth and recognition of the client as a worthwhile person indicate to the client that the staff are not merely trying to eradicate symptoms for their own convenience but are interested in helping the client to understand behaviors and feelings and to develop more satisfying patterns of interaction.[19] The nurse-client relationship allows the client to experience feelings and satisfactions which led to the development of more mature needs. This is particularly important for these clients, who have often exhausted the patience of relatives and friends with years of complaints and

anxieties. The disapproval and rejection they experience only confirm the feelings of low self-esteem and fear which originally led to the development of their neurotic responses.

Most clients do not understand or know why they behave as they do, so to ask them, "What is wrong?" or "Why are you acting this way?" is an exercise in futility. Rather, nurses need to label the emotion they sense the client to be expressing through his or her behavior. This forces the client to become consciously aware of what is being experienced by considering a specific feeling, which can then be expressed. If an accurate interpretation of client feelings has been made, the client will verbally validate it or respond with an appropriate change in behavior.[19] The excessive repression of feelings by these clients makes it most appropriate for the nurse to operate on a feeling level. The nurse acts as a role model, demonstrating that feelings need not be threatening and that verbal expression is an appropriate way of dealing with them.

Low Self-esteem

Many of these clients have low self-esteem, are indecisive, and avoid contact with others in the inpatient setting. On the other hand, their behavior may be so frustrating that mutual withdrawal occurs. When initiating social or sports activities, nurses should avoid making direct requests that these clients attend, since they are inclined to flatly refuse or to spend prolonged periods of time deciding what they will do. Instead, a more positive approach should be utilized to make clients feel wanted and needed and help them initiate movement toward the group. For example, the nurse may say, "We are going to play (ping-pong, shuffleboard, etc.) and we need you to complete the team," at the same time placing the appropriate playing equipment in the client's hand and gently guilding him or her toward the group.[16]

Another important principle is that of providing opportunities for the client to succeed. (It helps no one to ask clients to participate in activities beyond their capacity.) Activities and expectations should be structured in an incremental way, since small successes usually precede larger ones. Goal setting must be geared to this slow pace and related to the client, not to the success needs of the nurse.

Ritualistic Behavior

Clients who engage in ritualistic behavior must never have direct limits set on their ritualistic acts unless such intervention is specifically indicated. To forbid such behavior is to eliminate a defense which serves as a security operation for the client and possibly precipitate panic levels of anxiety. Instead, the following serves as a guide for intervention with the ritualistic client.

1 Use a quiet manner with the client, keeping the environment calm.

2 Reassure the client of your interest in him or her as an individual.

3 Don't be judgmental or verbalize disapproval of the client behavior.

4 Do not pressure the client to change.

5 Do not confront the client regarding ritualistic behavior. Instead, give reflective feedback, "I see you undress three times every morning. That must be tiring for you." This statement communicates empathy and understanding of the client's experience and may serve to lower the client's anxiety level, thus reducing the intensity of the ritualistic behavior.

6 Ritualistic clients have a low tolerance for change. Make only reasonable requests and always explain them. Logic and argument have no place here but only increase client anxiety, intensify the ritualistic behavior, and heighten the frustration of the nurse.

7 Engage the client in constructive activities which will leave less time for compulsive behavior. In ritualistic speech, for instance, it becomes obvious to the observant nurse that the client is ensnared in an exhausting compulsion to repeat the same litany over and over again. Nursing action involves planning situations—such as object-oriented activities, rather than interpersonal ones which require conversation—which help the client avoid constant verbal repetition. Examples of such activities are quiet games which require concentration, like checkers or chess, as well as arts and crafts such as needlework, woodwork, ceramics, and painting.

8 Give positive reinforcement for nonritualistic behavior. Avoid reinforcing ritualistic behavior, so that there are no secondary gains, such as attention and nurturing, for maladaptive behavior. For example, Mrs. S, a client who compulsively cleaned and recleaned her room many times a day, enjoyed talking with the staff about home decorating. Ms. D, a nurse on the unit, observed this pattern, and the staff decided that Ms. D would spend time with Mrs. S, during her nonritualistic periods, talking about decorating. When she was performing her cleaning and recleaning, Ms. D would spend time with her if necessary but without engaging her in talk about decorating. In this way positive reinforcement of an inappropriate activity would not be carried out by the nurse.

9 Help the clients to find ways of setting limits on their own behavior.

10 Support clients' efforts to explore the meaning and purpose of their behavior. Let them know that their feelings are understood and that you are willing to help them explore these feelings so as to become more comfortable with them. For example, John was okay eating unless someone approached his table, had a change of mind, and then sat elsewhere at another table in the dining room. When this happened, John would stop eating and ritualistically polish and repolish each eating utensil with his napkin. The nurse might say to him, "John, you were eating your dinner, but you seemed upset when David turned away and sat with somebody else. Can you tell me what that feeling was like?"

In managing ritualistic behavior, allow time in the day's routine for the rituals. The attempt to reduce them by not providing the necessary time only leads to the law of diminishing returns. As the client becomes more pressured and anxious, the probability of error within the ritual increases and the client will be more likely to have to start the ritual over again. On the other hand, when the nurse sets aside the necessary time needed for the ritual, the client is given to understand that the nurse accepts the client as a person along with the deviant behavior. For example, Mrs. K, the night nurse in a residential psychiatric unit, is in charge of Mrs. L, an obsessive-compulsive client with ritualistic behavior involving repetition of the morning toilette. Mrs. K awakens Mrs. L one-half hour earlier than the rest of the unit population. In planning her nursing care, Mrs. K informed Mrs. L that she would awaken her earlier "to give you plenty of time to finish dressing so that you won't be late for breakfast."

Due to the extremely resistant nature of the symptoms of obsessive-compulsive neurosis, the goal of therapy often is to confine the symptoms rather than eradicate them. Nurses play a significant role in supportive psychotherapy by assisting the client in limiting the undesired behaviors. There are no drugs currently known which alleviate the symptoms of obsessive-compulsive neurosis. Tranquilizers, in conjunction with psychotherapy, may afford the client some relief from the underlying anxiety.

Hysterical Behavior

Clients with conversion reactions are usually admitted to the medical-surgical unit of a general hospital for diagnostic evaluation of their physical symptoms. A complete physical history must be taken and tests carried out in order to make a valid differential diagnosis. When the outcome of the tests is negative, the staff are often frustrated and begin blaming and criticizing the client for laziness, malingering, and babyishness.

Intervention then becomes directed at understanding how emotional distress becomes converted into physical symptoms and what the meaning and purpose of the behavior is for the client. Nurses need to plan their intervention on the basis of the current level of need fulfillment; that is, existing needs must be met before more mature needs can emerge. The client's behavior is not consciously motivated and is an attempt to relieve anxiety and stress in a personally and socially acceptable way.[19] The symptoms are real to the client; the pain, if present, is real, and the need for intervention is real. The staff must share observations and feelings about the client so that effective intervention can proceed without interference from stereotyped images and feelings. Conversion symptoms usually have symbolic meaning which cover repressed feelings. The goal of intervention is to help clients become aware of what they are feeling, have greater acceptance of their feelings, and be able to deal with these feelings more effectively. Emphasis is on minimizing the sick role and behavior and on identifying and supporting client strengths and areas for growth.

For example, Gloria M, age 45, was admitted to the general hospital for treatment of paralysis of the lower extremities. The paralysis had appeared during the night prior to admission. Two days before that, Gloria's husband had been hospitalized in the same hospital with a myocardial infarction. The couple have no children and Gloria's mother, on interview, stated that "Gloria's husband treats her like a little doll. Now that he's sick, I would have been surprised if she had risen to the occasion to take care of him." A complete physical examination revealed no organic basis for the paralysis.

Gloria seemed submissive and talked very little when her mother was present. She did not ask about her husband, but she dramatically complained about her inability to move and was often irritable and demanding.

Ms. Brown, the nurse, recognized that Gloria enjoyed being the center of attention and being cared for. She sensed a constant undercurrent of anger in Gloria. One day, after visiting her husband on his unit, Gloria was observed curled up in bed, weeping, rubbing her legs. When Ms. Brown asked her if her legs hurt, she threw a book across the room and yelled loudly saying, "He's practically dying and he's still treating me like a baby." Ms. Brown listened quietly, and when Gloria had quieted down, she helped her to *talk* about her feelings. She told her it was normal to feel anger when others did not seem to understand what she was feeling or treated her as she may not have wanted to be treated. They discussed the role binds that people get into and do not know how to get out of because of an inability to communicate their feelings. Gloria stated that she feared that if she told her husband that she wanted to change, he would not understand, and that at this time it would be too much of a shock for him. Also, she was not sure that she knew how to change at this point in her life.

Ms. Brown said "Strong emotions and the need to change are often frightening feelings that a person may not be willing to acknowledge, much less communicate." As Gloria listened, she relaxed visibly. She said she had become convinced that she was stuck being a "Middle-aged doll" and that neither she nor her husband would be able to cope with a change. Ms. Brown said, "Your husband's heart attack will necessitate some changes anyway, so this may be a realistic time to start."

During subsequent sessions with the psychiatrist and the nurse, Gloria became more aware of her feelings and the connection between her husband's illness, her loss of dependency, her anger, and the subsequent paralysis. During her recovery, Gloria experimented with new feelings and behaviors, using Ms. Brown as a role model and testing ground.

Avoidance Behavior

Clients who displace their anxiety onto a particular object or situation will have varying degrees of restriction in their life-styles. Successful intervention with such clients has been limited. However, behavior modification seems to indicate more promise than traditional psychotherapeutic models of treatment (see Chap. 4 for a discussion of behavioral therapy). Behavior modification is ac-

companied by close contact and open communication with the client and consistency toward the client on the part of the staff. These techniques are often carried out in conjunction with the administration of tranquilizers to decrease the impact of the anxiety which might be experienced.

The Family

Discharge planning starts from the first day the client comes in contact with the nurse. In caring for persons with emotional disorders, the return of the client to an active, productive life within the family and the community is a major goal. Therefore, from the onset of treatment, the client's relationship with others is constantly monitored. Difficulties in relationships with family, friends, and coworkers should be explored by the client and nurse. Interventions are directed at readjusting and learning to cope with the reality setting. If the client has been hospitalized, the significant others must be included in the nursing process so that the family dynamics continue to include the client and the family does not relinquish responsibility for the client.

Evaluation

The effectiveness of nursing intervention is measured by comparing behavior indicated on admission to change in behaviors throughout the treatment program; achievement of the goals of therapy which the nurse and the client originally formulated is also considered.

For example, Mr. D was admitted to the psychiatric unit of the local general hospital. He was experiencing severe levels of anxiety accompanied by ritualistic cleaning of his room. On admission, the nursing assessment included the following observations:

Severe anxiety level
Decreased nutritional intake
Inability to concentrate

Difficulty falling asleep

Social isolation; withdrawal from family and peers

Ritualistic cleaning of room

Nursing observations made toward the end of Mr. D's hospital stay were:

Realistic apprehension regarding return to family and job

Concern about repetition of ritualistic behavior

Concern about how he relates in social situations

It is the responsibility of nurse practitioners to identify effective nursing interventions and thus acquire an individual store of empirical data. This constitutes additional resource material from which the practitioner can draw when making future nursing assessments.

References

1 Clarence L. Barnhart (ed.): *World Book Dictionary,* Field Enterprises, Chicago, 1968.

2 Gertrude B. Ujhely: *The Nurse and Her Problem Patients,* Springer, New York, 1963.

3 David Shapiro: *Neurotic Styles,* Basic Books, New York, 1965.

4 D. Wilfred Abse: "Hysterical Conversion and the Hysterical Character, In Silvano Arieti (ed.), *American Handbook of Psychiatry,* 2d ed., Basic Books, New York, 1974, vol. 3, chap. 8.

5 Pierre Janet: *The Major Symptoms of Hysteria,* Macmillan, New York, 1920.

6 Robert L. Stevenson: *The Strange Case of Dr. Jekyll and Mr. Hyde and Other Famous Tales,* Dodd, Mead, New York, 1961.

7 C. H. Thigpen and H. M. Cleckley: *The Three Faces of Eve,* McGraw-Hill, New York, 1957.

8 Flora Rheta Schreiber: *Sybil,* Regnery, Chicago, 1973.

9 John Nemiah: "Obsessive Compulsive Neurosis," in A. M. Friedman, H. I. Kaplan, and B. Saddock (eds.), *Comprehensive Textbook of Psychiatry,* 2d ed., Williams & Wilkins, Baltimore, 1975.

10 Lewis Linn: "Diagnosis and Psychiatry," in A. M. Freedman, H. I. Kaplan, and B. Saddock (eds.), *Comprehensive Textbook of Psychiatry,* 2d ed., Williams & Wilkins, Baltimore, 1975.

*11 J. P. Watson: "Phobic Disorders, Part I: Clinical Aspects," *Nursing Mirror,* vol. 134, pp. 22–23, March 3, 1972.

12 Sigmund Freud: *A General Introduction to Psychoanalysis,* Garden City Publishing Company, Garden City, N.Y., 1943.

13 J. Breuer and Sigmund Freud: *Studies on Hysteria (1893–1895),* J. Strachey (trans.), Basic Books, New York, 1957.

14 Erik Erikson: *Childhood and Society,* 2d ed., Norton, New York, 1963.

15 Lynn R. Bernstein: Unpublished case history from South Shore Mental Health Services, Wantagh, New York.

*16 Gladys Lipkin and Roberta Cohen: *Effective Approaches to Patients' Behavior,* Springer, New York, 1973.

17 Pamela Mitchell: *Concepts Basic to Nursing,* McGraw-Hill, New York, 1973.

*18 J. P. Watson: "Phobic Disorders, Part II: Management," *Nursing Mirror,* vol. 134, pp. 32–35, March 10, 1972.

19 Joan Kyes and Charles Hofling: *Basic Psychiatric Concepts in Nursing,* 3d ed., Lippincott, Philadelphia, 1974.

*Recommended reference by a nurse author.

17
The Client Who Generates Anger

Laura Coble Zamora

Learning Objectives

After studying this chapter, the student should be able to:

1 Describe how anger is learned developmentally
2 Differentiate between the functional and dysfunctional aspects of anger
3 Describe how anger in the nurse leads to countertherapeutic responses to client behaviors
4 Construct a plan of care for a client with delirium tremens, with attention to needs for rest, metabolic and nutritional equilibrium, physical safety, and psychological comfort
5 List five signs of heroin withdrawal
6 Describe how early interpersonal events predispose to the development of
   a substance-abusive behavior
   b psychopathic behavior

7 Identify four sociocultural factors that perpetuate substance abuse in the United States

8 List ten significant factors the nurse assesses in relation to substance abusers and psychopaths

9 Define operationally the following behavioral themes as they are manifested in substance abusers and psychopaths
   a manipulation
   b impulsiveness
   c withdrawal
   d grandiosity

10 Construct a plan of care for substance-abusive and psychopathic clients who are manipulative, impulsive, withdrawn, and grandiose, with attention to specific goals and communication skills

11 Identify three aspects of the nurse's role and responsibility in the community in relation to substance abuse and psychopathy

Anger is a human experience of great significance for nursing practice. The awareness of anger and related emotions such as hostility, resentment, and rage has been identified elsewhere as being of help to the nurse in explaining and intervening in certain client behaviors.[1,2,3] Equally important to the therapeutic nurse-client relationship is the study of those client behaviors which *generate* anger in others. The anger generated often interferes with the therapeutic aim of a mutual problem-solving process.

Anger

Anger is a feeling or emotion which has been defined as a learned means of neutralizing or avoiding the anxiety which arises in response to interpersonal threat.[4] Anger is "learned" in the sense that it is empathized from significant others during the process of socialization. Young children become alert to the fact that when they challenge the authority of significant adults, the most remarkable degrees of anger can be generat-

ed in the adults. Furthermore, children notice that anger seems to wield much more power than anxiety. Consequently, they begin to cope with their own anxiety by converting it into the more powerful feeling of anger. A typical example of this learning experience in our culture occurs during toilet training, the so-called battle of the pot. In that situation the child discovers that when demands by significant adults for the giving of feces and urine are met with rebellion and noncompliance, anger is generated in those adults. Although children may ultimately comply with adult demands, they begin to experiment with anger. They often act it out in play situations in response to imagined violations of their own authority.

Anger, then, is developed by people as an important, unrefined tool to be used in situations where they would otherwise feel anxious and powerless.[4] It can be seen from this model that one situation in which anger is typically engendered is when one's sense of authority or perceived right to exercise influence over another is challenged or doubted.

There are three points about anger which must

be emphasized as significant for interpersonal relationships and thus for nursing: (1) one becomes angry when one's sense of authority or influence is threatened in interpersonal situations; (2) anger can be more functional than anxiety for the *individual* in that its expression gives a person a sense of power and immediate relief rather than powerlessness and insecurity; (3) anger can be dysfunctional for *interpersonal relationships* in that its expression is more conducive to ridding oneself of anxiety than to mutual learning or problem solving.

Anger as a human response to anxiety finds fertile ground for development in nursing. Nurses are often confronted by clients and colleagues who challenge their competence and authority. Each time a nurse feels challenged in this way, the potential exists for a perceived attack on self-esteem and an angry reaction. The therapeutic use of this very human response is possible *only* if the nurse recognizes anger in self and others and understands its strength and limitation as an immediate defensive response to anxiety.

One's self-esteem rests upon a variety of factors, and these depend upon the degrees of anxiety associated with one's early interpersonal experiences. Although it is possible that any of a wide range of client behaviors will evoke anger, the feeling of being used, which results from manipulation, is what really generates anger in the nurse. The problem is complicated by the fact that the manipulative behaviors may be unwitting and passive in nature and so are not readily identifiable as anger-provoking by client or nurse.

The clients are persons who are continuing to enact the drama of early conflicts over trust, independence, and identity—conflicts during which expressions of anger were forbidden, ignored, or otherwise rendered ineffective as a means of relieving anxiety. Anger then becomes a source of tension for the client rather than a source of relief. Relationships with others are dominated by attempts to rid the self of these tensions in other ways. Such clients often appear to be "asking for it"; and yet almost any response elicits from the client contempt or repeated efforts to test. The client's behaviors become increasingly incompre-

hensible and exasperating to others in the continual testing and rejecting of others' responses. Eventually the client's behavior induces in the other a felt powerlessness to influence the client. Anger is thus generated in the other as a means of restoring a sense of power. Long-term problematic behavioral themes can be understood in part as cycles of testing, rejecting, and ultimately escaping from relationships with others. Figure 17-1 will help the reader to conceptualize the anger cycle as it applies to these clients. Clients to be discussed in this framework include substance abusers and antisocial persons or psychopaths.

Substance Abusers
The Alcoholic

Alcoholism is said to be the third major health problem in the United States.[5] Current estimates indicate that about 9 million people in this country are alcoholic or "problem drinkers."[6] Alcoholics adversely affect the mental health or functioning of another 30 million relatives and friends. While it is estimated that 70 percent of alcoholics are male, the number of known female alcoholics is rising. At least part of the difference between male and female alcoholism statistics is due to the more covert nature of problem drinking among women in our society. In addition to human suffering, the economic cost of alcoholism to America may be as much as $20 to $25 billion in medical expenses, lost wages, and reduced industrial productivity.[5] Another major impetus for the study and treatment of alcohol abuse during the past few years has been its rapid rise among children and teenagers.[5,7] The preceding factors combine to underline the continuing serious drain on the nation's health in terms of both its human and economic resources.

There is no precise agreement on the definition of alcoholism; distinctions between "alcoholic" and "problem drinker" are difficult to make. Broadly speaking, alcoholism is "any use of alcoholic beverages that causes any damage to the individual or society or both."[8] Most definitions of alcoholism refer to the following clinical features:

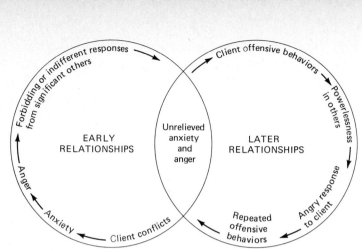

Figure 17-1 The problematic anger cycle.

(1) chronicity as a disease or disorder of behavior; (2) undue preoccupation with intake of ethyl alcohol; (3) loss of control over the drinking pattern itself; (4) use of alcohol in a way that is damaging to drinker's physical health, interpersonal relations, and/or economic functions; and (5) use of alcohol as a universal solution to problems.

Alcohol abuse can become a problem over a long or short period of time following the onset of excessive drinking. The progressive, untreated alcoholic may begin to develop an increasing tolerance for alcohol. Drinking behavior becomes surreptitious and uncontrollable. Periods of intoxication become prolonged, with loss of memory for the actual episodes. The alcoholic becomes guilty and persistently remorseful about drinking and this, of course, impels him or her to drink more in order to relieve such feelings. Relationships with others become dominated by feelings of self-pity and unreasonable resentment. Attention span and concentration ability are decreased. The client develops tremors, recurrent somatic symptoms, and insomnia.[9]

Despite the somewhat characteristic nature of the above clinical features, the reader should be cautioned against conceptualizing a "universal alcoholic profile." The stereotype of the alcoholic as a skid-row bum is applicable to only 5 percent of the alcoholic population. There are in practice wide individual variations in excessive drinking.

The excessive use of alcohol cuts across all personality and diagnostic categories. Therefore the abuse of alcohol must always be evaluated in the context of the total person and his or her environment. While the alcoholic is still viewed by some as one who is engaging in "criminal" behavior, the conscious attitude of most people is that alcoholism is an illness.

Dynamics

The forces which prompt alcoholic behavior have been studied from biological, psychological, and sociocultural points of view. At this time there is insufficient evidence to "prove" one causal theory over another. Rather, the evidence supports the argument that human behavior is multidetermined, and that a variety of biological, psychological, and sociocultural factors interrelate to produce and perpetuate alcoholic behavior. While the present discussion focuses on psychological and sociocultural factors, it should be noted that the major theories of *biological causes* have included genetic factors, allergic responses to food and chemicals, biochemical imbalances, central nervous system pathology, nutritional deficiencies, and endocrinological dysfunctions, particularly hyperadrenocorticism.[8]

Psychological explanations of drinking vary in detail but generally point to the use of alcohol as a means of escape or relief from anxiety. Some of the more common explanations for the existence of severe anxiety entail theories of oral and oedipal fixation. Orally, what is sought, via the bottle and oblivion, is a regressive reunion with the all-caring mother figure; oedipally, the fantasized reunion excludes such unwanted interlopers as fathers and siblings. This implies that the roots of alcoholism lie in anxiety-ridden early relationships with significant others.

For example, the family environment of the potential alcoholic may promote excessive dependency by depriving the child too abruptly and too soon in relation to normal dependency needs. Or parental overprotection may discourage the child from seeking self-dependence and encourage prolonged, sexualized dependence. Additionally, parental insecurity which takes the form of uncontrolled aggression, instability, or irresponsibility provides limited "healthiness" to emulate or with which to identify. A child in the above situations can develop a poor foundation for sexual identity and for responsible, mature behavior. Beyond that, the child is bound to feel resentful and then guilty for harboring unacceptable dependency feelings. Resultant rage, hostility, and mistrust are expressed and atoned for later in the guilt, low self-esteem, dependence, and self-destructiveness that characterize the alcoholic's relationships.

Unresolved conflicts in the early phases of development predispose to severe anxiety, confusion, and self-doubt during adolescence, when issues of sexual identity, independence, and relation to authority normally emerge and must be resolved. These, too, continue to be significant areas of conflict in many alcoholics.

Another way of understanding alcoholism is to view drinking behavior and attitudes as learned patterns within a given *sociocultural* context. In assessing alcoholism from this viewpoint, one must look at sociocultural patterns of drinking and at family operations which teach and reinforce excessive drinking. In this connection, it should be noted that drinking itself is a typical behavior in the United States.[10] The media bombard us with graphic representations of this fact through advertising and other portrayals of drinking as a socially approved behavior.

Beyond that, sociocultural data show, for example, that although most Jews drink occasionally, the incidence of alcoholism among Jews is low. More people in urban areas than in rural areas tend to drink. Although people in higher social classes drink more frequently than those in other social classes, they less often drink to excess. Within social classes, more men than women and more young people than old people drink.[10] These patterns are not static, of course, but they can be potentially influential in the "learning" of alcoholic behavior, since they tend to set models and expectations of drinking behaviors for families and individuals within a particular sociocultural environment.

Within the family, a developing child can be socialized into drinking as a means of relieving anxiety and releasing rage. For example, the child may observe and identify with this behavior in a significant adult. Family members may communicate conflicting messages about the acceptability and moral virtue of alcohol ingestion and thus indirectly encourage "forbidden" behavior in the form of alcoholism. That is, the child may be the recipient of double-bind communication regarding alcohol use and abuse (see Chaps. 4, 11, and 14). In this type of situation, the parents may overtly forbid the purchase or presence of alcohol within the home as being morally reprehensible; at the same time, they describe with relish how tipsy everyone was at the last office party. Children gradually discover that the "forbidden pleasure" is worth seeking, although it is simultaneously disapproved. In each of these cases, drinking behavior is learned from and/or reinforced by operations within the family system. The operations within the family are, in turn, influenced by the patterns and attitudes of the larger sociocultural system.

Treatment Approaches and Acute Care Aspects
Current approaches to the treatment of alcoholism encompass four aspects; (1) managing acute episodes of intoxication, (2) correcting the chronic health problems associated with alcoholism, (3)

changing the long-term behavior of alcoholic individuals,[6] and (4) assisting family systems to develop healthier patterns of relating.

Individual, group, and family treatment modalities are used with alcoholics. They aim for increased self-awareness, enhanced self-esteem, and improved interpersonal skills. Nurses may be involved directly in individual, group, or family treatment of alcoholics; or nursing roles may be more concerned with establishing a therapeutic milieu for alcoholic clients (see Chaps. 9, 10, and 11).

Behavior modification in the treatment of alcoholism is designed to modify and eliminate drinking behaviors by using basic principles of classical conditioning. The best-known aversive agent used in the treatment of alcoholism is Antabuse (disulfiram). Antabuse blocks the action of an enzyme required for the metabolism of alcohol. When Antabuse is taken on a regular basis, the result for the client who imbibes even small amounts of alcohol is nausea, vomiting, palpitations, and general prostration. The client is thus conditioned to avoid the use of alcohol. Antabuse has sometimes been used as an adjunct to other therapeutic approaches, such as individual, group, and family therapy.[11]

In addition to aversion therapy, recent innovative applications of the behavior modification approach have included use of avoidance procedures as well as positive reinforcement techniques.[12] Although an interpersonal relationship is not the major vehicle of this treatment modality, the accompanying elements of caring, emotional support, and encouragement are generally felt to be important for successful treatment.

Alcoholics Anonymous (AA) continues as one of the major traditional approaches to alcoholism. This group is composed entirely of former alcoholics. Through education, self-help, and supportive fellowship of a strongly religious nature, it aims for sobriety through total abstinence from alcohol. As the primary resource for the rehabilitation of alcoholics, AA has been most successful in helping clients who can identify with the socioeconomic background of a particular chapter's membership. Referrals are most effective when contact is established between client and AA prior to the client's discharge from an acute treatment setting. The AA program itself focuses on group meetings where members acknowledge their alcoholism and share their personal experiences of alcohol abuse and control.

In addition to AA, other groups such as *Al-Anon* and *Alateen* have been formed to assist family members with the problems of alcoholism. Al-Anon is an organization of spouses and Alateen an organization of teen-age children of alcoholics. The emphasis is on education, guidance in relating to the alcoholic family member, and the sharing of problems and experiences.

Detoxification entails withdrawing the client from alcohol in a controlled environment via one of several protocols for detoxification. The setting and the criteria for detoxification will depend upon the institution.

Clients who seek or require detoxification are not necessarily admitted directly to an acute treatment center. They are frequently found in hospital emergency rooms and on the various wards of general hospitals. The presenting complaint may be physical trauma as a result of an "accident," other physical illness which has interrupted alcohol ingestion, or emotional disturbance. Because of the emotional and behavioral aspects of alcohol abuse, such clients may be admitted to a psychiatric facility which is not equipped to deal with detoxification. For these reasons, nurses should be alert to a history of alcohol abuse or early signs of impending withdrawal. The potentially life-threatening consequences of withdrawal from excessive use of alcohol necessitate a well-monitored detoxification process (see Chap. 15).

In general, during detoxification, the nurse permits the client to rest as comfortably as possible. The client must be protected from injury and observed for any signs of psychological or physiological instability which suggest the development of complications such as delirium tremens. Detoxification is best handled in a quiet environment where lighting is adjusted to reduce shadows and distortions and thus to prevent anxiety or panic in the client.

While a client is still intoxicated, the introduction of other chemicals into the body should be avoided if possible. This is primarily because of the fact that alcohol may potentiate or compound the action of other drugs.[13] Alcohol (ethanol) acts pharmacologically as a central nervous system *depressant*. It acts to block synaptic transmission, retarding or preventing the stimulation of one neuron by another. In very large doses, alcohol apparently interferes directly with the oxygen metabolism of the cell bodies.[14] Excessive alcohol ingestion often appears to alter behavior in the direction of hilarity and high spirits or aggression and violence. This "stimulant" effect is more apparent than real. What happens is that alcohol depresses the highest cortical centers first; therefore, such altered behaviors can be understood as due to decreased cortical inhibition and control of behavior.

Due to the progressively depressant effects of alcohol, the problem of sedation during detoxification is a difficult one. In general, the aim should be to prevent acute withdrawal symptoms without immobilizing the client unduly with additional sedation. Agitation that interferes with rest, sleep, or physical safety should be controlled with sedatives such as paraldehyde or tranquilizers such as chlorpromazine or chlordiazepoxide.

Detoxification is *not* a cure; it is the first step in a treatment process that is often long and arduous for both client and health professional. Therefore, one difficult aspect of caring for clients who are acutely intoxicated and/or undergoing detoxification may be the nurse's task of dealing with his or her own attitudes toward "drunkenness." Awareness of such attitudes is particularly important for nurses who work in emergency rooms, walk-in clinics, or other facilities where they are likely to encounter the same client repeatedly. If any long-term treatment is to be instituted, it is often the nurse who can use these repeated encounters to encourage and coordinate such efforts; but negative or despairing attitudes will prevent these actions and will most likely be communicated to the client and family as well.

Delirium tremens (DTs) is an acute complication of alcoholism that constitutes a medical and nursing emergency. Treated, DTs carries a 5 per-cent mortality rate. Untreated, it carries a 15 percent mortality rate. The nurse is frequently in a position to note the signs or to pick up a history suggestive of impending DTs. (See Chap. 15.) The client with impending DTs may be found in any circumstance which has suddenly interrupted the excessive intake of alcohol. For example, a client may enter a general hospital for gallbladder surgery and, 2 to 4 days later, develop beginning signs of DTs. The challenge to the nurse is amplified in that the client often needs lifesaving measures at the same time that the mental status renders the client at best uncooperative and, at worst, actively resistive to treatment.

The etiology of DTs, although still not entirely clear, is thought to be sudden withdrawal from alcohol following a period of chronic intoxication. Other factors that can contribute to the development of DTs include physical trauma, infections, and metabolic disorders as well as anxiety-provoking stimuli. DTs at the beginning is an acute organic brain syndrome that comprises the following symptoms: increased psychomotor activity and tremulousness, confusion and disorientation, fearfulness, signs of vasomotor lability, tachycardia, temperature of 100 to 105°F., and illusions and hallucinations. The latter are most commonly visual and tactile, often consisting of terrifying animal images and crawling skin sensations. The onset of DTs is typically quite sudden and dramatic, and the condition usually lasts from 2 or 3 days to a week.[14]

The treatment aims in DTs customarily include rest, restoration of nutritional and metabolic equilibrium, prevention of seizures, reduction of fear and anxiety, and prevention of impulsive acts. Table 17-1 outlines the nursing care for the client in DTs.

One nursing measure that does not appear in Table 17-1 but deserves separate comment is the use of restraints for the patient in DTs. *If at all possible, the use of restraints should be avoided,* as restraint tends to agitate the client who is confused and disoriented. The client must, however, be protected from self-injury. If there is no one available to remain with him or her, then restraints may be necessary (see Chap. 15).

Table 17-1 Care of the Client with Delirium Tremens

Nursing diagnoses	Goals	Nursing intervention
Sleep disturbance	Restore normal sleep pattern	Assess effectiveness of chemical sedation (paraldehyde, chlordiazepoxide, chlorpromazine).
	Decrease agitation	Reduce external stimuli by speaking calmly and distinctly, adjusting lighting to prevent shadows and extremes of light and dark, restricting interpersonal contact to as few people as possible, adjusting room temperature, eliminating extraneous noises.
Metabolic and nutritional disequilibrium	Restore fluid and electrolyte balance.	Force fluids as ordered
		Monitor intake and output and record.
		Check bladder for distention.
	Restore nutritional balance.	Administer high-protein, high-carbohydrate, low-fat diet.
		Administer vitamins B complex and C.
Potential seizures	Prevent seizures.	Administer anticonvulsant medication as needed (diphenylhydantoin).
		Observe seizure precautions.
Fear, anxiety, panic; impulsive, self-destructive behaviors	Reduce fear, anxiety.	Note signs of anxiety, agitation.
	Prevent panic.	Reduce external stimuli (as above).
		Remain with client and inform him or her of your intent to do this.
	Prevent impulsive, self-destructive behaviors.	Orient client to situation by informing him or her where client is and what is happening.
		Respond to client's fright by acknowledging client's fearfulness and emphasizing your intention to remain present. Interpret the client's surroundings to him or her clearly.
		Respond to client's reports of illusions and hallucinations by telling him or her that these frightening sights, etc., are part of the illness and that, as improvement occurs, they will no longer bother the client.
		Use side rails.
		Assess effectiveness of chemical sedation (as above).

Another important nursing aim in the care of this client is to view the acute organic episode in the context of the client's overall, continuing needs. In other words, instead of allowing care to end with management of the acute episode, the nurse may be able at this critical point to influence the client to accept long-term therapy for the underlying chronic alcoholism. It is well within the nurse's province to take the initiative in discussing this with the client and the rest of the health team.

Korsakov's psychosis is a relatively rare syndrome which apparently results from vitamin B deficiency and is associated with longstanding use of alcohol and inattention to adequate diet. The symptoms include disorientation, memory impairment, and the fabrication of elaborate stories to fill the memory gaps (confabulation). The client may recover from a single episode, but irreversible damage to the cerebral cortex results from continued drinking. Treatment therefore entails strict abstinence from alcohol and the administration of large doses of B-complex and C vitamins. When there is severe brain damage, long-term custodial care may be required. In less severely impaired cases, family members may be willing to offer supervision. Nurses in the hospital and in the community may be called upon to assist this client and his or her family in coping with the responsibility and frustrations of long-term abstinence and care (see Chap. 30).

The Drug Abuser

Since alcohol is in itself a drug, "alcoholism" and "drug abuse" are not mutually exclusive terms.

Substance abusers often mix other drugs and alcohol in varying degrees, so that the problems of alcoholism and drug abuse cannot be viewed as entirely distinct. However, the following section on the drug abuser will speak primarily of the person who abuses drugs other than alcohol. The *drug abuser,* as defined in this chapter, is a person who repeatedly uses a chemical substance or substances other than alcohol in a way that is harmful to self and society. A variety of chemical substances have been included under the umbrella of "drug abuse," and the ever-changing drug scene makes it impractical and perhaps misleading to attempt a comprehensive listing. To help the nurse conceptualize the range of substances abused, however, there are eight major categories. These are outlined in Table 17-2.

Traditionally the terms "habituation" and "addiction" have been used by health-care professionals in defining the nature and extent of drug abuse. In essence, *drug habituation* involves repeated use of a drug to the point where there is psychological dependence. *Drug addiction* is more compulsive drug use which involves craving, psychological dependence, and physical dependence; it includes the development of tolerance for increasing doses and the appearance of withdrawal symptoms. Withdrawal symptoms may include: rhinorrhea; lacrimation; sweating; chills; elevated temperature; dilated, sluggish pupils; insomnia; restlessness; muscle and joint pain. In actual practice, the attempt to make such distinctions is often meaningless; therefore the World Health Organization's term of "drug dependence" has been adopted by many health workers. *Drug dependence* refers to a "psychological and/or physical dependence on a drug that is taken periodically or on a scheduled basis."[14] This term is then further clarified in relation to a given individual by specifying the drug or drugs involved.

Although the use of drugs does not receive the same overt moral and legal acceptance as drinking, Americans are drug-oriented in the sense that they often turn to these chemical means of resolving their problems in living. The actual extent to which drugs are abused in this country has been difficult to document. Burkhalter comments that the available statistics on heroin dependency, drug-related deaths, and the like "point to the existence of a fluctuating, pervasive health problem that is of vital concern to all health professionals."[14]

Drug abuse affects in varying degrees all strata of American society. Vulnerability to drug abuse is great among children who live in the low-income neighborhoods of large urban centers. On the other hand, the stereotype of the heroin addict as coming from a deprived background in the ghetto is invalid in light of the number of narcotics abusers also coming from middle- and upper-class backgrounds.[14]

Dynamics

A concise discussion of *the* drug abuser is impeded by a need not to overgeneralize about personality traits or to oversimply the complex interplay of forces which may lead to and then perpetuate the practice of drug abuse in any given individual. The clinical features present in many drug abusers,

Table 17-2 Drugs of Abuse

Category	Examples
Narcotics	Heroin, morphine, methadone, codeine
Stimulants	Amphetamines, cocaine, amyl nitrate
Sedatives	Barbiturates, methaqualone (Quaalude), glutethimide (Doriden)
Minor tranquilizers	Diazepam (Valium), chordiazepoxide (Librium)
Hallucinogens	LSD (lysergic acid diethylamide), marijuana, mescaline
Volatile substances	Hair sprays, insecticides, model-airplane glue, lighter fluid
Nonnarcotic analgesics	Darvon, Aspirin
Over-the-counter drugs	Antihistamines, cough syrups, sleeping medicines

however, are similar to some of those mentioned in relation to the alcoholic. Also present in many instances are some of the features to be discussed later in this chapter as psychopathic or antisocial.

The drug abuser is often described as an excessively dependent, passive person who has difficulty tolerating frustration and anxiety. Theoretically this occurs when one's very early emotional needs are not met. For example, Singer notes that the sense of competence and hope essential to emotional maturity derives from a normal progression through phases of symbiosis, individuation, and adolescence. Certain mothering behaviors—such as rigid feeding schedules and the restriction of children's efforts to move and explore—interfere with this normal progression and predispose children to addictive patterns.[15] Furthermore, punishment for normal expressions of anxiety and anger prevents children from learning how to express or cope with these feelings adequately. The development of the trust in self and others that is necessary to tolerate delays in gratification is thwarted. Such persons search instead for immediate ways of escaping rising tensions. Drugs become a means of escape through feelings of euphoria and/or oblivion. The use of "forbidden" drugs also allows one to express rebellion toward parents and society through the use of the drug itself and the crime that is often necessary to support the habit. Occasionally one finds that the drug abuser has followed the example of the parent in the use of drugs as a means of escape and expression of rebellion.

The euphoria or oblivion that is available through drugs becomes a potent factor itself in perpetuating drug abuse. The injection process and resultant "high" are similar to orgasmic sexual feelings. The behavior is also reinforced by the abusers' life-style, where distinctive language, customs, and mores afford abusers some sense of belonging to a special group—a feeling that would not be possible otherwise. The combination of drug effects, preoccupation with securing and administering the drug, and identification with a deviant subculture prevents drug abusers from viewing and testing out alternative solutions to their problems.

Treatment Approaches and Acute Care Aspects
Table 17-3 provides an overview of treatment approaches to drug abuse.

Physical problems related to drug abuse warrant the nurse's attention in terms of both direct care and health teaching. These problems are inevitably intertwined with the client's psychosocial status and most often emerge from three predisposing conditions: (1) the client's neglect of nutritional needs; (2) the client's administration of drugs by injection under septic conditions; and (3) the properties of the drug themselves. Table 17-4 provides an overview of the more common physical problems of drug abuse.

The Psychopath

In clinical settings, nurses will encounter clients who are charming but who continually make serious trouble for themselves and others. Such clients have long fascinated students of human behavior, and various labels have been applied to them—including "psychopath," "sociopath," "antisocial person," and "impulsive character."[16,17,18] In essence, psychopaths don't fit into any other diagnostic category and their behavior is offensive.[19] The term "psychopath" will be used in this chapter to refer to such clients. There is overlapping between psychopathic and substance-abusive behavior in that psychopaths often engage in drug or alcohol abuse.

The psychopath's interpersonal relations are chiefly characterized by manipulation, shallowness, and lack of duration. Since the psychopath's behavior is governed by an overwhelming need for immediate satisfaction of basic needs and desires, such a person views others primarily as sources of potential danger or gratification. Due to feelings of underlying powerlessness, these clients often seek out persons of power and status to manipulate for the fulfillment of their needs. It is as though, in this way, psychopaths achieve the power and control they do not possess themselves.

Psychopaths seem to have few scruples about how they achieve satisfaction. Thus their behavior

Table 17-3 Drug Abuse: Treatment Approaches

Program type	Goals	Special aspects of approach to client care
Uncontrolled withdrawal: an unexpected acute-care problem	Prevention of physiologic disequilibrium Reduction of psychomotor agitation Instigation of long-term treatment	Assessment for signs and history of drug abuse Assessment for signs of drug withdrawal Alteration of acute nursing and medical regimens in accordance with drug-withdrawal problem
Detoxification: controlled withdrawal from drugs of abuse	(Same as for uncontrolled withdrawal)	Awareness that tolerance phenomenon may (1) explain client's seeking detoxification as a means of reducing drug habit cost or (2) be unknown to staff and therefore potentiate overdose in client
Methadone maintenance: substitution of methadone (a synthetic narcotic) for heroin in order to block the euphoric effects of heroin	Elimination of craving for heroin Promotion of independent functioning in society	Awareness that substitution does not resolve underlying problems leading to drug abuse Awareness that the absence of accustomed euphoria may increase client need for psychiatric intervention
Drug-free programs: therapeutic communities which emphasize discipline, confrontation, and peer support (Synanon, Phoenix House, Odyssey House)	Abstinence from drugs Promotion of ability to delay gratification Promotion of altered attitudes toward self and society	Residential long term treatment setting

is often in direct conflict with accepted legal, social, and moral codes. They feel little responsibility or remorse for the trouble they cause, and it is sometimes appalling. Psychopaths seem unconcerned about the lies or self-contradictions which emerge in their glib attempts to smooth over rough situations. Although these clients usually try to avoid punishment, the threat of possible punishment does not serve as an effective deterrent to their behavior. In general, the psychopaths fail to profit from experience in the sense of learning, although there is nothing amiss with their basic intelligence.

What happens theoretically to this client's emotional equipment is highly controversial. One view holds that psychopaths are unable to feel anxiety and that their behavior is therefore virtually closed to modification. Another interpretation is that the psychopath has failed to develop the more common security operations in response to anxiety.[20] For example, such mechanisms as selective inattention, dissociation, or sublimation are not available to the psychopath as a means of reducing the impact of tensions or rechanneling them. The psychopathic individual thus has a peculiarly low tolerance for anxiety or any painful emotion; the slightest hint of pain calls for seemingly drastic action. On the surface, there seems to be little ability or desire to control this pattern.

Dynamics
The forces behind this client's behavior are unclear, but various theories exist; again they are biological, psychological, and sociocultural. As with the substance abusers, at the present time it is probably wisest to assume an interplay of the three forces.

The psychopath's history generally shows that his or her early needs for satisfaction and security were met with delay, indifference, and rejection on the part of significant others. Such neglect may be

Table 17-4 Physical Health Problems of Drug Abuse

Predisposing conditions	Problem areas	Nursing intervention*
Neglect of nutritional needs	Malnutrition, including vitamin deficiencies	Explain how the drug habit gives rise to problems.
	Dental caries and loss of teeth	Provide nutritional information, particularly about foods of high value that are easily available and require little preparation.
	Respiratory infections	
Administration of drugs by injection under septic conditions	Skin abscesses	Provide vitamin supplements.
	Cellulitis	Assess for signs of infection.
	Hepatitis	Refer for appropriate medical and dental treatment.
	Bacterial endocarditis	
Drug properties	Constipation	
	Amenorrhea	
	Impotence	
	Tolerance	
	Seizures (in cocaine sniffers and during barbiturate withdrawal)	

*Nursing interventions are for application in each of the problem areas.

due to some direct inaction on the part of the parenting ones or to the experience of rejection which accompanies abandonment and long-term institutional or foster care in childhood. In any case, people who later become psychopaths have, as children, had limited opportunities to trust that their needs will be met. The lack of relatively enduring, involved parental figures obliges these children to abandon any expectation of mutuality in relatedness. Consequently, at the time when a child normally internalizes the standards, values, and morals of significant authority, the potential psychopath is severely hampered by a basic lack of involvement with people who might serve as models. The development of a superego or conscience, which depends upon such identification and internalization, is arrested. Consequent to this impaired superego development, later psychopathic behavior may be explained in terms of lack of involvement and absence of guilt.

Family integrity in general and child-rearing practices in particular influence and are influenced by the prevailing sociocultural climate. In the case of psychopathy, social crises which are divisive and stressful to the culture may have a negative impact on parents' attitudes toward children and child-rearing practices. For example,

children may be seen as burdensome, and child-rearing practices may be erratic and inconsistent with regard to discipline. Parents whose behavior suggests conflict over moral values can confuse and alienate the growing child with regard to moral values and behavioral standards. Thus the child may "learn" from parents that deceit, superficiality of involvement, and self-centeredness are the models for survival. The child may also respond to covert messages within the family that one is expected to behave antisocially. Later reinforcement of the behavior by the attitudes of other persons in authority serves to predispose the child to a psychopathic life-style.

Nurses' Response to Substance Abusers and Psychopaths

On the mental health–mental illness continuum, it is doubtful that any clients evoke greater disapproval, intolerance, and generally moralistic condemnation than do substance abusers and psychopaths. Instead of being viewed as persons in need of help, they are frequently seen as morally weak or, on the other hand, as quite capable of putting a stop to their offensive or self-destructive behaviors if only they would use their "will power." Not too surprisingly, people find it difficult to understand why someone who is apparently capable of clear thinking repeatedly gets into trouble with self, family, friends, work, the law, and society in general.

Nurses are not exempt from such responses. They, like everyone else, wish to feel appreciated and successful. When confronted by clients who solicit and then abuse their help or who seem to resist or defy their influence, they become angry. If there is no satisfactory resolution of the interpersonal situation, increased anger, disappointment, helplessness, and despair may follow for the nurse. Under such battle conditions, both nurses and clients lose.

Out of the nurse's anger there often develops a tendency to view a client's return to drugs, alcohol, and antisocial acts as failures on the part of the client. Unlike other instances where client behaviors may be seen as understandable defenses to be explored in the therapeutic process, substance abusers and psychopaths are expected to abstain from their customary defenses. In fact, these clients are usually asked to give up their defensive behaviors as a *condition* of being treated. Considering the enormous needs for their particular defenses that these clients have developed, it is possible that in this respect we ask far more of them than we would ask of ourselves.

At the same time, it is not uncommon for nurses, especially students and beginning practitioners, to set extremely high standards for themselves in relating to these clients. In their desire to be helpful to the clients, nurses may mistake the clients' charm, intelligence, and promises for meaningful commitment to change. The nurse's response when clients' promises are not kept or their contempt surfaces may be self-blame and disillusionment.

Another problematic response by nurses may be an unwitting tendency on their part to foster the problematic behaviors in the client. For example, the skill with which the psychopath beats the system may give rise to admiration and envy. The psychopath's more rebellious behaviors may meet

some unconscious need in the nurse for complicity, vicarious enjoyment, or even punishment. Thus, instead of directing intervention toward behavioral change, the nurse and client become involved in an interaction that supports the pathological status quo.

Nurses' responses to substance abusers and psychopaths will be in part influenced by their own sociocultural backgrounds. Therefore they need to be aware of how their past and current environments may resemble or differ from those of the clients in their care.

Of particular significance are differences in their attitudes toward the two sexes. For instance, attitudes toward female alcoholics are generally quite different from attitudes toward male alcoholics—and these differing attitudes directly influence the judgments made about their behavior as well as the attention given their various problems. Gomberg reports that while male alcoholics tend to be viewed as amusing or pitiable, female alcoholics are viewed as disgusting or disgraceful.[21] These differing attitudes may be responsible for women's tendencies to conceal their problematic drinking behaviors far more frequently than men do. One possible implication, of course, is that women's alcoholic problems are not recognized, studied, or treated with the same frequency as are men's. On the other hand, stereotypes of alcoholism as a "male problem" may influence the frequency with which alcoholism becomes a defensive solution for males in our society.

It is obvious, then, that nurses need to be aware of their attitudes and feelings toward these clients and their families. Even more useful would be the development of respect for the peculiar struggles of clients whose so-called deviant behaviors are to some extent actually condoned and functional within the society.

Nursing Assessment

Nurses' knowledge of various theoretical explanations of substance abuse and psychopathy as well as nurses' examination of their own attitudes toward these clients will provide a basis from which an ongoing assessment of client and nurse behaviors can proceed. The following list of questions, although not exhaustive, will serve as a guide to nursing assessment:

General Factors

1 Who has defined the behavior as a problem?
2 What function does the problematic behavior serve for the client at the present time?
3 In what way and to what extent does the client perceive substance abuse or antisocial behavior as a problem?
4 What particular circumstances trigger the behavior?
5 Who and where are the significant others?
6 What is the client's developmental level?
7 How does the behavior influence (alter or maintain) family roles and behavior at home?
8 How does the behavior influence (alter or maintain) staff roles and behavior in the treatment setting?
9 Is the client employed? What is the pattern of employment?
10 How does the behavior affect job or role performance?
11 What are the realistic possibilities of altering the client's behavior in present environment (home or health facility)?
12 What is the philosophy of the treatment setting, particularly regarding substance abusers and antisocial persons?
13 Does the client have the resources (significant others' support, job training, skills, etc.) for an alternate life-style?
14 Is the client presently in trouble with school or police or other public agency?
15 Has the client been or is the client now in treatment elsewhere?

Specific Factors Relating to Substance Abuse

1 What function does the substance itself serve for the client?
2 What substance(s) is (are) abused? How much is taken and when?
3 How available is the substance? How is the source of supply controlled?
4 Is the client recently withdrawn from the substance?
5 Who in the client's environment also uses or abuses the substance?
6 What are family attitudes toward use of this substance?
7 What are the cultural attitudes toward use of this substance?
8 What is the client's physical condition?
9 What are the client's dietary habits?

Assessment of such factors is directed primarily toward diagnosing *for whom* a given behavior is a problem, the *extent* to which the behavior is a problem, and *why* the behavior is occurring within a given context of time, place, and persons.

Nursing Diagnoses: Behavior Problems—Long-Term and Recurrent

Clinically, nurses often identify an overlapping of substance-abusive and psychopathic traits; it is rare indeed to meet a "textbook case." There are also some common dynamic elements in that *mistrust, excessive dependency, faulty identification and learning, and low tolerance for the tensions of anxiety, guilt, and anger* have developed and persisted. These elements give rise to several behavioral problems with which nurses must be concerned in both substance abusers and psychopaths. These include *manipulation, impulsiveness, withdrawal,* and *grandiosity.* These behaviors are not in and of themselves pathological or maladaptive; in fact, circumstances may give rise to such behaviors in almost anyone at one time or another. What must concern the nurse, however, are repetitive patterns which emerge as obstacles to healthy interpersonal relations.

Manipulation

"Manipulation" is a term frequently used by health workers to label clients' offensive attempts to get something the worker does not wish to give. In order to intervene therapeutically, nurses need to recognize their own reactions and then apply "manipulation" as an explanatory concept rather than a disparaging label.

The process of manipulation begins with a conflict of needs or goals between client and nurse: the client wants something from the nurse, and the nurse cannot or will not give it. Because they have developed little self-esteem and trust, substance abusers and psychopaths are poorly equipped to cope with the tensions of their unmet needs. Their interpersonal experiences have severely limited their ability to consider any needs or goals the nurse may have. Consequently, instead of engaging in a mutual problem-solving process, these clients automatically increase their attempts to influence the nurse to meet their needs. These attempts almost inevitably include some element of deception—insincerity, fabrication, denial, or rationalization—all of which underline the uniquely offensive aspect of the interpersonal process. Although some of the process may remain unconscious, at least part of it is conscious and deliberate.[19,22]

The aim of the client may range from simply trying to avoid anxiety, to achieving pleasurable ends, to attempting to put something over on the nurse when there seems to be no real advantage. The net result for the nurse is a feeling of having been used.

In the case of substance abusers, the manipulative process often revolves around unmet dependency needs. This may appear in the client's deliberate maneuvers to get the forbidden substance itself, or it may appear more subtly in demands for the nurse's time or for physical contact, attention, permission, approval, or disapprov-al. Substance abusers manipulate the nurse via a sort of "taking in" process that reflects the infantile nature of their difficulties.

The manipulative maneuvers of psychopaths, on the other hand, seem related to frank mistrust and a contemptuous view of the motivations of others. In other words, because of life experience with rejection and deception, it is inconceivable to this client that the nurse could possibly relate honestly, sincerely, and directly. The psychopath therefore engages in games of outwitting the nurse, where the manipulation itself is the primary goal. In contrast to substance abusers, then, psychopaths seem to "take in" nurses in order to reject them.

In both instances, faulty identification and learning as well as low tolerance for anxiety have contributed to the use of manipulation as a survival technique.

Operational Definition of Manipulation:

1 Client wants (needs) something from nurse.	1 Client: "It's so nice out, how about letting me sit out on the bench?" (Client is on bed rest for infected leg.)
2 Nurse perceives client's want as pathological or unreasonable.	2–3 Nurse: "No, Mr. A, you have to stay in bed because of the infection."
3 Nurse does not fulfill client's want.	
4 Client's tension increases.	4 Client gets out of bed.
5 Client increases attempts to influence nurse to fulfill want by:	5 Client: "Aw, c'mon. It's *my* leg!
a Becoming dependent, clinging, demanding, helpless	This is ridiculous— I'll rest much better outside."
b Denying either the	Client to patient group: "That nurse is

meaning or mani-
festation of the
want

c Rationalizing the
want by supplying
logical reasons for
its appearance
and fulfillment

d Fabricating by
making false
statements and
promises about
his/her behavior

e Questioning or de-
fying the nurse's
competence and
authority

a stupid bitch. What
do you say we all re-
fuse to take our
meds until she lets
us out?''[23]

6 Nurse feels power-
less and angry.

6 Nurse: "I'm calling
the doctor. Then
we'll see who's
boss!''

Impulsiveness

Impulsiveness is a predominant theme in the behavior of substance abusers and psychopaths. In
fact, if nurses could find one word that would sum
up such clients' more trying attributes, it would be
this. "Impulsiveness" as used here refers to a
pattern of behavior which is directed toward immediate gains and gratification, with little time between thought and action.[23] Therefore clients experience a diminished feeling component of behavior. Guilt, anxiety, and anger as conscious
feelings are to some extent avoided. The brief time
between thought and action also prevents clients
from "thinking things through" or weighing consequences, particularly in relation to others. Actions
appear abrupt and unplanned in any long-term
sense, although considerable cleverness and
aplomb may be noted in their immediate execu-
tion.

The impulsiveness may be active or passive.
The "antisocial" acts of the psychopath, for example, often are dramatically active pursuit of some

spur-of-the-moment exploit, with blatant disregard
for others. The attitude is one of contempt. The
substance abuser, under the influence of a chemical, may behave similarly; but this client's basic
mode of impulsiveness is more passive, a sort of
giving in to temptation.[23] One senses here the
helpless, dependent, "I-have-no-control-over-it"
attitude, which is passive-manipulative.

Among alcoholics, impulsiveness must be
atoned for, which differentiates it from the impulsiveness of psychopaths and, to some extent, that
of other substance abusers. The guilt and anxiety
associated with forbidden oedipal sexual and aggressive urges are impulsively obliterated through
the use of alcohol. The intoxicated state permits
even greater impulsiveness, which subsequently
lowers self-esteem and gives rise to additional
guilt feelings. Alcohol abuse also takes a tremendous toll in physical suffering—hangovers, toxicity, damage to body organs. Thus, in one cycle of
impulsiveness, alcoholics achieve momentary release and gratification, feel guilty, and punish
themselves. Unfortunately, because of the underlying low self-esteem, the punishment aspect becomes a potent secondary source of gratification,
and so the cycle must be repeated.

Operational Definition of Impulsiveness

1 Client perceives
need for gratification
in a material or bod-
ily sense.

1 Client: "I need to
get out of here—a
night on the town!"

2 Nurse communicates
expectation of delay
in gratification and
focus on interperson-
al relatedness.

2 Nurse: "You and
I are scheduled
to talk for awhile
now."

3 Client experiences
slight but intolerable
rise in tension.

3 Client feels frus-
trated.

4 Client acts abruptly
and without reflec-
tion by:

4–7 Client walks away
from nurse; leaves
the unit with a

a Actively moving toward gratification

b Passively submitting to temptation of drugs, food, alcohol

5 Client thus avoids anxiety of nurse-client relatedness by

a Disregarding the nurse's significance and influence

b Blunting awareness of the nurse's significance and influence

6 Client's tension is decreased momentarily.

7 Nurse feels rejected, powerless, angry.

The essential difference between the impulsiveness described here and that of clients who generate fear has to do with the concept of "loss of control." Substance abusers and psychopaths who encounter serious obstacles to their goals are quite capable of the fear-generating kind of impulsiveness. (See Chap. 15.) However, the problems referred to in this chapter stem from lack of the usual controls refining the thinking process rather than from loss of control of aggressive feelings themselves. The nurse is more likely to view the resultant behaviors as maddeningly erratic, self-serving, thoughtless, and infantile than as rage-filled or frightening.

Withdrawal

"Withdrawal" refers to an extreme pattern of client behavior that facilitates escape from the real or

friend, saying to nurse, "We can talk tomorrow sometime!"

Nurse asks to have client assigned to another staff member.

anticipated anxiety of relatedness. Escape through withdrawal can occur only to the extent that others participate in the process.[26]

Withdrawal can be physical, but in the case of clients with problems of substance abuse and antisocial behavior, it is more likely to be emotional, and its manifestations rarely go unnoticed. The withdrawal process is usually provocative and infinitely exasperating to the nurse—it is by no means a simple fading into the woodwork.

For example, the excessive use of substances such as alcohol and drugs accomplishes "escape" by dulling the client's feelings of guilt, anger, or sexual insecurity. At the same time, the behavior at some point demands a response by the nurse, either for physical care, punishment, or forgiveness.

In psychopaths, withdrawal is seen in the withholding of emotional involvement—in the shallow, fleeting nature of relationships. It is as if this client were constantly escaping from *feeling* and thus always running away from people. The "running away," however, is often sensational in its style and certainly is hurtful to others.

Thus it can be seen that the process of withdrawal contains not only escape aspects but controlling aspects as well. The tragedy for the client is that such a form of escape often involves real loneliness. It is not by simple choice that the person is isolated and distant. It is from his or her inability to tolerate the anxiety and anticipated emotional demands of interpersonal relatedness. In effect, the client has been sensitized to threatening or indifferent interpersonal relationships in the past; therefore he or she mistrusts the present experience.

Operational Definition of Withdrawal:

1 Nurse communicates an expectation of interpersonal relatedness.

2 Client is fearful, mistrustful, or contemp-

1 Nurse asks client to join a client group for discussion of problems.

2–4 Client readily goes to the dis-

tuous of the intentions or actions of the nurse.

3 Client escapes from anxiety of interpersonal demands by:

   a Physically removing self from nurse

   b Blunting awareness of feelings associated with relatedness through drug, or alcohol abuse

   c Keeping relatedness at a superficial, pleasant "chit-chat" level

   d Maintaining an "as if" involvement in nurse-client relationship

4 Client maintains distance by controlling access to the self.

5 Nurse feels rejected, powerless, angry.

cussion group with nurse, smiles pleasantly, comments and looks interested, responds to question about self with: "Oh, I'm working things out, you know; it takes time to develop insight." In middle of nurse's response, suddenly excuses self to attend to something "important."

5 Nurse begins to have difficulty focusing on group process.

Grandiosity

Another common and problematic behavioral theme encountered in substance abusers and psychopaths is grandiosity. According to Salzman, "grandiosity is the assumption of an exalted, superior state which is beyond realistic possibility of actuality."[25] Specifically in relation to substance abuse and psychopathy, one finds that such clients manifest remarkable denial and rationalization of, as well as arrogance and irresponsibility toward, the consequences of their behaviors. It is as though the rules that apply to people in general bore no relation to the client. In effect, then, the client maintains a "privileged status."[25]

Substance abusers often reveal grandiosity in their beliefs or fantasies about giving up alcohol or drugs. They may, for example, boast of being able to give up the substance any time they feel like it; or they may refer to elaborate and patently unrealistic plans for becoming functional within the society. Grandiosity is also apparent in the suffering of alcoholics: they see their sins and guilt as being much blacker than those of ordinary people; nobody else could possibly be so awful.

Psychopaths demonstrate grandiosity in their unshakable belief in their own perfect cleverness. Such clients are convinced of their faultless abilities to outwit those in authority. The client "invariably overestimates his cunning and underestimates the capacities of the police and all others."[25]

Unfortunately for the clients, grandiose patterns are based on extremely shaky foundations of low self-esteem, powerlessness, and inadequacy. In a sense, clients' felt powerlessness to influence others is compensated for in the opposite views they take of their behavior, its motivations, and its consequences. The false view of self in relation to others is doubly unfortunate in that it obscures the clients' real assets and interpersonal potential, leaving these undeveloped.

Operational Definition of Grandiosity

1 Nurse communicates expectation for human relatedness.

2 Client tension rises, due to underlying view of self as worthless, inadequate, powerless (inhuman).

3 Client defends against anxiety by adopting a superior and exalted attitude toward nurse.

4 Client reacts overtly to nurse's expectations by:

1 Nurse asks client how job interview went.

2–4 Client flippantly responds that interview went "right down the drain—right where you'd expect it to go, considering the fact that I'm over-qualified!" Then: "It was your idea anyway—and obviously a poor one." Then: "I don't need the job

a Disclaiming knowledge of or responsibility for behavior and its consequences

b Arrogant, derogatory attitudes toward rules and expectations

c Exaggerated self-pity and resentment of demands by others

5 Client avoids anxiety at the expense of failing to develop real abilities.

6 Nurse feels rejected, powerless, angry.

anyway, so it doesn't really matter."

5 Client refuses to discuss incident further.

6 Nurse reminds client that he'd better get a job soon, as he's up for discharge.

Nursing Goals and Intervention: Manipulation

Nursing intervention when the client engages in manipulative behavior is directed toward defining a relationship in terms of a mutual experience in learning and trust rather than a struggle for power and control. This involves goals which assist clients to (1) increase their awareness of manipulative behavior as a problem which *curtails* their experience; (2) recognize the feelings and thoughts which prompt the behavior; (3) lessen the need for exploitative, deceptive, and self-destructive maneuvers; and (4) discover and test alternative ways of relating to their interpersonal environments.

In the nurse's endeavors to assist substance-abusive or psychopathic clients, it is well to remember that they are often operating at a "pretrust" level. Early expectations of solid confidence or trust are unrealistic, although the client's superficial behavior may suggest that such a level has been reached. The pretrust nature of the clients' behavior means that they cannot deal effectively with other people's expectations. In particular, their manipulative tactics are exacerbated by excessive rigidity or permissiveness, inconsistencies, or ambiguities in environmental expectations. Therefore, nursing actions in response to manipulation often take the form of *setting limits, acting as a role model, and providing learning experiences.* The rationale is that the client needs from a person in authority a reasonable, consistent, and clearly defined framework within which to learn and grow interpersonally.[22,26,27] The nurse operates on the basis of open, clear, self-actualized communication.

Setting limits

In setting limits, the nurse:

1 Defines clear expectations for the client and communicates these positively and firmly.

2 Limits only those behaviors which clearly impinge upon the health of the client and/or the rights and interests of others; automatic opposition to all client behavior does not allow clients the opportunity to discriminate among various behaviors in self or others.

3 Confines the *means* of limiting client behavior to those actions which feasibly can be carried through; empty threats or promises only reinforce the client's idea that he or she cannot depend upon others.

4 Offers the client an alternative; often this entails encouraging the client to use the nurse to review problem episodes.

5 Avoids making a public issue out of manipulative behavior; bringing it up for discussion in a community meeting, for example, may revive the "contest" and, in a sense, reward the client for the manipulative behavior.

6 Does *not* engage in accusations, arguments,

and demands for justification from client; again this only exacerbates the power struggle, which is fatiguing and futile.

7 Collaborates with all involved health staff in achieving a consensus about client behavior expectations and the means of approach; conflicts among staff members in regard to limit setting almost guarantee that the client's manipulations will thrive; the need is to maximize clear, direct communication (see also Chap. 19).

One complex issue the nurse must confront in setting limits is whether it is the client's initial need or want, the manipulative process itself, or both that are truly pathological or unreasonable.[19] In some instances, a little reflection on what has occurred will show that while the want was valid, the method of expressing it was offensive and disruptive.

Common manipulations which these clients present early in a therapeutic relationship are those of seizing the initiative and focusing on the helper's "flaws."[20] There is an element of role reversal in these behaviors which can easily put the nurse on the defensive.

For example, such a client often will ask nurses how they are feeling or how their day has been. The client may express an interest in the personal life and qualifications of the nurse: "I notice your pin is from _____ University" or "I see that you're wearing a wedding band." While on one level these behaviors may seem sociable, they are often attempts on the part of clients to avoid discussing their own difficulties. Beyond that, they may represent clients' efforts to prove that the nurse, like everyone else, is not really concerned about anyone but self; or that the client is not worthy of the nurse's interest or respect.

Limit setting in response to these initial behaviors is an important but delicate issue. If the nurse becomes immediately bogged down in conflicts between the client's possible motivations and how much personal information the nurse should reveal, the chances are that initial steps toward rapport and respect will be impeded by defensiveness. It is probably wiser for the nurse to *notice* the client's behavior, to answer questions or comments briefly, and then to refocus on some aspect of the client's day without confronting the manipulation directly at this point. If the client's maneuvers continue, it may help for the nurse to reclarify the purpose of the interaction: "Use the time to talk about yourself," or "I'm here for you to talk with about whatever difficulties *you're* having." In this regard, nurses often state their purposes erroneously by saying, "I'm here to talk with you." Such words convey that the *nurse* will do the talking—the client is provided with a means of avoiding talk!

Role Modeling

As a corollary to limit setting, the nurse acts as a role model. First, this means that the nurse is ready to give up the functions of authority when relevant.[22] Second, it implies that in representing rational authority through knowledge and competence, the nurse also has the human capacity to be fallible.

While it is important for nurses not to be naïve or gullible in relation to manipulative clients, it is equally important that they demonstrate how one deals with mistakes or "imperfections" in self. Probably the only way to communicate to these clients that such aspects of the self are human—and therefore tolerable—is to admit any obvious errors that may occur in relation to the client. For example, when a client boasts of successfully outwitting the nurse, the nurse might reply casually that indeed the situation has been misjudged, but that in any case something has been learned. The message is that it is neither shameful nor virtuous to admit one's mistakes but rather a sign of mature responsibility.[19]

Providing Learning Opportunities

The third general approach to manipulative behavior which is correlated with limit setting is providing learning opportunities for clients. For an explanation of the therapeutic learning process, see Chap. 6.

Nursing Goals and Intervention: Impulsiveness

Nursing intervention when the client engages in impulsive behavior is directed toward defining a relationship in terms of opportunity for long-term mutual satisfaction rather than as a source of immediate pain or pleasure. The goals involve assisting clients to (1) spend time "thinking through" and talking out rather than acting out, (2) increase awareness of and tolerance for feelings as "danger signals" which precede impulsive acts, (3) recognize the ways in which impulsive behavior hurts oneself, (4) develop self-control and self-responsibility.

Setting Limits

One emphasis is on providing more concrete external controls while the client learns internal control. For example, the client may require a structured setting such as a day hospital where behavioral regulations restrict substance abuse and harm to others.[28] It also may be necessary to convey limits on impulsive behavior in a more authoritative, direct manner. This is because impulsive behavior by its very nature does not permit "thinking through." There may be no opportunity to reason with the client while at the same time protecting clients and others from the consequences of impulsive acts. (See Chap. 15.)

Providing Learning Opportunities and Role Modeling

Extremely important is providing impulsive clients with regular opportunities to apply problem solving to their life experiences. Such persons generally require a great deal of patience and practice as they teach themselves to feel and to think. They have no faith in the validity of talk unless that talk leads to an immediate, concrete gain.[20] The nurse

will be confronted repeatedly with evidence of resentment or distrust. Such remarks as "You're *supposed* to help me, but I still don't have a job" may reflect this distrust. Such attitudes can easily tempt the nurse to become defensive or disillusioned. If, however, the nurse can overcome such reactions and recognize that the behavior is prompted by the client's tension rather than the nurse's failure to help, it may be possible to elicit more of the client's thoughts and feelings. In the above example, the nurse might respond by asking the client to share his or her thinking about their talks leading to a job; or the nurse might comment on the client's frustration with the perceived lack of help. The nurse thus invites the client to learn and, at the same time, role models as a problem solver.

Nursing Goals and Intervention: Withdrawal

Nursing intervention when the client is withdrawn is directed toward defining a relationship as an opportunity to experience feelings directly and safely with another person rather than as a signal for escaping feeling. The goals involve assisting clients to (1) recognize and label feelings of anxiety, anger, guilt; (2) tolerate interpersonal contact, with its attendant levels of feeling; (3) express thoughts and feelings in ways that are gratifying to themselves and productive for interpersonal relatedness.

Providing Interpersonal Contact

Nursing actions frequently center around providing opportunities for interpersonal contact while at the same time respecting the client's needs for privacy and distance. Attention should not be limited to the client's "bad" moments, moments when the client has physically or emotionally withdrawn. This has the effect of rewarding the withdrawn, withholding, controlling aspects of behavior. Rather, the nurse conveys an expectation that the client will at some point wish to relate in a different way.

For example, client M is undergoing long-term hospitalization for peripherovascular disease. He has a history of alcohol and drug abuse and a long criminal record. On the ward his behavior shifts between charming concern for other clients; loud, angry demands for improved care and attention; and episodes of withdrawal. During one of the latter episodes, Mr. M draws the curtains around his bed, posts signs warning others not to disturb him, and, to all appearances, is asleep. As a "care giver" in the situation, the nurse feels concern and yet wonders about the wisdom of intruding on Mr. M's territory. The nurse finally speaks to Mr. M, who barely responds, and asks him what the trouble is. When Mr. M does not reply, the nurse says that she will return in an hour and perhaps Mr. M would like to share his thoughts then. When the nurse returns, Mr. M is sitting up and talks for awhile, although the curtains remain closed. The nurse was primarily concerned here with providing contact and communicating some expectation that the client would make use of the contact.

Facilitating Recognition and Expression of Feelings

When nurses observe signs of mood change or withdrawal, they ask clients what they are feeling. Often the response will be noncommittal, a denial of feeling, or a response that does not answer the question. "Try talking about what you're feeling," and "If you're upset it would be useful to talk about it," suggest that it's human to feel and that verbal expressions of feelings are more comprehensible interpersonally than unverbalized, acted-out feelings.

Setting Limits

In the case of seeking withdrawal through the use of substances, of course, limits are usually set on access to the substance as well as on behaviors associated with securing and administering the substance. These limits are implemented via mi-

lieu controls, such as peer pressures, and rules and regulations of the treatment setting. Such environmental limitations may indeed increase anger and anxiety, but the clients are thereby faced with an opportunity to recognize these feelings and cope in ways other than chemically induced euphoria or oblivion. Structure for clients that specifies regular one-to-one and group interaction sessions calls for adherence to others' expectations and increasing one's levels of tolerance for involvement and anxiety.

Nursing Goals and Intervention: Grandiosity

Nursing intervention with the client who is grandiose is directed toward defining a relationship as an opportunity for recognizing and developing one's real competencies, worth, and responsibilities—not as a signal for demonstrating one's superiority or unconcern for the real effects of one's behavior on self and others. The goals involve assisting clients to (1) use those attributes within themselves that are positive, (2) act with increased sense of responsibility for their own behaviors, (3) recognize realistic limitations to their powers of influence over people and situations.

The nursing actions, as with diagnoses of manipulation and impulsiveness, often involve setting limits, role modeling, and providing learning opportunities. These actions are often integrated in actual practice and will be so presented here.

Setting Limits, Role Modeling, and Providing Learning Opportunities

Substance abusers' and psychopaths' tendencies to be unrealistic about their motivations and behaviors—as well as the consequences of their acts—are often manifested in denial, rationalization, arrogance, or irresponsibility. Nurses have to determine to what extent and when they should set limits by "pointing out reality" to such clients. Considerable controversy exists as to whether it is wise to confront a client's defenses directly. The ability of these clients to cope with confrontation in relation to their grandiose themes is largely dependent upon the confronter's relationship with that client. This may be so for two reasons: first, the client may have developed some degree of rapport or trust with a given nurse, which allows that client to respect that nurse's judgment; second, the particular nurse may have developed a sensitivity that allows for an accurate clinical judgment as to that particular client's ability to cope at a given time.

At the root of the decision are the following questions: To what extent is the behavior interfering with the client's physical and psychosocial adaptation at this time? To what extent does the client need this defense at this moment in order to survive? The nurse does not have to make the decision alone; it is often valuable to consult with colleagues for validation.

Denial and rationalization of feelings and behaviors characterize stages that the particular client is going through.[14] Alcoholics, for example, may gradually give up these behaviors as they discover an ability to be trusting and to tolerate anxiety. There is, however, some agreement that substance abusers need to be dealt with directly regarding their habits of substance abuse.

Another way the grandiose theme manifests itself is in clients' elaborate or vague plans for the future. It is well to question, through a mutual problem-solving process, some of the clients' conclusions about themselves. For example, a male client mentions that he's going to get a job and everything will be OK. The nurse responds by asking the client when he began to think about getting a job. The focus is on the thinking aspect; there is no direct attack on the client's capabilities or his real situation.

Psychopaths' unconcern for the consequences of their actions is often blatant. The question with regard to confrontation here is not so much whether the client can *tolerate* it but to what extent confrontation will reinforce the client's familiar "bad-me" self-concept and thereby exacerbate irresponsibility and arrogance. Again, to reduce the latter "gain" aspect, it is probably better for the nurse to handle necessary limit setting as directly, quickly, and *privately* as possible. The more noise, attention, and people are involved, the more likely the psychopath is to retain dreams of superior influence.

In relation to both psychopaths and substance abusers, it is useful for nurses to demonstrate acceptance of responsibility for their own behavior. If nurses present themselves as nondefensive in the face of errors in judgment and other "imperfections," the clients may observe that the outcome for the nurses is not catastrophic.

Evaluation

In order to make judgments about the effectiveness of their interventions in clients' manipulation, impulsiveness, withdrawal, and grandiosity, nurses must constantly evaluate the significance of any behavior changes manifested by the client. How do these changes relate to the expected outcomes or goals of intervention which were established initially? For example, in the impulsive client, have there been fewer instances of interruption of others' conversations and activities? Does this client use more time in problem solving? Does he or she carry out plans that are verbalized? What do these changes mean? The nurse analyzes the behavioral outcomes so that nursing intervention may be altered appropriately.

The Family

Nurses in community health agencies can assess communication patterns and child-rearing practices. They can identify early patterns of parental rejection, indifference, and inconsistency. Nurses may then be able to assist families in adopting more effective parenting roles. (See Chap. 33.)

Assessment of family dynamics may also lead to early counseling of parents with regard to children's problems. For example, a parent who complains that her child is "too dependent" or "unmanageable" may offer the nurse an opportunity to explore developmental behaviors that tend to generate anger in others. Specifically, parents may need assistance in handling such behaviors as tantrums, food fads, hunger strikes, separation anxiety, and the like.

Another way a nurse intervenes is by assessing problem behaviors *before* alcoholism, drug abuse, or psychopathy becomes chronic and disruptive. Listening for clues to anxiety, depression, frustration, and conflict is an important tactic. When such feelings within the family are elicited, the nurse should encourage clients to tell how they seek relief. If the "relief" is problematic, then nurse and clients can explore alternatives.

Actions and comments by all family members are significant in that they convey information about family problems. For example, one might question why a teen-ager does not come home at night or why a child spends too much time at home. The stresses to which the children are responding may be substance abuse or psychopathy in another member of the family (see Chap. 35).

Nurses who view the family rather than the individual as "the client" will be more attuned to the effects of parental substance abuse on other members of the family. For instance, a woman who is married to an alcoholic who experiences uncontrolled rages may unwittingly provoke her husband's drinking bouts because of her own unconscious needs. On the other hand, an alcoholic spouse may look for external sources of blame and rationalization for his or her drinking. The familiar refrain "You're driving me to drink" can be used as a threat to increase the guilt and discomfort of the nonalcoholic spouse. Often the nonalcoholic spouse becomes frustrated and desperate for assistance while the alcoholic partner is still resisting help. In these instances it is useful to counsel the nonalcoholic spouse. The major goals of this process as delineated by Estes include helping the spouse to (1) learn about alcoholism, (2) recognize and alter his or her own problematic coping behaviors, and (3) formulate wise decisions regarding his or her own present and future welfare.[29]

What begins as a counseling process for the nonalcoholic spouse may develop into a marital or family counseling situation. In addition, referrals to such groups as Al-Anon or Alateen may be indicated for the support and education of the family. Specifically children of substance abusive parents need assistance in dealing with the shame, guilt, anger, and unrealistic sense of responsibility that they feel.[30]

In assisting substance-abusive and psychopathic clients and their families to identify and use resources, the nurse can be most helpful if he or she is immediate, concrete, and direct. For example, the nurse should make the referral appointment rather than leave it up to the client to follow through. Or the nurse may accompany the client directly to the service or agency. If the decision about referral *must* be delayed or deferred for some reason, the nurse should give the client a telephone number and the name of a person to contact. Such specific actions may help to communicate the concern and seriousness of purpose which is crucial to getting started with such clients.

The Community

One area where professional influence in the community could be significant is that of industrial health. A number of companies in the United States have been effective in developing programs that identify and treat their alcoholic employees or refer such employees for appropriate treatment. These programs often involve educating supervisory personnel to recognize early warning signs of alcohol abuse and to overcome prejudices about alcoholism. In addition to providing such training, industrial health personnel—physicians and nurses—are in a position to detect alcohol abuse directly, particularly during physical examinations.

Another significant community need which involves nurses is the need for rehabilitation resources for those individuals who no longer have support systems, such as family or fellow employees, upon whom they can depend. Substance abusers and psychopaths are clients who succeed so well, via their offensive behaviors, in alienating family and community that they frequently are in need of such a service. The halfway house is an example of a resource which offers group living, referral for ongoing treatment, and, in some cases, close health supervision. Nurses can also assist such clients by referring them for vocational rehabilitation. This type of referral may be done through private programs or through the Division of Vocational Rehabilitation, a public service.

Finally, nurses can use their expertise to influence the systematic study of the problems of substance abuse and psychopathy. Clearly, the nature of these difficulties is not thoroughly understood; until such time as our body of knowledge is more complete, results of intervention often will be limited. Considering the numbers of such clients who populate our corrections systems as well as our health agencies—not to mention the human suffering involved *wherever* they may be found— the problems of substance abuse and psychopathy deserve our continued research.

References

1 Karen Gahan: "Everybody Gets Angry Sometime," *Journal of Psychiatric Nursing and Mental Health Services,* vol. 12, no. 3, pp. 27–33, May–June 1974.

*2 Dorothea R. Hays: "Anger: A Clinical Problem," in Shirley F. Burd and Margaret A. Marshall (eds.), *Some Clinical Approaches to Psychiatric Nursing,* Macmillan, New York, 1963, pp. 110–115.

3 Mary Martha Kiening: "Hostility," in Carolyn E. Carlson (ed.), *Behavioral Concepts and Nursing Intervention,* Lippincott, Philadelphia, 1970, pp. 187–205.

4 Harry Stack Sullivan: *Interpersonal Theory of Psychiatry,* Norton, New York, 1953.

5 "Teen-age Drinking Rising Sharply," *American Medical News,* vol. 1, July 22, 1974.

6 National Institute of Alcohol Abuse and Alcoholism: *Facts About Alcohol and Alcoholism,* U.S. Department of Health, Education, and Welfare, Washington, D.C., 1974.

*Recommended reference by nurse author.

7 "Rising Toll of Alcoholism: New Steps to Combat It," *U.S. News and World Report,* October 29, 1973, pp. 45–48.

9 E. M. Jellinek: "Phases of Alcohol Addiction," in D. J. Pittman and C. R. Snyder (eds.), *Society, Culture and Drinking Patterns,* Wiley, New York, 1962, pp. 356–368.

10 Gary Albrecht: "The Alcoholism Process: A Social Learning Viewpoint," in Peter G. Bourne and Ruth Fox (eds.), *Alcoholism: Progress in Treatment and Research,* Academic Press, New York, 1973, pp. 11–42.

11 Ruth Fox: *Alcoholism: Behavioral Research and Therapeutic Approaches,* Spring, New York, 1967, pp. 242–255.

12 Halmuth H. Schafer and Patrick Martin: *Behavioral Therapy,* McGraw-Hill, New York, 1975.

13 James H. Coleman and William Evans: "Drug Interactions With Alcohol," *Alcohol Health and Research World,* Winter 1975/76, pp. 16–19.

*14 Pamela K. Burkhalter: *Nursing Care of the Alcoholic and Drug Abuser,* McGraw-Hill, New York, 1975.

*15 Ann Singer: "Mothering Practices and Heroin Addiction," *American Journal of Nursing,* vol. 74, no. 1, pp. 77–82, January 1974.

16 Hervey Cleckley: *The Mask of Sanity,* Mosby, St. Louis, 1941.

17 Otto Fenichel: The Psychoanalytic Theory of Neurosis, Norton, New York, 1945.

18 William McCord and Joan McCord: *The Psychopath: An Essay on The Criminal Mind,* Van Nostrand, Princeton, N.J., 1964.

19 Ben Bersten: *The Manipulator: A Psychoanalytic View,* Yale University Press, New Haven, Conn., 1973.

20 Roger A. MacKinnon and Robert Michels: *The Psychiatric Interview in Clinical Practice,* Saunders, Philadelphia, 1971, pp. 297–338.

21 Edith Gomberg: "Women and Alcoholism," in Violet Franks and Vasanti Burtle (eds.), *Women In Therapy,* Brunner/Mazel, New York, 1974, pp. 169–190.

*22 Fern Kumler: "An Interpersonal Interpretation of Manipulation," in Shirley F. Burd and Margaret A. Marshall (eds.), *Some Clinical Approaches to Psychiatric Nursing,* Macmillan, New York, 1963, pp. 166–124.

23 David Shapiro: *Neurotic Styles,* Basic Books, New York, 1965, pp. 134–175.

*24 Gwen E. Tudor: "A Sociopsychiatric Nursing Approach to Intervention in a Problem of Mutual Withdrawal on a Mental Hospital Ward," *Psychiatry,* vol. 15, p. 2, May 1952.

25 Leon Salzman: *The Obsessive Personality*, Aronson, New York, 1973, pp. 162–236.

*26 Maxine E. Loomis: "Nursing Management of Acting-out Behavior," *Perspectives in Psychiatric Care*, vol. 8, no. 4, pp. 168–173, 1970.

*27 Glee Gamble Lyon: "Limit Setting as a Therapeutic Tool," *Journal of Psychiatric Nursing and Mental Health Services*, vol. 8, no. 6, pp. 17–24, November–December, 1970.

*28 Rita Sue Henschen: "Learning Impulse Control through Day Care," *Perspectives in Psychiatric Care*, vol. 9, no. 5, pp. 218–224, 1971.

*29 Nada J. Estes: "Counseling the Wife of an Alcoholic," *American Journal of Nursing*, vol. 74, no. 7, pp. 1251–1255, July 1974.

30 Margaret Hindman: "Children of Alcoholic Parents," *Alcohol Health and Research World*, Winter 1975/76, pp. 2–6.

18
The Client Who Generates Depression

Ardis R. Swanson

Learning Objectives

After studying this chapter, the student should be able to:

1 Identify the behavioral manifestations of depression
2 Describe the dynamics of depression
3 Utilize self-awareness in the therapeutic use of self when interacting with depressed clients
4 Apply the nursing process in planning care for depressed clients and their families
5 Identify nursing interventions for depressed clients
6 Evaluate nursing intervention

The Prevalence of Depression

The existentialists identify two kinds of anxiety and depression: that which is an integral part of human existence and that which is attributable to the circumstances of time and place.[1] The first is omnipresent, perpetual, and governed by the laws of nature; the second is "the human condition," the epiphenomenon of technological growth. In this view, depression is a universal human phenomenon which every person experiences at some level in the course of a lifetime. To live is to experience anxiety and depression; to live with growing technology is to experience these emotions increasingly.

Technology has brought about rapid and profound changes in life-styles and relationships among people. Human beings are becoming aware of the limitations of resources on the planet and of what they are doing to their environment and to themselves. In the context of these changes, depression may become the most prevalent of all mental health problems if indeed it is not already.

In statistical terms, the prevalence of depression is hard to estimate. The difficulties of estimation arise largely from the problems of definition and diagnosis. Depression is manifested in many ways and appears in varying degrees of intensity and duration. In a given person, depression may be the predominant problem; in another person or the same person at another time, depression may be one feature in a constellation of physical and emotional symptoms. The person may be given a diagnostic label which does not even carry the word "depression," and yet he or she may be decidedly depressed.

Statistics from hospitals and clinics indicate only a fraction of the incidence of depression in the population at a given time. Findings from surveys of a population in a defined geographical area for manifestations of depression (such as tiredness, sadness, sleep difficulties, or weight problems) can be compared with responses from identified cases of depression to determine prevalence. Such field studies have the potential for a more accurate index of the prevalence of depression in the total population.

The available statistical data indicate that depression is a significant mental health problem. These data show that:

1. In 1970, the admission rate for the major affective disorders (*Diagnostic Nomenclature of the APA*, 296) to hospitals and psychiatric clinics in the United States was 31.7 per 100,000 population, according to the Biometrics Division of the National Institute of Mental Health.

2. If the number of clients seen for depression in outpatient clinics is added to the figure given above, the latter is multiplied (approximately) by three.[2]

3. The number of those in the general population who suffer from affective disorders is estimated to be several times greater than the number seen in clinics; it is believed to represent approximately 15 percent of the population.[3] Variations according to geographic area may actually exist or may be only apparent, stemming from defects in the methods used to gather the figures.

4. The incidence of depression is higher among women than among men.

5. Depression is positively correlated with age in most studies. However, in a recent field study in the United States, young people showed at least as much depression as the middle-aged group and possibly more.[3]

Behaviors of Depression on Continuum

The behaviors of depression may be placed on a continuum from the mild transitory affects of feeling low to a severe, psychotic depressive state. Other approaches to conceptualization, such as the identification of separate and distinct diagnostic categories of depression, tend to ignore the dynamic nature of the human personality and the fact that the person as a whole is constantly changing. Affects, thoughts, somatic experiences, and interpersonal behaviors are delineated separately according to these approaches; however, in real life these dimensions of depression cannot be seen in isolation. A depressed person experiences them all simultaneously.

Any systematic presentation of depression calls for an organized framework of thought, and this organization is inevitably somewhat arbitrary. The concept of a continuum of depression, however, has these advantages: (1) it does not deny that depression changes in quality as it becomes deeper and (2) it respects the wholeness of a person's experience at any one level. Labels and descriptions, though they are also less than exact, are needed to enable professionals to acquire and exchange information and to identify behaviors.

Transitory Depression

Sadness, dejection, and downheartedness are affects which all people experience from time to time. They may be appropriate to the realities of the present and are not necessarily persistent or dysfunctional. One may feel let down after a busy and exciting weekend, discouraged after a disappointing outcome has followed hard work, downcast because of the loss of some meaningful possession, or even sad—temporarily—for no clearly definable reason. These experiences are referred to as mild, temporary, or first-level behaviors of depression, from which recovery occurs within a relatively short time.

The loss of something or someone particularly meaningful and highly valued—such as a friend, or family member, one's home or job—ordinarily brings on deep sadness of limited duration. Such an experience is a normal grief reaction. (See Chap. 23.) Grief tends to be transitory when the loss is acknowledged, the accompanying feelings are fully expressed, and interaction with others permits a repatterning of life. Without these responses to loss, grieving is distorted and tends to evolve into depression. Then sadness, dejection, and downheartedness persist and intensify. Changes in thought and body sensation occur, forming a constellation of behaviors that belong further along the continuum of depression.

Middle-Level Depressions

Middle-level behaviors of depression, which are more problematic, involve affects, thoughts, somatic sensations, motor activity, communication, and social participation. One or more of the listed behaviors may plague the person affected and thus characterize his or her depressive state. The depressive states at this middle level of the continuum of depression are often referred to as *reactive depressions* or *neurotic depressions*. (See App. A.)

Affects

Depressed people find themselves unable to experience pleasure from activities which are ordinarily enjoyed; their *joie de vivre* seems to vanish. Their low self-esteem is reflected in the feeling of being ineffective, powerless, or helpless. Their outlook is one of gloom and pessimism. Tears and crying may be evident. Anxiety may or may not be felt; if it is, it may be intensely experienced. Hostility and anger are believed to be present whether or not they are directly experienced as such. Feelings that are suppressed or repressed tend to manifest themselves in other behaviors.

Thoughts

Thoughts tend to be slowed and interests narrowed in the middle level of depression. There is a loss of perspective, and concentration becomes difficult. Doubt and indecisiveness are common. Life seems to have no meaning and no future. Thoughts tend to be ruminative, going over and over the same issues and content with no movement toward or recognition of alternative solutions. Such thoughts, which repetitively and insistently force themselves into consciousness, are known as *obsessional* thoughts. For example, the depressed person at this point on the continuum, preoccupied with questions concerning the purpose of life or ultimate destiny, may be unable to clear his or her mind of these matters or to focus on the more pressing matters of daily living (see Chap. 16).

Sleep disturbances are common. Sleep is

desired but not satisfying. Mildly depressed persons may sleep a great deal; others, who are anxious as well, may have difficulty falling asleep at night (DFA). They also feel worse as the day progresses. The still more depressed and anxious may suffer from insomnia or may sleep for only short periods of time. Suicidal ideas may then occur to them (see Chap. 20).

Somatic Sensations and Motor Activity

The depressed person feels empty. Somewhat paradoxically, there is also a feeling of great heaviness. Movement and speech are slow (psychomotor retardation) and every task is a burden. Every fiber of the body may ache. Weakness and fatigue persist despite rest. There is little energy available for grooming and self-care. Frequently, there is high sensitivity and concern over organ functioning. For example, a person may experience something disordered about the heartbeat or about breathing, digestion, elimination, or any other organic function, while health professionals are unable to find clinical evidence of anything wrong. Oral intake varies, with some inclined toward excessive eating and drinking, others toward anorexia and weight loss. There is usually a decrease in sexual interest. In some cases motor activity is considerable, as seen in constant walking, repetitive cleaning, or some other seemingly purposeless activity. The motor activity may arise from obsessional thoughts which intrude and persist with increased anxiety. The patient's constant activity then serves to decrease tension.

Communication

The depressed person tends to be slow in speech and to have a paucity of verbal output. The limited verbalizations are generally self-deprecatory and ruminative. The communication of depressed people may center around the constant repetition of a given life experience. Each time these people seek evaluation from others they reject any positive assessment, maintaining that the experience was an example of personal inadequacy and failure. In relating events, depressed persons may manifest a kind of inflexible, unyielding attachment to their self-deprecation. For example, one man related that he had been silent about the illegal act of a friend. The act allegedly cost both of them their jobs when the act and his knowledge of it were discovered. The man also went on to talk obsessively about morality in general. He asked for reactions from others but was unable to accept either a positive or a nonjudgmental acknowledgement of his experience. He then repeated all his previous remarks, and tenaciously held to his self-deprecatory view.

Speech is only one means of communication. Depressed persons also communicate their inner state through posture and motor activity, as described above.

Social Participation

Depressed persons tend to withdraw from social participation. Early in the development of a depressive state, the withdrawal may be seen simply as a reluctance to go out, to go to work, to socialize, or to be with others. The depressed tend to focus on self rather than on relationships with others. Their egocentricity and narcissism diminishes their sensitivity to the rights and needs of others. This inward focus and tendency to isolate oneself creates a climate which others may perceive as hostile. Therefore those who might attempt to establish a relationship with the depressed person are discouraged from doing so, and the isolation is heightened. In the more severely depressed, anxiety, anger, and aggression interfere with social intercourse more overtly and observably.

Severe Depression

People who manifest the behaviors of severe depression are frequently labeled as *psychotically* or *endogenously depressed*. (See App. A.)

Affects

The severely depressed seem to be without affect. They experience nothingness, a feeling of bottomless emptiness. They are despondent and despairing; feelings of futility, helplessness, and worthlessness prevail. They have little life energy available, so that there is none for self-initiative and rarely enough for self-harm.

Thoughts

The thoughts revealed through the depressed person's limited verbalizations may contain gross misinterpretations of reality. *Delusional thinking* may be present and generally categorizes an individual as psychotic. The delusions confirm the person's feelings of worthlessness, guilt, and powerlessness. They punish the person and defend against a pleasant reality. For example, a deeply depressed person may believe that a body organ is missing or malignantly diseased. This thought is in contrast to the mildly depressed person's experience of heightened sensitivity to body function.

Somatic and Motor Activity

The motor activity and body movement of the severely depressed may be at a standstill (vegetative) or may consist of rapid, agitated, purposeless movement. These clients do not maintain self-care or provide self-nurturance. Without intervention, there may be a marked loss of weight because the clients do not initiate eating activities. Digestion is sluggish, constipation common. There may be urinary retention. Early-morning awakening (EMA) from sleep is common and the morning thought pattern may be severely despondent. The client often feels worse in the morning but better as the day progresses. Posture is poor; when resting, clients often sit slumped or curled up. There is an inclination to stay in bed and to avoid social relationships. What appears to the onlooker to be a simple task is viewed by the depressed person as very complex and insurmountable.

Overall, depression is a distinctly unpleasant experience. Throughout history, it has defied adequate description, though artists have often come closer to depicting its essence than clinicians have done. For example, Burton, in 1628, delineated depression in his classic paper *The Anatomy of*

Melancholy.[4] He drew from the poets to help him describe the indescribable:

> For that deep torture may be call'd a hell,
> When more is felt than one hath power to tell.

Psychodynamics

There is no one universally accepted theory explaining depression. There is, however, a great body of literature from which may be selected those relationships which have proved most useful over the decades and which provide the building blocks for nursing theory and intervention.

Psychoanalytic Theory

Years ago the observation was made that a person in a depressed state manifests many of the features of a person who is grieving. This insight provided an important foundation stone for the psychoanalytic explanation of depression. In grief there is a real, known, and current loss. In depression, it was postulated, there is a real or *symbolic* loss which reactivates the feelings that attended a much earlier loss. It was theorized that people who experience depression carry with them the seeds of unresolved grief. The first experience of loss was loss of the original love object. Freud elaborated that the original love object, the parent, is both loved and hated, and that this ambivalently regarded object is incorporated into self.[5] The assimilation of the hate component explained the self-hatred which is manifest in the depressive state. Detachment of interest from the external world, accompanied by a manifest self-interest, was explained as withdrawal of libido from the lost love object and the redirection of libido toward the internalized love object.

Spitz studied the separation of infants from their mothers in war-torn England in the early 1940s and interpreted the sequential behaviors he identified in them as supportive of psychoanalytic theory.[6] In the studies, the infants' initial response to separation from their mothers was characterized by distress and weeping, which subsided in time to be replaced by expressionless eyes and frozen, immobile faces. The syndrome was labeled *anaclitic depression.*

Bibring points out that, at any stage of development, the ego may fail to achieve its "narcissistic goals," and that this loss or failure impairs development of self-esteem.[7] According to Bibring, the most characteristic features of depression are low self-esteem and helplessness. Since an infant is rendered helpless in a very real way when its needs are unmet, Bibring found it logical to assume that many depressions have their predisposing roots in trauma during the oral phase of development. As a result of early trauma, the person has a residual, excessive hunger for *affection, warmth,* and *appreciation.* Any failure or loss to the fulfillment of affection and being loved in later life reactivates the earlier feelings of helplessness. Bibring extended the theory with the view that depressions may have their predisposing roots in other phases of development as well. He pointed out relationships between blows to the ego during other developmental stages and the specific depressive affects that accompany them. For example, failures in tasks usually associated with the anal phase of development—i.e., to be good, not hostile; clean, not dirty; etc.—predispose a person to depression characterized by feelings of inadequacy and inferiority. Table 18-1 illustrates the development of depression according to Bibring.

Bibring's theory provides a framework for understanding and working with clients who differ in their depression. Consider three clients in the same treatment setting who were notably different in the manifestations of their depression and in the nature of the precipitating events.

1 Client A's predominant behavior was helplessness and a chronic hunger for affection. This woman had never known her family of origin. A widow and childless, her depression seemed to be precipitated by the death of her husband some 5 months earlier.

2 Client B's predominant symptom was an overwhelming guilt that he had not been a good father to his children or a faithful husband to his first wife. He had remained unmarried for 10 years following the death of his wife, spending most of his time in building up an already successful business. Recently, he had remarried and retired despite the objections of his children. Shortly thereafter, he suffered a depressive reaction.

3 Client C, an emergency admission, expressed feelings of inadequacy, having recently failed an important examination. This failure contrasted sharply with a prior, superior academic record and evidence of overachievement.

These three people exemplify Bibring's groupings. Whenever a parallel is observed, the theory can be used as a guidepost for further

Table 18-1 The Development of Depression*

Developmental phase	Wish or goal that failed	Affects
Oral	"To get affection, to be loved, to be taken care of, to get 'the supplies'."	Chronic hunger for affection, warmth, appreciation
Anal	"To be good; not to be resentful, hostile, defiant but to be loving; not to be dirty but to be clean."	Lack of control, weakness, guilt
Phallic	"To be strong, superior, great, secure, not to be weak and insecure."	Inadequacy, inferiority
Any phase	Any narcissistic goal.	Helplessness, powerlessness, low self-esteem

*Adapted from Bibring.[7]

exploration and understanding. A misuse of theory occurs when it leads to premature conclusions on the stereotyping of individuals. Good theory also helps to identify those who are more vulnerable to depression, so that efforts toward health promotion and remediation of problems can begin earlier.

The term *narcissistic* was first applied to infants, whose behavior is naturally self-loving and self-serving. Later, the term came to be applied to depressed persons whose behavior suggested a similar orientation to self and world. *Negative narcissism* may be the better term for what is seen in the depressed. A sense of omnipotence characterizes simple narcissism, whereas feelings of inadequacy and self-accusation characterize the negatively narcissistic depressed person. The depressed person doubts that there is anything within the self for another to care about, so the person alone is left to care for self. The depressed person may pull in all resources and defenses close to self, in an effort to concentrate that which is perceived to be limited and fragile. Self-service is essential for survival, the person feels, while both the desire and the ability to survive remain in doubt. Such depressed persons tend not to allow other human beings into this encampment; they are wary of being influenced. To avoid involvement with another person avoids another possible loss of failure. The result is isolation. Expectations and needs have not been met in the past, and the person feels this will occur again and again. Consequently depressive behaviors are adopted and defended.

Interpersonal Theory

Interpersonal theory holds that depressive persons as infants had been accepted and fulfilled in their earliest needs. This total nurturance was later withdrawn and care was given provisionally; it became contingent upon the child's fulfillment of the needs and expectations of the parents.[8] Such a duty-bound child feels a lack of gratification in the now. Fulfillment has been extrapolated to the future and seems to remain forever beyond grasp.

Interpersonal theory also emphasizes the subtle forms of loss that occur in childhood despite the physical presence of a significant adult. Such "loss" includes the failure to receive positive validation from significant others for natural aliveness and spontaneity. The early loss was, then, a failure to receive satisfactory responses in return for efforts to reach out. This sets up a dynamic of expectations in adulthood which rests on the maintenance of that early position and blocks the capacity to establish relationships. The person concludes in advance that efforts to reach out will fail; therefore he or she no longer continues to try.[9]

Communication Theory

Communication theory offers further explanation of the depressive position. *Information,* a central concept in communication theory, reduces uncertainty for a receiver confronted by alternatives. Information is used as a measure of order, reducing uncertainty and providing readiness for action. Basch, using communication theory, offers a revision of the psychoanalytic explanation of anaclitic depression.[10] In a mother-infant relationship, the rhythmic behaviors (heartbeat and rhythmic caring behaviors) provide the infant with feedback and convey ordering rhythmicity. Separation interrupts this ordering and disorganizes the infant. The infant is then left out of the mother's meaningful ordering system. After a period of protest (disorganization), mental and motor retardation are seen as a consequence of understimulation—particularly the absence of *rhythmic* stimulation. Depression, then, designates "a particular sort of malfunction in the ordering process that can be precipitated by a variety of disturbances in communication on the symbolic, sign, or signal transmission level."[10]

Communication theory, with its concepts of verbal (digital) and nonverbal (analogic) codes, helps one understand the frustration, anger, and anxiety of depression. Like an aphasic person, a depressed person cannot speak in verbal codes that match the nonverbal codes of thoughts and feelings he or she experiences. The reason may rest in a developmental failure to experience organizing rhythmicity, as described by Basch. Depressed persons are frustrated by the lack of synchronization in their codification.[11] Failing to communicate well evokes more frustration and anxiety in a circular fashion, thus inhibiting communication further. Yet the depressed person cannot avoid communication by silence, because even in silence one inevitably communicates. It is an axiom in communication theory that one "cannot *not* communicate."[12]

Systems Theory

Systems theory unifies these various theoretical contributions. The human being is a system of interrelated subsystems and of larger systems, all of which are open; a change in one part is accompanied by a change somewhere else. Accordingly, arguments as to whether depression is a chemical, neurophysiological, or psychological illness miss the point, and single theories are inadequate. Mutual interaction between peoples, subsystems, and the environment is a more logical interpretation. Individuals cannot create total isolation or isolate their depression in one part of the body, nor can one person in a family encapsulate the family's depression indefinitely and not have an impact on the other members' functioning. A depressed family member may for a time embody this depression, but it will eventually move about to different members within the family system. Thus, depression becomes comprehensible as a general systems phenomenon rather than a disease entity. Paul has shown that, in many troubled families, depression in the form of unresolved grief is threaded throughout the family system, manifesting itself in different ways in various members.[13] An outside agent, the nurse, can effect a dramatic relief of the depression by working with the family system as the client.

Primary Prevention

The promotion of mental health begins with the facilitation of mothering behaviors that are responsive to infants. Responsiveness requires the presence of a mothering figure not only physically but also emotionally.[14] The mother who is depressed herself, or highly anxious, or otherwise preoccu-pied and detached finds it difficult to be totally present and responsive to her infant. She may not be able to tune in to her infant's wavelength, being too closed up in her own. Thus the health of mothers is inevitably linked to the health of developing children. (See Chap. 31.)

When a child fails to receive positive emotional responses from a significant adult, the experience for the child is the emotional equivalent of parental loss or absence. Thus the seeds of depression are planted. Responses that are unaccepting of a child's natural spontaneity and aliveness begin the depressive life-style. Children need to be active, to explore, and to experience pleasure in relation to their environment. Therefore, positive parental behaviors (those that help to prevent future depression) include the acceptance and fostering of spontaneity, aliveness, exploration, the development of skill in relation to environment, and pleasure in present action. There ought not to be too many frustrations in the present for the sake of the future. As Ruesch has pointed out, children whose parents place great emphasis on end results rather than the pleasures of attaining short-term goals learn to project their goals more and more to the future, and their goals and satisfactions become more and more difficult to attain.[11]

The trauma of physical loss or lengthy separation of infant and mother can be mitigated by good surrogate mothering. From developmental studies, it is known that a child between the ages of 5 and 12 months, is particularly sensitive to separation.[15] After the child is 2 or 3 years old, verbal communication can be used to help the child understand and cope. The child of 2 or 3 has a new and useful mode for expression—verbal communication—and increased access to persons through language and mobility to help in replacing a lost relationship.

As children move through their early years, the significant adults in their lives can help equip them for disappointments later in life. If children are allowed considerable freedom to act and affect their environment and if the presence and emotional responsiveness of adults is accompanied by an abundance of positive appraisals of the child, then the child has a greater opportunity to develop self acceptance and self-esteem.[9] Without a positive self-view, later losses or failures tend only to confirm and accentuate low self-esteem.

The Nurse's Response to Client Behavior

One of the most interesting and at the same time potentially problematic aspects of working with depressed persons is the response in oneself that the depressed person tends to evoke. In the presence of a depressed person, it is not at all uncommon to find oneself feeling sad, low, and irritable or somewhat hostile, frustrated, and helpless. Through voice, body posture, movement, and probably other subtle modalities not yet even identified, the depressed person's dejection, boredom, and emptiness are communicated. Under ordinary circumstances, feelings that have come to one through nonverbal means remain below cognitive awareness. To a therapist, feelings that are peripheral to awareness are potentially problematic. When he or she is only marginally aware of such feelings, the nurse is likely to fall into feelings of gloom, irritability, or helplessness. Feeling ineffective, the person who *could* be helpful then tends to respond automatically in less useful ways. For example, one may tend to avoid the depressed person, setting up a circular rejection cycle. A helping person who is unaware of the interpersonal dynamics tends to make naive efforts to be helpful. Efforts such as trying simply to cheer up the depressed person or to talk him or her out of their expressions of helplessness, inadequacy, or whatever result in frustration and failure and only circularize the helplessness. Self-aware helpers use their feelings as data in the recognition of depression and in making constructive interventions. For example, during intake evaluations in a general health service, these feelings within self may be the first clues to mild to moderate depression in the client. For persons already diagnosed as depressed, these feelings can indicate the depth of the depression. One may, for example, feel the client's powerlessness or sense of failure. When depression is evident in a general way but the problems have not yet been clearly differentiated, these feelings in the nurse can provide important clues for the identification of particular feeling states that the client is, as yet, unable to verbalize. Awareness of specific responses in the self increases learning about both the client and oneself as well as growth in the therapeutic use of self. Awareness, then, can transform a potentially problematic phenomenon into a useful tool of observation, assessment, and growth as a therapist.

Some persons, including professionals, are more susceptible and vulnerable than others to messages of depression. In some, a depressed person triggers off latent feelings of depression in themselves. Depressive elements that the helping person has not resolved are reactivated. Perhaps the helping person has coped with these depressive elements fairly well when not confronted with another's depression. Now, however, the helping person may empathize with the depressed person too readily and completely to be useful. Others may defend strongly against the depression by fight or flight. (One cannot at the same time defend against depression and relate genuinely and openly to the depressed person.) These phenomena account for the inability or reluctance of some personnel to work with the depressed.

Those who work with depressed people need working structures through which they can obtain validation of their experiences with clients and express concerns about their responses to clients. Structures for this include skilled clinical supervision and team meetings wherein the aim is staff development.

The helping person who is not too vulnerable to depression can put sensitivity and empathy to good use. An empathic response, neither detached nor overtly responsive, that is coupled with a knowledge of the dynamics of depression provides the foundation for an effective therapeutic stance.

In short, nonverbal messages may be received out of conscious awareness; if they remain unrecognized at that level, they will only cause problems for the potential helper. When there is knowledge of the phenomenon and an effort to increase awareness, the same circumstance can provide valuable information and service to the helping relationship.

Assessment and Diagnosis of Client and Family

Assessment and diagnosis are prerequisite to the design of an appropriate nursing-care plan. The data are obtained through three processes: (1) observation while in interaction with the client; (2) observation while in interaction with the client's family and/or significant others, with and without the client; and (3) contact with other sources. The latter may include sources at home, work, or school and/or other relevant systems in the client's community, provided that the client approves of such contacts. It is generally better to place the emphasis on the client's own behavior and self-report, since the client is, after all, the most involved person, and the nurse-client relationship should be directed toward the development of a mutually trusting relationship. Sometimes family members or other significant persons must necessarily provide information if the client is altogether unable to do so or if this is necessary for the sake of the client's safety.

The data should include three kinds of content: (1) the client's and family's perception of the problems, (2) the extent of existing interpersonal and situational supports, and (3) the adequacy of the client's coping patterns.

The Problems

The identification of depressive behaviors begins in the initial interview and is based on what is observed, what the client and family describe, and the feelings generated in the interview. The interviewer is alert to affects, somatic reports, motor activity, and thought and communication patterns. For example, a client who appears unremarkable in the initial introduction might begin to weep as the family complains of her neglect of her baby,

and the interviewer may feel increasingly anxious as more information unfolds. Anger, anxiety, dependency, and helplessness are all seen as tentative problem choices which more data would either support or reject. The affective behaviors which are associated with depression are emphasized below. Each is briefly defined, its origin is suggested, and the automatic responses that each tends to generate in others are identified.

Ambivalence

When opposing emotions toward a person, object, or situation coexist, there is ambivalence. It is believed to make its first appearance in the oral stage of development in the form of simultaneous feelings of love and hate. In adulthood, it may take this same form or appear under the guise of antithetical emotions. An example of the concurrent experiencing of pleasant and unpleasant feelings is the pain and pleasure that often accompany adult human relationships. The self-hatred and self-concern so characteristic of the depressed is also understandable through the concept of ambivalence. Ambivalence tends to generate confusion in others. People do not know where they stand in the relationship and cannot understand what they are doing to provoke a particular response, since there is actually no direct and simple connection between the client's emotion and the other's behavior.

Anger

The feeling of intense displeasure and tension one feels on encountering an obstacle to a goal is anger. Anger and anxiety are closely related since both produce discomfort and a sense of threat to self. However, anger leans toward fight, anxiety toward flight. The depressed person may not know the source or object of the anger. Ordinarily, a person knows at whom or about what he or she is angry, but the depressed person tries to avoid confronting feelings of anger. An automatic response to the anger of others is anxiety. Many persons are fearful of or intimidated by a sense of anger in another (see Chap. 17).

Anxiety

This may be defined as a distinctly unpleasant sense of tension and danger without any special source—that is, no awareness of a specific object or situation that is threatening to the self. Although anxiety is not limited to depressed persons, it may nevertheless be a major affect in depression. *Depressive anxiety* has been explained as the striving to save the good objects that the person senses may be destroyed along with the bad. Anxiety tends to generate anxiety or helplessness in others, who may respond with a strong desire to reduce the other's anxiety or to distance themselves (see Chap. 14).

Dependency and Demandingness

Dependency is a tendency to rely on others for advice, guidance, support, and care; it may extend to asking, imploring, or even requiring these supports from others. Dependency and demandingness have their origins in the individual's development, when the need to "take in" was paramount and eventually frustrated. People with unresolved dependency needs often had little experience, as children, of securing the needed "supplies" directly through actions of self. Demanding and manipulative behavior indicates a strong and persistent struggle to obtain satisfaction literally "on demand." Client dependency evokes, in some caretakers, feelings of caring and protectiveness, which are usually not in the client's best interest. In other persons, annoyance and fatigue are evoked. As an analogy, observe any female mammal that is trying to move away from her hungry, breast-clinging offspring. Demandingness evokes resistance and avoidance from most persons; others may be intimidated and therefore comply under duress.

Self-doubt

When a person is unsure about personally possessing the resources, abilities or power needed for performing a given task or role, he or she suffers from self-doubt, which is generally accompanied by anxiety. Self-doubt is an inhibitor to self-action, a defense against personal failure. It is related to dependency in the sense that self-doubting people are not confident of their own resources and abilities and are inclined to rely on others rather than themselves. Self-doubt can be differentiated from two other concepts that appear in this listing: helplessness and hopelessness. If people have no self-confidence, they feel helpless; if they feel no confidence in others either, they feel hopeless.

An automatic response tendency of caretakers is to fill in for the victim of self-doubt, much as one may feel tempted to finish sentences for a stutterer. Obviously this is not the most helpful response for the depressed person in the long run. All response tendencies must be brought into awareness, where they can be evaluated as to whether they are growth-facilitating or whether they merely tend to satisfy one's own needs.

Guilt

A feeling of distinct displeasure with self accompanied by the thought that one has done wrong and ought to be punished constitutes guilt. In the severely depressed, it becomes a desire for complete annihilation (see Chap. 20). Guilt may arise from the conviction that one has failed to do that which is morally right. In the eyes of others, however, the person who feels this way may seem to be inappropriately self-condemning. Guilt may be understood as a kind of fixation at or reactivation of the developmental stage when the sense of right or wrong began to arise. The incident precipitating the guilt may have been some violation of a principle of conscience or another action unacceptable to self. Expressions of guilt may lead others to express sympathy and the hope that the sufferer will find a way to make good the loss. Persistent or unremitting verbalizations of apparently inappropriate guilt tend to evoke annoyance and a desire to avoid the guilt-ridden person.

Helplessness

The discomfort of an unfulfilled need combined with the anxiety of feeling unable to act to relieve the discomfort defines the feeling of helplessness. It is closely akin to anxiety; the two probably have a common origin in the experience of the infant whose basic need is unsatisfied and whose efforts to fulfill the need or to induce someone else to fill it are unsuccessful. The helpless person is uncomfortably aware of a discrepancy between the actual and the ideal, between the obtained and the desired. Helpless people are unable to mobilize energy for effecting a change. They are persuaded that no effort on their part could change the situation. They feel powerless. Helplessness tends to generate helplessness—as well as anxiety, annoyance, or withdrawal—in others. Shea and Hurley[16] found that staff who spontaneously invent rules, regulations, and policies restricting client expressions of helplessness avoid the anxiety of dealing with clients who try to act on behalf of themselves and fail.

Hopelessness

When helplessness is deepened due to the conviction that all efforts by anyone to improve the situation are doomed to failure, one arrives at hopelessness. Persons who *say* that their situation is "hopeless" reveal some ray of hope just by the very expression of their feeling to another person. The most deeply felt hopelessness is not verbalized. Expressions of hopelessness tend to elicit anxiety—as well as defenses such as denial and withdrawal—in others. In contrast, anxiety can also be utilized constructively by the caretaker. Anxiety can be used as a motivating factor to initiate efforts at problem solving. Anxiety is not a totally negative thing; it indicates a striving for life and often evokes a schema of hopefulness in the caretaker.

Every person develops an individual schema of hopefulness.[17] This schema is a cognitive, symbolic, unconscious structure which emerges as the individual encounters and deals with ambiguous situations in the environment. Success or failure in the resolution of these situations contributes to the person's perception of his or her ability to modify or change the environment. The schema is constructed from these experiences and communications from others. Consistent, persistent encour-

agement and expectations by authoritative persons that the other person can and will succeed in mastering and solving problems contribute to the development of a high-order schema of hopefulness in which the person confronts problematic issues with the perceptual framework, "I can affect the environment. . . . I can succeed." When the nurse evokes this high-order schema in the face of the most difficult circumstances presented by the client, the therapist's hopefulness can influence the client to act. This in itself evokes a hopeful schema in the client. The nursing staff may structure controlled situations in which clients experience small successes for which they are praised; this further enhances the development of hopefulness.

Low Self-esteem

The low self-regard so characteristic of depressive states is also called low self-esteem. The low self-esteem of depression is rarely confused with a mature humility, which tends to evoke respect from others. A guilt component frequently accompanies low self-esteem and has led to the view that this condition occurs when one is on bad terms with one's superego. In ego terms, low self-esteem is an outcome of a poorly developed ego which has been additionally traumatized by the blow of a failure or loss. Very low self-esteem is equivalent to feeling worthless. Caretaker responses to a person who is experiencing low self-esteem are varied in their possibilities. The helper whose own self-esteem is none too strong may feel more secure and comfortable in the presence of a client who feels still lower in self-esteem. Such feelings will contribute to maintaining the client's status quo unless there is awareness and effort directed toward change. Any lift in the client's self-esteem will reactivate the helper's anxieties and uncertainties about self and may elicit behavior which will be directed at deflating the client's self-esteem. The helper whose self-view is moderate or strong is vulnerable to other feelings and responses that may, if unnoticed and unattended, be equally untherapeutic. A helper's efforts to talk the client out of his or her low self-esteem can only result in failure or minimal success followed by frustration and possibly mutual withdrawal.

Worthlessness
This is the feeling of uselessness which is a component of low self-esteem. See "Self-Doubt" and "Low Self-Esteem," above.

Powerlessness
The feeling of being unable to effect any change in self or the environment—powerlessness—is a component of self-doubt and helplessness, as previously discussed.

Interpersonal and Situational Factors
Seeing the client in the context of the family, home, community, and/or work setting can help to refine the accuracy and completeness of the total evaluation. The behaviors of a depressed person will be relatively the same from one setting to another, but this cannot be taken for granted. For example, a client's behavior in the clinic during intake may be more active than behavior observed in the home. The environment may, in fact, shed light on the client's predicament. Since depressions are precipitated by the real or symbolic loss of a person, material goods, status, position, or anything that has meaning for the person, the environment may provide clues to the loss. For example, the material comforts in the home of one woman only served to depress her further, to remind her of the disparity between her home and that of her invalid husband, now in a nursing home. Her loss was the loss of his presence and a loss of her self-esteem because she could no longer take care of him. One must refrain from judgments on what is observed in the environment until its meaning to the client can be ascertained. A client may have unrealistic expectations of the environment. The nurse assesses whether the environment has the potential for meeting these needs.

The family interview is a modality for both assessment and treatment. In the family context, one can see the familial ties and commands that the depressed person automatically obeys. For example, parental assertions of love and caring may be coupled with exhortation to try harder, pull oneself up, and become a successful person of whom the parents can be proud. Or one may see the client practice an inverted version of the golden rule: "Do unto others as I have been done unto." What clients demand of others, others once asked of them. In the family, one can see the acting out of behavior that reinforces the client's depression. For example, familial denial of the client's felt experience can only reaffirm his or her feelings of isolation and helplessness.

Coping Patterns
Assessment includes noting the patterns of behavior that have given the client some measure of success, pleasure, or relief from anxiety and have enabled him or her to go on living. These may include ways of staying in school, holding a job, or dealing with earlier loss or defeat.

For the moderately depressed, residual sources of pleasure will indicate ways in which they defensively isolate or comfort themselves. A bed, a chair, a corner, or a given room may be the consistent choice.

Assessment includes noting the availability of environmental factors which are ordinarily pleasurable when one is not depressed. These may include colors, sounds, fragrances, textures, pets, and opportunities for human interaction. For example, it may be determined that the depressed person had enjoyed little in the way of sensory inputs except to take pleasure in flowering plants. This could be valuable data for planning intervention. Making this one-time pleasure available again—as well as a willingness to share this interest—would provide an opportunity for reinvestment in life and living things.

Nursing Diagnosis
Assessment flows into nursing diagnosis and the planning of care as a total process. The problem list may be made up of any or many of the behaviors referred to in the earlier sections of this chapter. The full diagnosis may also include the

automatic response tendencies associated with each problem or group of problems. For example, along with identifying a paucity of verbal expression, one might identify the tendency to feel frustrated when efforts to engage the patient in verbal communication are rejected. It is also useful to note a response tendency to avoid the patient or to try to guess, without validation, what the patient is thinking or feeling. Having listed as many problems and response tendencies as possible, the nurse is on the threshold of planning care which specifically includes the consideration of goals and selection of interventions. How the process might evolve for one patient on one particular behavior can be seen from Table 18-2.

Table 18-2 The Process of Planning: From the Diagnosis of a Problem to the Evaluation of Change—An Example

1 *Behavior:* Paucity of verbal expression.

2 *Nurse's automatic response tendencies:* To feel frustration and annoyance when ordinary efforts to communicate verbally are unsuccessful; to guess what the client is thinking and feeling and let it go at that; to avoid the client or at least to avoid efforts at communication.

3 *Goal Selection: Short-term goals and long term goals. Short term:* Client inserts names and places into brief and generalized statements. Makes movement toward fleshing out skeletal descriptions of family relationships. *Long-term:* Client verbally expresses life experiences, thoughts, and feelings, including aspirations in life and anger at obstacles to success. Greater mobility in facial expression and body movement, coordination of thoughts with feelings.

4 *Interventions:* (*a*) Ask for names and places, then gradually ask for thoughts and feelings about the people, places, and activities named in the client's verbalizations; (*b*) attend to the nonverbal messages and ask for validation (e.g., "I sense you felt relieved when Mr. John left just now. You appeared to be.

Was that in fact your feeling?"); (*c*) arrange for opportunities for interchange, including both concretely planned times and informally available times with professional staff, with family and loved ones, and with other clients; (*d*) maximize opportunities for verbalizations by providing a physical environment comfortable for talk. Provide activities which lend themselves to discussion afterwards.

5 *Evaluation of change:* At a preplanned time—for example, after 2 weeks—assess where the problem then stands along the goal continuum. Has the first short term goal been met? Use the data to revise the plan for the next period of time. *Example of data gathered at end of a time period:* "On request, client will flesh out a brief description with some detail. On occasion, client appeared annoyed at the expectation of staff. Staff not put off. Client denies feeling annoyed about anything. Refusing many of the arranged opportunities for interchange. Approaches night staff for interchange in the early morning hours. Among relatives, engages in walks and talks best with Al, the youngest brother." *Example of modification of original plan:* (*a*) Behavior—denial of any negative affect, even in response to delays or obstacles to goals on the ward; (*b*) Automatic tendency is to accept the denial, since few enjoy being recipients of negative affects. *Short-term goal:* the acknowledgement of minor annoyance. *Intervention:* seek opportunity to be a role model on relatively minor irritations to begin with, which illustrates that client's expression of annoyance is OK and no one is hurt.

Planning Nursing Care

Goals

One approach to the setting of goals is to select for each identified behavior or problem of depression an alternate behavior that would characterize the same person en route to feeling free of depression. Each is a short term goal which stands between behavior and long term goal. For example:

Behavior	Short-term goal	Long-term goal
Insomnia	To be less concerned with needing sleep	To fall asleep within an hour after bedtime without medication
	To sleep some, in the night	To feel relatively rested and without need of sleep during the day

This approach leads to considerable specificity and detail in a total plan of care. Each short term goal is preceded by the identification of the behavior and the automatic response tendency, and each is followed by listing interventions, both personal and environmental, for each short term goal (see Table 18-2).

There are several dilemmas in regard to goal setting that need attention. One is the question of client participation in the selection of goals. On the one hand, there is advantage to client involvement. The client may be helped to break down, to a point where it appears realizable, a goal that seems hopelessly unattainable. The process may not only serve the client as a means to an end but may be an end in itself. That is, the client is included, heard, and respected for his or her thoughts and feelings and thus does not escape being effective before the plan even begins. On the other hand, a problem that arises when clients participate in goal setting is that goals for the depressed can reinforce their problematic tendencies. As Ruesch[11] points out, the depressed person has been trained all too well for goal achievement, to the detriment of pleasures of the moment. There is an arbitrary end-state quality about goals to which depressives all too readily attach themselves—as against seeing life as an ongoing process to be experienced in the present.

A second problem of goal setting rests in the itemization of behaviors and goals as if they existed in isolation one from another. All behaviors are interrelated, and a person is a unitary whole. When behaviors are viewed as varied manifestations of a dynamic state, then overall goals aimed at the dynamic state seem most appropriate. From this point of view, one would select from the more central goals: (1) to help the client feel accepted despite symptoms, not because of them; (2) to help the client identify the loss of or wound to self-esteem and to get in touch with its full meaning; (3) to begin to find some replacement for the loss; (4) to differentiate between past, present, and future and to expand the dimensions of the client's present; (5) to find ways in which the client can be effective once again and regain self-esteem. When these goals are achieved, the characteristic de-pressive behaviors inevitably change and fade away.

Whatever the form in which goals are stated, their clear expression will facilitate the choice of interventions and modalities through which the goals can be achieved.

Nursing Intervention

There are currently a wide variety of modalities for the management and treatment of depression. Nurses collaborate with peers of other disciplines in various efforts directed at alleviating depression. Nurses are not disinterested in any of the efforts to relieve the painful experience of depression; however, nursing is uniquely committed to the whole person and to the use of self as the nurse's most valuable and potentially therapeutic tool. In identifying the nursing intervention for the depressed person, the use of self through communication is of central importance.[18]

A detailed plan of care has particular usefulness in a residential treatment setting, where multiple changes of staff occur during each day, 7 days a week, and where many of the staff may be paraprofessionals. Discussion which includes all staff levels can generate ideas for creative plans in addition to more standard procedures. For example, intervention for insomnia might include not only the measures used in general nursing to facilitate relaxation and sleep but also individualized planning of daytime activity, exercise, and the provision of a person to respond to the client when he or she is anxious and wakeful during the night. Similar measures can be taken for each identified problem. The selection of interventions should be individualized for each patient. The following, then, is best viewed as an inventory of problems and interventions from which to select in the process of detailing the plan of care for a particular depressed person.

Ambivalence
The nurse should acknowledge the coexistence of antithetical emotions. Remember that neither ex-

treme represents the person's overall feeling. A depressed person's ambivalence includes mixed feelings about relating to another—both wanting it and not wanting it. Apparent disinterest ought not to be taken as conclusive proof of an overall wish to be left alone. For example, a response to a client's retreat from others might be, "It seems you want to be with us and yet to be alone. I will come to be with you for a while before lunch."

Anger and Anxiety

Having provided appropriate safeguards against any real danger, do not show fright or intimidation. Encourage the client to verbalize his or her emotion. Allow and sometimes arrange for physical activity that gives expression to the client's emotion without harm to anyone. Appropriate safeguards include sufficient staff who are prepared to accept verbal anger and to restrain, firmly but kindly, violent outbursts against self and others.

Utilize simple, direct explanations and speech that is clear and honest, as opposed to any containing trickery and manipulation. Depressed people may fear communication because of a deep-seated fear of their own anger and its effect on others. It can be a great relief to a depressed person to find a caretaker who is not frightened or intimidated by irritability or anger.[11] This will also decrease the client's anxiety regarding his or her ability or tendency to destroy both good and bad objects in the environment. Direct provocation of a depressed person's repressed anger, simply to get it expressed, is not recommended. There is probably less opportunity for a person to grow through provoked outbursts than through the day-to-day expression and exploration of irritations. Expressions of the less threatening day-to-day irritations can be encouraged by a generally permissive attitude and through the expressiveness of staff as role models. These responses can be explored and discussed, facilitating the growth of staff and patients alike. If an outburst does occur, it can be a profound learning experience for a client to see that no one was destroyed by the anger and that there are still those who remain open and interested in the person beneath the anger.

Self-doubt and Indecision

Acknowledge and encourage assertions of likes and dislikes. Support those assertions and decisions that are expressed and help to make their expression a positive experience. (See discussion of dependency, below.)

Dependency and Demandingness

Expect depressed clients to take the position that they are incompetent and you are the able one in regard to almost any task to be performed. Assess clients' ability to do for themselves. Provide help where client is clearly unable to manage alone. In most instances, take the stance that the client *is* able to act, and assume an attitude of firmness, calm, and patience, reflecting your confidence in the client's ability. With alertness, one is not drawn into reinforcing the client's weakness. In some instances, the best therapeutic stance may be to do a task along with a client; at other times, it may be best simply to wait for clients to help themselves. Irrational demands ought to be recognized as such, brought into the open, discussed with the patient, and refused.[19]

Guilt

Acknowledge the expressed self-view as the patient's view, not your own, without arguing about it. Avoid participating in the client's system of shoulds and shouldn'ts. When the client has ruminations that derogate self, resist the automatic response of cutting off the repetitions and, more usefully, help the client to go beyond the present story. For example, a client who has told you for the hundredth time, it seems, of doubts about doing the right thing, could be asked for further details about the circumstances surrounding the event that preoccupies him or her.

Helplessness and Hopelessness

For helplessness, see the discussion of dependency, above. For hopelessness, help build a new schema of hopefulness by building a new set of successes and gratifications. It is possible to maintain one's own stance of hopefulness in respect to the client's future without negating the client's right to have negative feelings.

Low Self-esteem (Including Worthlessness and Withdrawal)

Grade goals and tasks to manageable sizes so as to increase the probability of successful experiences. Disallow total isolation from others. Maintain contact but provide the dignities of such personal privacy as can be safely allowed. When worthlessness is expressed in total immobility, provide the nourishment, cleanliness, elimination, etc., necessary for life and a sense of humanness. Cast doubt upon the validity of statements of low self-worth in ways that do not reject the person. Sometimes simply present another set of facts, but avoid a power struggle (which never persuades and only puts distance between therapist and the depressed person). Above all, the depressed person needs to feel accepted—not because of the symptoms but despite them.

Nonexpressiveness

(See Table 18-2.) Act as a role model in the expression of thoughts and feelings and in permissiveness toward expressive behavior. Arrange and facilitate activities that provide opportunities for physical and verbal expression, e.g., occupational therapy, art therapy, recreational therapy, etc. (see Chap. 9).

Any of the responses above can occur informally in the activities of daily living. They can also be introduced into more formally arranged one-to-one relationships or into group or family sessions.

Remediation through Group Therapies

Although depressed persons do not readily participate in group experience, this therapeutic modality is one avenue through which they can gain a new perspective on self and others. A group of depressed persons can exude a depressive and hostile atmosphere. Nevertheless, some helping persons achieve considerable expertise in helping the depressed through groups. As in an individual relationship with a depressed person, the group therapist ought not to be surprised or unduly affected by the depressed person's needs, frustrations, and anger. Effective therapists know that they are neither mother nor God and do not need to be needed in a manner that fosters dependence. The therapist believes in the human potential of each person in the group and has learned that interaction and responsiveness facilitate growth. The depressed person's most compelling need is to feel accepted. Transference phenomena are multiple and rich in the group setting (see Chap. 10). With a skillful exposure of transference, the depressed person comes to realize that some of what is experienced with others as problematic or painful today belongs to times past. One client's expectation, for example, was that others would laugh at her views. In the group experience, the client discovered important differences between the past and the present. Released from the past, one finds that today is a new day with opportunities for new ways of relating.

Groups range widely, from supportive types to analytic types. For change to occur in any type of group, facilitative leadership is more than warmth and caring. Warm, motherly qualities alone may do little more than reinforce dependency. Leadership includes understanding of the depressed person's predicament, sensitivity to nonverbal communication, and facilitation of growth. When the leader comments on what is communicated nonverbally, members may accept or deny, be silent or revise the observation, but in no way can they *not* communicate.

Remediation through Family Sessions

Hospitalization of the depressed client disrupts the family's homeodynamic mechanism. Other family members may begin exhibiting symptoms of the family's distress. Family group sessions are utilized to observe family interactional patterns. Family members are helped to notice and change problematic patterns. In family therapy, the focus is shifted from the client to the family as a unit—a family with whom the depressed person was unable to find a solution other than to be depressed. The family needs help to observe themselves and to evolve new patterns of relating.

Whether or not family sessions are utilized, an individual member of the family often needs special help. The family member or other significant loved one who has loved the depressed person the most may now experience intense pain, frustration, or anger, quickly followed by guilt and confusion when the client is hospitalized. This pattern also occurs frequently as the client demonstrates progress.

Frustration is evoked when an effort is made to express love and caring and the efforts are seemingly not appreciated. Guilt over the angry feelings adds weight to the burden. The depressed person responds to expressions of love negatively, feeling both needing and undeserving, both demanding and unable to receive. A depressed person may try to respond in a reciprocal, loving way but is unable to do so. The caring one thus feels drained and rejected. If the caring person succumbs totally to the needs of the one who is depressed, as by retreating from day-to-day obligations, another burden will be added to the depressed person's array of guilts and humiliations. Therefore those close to depressed persons need help themselves—to grow in understanding and to maintain an ongoing life as best they can.

Other Remediations

As long as nurses are participants in the dispensing of drugs, a dependent function, they must of course be guided by the same care and precaution that applies to the giving of medication in general. Currently the drug therapy of choice is imipramine or amitriptyline, but this may change. The nurse must, therefore, be knowledgeable about each drug's action, dosage, side effects, and contraindications. The nurse must exercise observational skills in assessing the drug's efficacy and monitoring the client for side effects. (See Chap. 8.)

One of the peculiar problems in the management of a depressed person on drug treatment is that in some cases an antidepressant will exacerbate the patient's anxiety and/or depression instead of lessening it. A drug may also have an idiosyncratic effect that is falsely attributed to the person's drug-free experience. Without careful reporting and assessment, a drug dosage may be continued inappropriately or increased instead of discontinued.

A nurse may be expected to care for a patient whose severe depression is being treated with electroshock. For nursing care of the person under these special circumstances, see Chap. 8.

Evaluation

Evaluative structures are introduced with the design of the nursing care plan. Specifically, these are the identification of behaviors and the setting of short- and long-term goals. In the evaluative process, they are important reference points against which one notes what behaviors have dropped away, what new behavior has emerged, and what behavior has been modified. The evaluation ought to be based on both observation of behaviors and client self-reports. It should be kept in mind, however, that the depressed are particularly disinclined to acknowledge in themselves progress that appears manifest to others.[20] The nurse should also realize that the initiation of interventions into depression may elicit anxiety, irritability, and sometimes anger before it leads to the desired end results.

Because of the interpersonal aspects of depression, evaluation will include an assessment of change in self. As mentioned earlier, skilled and sensitive supervision and/or staff discussion are processes that can supplement a nurse's own private process of self-evaluation and personal growth.

Prospects

The overwhelming majority of persons who suffer from depression recover and, indeed, are better off afterwards than before.[21] Flach emphasizes that a depressive episode is a way of letting go of old attitudes that no longer serve the person well—a signal that something is wrong in self or environment that demands change—and that afterwards if depression was used as an opportunity to achieve insight and growth, the person is often stronger, freer, better put together, more creative, and more effective as a person.[21]

References

1 E. James Anthony and Therese Benedek (eds.), *Depression and Human Existence*, Little, Brown, Boston, 1975.

2 H. E. Lehmann: "Epidemiology of Depressive Disorders," in *Depression in the 1970s*, Elsevier–Excerpta Medica, Amsterdam, 1971.

3 Steven K. Secunda: *The Depressive Disorders: Special Report*, Department of Health, Education, and Welfare, Washington, D.C., 1973.

4 Robert Burton: "Prognostics of Melancholy," *Anatomy of Melancholy* (1628); reproduced in *Suicide*, vol. 1, no. 5, pp. 47–55, Spring 1975.

5 Sigmund Freud: "Mourning and Melancholia," 1917; in *The Standard Edition of the Complete Psychological Works of Sigmund Freud*, Hogarth, London, 1957, vol 14.

6 Rene Spitz and K. M. Wold: "Anaclitic Depression," in *The Psychoanalytic Study of the Child*, International Universities Press, New York, 1946, vol. 2.

7 Edward Bibring: "The Mechanism of Depression," in P. Greenacre (ed.), *Affective Disorders*, International Universities Press, New York, 1953.

8 Silvano Arieti: "Affective Disorders: Manic-Depressive Psychosis and Psychotic Depression," in Silvano Arieti (ed.), *American Handbook of Psychiatry*, Basic Books, New York, 1974, vol. 3.

9 Harry S. Sullivan: *Clinical Studies*, Norton, New York, 1956.

10 Michael Basch: "Toward a Theory that Encompasses Depression: A Revision of Existing Causal Hypotheses in Psychoanalysis," in E. James Anthony and Therese Benedek (eds.), *Depression and Human Existence*, Little, Brown, Boston, 1975.

11 Jurgen Ruesch: *Disturbed Communication*, Norton, New York, 1959.

12 Paul Watzlawick, Janet Beaven, and Don Jackson: *Pragmatics of Human Communication*, Norton, New York, 1967.

13 Norman Paul: The Use of Empathy in the Resolution of Grief, *Perspectives in Biological Medicine*, vol. 11, pp. 153–169, 1967.

14 John Bowlby: *Separation, Anxiety and Anger*, Basic Books, New York, 1973; vol II.

15 Maragret Mahler, et al.: *The Psychological Birth of the Human Infant*, Basic Books, New York, 1975.

*16 Frank Shea and Elizabeth Hurley: "Hopelessness and Helplessness," *Perspectives in Psychiatric Care*, vol. 2, no. 1, pp. 32–38, 1964.

17 Ezra Stotland: *The Psychology of Hope*, Jossey-Bass, San Francisco, 1969.

*18 Ardis Swanson: "Communicating with Depressed Persons," *Perspectives in Psychiatric Care*, vol. 13, no. 2, pp. 63–67.

19 Myer Mendelson: *Psychoanalytic Concepts of Depression*, 2d ed., Spectrum Publications, New York, 1974.

20 Frederick W. Crumb: "A Behavioral Pattern of Depressed Patients," *Perspectives in Psychiatric Care*, vol. 2, p. 40, 1964.

21 Frederic Flach: "What Is Depression?" transcript of program #129-S produced by Life Science Advisory Group, 420 E. 51 St., New York, N. Y. 10022.

*Recommended reference by a nurse author.

Chapter

19
The Client Who Threatens the Self-Concept

Judith Haber

Learning Objectives

After studying this chapter, the student should be able to:

1 Recognize the characteristics of elation
2 Discuss the psychodynamic issues that contribute to the development of the manic process
3 Identify four ways in which manic clients threaten the self-concept of others
4 Assess the dynamics of the family system
5 Identify assessment factors in relation to manic clients
6 Identify goals for manic clients
7 Plan nursing intervention for manic clients
8 Evaluate the effectiveness of the plan of intervention

Clients who threaten the self-concept of others appear to be self-sufficient, know-it-all types of people. They frequently take command in an interpersonal situation and are skillful in evoking and utilizing the feelings of others.[1] Fromm-Reichman has described such clients as being particularly successful in finding weak spots in the self-systems of others, making them feel exposed, undermined, and vulnerable. Levels of anxiety rise as a result of the attack on needs for self-esteem, prestige, and power. The ability to respond therapeutically in such situations is inhibited and problems in the nurse-client relationship follow.

To understand the client who threatens the self-concept of others, it is necessary to understand something about the self-concept. The self-concept is a cognitive and affective picture that is determined by the way in which satisfaction and security needs have been met throughout the developmental process (see Chaps. 4 and 5). The view of self as good or bad is derived from the reflected appraisals of significant others in a person's life. The predominant mode experienced throughout the growing-up years will help to determine whether the primary concept of self is good or bad. All people want to view themselves as being good, approved of, successful, and liked.[2] To maintain such a positive view of self, people utilize coping mechanisms to defend against anxiety-producing experiences of disapproval and shame and to maintain self-esteem.

Thus, it is the core of a person's being, the self, and its attendant needs for approval, praise, and competence that is being threatened by the clients to be discussed in this chapter.

Selected Client Behaviors

Clients who threaten the self-concept of others are mainly those whose primary affective modes are *elation* and *euphoria*. The mood state varies and can range from what is perceived as normal liveliness to extreme stages of excitement. Such episodes can occur as isolated incidents or in a cyclical, repetitive pattern alternating between elation and depression (see App. A for diagnostic classifications). Manic episodes can also occur in the course of acute and chronic brain disease (see Chap. 30) or can be exhibited in the early stages of acute alcohol intoxication (see Chap. 17).[3,4] The incidence and prevalence of these behaviors as emotional problems is not reliably known. However, in the United States in 1970, an estimated 52.2 persons per 100,000 population experienced manic episodes.[5] This represents only 3.5 percent of all admissions to inpatient and outpatient mental health facilities.

The condition appears twice as frequently in females as in males. Genetic research studies suggest that there is a dominant x-linked factor present for the transmission of manic-depressive illness in families in which one or more members have had manic as well as depressive episodes. Maternal relatives are affected twice as frequently as paternal. The incidence of manic-depressive episodes is 25 times as high among siblings of manic-depressive clients as in the average population.[3]

Biochemically, a relationship seems to exist between catecholamine metabolism and the production of norepinephrine. Drugs which stimulate the production of norepinephrine produce behavioral expressions of excitement. A depletion or inactivation of norepinephrine seems to potentiate sedation and depression. Therefore, an excess of amines, specifically norepinephrine, at the adrenergic receptor sites in the brain seems to play a significant role in the behavioral state of elation.[3] Additionally, the intracellular distribution of sodium is lowered during manic states and appears to return to normal levels as the manic episode is resolved.[6]

However small their actual numbers may be, manic clients make up for this in the havoc they can cause and the difficulty that arises in implementing an effective therapeutic program. They exhibit affective changes. Their behavior is characterized by increased activity. They exhibit thought disorders including distractibility, flight of ideas, and delusions of grandeur, as shown in the following stages.[3,7,8,9]

Mild Elation—Stage 1

This stage is often difficult to detect. Many people exhibiting behaviors characteristic of this stage never become clients. They are often referred to as *hypomanic* and lead overtly successful and productive lives in the community. Perceptions of them will include the following features:[3]

Affect

1 Lively mood, happy, free of worry, unconcerned.
2 Extroverted personality, witty, joker, life of the party. These behaviors are exhibited without concern for reality or the feelings of others.
3 Confident, uninhibited.
4 Often, indifference to events which would normally make a person sad.
5 Variable mood, changing easily to one of irritation and anger, especially when others do not respond enthusiastically or are critical of them.

Thoughts

1 Content of thought often reveals an exalted opinion of self as a great lover and/or person of great wealth and ability.
2 Ideas move quickly from one subject to another, with poor ability to concentrate and pursue an idea to a goal-directed end.
3 The person has the ability to associate ideas rapidly. This enables him or her to grasp aspects of the environment which would otherwise go unnoticed. However, because of increased distractibility, the person is unable to utilize the perceptions in a meaningful way. For example, elaborate business schemes are devised, but they either fail or are never implemented.
4 Little evidence of introspection.

Behavior

1 Motor activity is increased. These are people who are always on the go. They talk, tease,

and joke excessively. They may sing walking down the street, dance as they walk, and laugh when others would find this inappropriate.
2 They may periodically experience loss of appetite, loss of weight, constipation, insomnia, and irregular menstrual periods. The sexual drive may increase.
3 Activity is not always appropriate for age and place. They may engage in a great deal of purposeless activity or in activities aimed at irrelevant goals. For example, such people may write numerous unnecessary letters or go on spending sprees to purchase unneeded items. Frequently, one will observe a rapid changing of activity.
4 Superficial relationships; many acquaintances, few close friends.

Acute Elation—Stage 2

Symptoms are more pronounced during this stage. They have either intensified from those manifested in stage 1 or have appeared suddenly. Most individuals appear in the treatment setting as clients at this point.

Affect

1 The affect is characterized by feelings of exaltation and expansiveness. The client appears to be on a real "high."
2 The expansiveness turns rapidly to anger when attempts are made to control the person. He or she reacts to provocations with fury and may scream, curse, or strike out violently at others or the environment.
3 The affect may be labile. A client may be happily talking about the success of a recent business venture, then may suddenly burst into tears and begin dwelling on what a failure he or she has been.

Thought

1 The thought process at this time is characterized by flight of ideas and

loquaciousness. *Flight of ideas* is a sudden, continuous, and rapid shift in topics. *Loquaciousness* is often referred to as *pressure of speech*. It is difficult to interrupt the client to get a word in edgewise. Communication patterns also include rhyming, playing on words, and making associations of words having similar sounds but no relationship in meaning.[3] An example of the above characteristics occurred during an early interview with a client.

Nurse: Mr. D, how do you like it at the hospital?

Client: Fine, fine, good . . . good looking women, I say women because they're different from the men at home. Home is a place to roam, place the food on the table . . . I want to place first in the stable.

The ideas and associations seem illogical, but the content and underlying message usually relate to an overvalued idea or egocentric interest of the client's which directs the stream of thought. Clients, not realizing the significance of their statements, often give information as to the unconscious motivation of their ideas.[10]

2 The thought content also includes grandiose and persecutory delusions (see Chap. 14). Clients may think they have x-ray vision or that the wrath of Satan is upon them and is making them destroy self and family to escape from Satan's wrath.[10]

Behavior

1 Inappropriate dress may be evident. Female clients may dress as if in costume, wearing excessive makeup, too much jewelry, and brightly colored, poorly matching outfits. Their hair may be decorated with beads or flowers. Male clients may also wear bizarre outfits. Clothing may be inappropriate for the weather and grooming may be poor.

2 Motor activity increases to a constant, urgent rate. Clients continuously meddle with others in ward or family activities. They may suggest numerous ways in which people should conduct themselves. Constant rearrangement of furniture, making and remaking beds, and frequent changing of clothing is also prompted by this activity drive.

3 Despite increased activity, there is little or no appetite, and the client does not want to stop moving to eat. Sleep patterns are disrupted and the client may go for days without sleep or without exhibiting signs of exhaustion. Even when objective signs of exhaustion are evident in eyes and body posture, clients continue to move about in random fashion.

4 Normal inhibitions may decrease and normally modest clients may engage in sexually indiscreet acts or use profane language.

5 The attention span is disturbed and the client is easily distracted. Environmental stimuli such as noises, movement, or changes in temperature constantly divert attention. People are sometimes misidentified because they present some slight similarity to persons the client knows well. The client seizes upon similarities without examining the differences. For example, when a short, chubby female nurse walked onto the unit, Susan, a client, ran over to her shouting, "Mary Mary, you bitch, why didn't you visit me yesterday?" The nurse, Ms. Jones, identified herself saying, "Susan, I'm Ms. Jones, the nurse on the unit." Susan replied, "You are? Yes, I guess you are, but you're short and chubby just like Mary."

Delirium—Stage 3

The client is in a state of extreme excitement. Feelings, thoughts, and behavior patterns observed are intensifications of those previously described. Clients appear disoriented, incoherent, and agitated. There is a frenetic quality to their behavior. They may injure themselves and others with their increasing, frantic, aimless activity. They exhibit delusions and sometimes visual or olfactory hallucinations (see Chap. 14).[11] Exhaustion, injury, and death are real possibilities. These clients must be protected against themselves.

Psychodynamics

A variety of dynamic factors lead to the development of manic or manic-depressive episodes. The influences of childhood and adult life will be explored.

Early Developmental Patterns

Infancy appears to be a time when the manic client feels loved and accepted. The complete dependence of the infant seems to be pleasurable to the mother. (Schizophrenics and their mothers, on the other hand, perceive all parenting and nurturing experiences as anxiety-provoking.) The infant offers little resistance to her care. The mother is generally described as one who feels "duty bound" to provide everything the child needs. The image of mother is incorporated by the child as good. As the infant begins to separate from the mother and reach out to explore the environment actively, his or her growing independence and rebelliousness is perceived by the mother as threatening. Unconforming or unconventional behavior on the part of the child is labeled "bad" by the mother, and every effort is made to eliminate it. Toward the end of the infant's first year of life, the previously loving and tender mother abruptly changes into a harsh, punitive figure.[8]

The small child's ability to integrate a unified image from the tender mother and the harsh mother is impaired by the anxiety accompanying the conflicting images. Opposing parental images exist to some extent for all children and are normally resolved and incorporated as one as the ego matures. However, these children wish to maintain only the good-mother image. They do this through compliance and conformity. The harsh mother is repressed. This dichotomy sets the stage for ambivalence toward others in later life.

During the second year there is a continued change in parenting patterns. Not only is direct care decreased but demands for independence and self-sufficiency are made. The child continues to receive some love and affection if parental expectations, no matter how unrealistic, are accepted and fulfilled. One client recalls that as a child she was expected to learn to ride a two-wheeled bike at age 3, but was not allowed to fall while learning. The bike was taken away when this expectation was not fulfilled. The attitude that "what is obtained is deserved" evokes an early sense of duty and responsibility.[9]

The child adapts by:

1 Accepting and trying to live up to parental expectations at all costs.
2 Consciously accepting the values and symbols of significant others without attending to his or her own wishes, feelings, and desires.
3 Complying, obeying, and working hard in an effort to recapture the early tenderness from mother and to maintain the love that does exist.
4 Harboring strong resentment against parents who have made so many demands and have not given enough. This can result in temper tantrums and apparently unprovoked rage, which is an outcome of bottling up feelings until they bubble over. These episodes end quickly because of the fear of loss of love. The feelings are repressed and retained unconsciously. They may reappear in dreams.
5 Acting rebellious and becoming the incorrigible child, exhibiting self-defeating behavior and fulfilling negative parental perceptions.

Children who conform to the directions and demands of others have several problems which follow them in later life. First, they do not learn to rely on their own problem-solving resources or perceptions of the environment. Second, trust in self and others is poorly developed because they have had minimal consistent, unconditional caring experiences. Third, anxiety is always present because these children live in fear of losing love and approval from significant others. Fourth, the parents continue to be viewed as good. The child's self-image is that of the "wayward lamb." The parents are seen as attempting to salvage the child through direction and punishment. Unlike the preschizophrenic, this child is not felt to be unsalvageable. Additionally, the child is often dethroned at this point by the birth of a sibling to whom the mother must "give her all."[9]

Family Social Network

The family of origin is often socially, economically, or religiously marginal. It is often unified in its wish to elevate the family prestige within their own social group as well as the larger society. The client is often the specially endowed family member in whom rests all hope of family salvation.[8] One client related the following:

> My mother would not let me go to our neighborhood high school. It was not good enough for me. She obtained special permission for me to go to another school on the other side of town where all the "right" kids went to school. She felt I would have a chance to meet Mr. Rich and make the right career connections. This would save my family from their genteel poverty. The kids' lives seemed so effortless to me, who had to struggle for everything. I never felt I made it despite all the clothes and things mother worked so hard to give me.

This feeling existed despite the fact that the client graduated with honors, belonged to many clubs, and had many friends.

The client's special position often arouses envy and jealousy in the siblings. As the clients grew up, they remained sensitive to envy and competition, often negating it by underselling themselves to hide the full extent of their abilities. Paradoxically, they dislike themselves for not actualizing their abilities and hate others for their demands and envy.[18] The family is viewed as having a fused and undifferentiated ego mass where the individuating experiences of the separate family members are not considered as important as the common good of the family as a whole (see Chap. 10). A kinship clan of several generations results in role blurring and multiple authority figures. Relinquished by the mother, the child is often at a loss as to who is really significant and to be looked to for sustained support, guidance, and approval. Consequently, the child never develops a reliable relationship with anybody where communication is open, free, and genuine. Additionally, stereotyped family rules and myths govern relationships within the clan.[8] The pattern of communication learned in the family is perpetuated in limited relationships outside the family. Essentially, the child and family are lonely and have few ties outside the family.

Later Developmental Patterns

Loss

The manic state is often referred to as a mirror image of depression. It is held that the elation represents a massive denial of underlying depression (see Chap. 18).[9] Clients deny the feelings of actual, threatened, or symbolic loss of love that are seen in depression. Such feelings have their roots in the helpless infantile response to separation that occurs around the time that personal differentiation takes place—a response that leads to loss of self-esteem. To counteract this state, manic clients act out with intense drive the fantasies of strength which enable them to feel liberated from their depression. Heightened activity levels and thought processes enable the client to avoid or escape the omnipresent depressive thoughts or activities. Joviality is a mask for the client, who states that "I am crying beneath the laughter and jokes." The loss is often not apparent to the onlooker. The client may, in fact, have recently received a promotion. The promotion, however, is unconsciously perceived by the client as a loss of dependency or as a loss of available support from a superior.

Superficial Relationships

Manic clients defensively present themselves to themselves and others as lively, hearty, and friendly. They characteristically have many acquaintances with whom they appear to be on excellent terms. On closer inspection, it becomes apparent that these relationships are very superficial and are not at all suggestive of intimacy, especially since the communications of these clients have little or no depth. The person suffering from mania carries out stereotyped social performances in which the other person's traits or needs are not considered. Relatedness always remains superficial, so that envy, competitiveness, and dislike will not be accurately perceived and acted upon by others. This adaptive position protects clients from the realization that people might like and accept them despite transitory lapses in behavior. Having never learned to consider their own feelings in a relationship, they are unable to relate to others on an open, actualized feeling level. They have never learned to put themselves in another's place and thus try to feel what is actually going on. They are afraid that real closeness will lead to rejection, afraid of knowing themselves, they are therefore unwilling to know others.[3]

Dependency

The manic client projects an air of pseudoindependence in an attempt to mask underlying wishes for dependency. The client's principal source of anxiety is the fear of abandonment. He or she perceives danger and threat in acknowledging the dependent need to be cared for by others.[8] This evolves from earlier experiences relating to premature separation and withdrawal of love. To maintain self-esteem and the feeling of power and strength, the client presents a repertoire of behavior that suggests omnipotent independence. These ideas of grandeur indicate that not only do they not need to be cared for but that instead they care for others. A common remark from such a client is "I don't need anybody." Such egocentricity is suggestive of narcissism, but the underlying dynamic is negative narcissism. (See Chap. 18.) While appearing jovial, outgoing, and friendly, such people are actually self-centered, controlling, and manipulative. They repeatedly attempt to test, manipulate, and over-commit people into involvement with them so that others will actually be caring for them. Those dependent relationships that do exist are usually of a demanding nature. These relationships provide the praise and approval that such clients need to maintain their fragile self-esteem.[3] The needs of the significant other, usually a spouse, are negated, and the relationship becomes a one-way street. When the client's demands on the significant other are frustrated, the client becomes angry and expresses hostility, thus further jeopardizing the desperately desired ties to others.

Anxiety

Increased physical activity is an attempt to escape the anxiety aroused by a punitive superego. The frenzied activity allows the client to be selectively inattentive to messages that are unacknowledgeable as components of awareness. Thus feelings of helplessness, worthlessness, and guilt are temporarily avoided.[9]

The psychotic attack occurs when the mask of joviality, manipulativeness, and demandingness no longer serves its defensive purpose. Emptiness is felt, anxiety rises, and behavior becomes more disorganized. The experience of elation may occur in isolation or occur preceding or following a period of depression.

The Nurse's Response to Client Behavior

Aggression and hostility are defensive maneuvers designed to elevate the client's self-esteem and place others in positions of embarrassment, self-doubt, and low self-esteem. Caretakers dealing with manic clients often find themselves responding defensively and attempting to justify their actions and motivations. It is not uncommon for nurses to feel outsmarted and outmaneuvered while knowing that their judgments and actions were appropriate. The client's interpersonal patterns revolve around four areas: (1) manipulation of the self-esteem of others, (2) sensitivity to potential conflict and to the vulnerability of others, (3) projection of responsibility onto others, and (4) progressive testing of limits.[1]

The manic client is adept at rapidly engaging

staff in seemingly genuine relationships. Such clients seem friendly, resourceful, and entertaining. They are quick to sense the form of flattery that will appeal the most to a given person. The good reality orientation of this client makes the flattery seem sincere and appropriate. The nurse is often told, "You are the first person who has really understood me. I really think I'll be able to make a lot of progress." This behavior increases the self-esteem of the nurse; the client becomes a source of gratification. The nurse, in turn, is led to entertain rescue fantasies. But this interaction pattern is disrupted as the relationship develops. The client, unable to continue utilizing denial to mask feelings of dependency, emptiness, and worthlessness, suddenly turns on the nurse in a demeaning, degrading way. The nurse is told that "My lack of progress in therapy is due to your ineffectiveness." The nurse's self-concept is, of course, tied up with being an effective practitioner. Thus, when the client threatens this self-concept with resistance and hostility, feelings of anxiety and anger rise in the nurse, who withdraws emotionally to protect self-esteem. The nurse may also respond by viewing the client as spiteful and uncooperative rather than looking at the purpose served by the defensive behavior. Additionally the nurse's reaction may be influenced by prior experiences of rejection.[1,12]

Closely related to self-esteem is the client's ability to perceive an individual's or group's area of vulnerability.[8] The client utilizes this vulnerability in an exploitative way, making covert conflict overt and causing anxiety in others. Often, the picture created by the client is not an accurate representation but contains elements of truth that may have previously been suppressed. Examples of such areas of vulnerability include issues related to sexuality, prejudice, aggressiveness, and self-esteem.[1] For example, a male client requested a weekend pass and permission was refused by the nurse. The client was on ward restrictions after having set fire to several bedrooms. The client did not accept the answer and went to the ward psychiatrist, complaining that the nurse was a rigid, authoritarian "witch" and repeated his request. The nurse, who considered herself to be understanding, objective, and, in fact, hesitant about being authoritative, began to think that perhaps she did have some negative feelings about authority. She began to question her decision despite objective data indicating that she was correct.

The result of this sort of maneuvering is that the staff member feels exposed, insulted, and put down. The immediate response is to deny the allegation, not to look at how it was arrived at or at its validity. The nurse becomes wrapped up in restoring self-esteem and objectivity is sharply reduced.

The client also uses this technique to divide staff members by complaining about the ineffectiveness of one group versus another. Some staff members may consent to privileges and activities that have been realistically refused by other staff members. This leads the latter staff group to feel attacked by their own peers, causing them to feel angry and resentful. The client's purpose in using this tactic is to keep the therapeutic focus away from meaningful consensus and action. Divisiveness among the staff allows the client to perpetuate pathological patterns of interaction.[12]

The manic client makes others feel responsible for client actions and forces others to accept blame when plans go awry. Thus dependency is perpetuated. For example, a client on a one-day pass was returned to the hospital by the police after the client had undressed on the main street of town. The staff blamed themselves for not having anticipated that this or something else could happen. Staff members tend to become committed to seeing that things do not go wrong with the client.[1] Again, this relates to the therapist's self-concept—the need to see efforts result in positive outcomes. Clients who forever "mess up" reflect badly on the staff's effectiveness.

The client often tests and violates limits set by the staff.[8,12] This generates feelings of powerlessness and helplessness. An example of this occurred with a female client who returned 8 hours late, roaring drunk, from an all-day pass. The limits had been "No drinking" and "Be back on time." In response to staff inquiries as to where she had been and why was she drunk, the client responded, "I'm back aren't I? Stop making a mountain out of a molehill." The client's superficial reasonableness made the staff begin to feel that *they* were wrong, not the client, and that maybe they were "nit-picking."

The preceding interpersonal patterns of behavior attempt to undermine the self-concepts of the nurse and staff. Self-assessment is essential to remaining aware of the dynamics underlying client behavior. The feelings of anxiety, anger, and powerlessness generated by this type of client can lead to a therapeutic stalemate. Open communication among staff must be maintained if therapeutic effectiveness is to exist.

The Family System

The patterns of communication and the quality of relationships previously described were learned in the family and continue to be played out until interventions through therapy are effected.

Relationships within the family system are closely related to the fulfillment of dependency needs. The client simultaneously feels that it is unsafe to rely on others and unacceptable to want to be cared for. The dependency role is assumed by default; the client resists and fails to acknowledge the loss of control. Hyperactivity, overcommitment, and exhaustion ultimately require that others assume responsibility for the client's care. Such clients appear to be searching for a relationship with the perfect other who will not be put off by the client's charade[9] and who will supply needed controls without making demands for reciprocity. The client uses the spouse to meet ungratified dependency needs without consideration of or attention to the needs of others. The narcissistic "I" is all important. The client will also shift responsibility for behavioral outcomes onto the family. The male client who loses a job after mouthing off to

the boss might blame his spouse for encouraging him to be assertive. When the client fails to carry out agreed-upon plans, the spouse feels betrayed.

Manic behavior tends to be cyclical, and the client may be highly productive and good company when the problem is not manifest. At these times, the family is lulled by a feeling that all is well; or else they may feel that they are sitting on a powder keg, waiting for the next explosion. Because of the client's manipulativeness, it is difficult to determine the point at which irrational, unreasonable behavior takes over. As the pathological behavior becomes more evident, marital discord is more frequent. The state of elation is perceived as threatening and exasperating. At some point, the spouse and children often feel "they've had it." Then, as normalcy returns, they are usually tempted to give the client one more chance.

Assessment

Nursing assessment must encompass the emotional and behavioral manifestations of elation and its consequences for the client. The interpersonal maneuvers must be identified. The family support system and safety needs must be assessed. The nurse should consider the items in Table 19-1 as assessment criteria from which to make the nursing diagnosis.

Manic behavior must be differentiated from schizophrenic behavior so that an appropriate therapeutic plan may be formulated. Most manic clients have had fairly successful interpersonal relationships. They relate easily, if dependently— as opposed to schizophrenic clients, who are withdrawn and aloof in relationships.[5] Periodicity is another important difference. Manic behavior is characterized by its episodic nature and symptom-free intervals. Schizophrenic reactions are either single experiences or tend to leave a distinct, enduring trace despite a relatively stable reconstitution.

The emotional response to manic clients

Table 19-1 Nursing Assessment

Assessment questions	Responses of client (C) and family (F)
1 Why has the client been hospitalized?	C: "Nothing's wrong . . . I'm fine ... fine a cop a thousand dollars." F: "During last 2 weeks he hasn't slept or eaten, is writing bad checks, is calling the White House collect 3 times a day."
2 What is the client's life-style?	C: "I winter in Palm Beach with the jet set, I summer in Spain with the best people. You can reach me through my private secretary." F: "When he's not 'up' he's a terrific insurance salesman, wins awards for sales records."
3 What were the precipitating factors? Has there been a change in lifestyle, an upset in structure, a recent loss, or is this the anniversary of a previous loss?	C: "No change . . . change is money . . . when you have money you make the change." F: "There hasn't been any real change except for his new promotion. He's had to travel a lot more and work longer hours seeing important clients at night. It was also at this time last year that he refused a promotion and became ill.
4 What have previous patterns of elation been like in terms of intensity, duration, and periodicity?	C: "It happens not often enough, I'm at my best, put others to the test. Being singled out from the rest really puts you over the crest. . . ." F: "He's been having these mood swings for about the last 6 years. They started after we got married and come about almost every spring. I can see him getting higher and higher, wanting to party, travel, and buy everything in sight. I take the checkbook and credit cards away or we'd be bankrupt. He's so clever he even ends up charging things where we have no accounts, and then I have to deal with the telephone complaints. As soon as he's hospitalized and medicated, he comes down and seems ready to go home."
5 What is the family history? a History of affective disorder in family of origin	F: "His grandmother had mood swings all her adult life. They began coming closer together as she got older. She died in a mental institution."
b Parenting patterns	C: "My mother was a cold fish, literally threw us out on our own as tiny kids . . . always expected me to be able to do everything perfectly the first time."
c Family structure	C: "My grandparents lived with us. There were lots of bosses in the house. We lived on the fringes of the 'right' neighborhood—I was to bring the family fame and fortune. Mom and Dad had very few friends outside the family, and we never quite fit in with the neighbors."
d Present family relationships	C: "She's the perfect soul mate for me, always saving my skin." F: "We have no children. He doesn't want any. If he weren't so independent most of the time, I'd say he's my baby. I always end up bailing him out of scrapes, cleaning up his mess, and taking the blame for his misfortunes. Between episodes it's great, but I am getting weary."
6 What effect does client's behavior have on work relationship and performance?	C: "I'm the best; they couldn't do without me." F: "He's such a supersalesman that they take him back after each hospitalization. They think he's a great guy—funny, witty, and effective."
7 What is the client's physiological level of functioning? What has it been? How has it changed? a Activity level b Sleep patterns c Appetite d Grooming e Medication status	F: "Activity! He's off the wall. . . . Now he never stops, up all night roaming around, no food, lost about 18 pounds in the last 2 weeks. And lithium—if he'd only take it, this might stop."

Table 19-1 Nursing Assessment (continued)

Assessment questions	Responses of client (C) and family (F)

8 What interpersonal maneuvers are utilized by the client?
  a Testing
  b Manipulation
  c Denial, etc.
	Client makes 10 phone calls when only allowed to make 2.
	C: "I don't have to do this, the other nurse said I don't have to."
	C: "Problems—I don't have any problems."

9 What is the impact of client's behavior on staff and other clients in the treatment setting?	The staff avoids the client because he is always telling them that they don't know anything.
10 What is the probability of effecting change in the client's interpersonal relationships and life-style?	Good, if the client's patterns of denial and superficiality can be decreased.

tends to be warm and humorous, as opposed to the sense of distaste and puzzlement the schizophrenic may evoke in others. Delusions and pathological communications are similar to those of schizophrenia but do not display the highly symbolic looseness of schizophrenic associations.[11]

Nursing Diagnosis and Goals

The nursing diagnosis and goals are formulated on the basis of data collection. Table 19-2 indicates examples of nursing diagnoses and goals applicable to the manic client.

Nursing Intervention

The client usually arrives at the treatment facility in a highly excited state. His or her boisterous, jovial facade may mask the feelings of anxiety, worthlessness, and isolation the client is actually experiencing. This makes it difficult for the staff to decide on appropriate nursing interventions. Understanding the underlying dynamics of the client's behavior is essential to implementing effective nursing intervention.

Increased Physical Activity

Hyperactivity requires decisive nursing intervention because the consequences of the activity can be life-threatening. The following guidelines are directed toward restoring and maintaining a homeodynamic state.

Decrease Environmental Stimuli

Decreasing environmental stimuli can be accomplished by means of soft lighting, low noise level, and simple room decorations. There should be as few people as possible in the client's environment. A consistent caretaker becomes the agent for supplying external controls on physical activity. Firm, clearly stated instructions will facilitate transitions from one activity to another. Hazardous objects and substances should be removed from the environment to protect the client from uncontrollable impulsivity.

Adequate Hygiene, Nutrition, and Rest

Provide the client with flexible opportunities to shower and change clothing. Loose, comfortable clothing is preferred. High-calorie finger foods and drinks that can be consumed quickly, standing and on the run, are suggested. A quiet environment, sedation, and opportunities for frequent

Table 19-2 Nursing Diagnosis and Goals

Nursing Diagnosis	Goals
1 The client denies underlying feelings of anxiety, dependency, worthlessness, powerlessness, and loneliness by maintaining a facade of joviality, competence, and independence.	1 To have client verbally acknowledge and explore feelings.
a Difficulty accepting client status.	a To have client acknowledge need for help.
b Resistance—the client is unwilling to engage in the problem-solving process.	b To have client utilize cognitive skills to identify sources of anxiety and worthlessness.
2 Lack of confidence in own abilities.	2 Increase client's ability to identify own strengths and weaknesses.
3 Pseudo independence.	3 Increase client's trust in others.
4 Superficial relationships that are carried out in a stereotyped manner without consideration of the needs of others.	4 Increase client's ability to identify the needs of self and others in a relationship.
5 Demanding behavior which attempts to obtain caring, approval, and advice.	5 Increase client's recognition of demanding behavior and its onset. Increase client's ability to set limits on own demanding behavior, and verbally articulate needs in an open direct manner.
6 Manipulative behavior directed toward maintaining power and control of others and the environment.	6 Increase client's recognition of manipulative patterns of interaction. Increase open, direct communication patterns.
7 Verbal hostility toward others that arises when attempts to manipulate fail.	7 Decrease verbal hostility and increase client's ability to express feelings in an appropriate manner.
8 Inadequate nutritional intake.	8 Restore normal eating patterns.
9 Weight loss.	9 Increase caloric intake to 3000 cal/day.
10 Inadequate hydration.	10 Increase fluid intake to 2000 ml/24 h.
11 Sleep disturbance.	11 To have client sleep 4—6 h without waking.
12 Agitation and hyperactivity.	12 Increase client's ability to mediate sensory input.

short naps will facilitate restoration of a regular sleep pattern.

Activities

Large motor skill activities that provide for appropriate discharge of energy and tension are walks, housekeeping chores, painting, and movement therapy. Choice of activities should consider the client's short attention span and easy distractibility.

Monitoring Medications

Lithium carbonate is the drug of choice in preventing and alleviating manic and manic-depressive episodes.[5,6,9] Nursing intervention is directed toward assessing the effectiveness of the medication and identifying the occurrence of side and toxic effects (see Chap. 8).

Denial

The first step in intervening to counteract denial should be the establishment of an open nurse-client relationship in which thoughts, feelings, and meanings are discussed.[8] The nurse should focus and comment on themes, nonverbal gestures, and tone of voice rather than verbal content. This facilitates recognition of what is actually occurring rather than what the client would like the nurse to believe is occurring. The client, unable to confront feelings, needs assistance to bring them into awareness and engage in the problem-solving process. An example of this process occurred between Ms. B. and her nurse.

Ms. B.: I think I'll leave the hospital, nobody here can help me. You're all just a bunch of no-good do-nothings. I'm going to get Satan after all of you (voice rising, wringing her hands).

Nurse: You sound upset Ms. B, your voice is rising and you're wringing your hands. I sense that you're feeling alone and perhaps unloved.

Ms. B.: Alone, alone . . . I'm never alone. I'm the most loved person around here (starts crying and laughing).

Nurse: You say you're never alone or unloved. Yet you're laughing and crying. Most people feel alone or unloved sometimes. It's all right to feel that way and it's OK to share the feeling with someone.

Another approach is to introduce startle experiences to undermine the client's stereotyped response patterns. For example, a very witty male client continuously entertained other clients on the unit. His jokes persisted even in light of a discussion about death and loss. In an effort to dislodge the facade of humor, the nurse said, "Tom, you were talking about your father's death, why don't you have a good cry now? It's OK; we can bear your painful feelings."

Role modeling can be a valuable tool for the nurse-client relationship. The nurse acts in an open way that demonstrates how one communicates feelings without making oneself vulnerable. The client can then see that his or her real self, which the client perceives as terrible, is not in danger of rejection (see Chap. 17).[8] The nurse should not assume that the client is finally engaging in meaningful communication when the client's reality orientation is good and data are offered about self. The client has the ability to maintain the flow of information on a superficial level. The nurse must frequently reassess the level of denial and the depth of the relationship.

Dependency

The clients' dependency needs are strong, yet clients feel that they are unacceptable and act pseudoindependently.[8] The nurse may be presented with a client who states "I don't need you," and "I don't need therapy." The client may miss appointments, arrive late, or discuss superficial trivia during the hour. In dealing with such *resistance,* the nurse should clearly state the time and frequency of the therapeutic sessions. The nurse must verbally acknowledge the dynamic of the *resistance* that is occurring and state that people sometimes need others to lean on for awhile, pointing out that the client can use the therapeutic sessions to learn how to deal with these feelings.[13]

Irrational demands should be firmly and consistently refused.[12] The nurse must be careful that in saying no to one request, he or she is not fulfilling another. One nurse refused permission for a client to go to a friend's house for Christmas day but ended up taking the client to her own home for Christmas dinner. Demands for advice and answers to problems are common examples of dependency. The client exhibits lack of faith in his or her ability to work out problems independently or interdependently. As soon as the nurse begins to provide guidance for the client, one of the client's most basic demands is being met and the stage is set for the client to make more and more demands for salvation. The effectiveness of the problem-solving process is thus inhibited and the client is allowed to maintain maladaptive response patterns.

Guidelines for dealing with dependency are as follows:

1 Be aware of when demands are being made.
2 Convey acceptance of the client while refusing to comply with excessive, irrational demands.
3 State observations and theme about the dynamic of the behavior. "I sense that you are attempting to have me guide your life and to take responsibility for mistakes that occur."
4 State reaction to interpersonal maneuvers: "I

am really ticked off" or "That really makes me angry."

5 State how behavior can be utilized in the therapeutic process. Help client to identify feelings, acknowledge them, analyze them, and learn how to develop alternate ways of seeking gratification.[8]

6 Reinforce client's self-esteem: "You have the ability to do it, let's work together."

7 Engage client in learning how to make decisions and accept responsibility.

Manipulation, Testing, and Acting-Out Behavior

The client, feeling alone and unloved, manipulates and acts out to test the caring and limits that are conveyed by others. Paradoxically, clients perceive that "giving in" to the unacceptable activity is equivalent to rejection. Escalation of manic activity usually follows; it is an attempt to elicit caring and controls from others. Thus, the fear that many caretakers have about provoking rage reactions when setting limits is unfounded. The client really welcomes such controls, even though he or she may protest loudly and violently.[12] The following guidelines are suggested for helping the staff set limits on manipulation, testing, and acting-out behavior.[14,15]

1 Identify the need for a limit; the client is unable to exercise self-control and needs external controls. For example, John is making twenty collect phone calls a day. Phone privileges are restricted for a week.

2 The decision on setting limits and what these are to be must be agreed upon and understood by *all* staff and shifts. Care plans must be *written* and posted clearly so that problems, goals, and interventions are clearly understood by all.

3 Communicate the limits to the client in clear language. For example "Mr. Jones, you cannot undress in the dayroom. If you want to remain undressed, you must stay in your room."

4 Enforce the limits in an unambivalent, firm manner. The eventual relaxation of restrictive rules will depend on what the client is *doing,* not on what he or she is *saying.* The client's demands for greater freedom are usually connected with a continued need to act out. For example, as soon as John's request was complied with, he was back to making twenty-five phone calls a day to "old friends." Clients who are effectively engaged in problem solving will have little time for testing and manipulation.

5 Reevaluate the need for the limit at regular intervals and also review the impact of the inappropriate behavior on others.

6 It is essential to have clear communication channels among team members in order to provide a consistent approach to the client. Sometimes dual therapists are utilized. One is the just disciplinarian and the other is the loving, accepting person. The objective splitting of roles minimizes the ability of the client to divide and conquer the staff. Limits may also have to be set on general meddling and advice giving to prevent further isolation and decreased self-esteem. For example, Jean, a manic client, was constantly going over to other unit members, giving directions for a crafts project that she had tossed aside. She also gave them advice about boyfriends and showered them with jewelry from her pocketbook. This behavior was initially received positively by them. Then their reaction turned to annoyance and anger. They said, "Jean, why don't you just get lost?" Limits may also have to be set on grandiose plans such as business deals and spending sprees.

Hostility and Aggression

These are defensive responses to both anxiety and loss of self-esteem and power; they are utilized by the client as "as if" behaviors to enhance control.[8,9] Nursing actions are directed toward:

1 Recognizing the purpose the behavior serves for the client.

2 Nonjudgmentally stating your observations about the behavior.

3 Refraining from any personal response to criticism, physical attack, or profanity.

4 Setting limits on the behavior. For example, "Barbara, I cannot allow you to hit the other patients—you'll have to go to the quiet room for 30 minutes."

5 Avoiding positive reinforcement of negative behavior.

6 After the episode is over, giving the client an opportunity to discuss feelings experienced prior to, during, and after the episode. Alternate coping patterns can then be explored.

Evaluation

Clients who experience periods of elation have the potential to relate to others in a self-actualized way. Criteria for evaluation are based on anticipated behavioral changes. The client who has shown improvement

1 Recognizes and acknowledges feelings of self and significant others

2 Is able to talk about areas of competence and self-worth

3 Is able to recognize the need for limit setting and sets his or her own limits on manipulative and acting-out behavior

4 Is able to engage in a mutual problem-solving process

References

1 D. M. Janowsky et al.: "Playing the Manic Game," *Archives of General Psychiatry,* vol. 22, pp. 252–261, March 1970.

2 Harry S. Sullivan: "The Interpersonal Theory of Psychiatry," in Helen S. Perry and Mary L. Gowel (eds.), *The Collected Works of Harry Stack Sullivan,* Norton, New York, 1953.

3 Lawrence C. Kolb: *Modern Clinical Psychiatry,* Saunders, Philadelphia, 1973, pp. 357–386.

4 G. Winokur: *Manic-Depressive Illness,* Mosby, St. Louis, 1969.

5 Alfred M. Freedman, Harold I. Kaplan, and Benjamin J. Sadock (eds.): *Comprehensive Textbook of Psychiatry,* 2d ed., Williams & Wilkins, Baltimore, 1975.

6 A. I. M. Glenn and H. W. Reading: "Regulatory Action of Lithium in Manic-Depressive Illness," *Lancet,* vol. 2, pp. 1239–1241, December 1973.

7 F. C. Redlich and D. X. Freedman: *The Theory and Practice of Psychiatry,* Basic Books, New York, 1966.

8 Freida Fromm-Reichmann: in Dexter M. Bullard (ed.), *Psychoanalysis and Psychotherapy,* University of Chicago Press, Chicago, 1969.

9 Silvano Arieti: "Affective Disorders: Manic-Depressive Psychosis and Psychotic Depression," in Silvano Arieti (ed.), *American Handbook of Psychiatry,* Basic Books, New York, 1975, chap. 21.

10 K. M Lipkin et al.: "The Many Faces of Mania," *Archives of General Psychiatry,* vol. 22, pp. 262–267, March 1970.

11 Gabriel Carlson and F. K. Goodwin: "The Stages of Mania," *Archives of General Psychiatry,* vol. 28, pp. 221–228, February 1973.

12 John G. Gunderson: "Management of Manic States: The Problem of Fire Setting," *Psychiatry,* vol. 37, pp. 137–146, May 1974.

13 H. S. Klein: "Transference and Defense in Manic States," *International Journal of Psychoanalysis,* vol. 55, pp. 261–268, 1974.

*14 Maxine E. Loomis: "Nursing Management of Acting-Out Behavior," *Perspectives in Psychiatric Care,* vol. 8, no. 4, pp. 168–173, 1970.

*15 Glee Gamble Lyon: "Limit Setting as a Therapeutic Tool," *Journal of Psychiatric Nursing and Mental Health Services,* vol. 8, no. 6, pp. 17–24, November-December 1970.

*Recommended reading by a nurse author.

20

The Client Who Generates Guilt and Rejecting Behavior

Lenora J. McClean

Learning Objectives

After studying this chapter, the student should be able to:

1 See in historical perspective the development of the theory of self-destructiveness

2 Discuss the dynamics of self-destructive behavior

3 Verbalize the interpersonal dynamics of a client-treater dyad

4 Review guidelines for introspection about personal responses to self-destructive clients

5 Outline a conceptual framework for the assessment of self-destructive clients

6 Define the therapeutic principles from which clinical intervention skills are derived

Let us begin from the point of view of someone who is feeling guilty and describe that feeling as a pervasive sense of being wrong or of having committed a wrong. It may be the awful awareness of having behaved despicably toward another person or of having transgressed one's own principles. The definition of guilt in personal experience is usually far more monstrous than the theoretical or psychodynamic definition. Yet the former definition is one that professionals who work with suicidal clients must learn and come to terms with as an aspect of human experience.

The personal identification and involvement with clients is never more dramatic and important than it is with those who are suicidal. Perhaps the main reason for this is that there is no clear-cut profile of a suicidal person. It is the work of this chapter to gain a better understanding of people who are self-destructive and the people who attempt to help them.

A National Health Problem

Of those who are known to have attempted suicide in the United States in 1974, 12 percent succeeded. Mortality rates have been surprisingly consistent during this century in spite of wars, slowly changing attitudes about suicide, and the rapid growth, in the last two decades, of suicide prevention centers. Among those who commit suicide, about three times as many men die as women; although women more often attempt to kill themselves, they typically choose less effective means. Rates are higher among certain sectors of the population: black youths and males, alcoholics, and American Indians. Rates also vary by age group. Adolescent suicide has increased in the past 20 years along with the rate among people over 50 years of age. With the more recent awareness of the relationship between lethal accidents and self-destructive feelings experienced by children, statistics in the future may also reveal a surprising number of suicides among the very young.

Shneidman emphasizes that the extent of the human problem of suicide is far greater than a count of actual deaths would indicate.[1] Statistics reflect incomplete reporting of suicides. High-risk behavior—for example, that involving alcoholism and accidents—is also an indicator of destructive behavior. Those who are family members and loved ones of the person who commits suicide are also considered victims of the suicide. Multiply the 22,000 actual suicide deaths in 1973 by as few as three family members or close friends, and you have 66,000 people who suffer unusual and terrible grief and whose lives are forever influenced by their loss.

Origins of Suicide

Suicide is a perplexing problem in a culture which teaches the value of life and abhors death. Regardless of one's philosophy and value system, it may be difficult to understand and accept suicidal behavior in either a historical, sociological, or psychodynamic context.

Three major theories on the origins of suicide will be briefly mentioned by way of historical perspective; however, none is offered as more correct than another. No one explanation has yet provided answers to the myriad of questions about people who kill themselves.

The Genetic Theory

During the first decade of this century, George Mudge was fascinated by the frequent occurrence of suicide in some families and sought to explain these events on the basis of genetic transmission via a mendelian ratio.[2]

In 1935, Louis Shapiro avoided advocating a hereditary theory but studied certain family tendencies that seemed to lead to suicide.[3]

The Sociological Theory

Émile Durkheim disposed of the genetic theory as a cause of suicide by observing that if heredity determined the suicide rate, then males and females would kill themselves with equal frequency.[4] Durkheim's interest focused on the characteristics of an individual's integration with social forces. Conceptualizing society as a dynamic integration of forces larger than the sum of individuals in the population, he hypothesized that suicide varies immensely with the degree of integration of religious, domestic, and political society.[4] In his theory, suicide takes one of four forms: (1) egoistic suicide, which is brought about by separateness, "excessive individualization," or lack of relatedness to others in society; (2) altruistic suicide, the reverse of the egoistic, which may occur when the individual's identity is insufficiently developed apart from the social group; (3) anomic suicide, which is brought about by abrupt changes in social norms, even though these may be time-limited (Durkheim defined *anomie* as "normlessness" or "deregulation"[4]); (4) fatalistic suicide, which is the reverse of the anomic type and is brought about by the imposition of excessive demands or structures on an individual by external forces.

Psychodynamics of Suicidal Behavior

A new era of progress in understanding self-destructive behavior began in the early 1950s with unprecedented empirical study as well as theory development. Research and simple logic have demonstrated that suicide is caused by many different combinations of factors. However, suicidal people have certain characteristics in common regardless of the factors which brought them to that state.

Ambivalence

One of the most common features of suicidal people is that they are ambivalent.[5] Within them there is a struggle between self-preserving forces and self-destructive forces. Ambivalence is apparent when people threaten or attempt suicide and then try to get help to be saved. When the possible outcomes of suicide are discussed with clients, it is remarkable how often the client talks of life-related outcomes such as relief from an unhappy situation or revenge. Although many people ponder suicide as an alternative to the way they are living, they may not consider the outcome of not living. For example, it is incongruous for a woman to do her laundry in the morning and then to attempt suicide. If she will be dead by evening, what difference does it make if some of her clothes are not clean? It *would* make a difference if she survived to feel more like wearing the clothes or if she died but somehow remained vulnerable to embarrassment from comments about the dirty laundry she left behind. The frequency with which this kind of incongruity is evident in the behavior of suicidal persons makes it impossible to assume that suicide is necessarily consciously equated with death in a person's mind. But whether or not an attempted suicide leads to a death is unlikely to rest upon the client's unconscious expectations.

Helplessness and Hopelessness

When attempts to cope with problems fail, not only do the problems remain or worsen as stressors but the client is left without the coping mechanisms that previously helped to protect and enhance the image of self as a capable being. Diminished self-esteem leaves one less able to develop new coping mechanisms, and the snowball effect eventually brings the client to feel not only that he or she is helpless to change things but also that there is no hope of change or relief.

Helplessness and hopelessness are frequently related to the torturous feelings of worthlessness and guilt in depression. (See Chap. 18.) It is difficult to tell which of these feelings develops first, but in combination they pose difficult problems in intervention. When clients feel that they have no right to feel better, it is difficult to help them develop new interpersonal behaviors that may relieve some of the stress.

Guilt

Clients frequently claim responsibility for vast difficulties and misfortunes, far beyond the capacity of one person to generate, in addition to the guilt they feel for their personal dilemmas. The client's guilt may be seen as a subjective explanation for his or her sorrow or melancholy.

Aggression

While it is a widely held notion that suicidal people turn their aggression against themselves rather than other people, there is strong clinical evidence that outward-directed aggression is often characteristic also.[6] Newspaper accounts of combined homicide and suicide are not uncommon. Some callers to crisis centers either threaten to kill or express a fear of killing another person, saying: "I'm going to kill my children," or "I'm afraid I may kill my mother." Aggression is more subtle in the manipulative behavior of people who use threats of suicide to rule the lives of others. The following note was found by a man who was the youngest child and last to be married: "Charles, darling— Tomorrow you will marry the woman you love and my life is over. I have lived for my children and you are my last reason to go on.—Love, Mother."

It is doubtful whether the woman who wrote this note would have committed suicide, because she achieved her objective in stopping her son's wedding. Charles and his future wife postponed their wedding and sought counseling because they realized Charles's mother's motives. They wanted to work through their own feelings of responsibility toward her vis-a-vis their own relationship. They did not want their hopes for a marriage relationship sabotaged by their own guilt, regardless of what Charles's mother did. By the time Charles did marry, his sister had given birth to the first grandchild; the mother was happy about that and had a new reason to live. However, the note clearly communicates hostility and aggression toward others.

Suicide is clearly not a simple question of living or dying but has several identifiable components related not only to onself but also to other people: the wish to kill, stemming from aggression and rage; the wish to be killed, stemming from guilt and a feeling of worthlessness; and the wish to die, stemming from fear and helplessness.[7] People who are suicidal are focusing their vio-

lence on themselves. Overt murder is an option, but suicide accomplishes at least three objectives: it destroys that part of the self that is made up of the self's experience of another person; it destroys the self that is experienced as an identity; and it achieves death and release from intolerable stress. It is not unusual to see another person implicated or blamed in suicide notes. Such a note becomes a document of the rage the suicidal person felt toward another but expressed toward the self.[8]

The Appeal and Ordeal

Shneidman and Farberow have observed at least two types of suicidal behavior. The attempt to commit suicide can most often be seen as an appeal, a "cry for help."[9] It is a desperate way of saying "I no longer know of a way to live, therefore I shall die—unless someone can help me." Another type of attempt is more of an ordeal, or a test of ability to survive an extremely dangerous situation. A person whose attempt seems to have an appeal element may be terrified of dying and may be very responsive to therapeutic intervention in the suicidal crisis. People who have survived Russian-roulette-type risks sometimes feel a release of tension by having put themselves through the ordeal; they feel more able to live afterwards. For others, the survival of an ordeal may provide reaffirmation of a fantasy of immortality. Such a fantasy may be a defense against self-destructive feelings.

Levels of Consciousness and Suicidal Behavior

Myths about suicide have, over the years, perpetuated some interesting myths which appear to have served as good excuses for avoiding involvement with suicidal people. These run as follows: "Once someone has decided to commit suicide, there is nothing anyone can do to stop it," or "If someone is really despondent, you should not mention suicide or that will give them the idea," or "People who talk about killing themselves will never do it." Such statements are untrue, but myths frequently suggest an element of truth and embellish it with fancy. When people are extremely depressed and decide on some level of consciousness to die, there is often an apparent improvement in their condition because a conflict has been resolved. A decision has been made to die, and therefore the client has nothing at stake. The apparent improvement may mean that a client who has been indecisive about everything makes decisions and may gain new stature in a group. The client may sleep better, eat better, work better, and generally venture into activity and relationships that were previously threatening or even immobilizing. For many reasons, it is difficult to prevent such people from committing suicide. First, it is difficult to know how and when such decisions are reached if they are made subconsciously. Second, professionals whose own egos have taken a beating in working with chronically depressed people may allow themselves to stop looking for clues in the belief that an improvement in a client's condition has lessened the danger of suicide.

Another approach to understanding suicidal decision making is Shneidman's concept of intention.[10] Shneidman believes there are levels of *intentionality* which are related to levels of consciousness. Suicide is intentioned when an individual takes a direct, conscious part in the self-destructive behavior, such as taking his or her life by hanging. Suicide is subintentioned where an individual plays an important indirect role in bringing about death. Subintentioned behavior shows evidence of bringing about both conscious and unconscious wishes. For example, high-speed driving on dangerous roads may result in a fatal accident which may be the equivalent of suicide.

Further evidence that self-destructiveness may be present in unconscious life, without an individual's awareness of it, is demonstrated by the different ways in which people experience self-destructiveness. It is most common for clients to relate that they have been thinking about suicide off and on for some time, but that lately, due to stressful circumstances which they have tried but failed to cope with, they can think of nothing else but misery and suicide. They are *perseverating*.

Other clients, however, terrified at what they have done, may seek help immediately after a suicide attempt. These clients may liken their suicidal experiences to being hit by a bolt of lightning in the form of a sudden, uncontrollable impulse to destroy themselves. They are frightened because they have lost control of their own behavior, because they might have killed themselves, because of the sudden and continuing awareness that they became suicidal and that if it happened again they might not survive. Clients who experience self-destructiveness in this fashion desperately need information about what is happening to them and help in coping with that experience in the likely event that it will happen again. The nurse may explain it to the client as a partial breakdown in the personality's defense system—not an indication of doom but rather a positive event that brought some dangerous feelings into consciousness—feelings with which the client may now deal.

The Suicidal Crisis

Nurses typically meet suicidal clients after a crisis has been precipitated and an attempt has perhaps been made. However, the client may still be in crisis, which Gerald Caplan maintains may last from 1 to 6 weeks. Crisis is not a pathophysiologic concept but a phenomenon which occurs in most people who experience three sets of interrelated factors which can produce a state of crisis: (1) a disastrous event, such as the loss of a loved one; (2) threatened loss of a basic gratification, as when loneliness, for example, seems to signify a loss of human relationship; (3) failure to cope with the stress of the first two,[11] and in addition (4) perceived absence of situational support from significant others.

The onset of the crisis is characterized by increased tension. The client attempts to deal with it by using every kind of coping strategy in the repertoire of personality. All efforts prove futile, and the *impact phase* of the crisis begins. Disorganization, confusion, frantic activity, and increased anxiety are present. Clients are cognitively impaired. They cannot speak accurately or confidently about the causes of the crisis or identify the real problem. This phase may allow for a catharsis of feelings which the client has not been able to express before.

As a response to the discomfort of extreme anxiety and stress, the client passes into the *recoil stage*. The client literally pulls away from the pain of open confrontation. Coping mechanisms are mobilized as the anxiety diminishes, and logical thinking is restored. The chaotic state of his or her life is still difficult for the client to understand. The *reorganization stage* begins as the client starts to organize the chaos and develop alternative ways of coping in similar situations.[11]

The Nurse's Response to a Suicidal Client

Nurses who work with the suicidal must recognize their negative as well as their positive responses. The nurse's feelings are important in any relationship, but here they can also serve as a good barometer of what is going on in an interaction. Further, it behooves the nurse to engage in an ongoing examination of relationships with clients to identify covert, tacit agreements which may develop in the course of treatment.

Mr. J, age 24, was admitted to the psychiatric inpatient unit of a general hospital after having attempted suicide by slashing his throat with a razor blade. Prior to his attempt, Mr. J had been embattled with his family over some personal decisions he had made, one of which was to live with a woman his parents disliked. Immediately prior to his attempt, family attorneys informed Mr. J that he had been disinherited and his name was being removed from all family documents. Mr. J stood to lose several million dollars and his identity as a member of that family.

Mrs. B, a registered nurse, admitted Mr. J after his wound had been repaired. As she learned fragments of his personal history, she became angry. Mrs. B told her client that he was a fool for attempting suicide; after all, a lot of people would love to have the problem of losing a million dollars. Beside, he had the better part of his life ahead of him.

The nurse in this situation rejected her client because his situation was so offensive to her. Mrs. B's husband was dead; she supported four children on her salary and had all the problems that go with being a single parent of four. Mrs. B felt that there was some basic injustice in the fact that she had to work so hard to cope with her responsibilities while this young man was trying to escape. To make matters worse, his problems would be the solution to her problems. Because of her own frustrations, Mrs. B evaluated Mr. J's problems and judged his behaviors in the context of her own life, not his.

Relationships with clients who are suicidal are extremely taxing to the mental and emotional resources of the nurse and other team members. Whenever possible it is desirable to limit the number of suicidal clients on any one caseload so that the professional person may be accessible to clients. Accessibility in a supportive relationship means that clients may need assistance in problem solving, decision making, or when anxiety is increasing. It is impossible to confine the needs of suicidal clients to a therapeutic hour or a particular hospital shift. It is difficult to explain to the client what "accessibility" means in practice: how much access and when is access a priority? The nurse and other team members must continually evaluate the client's current ability to cope with anxiety. They must establish guidelines by which each can respond consistently. Excessive "support" of a client may begin to substitute the nurse's problem-solving ability for the client's, making the client so dependent that she or he cannot solve problems or make simple decisions without the nurse. The dependency becomes so frustrating to the nurse who encourages it that the patient is eventually rejected because of it. Ideally, the client should have easy access to therapists as needed in the early phase of treatment; then accessibility should gradually be diminished as the client learns to manage stress more effectively.

In the course of treatment, many conflicts

between the nurse and the suicidal client are negotiated, and the client also learns to resolve problems alone. The most basic conflict between the nurse and client stems from the fact that the nurse defends life over death while the client takes the opposite position. In reality, neither the nurse nor the client can justify their positions and both could line up legions of people for theoretical debate. Both nurse and client have their own fantasies, as well as abstract rationales, and both are faced with certain indisputable facts about their respective roles. In their negotiations, all levels of logic and paralogic are in play, from the most primitive to the most sophisticated, and feelings of anger and guilt are intensely felt. The nonverbal, implicit transactions and feelings are as natural and predictable as the script of a well-known play. Telescoped in time, the script for alter egos would read approximately like this:

Client: By seeking help I am saying that life is too difficult to cope with. I need to be cared for or I will die.

Nurse: I see that you are helpless right now, but I understand that. I care about you as a human being. (Reaches out.) I can help you.

Client: Stop! You're so sure you can solve problems that I can't; that means I'm incompetent (pulls away) and worthless.

Nurse: (Keeps distance.) I see I've just confirmed your worst fear. But it is not true. My team members and I believe in better options for people who are suicidal.

Client: I can see you mean well. Perhaps I'll try to work with you.

Nurse: Shall we proceed?

Client: Not so fast! I have needs I don't trust you to meet. I'm conflicted about this. I really must die.

Nurse: I'll save you!

Client: What about the others? They don't care.

Nurse: Never mind the others . . . I feel omnipotent now; it's the Jehovah complex.

Client: My problem-solving is not improving. I feel worse and I need more resources.

Nurse: What do you mean "more resources"? I'll

try harder and you try. . . . Stop! How dare you attempt suicide again!

Client: This isn't working. You're not helping me. I need more help.

Nurse: You've disappointed me. You're supposed to get better—to want to live—after all I've done for you.

Client: You're treating me like an infant. How can I have any respect for myself?

Nurse: I see what I've done. Please forgive me! How could I have been so stupid? I'm guilty of everything a professional person should not do. I took responsibility for and control of your life.

Client: I'm afraid to go on living.

Nurse: You're disgusting, and you won't try to get better.

Client: You're right. I shouldn't go on living.

Nurse: I'm angry at you for making me feel incompetent and guilty. Maybe you're right. Maybe you shouldn't go on living.

Negative feelings are responses to conflicts, frustrations, and loss of self-esteem which occur in relationships with self-destructive people. The client presents the nurse with a dramatic challenge—that is, to help the client live out a natural life. However "professionally objective" the nurse may have the illusion of being, subjectivity and personal involvement are real and painful.

Members of helping professions tend to have rescue fantasies when working with suicidal people. When clients resist being rescued and act out to sabotage therapeutic efforts, the nurse is frustrated and becomes angry. After realizing the basis of this anger, the nurse is likely to feel incompetent and guilty for rejecting the client. Because the needs of suicidal clients are so great, it is important for nurses to maintain supportive relationships with professional colleagues. It is also important for the nurse to work closely with the health team in the care and treatment of clients. Team members are mutually supportive and they also assist in reality testing. Finally, a multidisciplinary approach provides the client with access to a greater number of helping resources.

The Nurse's Response to the Family of the Suicidal Client

Family members of the suicidal client may see themselves as victims, bystanders, or perpetrators. Richman has observed that the suicidal person may be acting out a family drama. He identified characteristic family dynamics that appeared when a member became suicidal, including scapegoating, family depression, intolerance for separation, and sadomasochistic relationships.[1,2] Not all families were characterized by the same set of features, but it was apparent that family members were deeply involved in the destructive phenomenon. In some complex way, a particular family member is either appointed, or self-chosen to act out the destructiveness or "bad self" of the family. During the crisis of the suicide attempt and the client's rescue, the family members who are available must also receive professional attention and assessment. Judgmental and hostile attitudes toward the family are pitfalls to be avoided. The family does not "cause" someone to become suicidal; rather, the relationship builds up in a mutually interactive way. In families where suicidal behavior has an established precedent as a way of dealing with aggression, the suicide attempt may be a first option rather than the last desperate effort it looks like to us.

The family of a suicidal person figures prominently in the treatment process. The professional initially collects data about family members from the client, whose perception may be either positive or negative. It is thus important to collect first-hand data from the whole family in order to have a complete, objective picture. It is sometimes tempting to align oneself with the client against a ruthless, punitive parent. If this happens, the client may become further alienated from the family support system. While some family members may be disturbed or otherwise quite destructive, an objective of treatment is to help clients claim some responsibility for what happens to them and take control of their own destiny. As clients feel better about themselves, they are sometimes astonished to realize that they have attributed far more destructive influence to another person than that person actually had. As clients act more on their own behalf, other people act less for them. This may not be acceptable to the family, causing disequilibrium in the system which must be worked through; otherwise another family member may emerge as the focus of bad family feelings.

Another kind of response is when the nurse identifies with and takes the role of one of the family members in the relationship with the client. The client is familiar with certain role relationships—whether they are punitive, supportive, or otherwise—and may test out complementary relationships with therapists. For example, nurses may be shocked to hear themselves using words and phrases that are not commonly used in their own communication but which are common to the father of the client. This may be a clue that the nurse is taking on role characteristics which have been in some way suggested by the client.

Assessment of the Suicidal Client

Intervention actually begins with the first contact between client and the helping person. Therefore, it is difficult to separate assessment and intervention. The commonly used conceptual framework in which therapeutic strategy is developed is primary, secondary, and tertiary prevention.[13]

Primary prevention involves the identification of health and adjustment needs or risk factors in groups of people. Intervention through health education or couseling strategies prevents the occurrence of self-destructive behavior.

The nurse assesses the community—the life context of an individual client who lives, works, and functions within a given ecological and demographic area. For example, population density is a factor which correlates with higher suicide rates. In urban neighborhoods, many people live close together but are emotionally distant; such people may not be resources to one another. Where poverty is pervasive, there will be people who have so few alternatives in coping with problems that suicide is a likely event. Conversely, there are the densely populated urban neighborhoods in the middle- to upper-income areas where people are alienated from each other by pressures of work and the demands for achievement in a vastly complex and competitive world. Again, suicide is a likely option for many such people.

The nurse can use strategies of primary prevention by assessing a given community to identify risk factors relating to health problems. Equally important is identifying the strengths and resources present in the area. This important information must be communicable to residents of the community. Social "consciousness raising" involves working with community people to identify the "how tos" of using resources (or obtaining more) to diminish the incidence of health problems and improve the quality of residents' lives.

Secondary prevention focuses more on identifying those who may be "at risk" in a given population and who show a degree of disorganization. Hypertension screening programs serve as excellent examples of follow-through of primary and secondary prevention. The public is constantly being informed by the mass media about risk factors related to hypertension. As health and special-interest groups relate these data to a given population, a special effort is organized to get as many people as possible out to have their blood pressure taken. Those who have elevated blood pressures are referred to physicians for diagnosis and treatment. Nurses and other health professionals need to rely on community residents as workers in health programs insofar as these people have time and talents to offer. In working with suicide as a health problem, volunteers from the community are trained in crisis counseling and constitute a significant portion of the staff of almost every crisis center and hot line in the United States.

Tertiary prevention addresses serious health and adjustment problems already in progress. Intervention in suicidal crisis is tertiary prevention, while work with the client's family members may be secondary prevention. When a suicide has been committed, the work that is done with the family and other survivors is primary prevention because survivors are at risk.

The immediate objective of assessment is to determine how likely the suicidal client is to die in the immediate future. At best, one can do no more than make an educated guess about the relative *lethality* of the client's self-destructive intent and the relative strength of his or her will to preserve life. It is an assessment of ambivalence.

In the initial contact with a suicidal client, the nurse must recognize that there is a clear order of business to be conducted and that it is helpful to get started as soon as possible. Suicidal clients are not people to be kept waiting, either for an appointment or in emergency rooms or clinics, regardless of a lack of physical evidence of impending disaster. Only a small fraction of people who are suicidal are able to verbalize their discomfort in such a way that others will know they are suicidal. Some people give clues by giving away some of their prized possessions, while others may visit their family doctors with vague somatic complaints. Many of the latter eventually kill themselves with an overdose of the sedative or tranquilizer prescribed by their physician.

The first step in intervention with suicidal clients is to establish a relationship in which the nurse assumes an authoritative role. The client does not want to ask a stranger, who is going to cringe at the word "suicide," for help. The nurse needs to be matter of fact *and* caring about what the client is relating. The relationship is helped along if the nurse communicates that the client's complaints are legitimate. Many people still believe that only physical complaints are worthy of attention in health-care facilities. Some clients may feel embarrassment at being unable to cope with their problems. A comment from the nurse, such as "I see you're really upset. You've done the right thing in coming for help," may serve to lessen the embarrassment a client may feel.

The client needs to know from the outset that the nurse will assist the client in seeking every possible resource for problems, but no promises should be made. False assurances are dangerous not only because they may promise the impossible but also because, since the client knows that there are no easy answers, this diminishes the credibility of the nurse. Most clients allow treating persons some communication errors, but adolescents are particularly sensitive to unrealistic or condescending communications.[14]

Many clients who have the ego strength to ask for help are still ambivalent about getting it. Crying, profuse profane language, arrogance, and silence are obstacles to effective communication. Clients who are arrogant and condescending are particularly anxiety-provoking. For example, Mrs. A called a suicide prevention center for help, and when a young man answered, she began badgering him with questions, including, "What are your credentials that you presume to hold this position?" and "My problems are very complex, I need to talk to your best psychiatrist immediately." Some clients are best seen by someone who more closely meets their needs for self-esteem, even though the nurse may be very capable. Knowing when to refer is important, and failure to refer a difficult client is sometimes an effort to overcome feelings of rejection and anger.

The nurse may see that an adversary relationship is developing when a client asks for help but maintains the right to die. In their zeal to rescue clients, nurses sometimes try to remove the option of suicide immediately. It is not possible and not wise on the nurse's part to deny the reality of the client's option. Maintaining this option may be one way for the client to control the situation. Suicide may be a last-straw act of desperation for some, but it is an act of courage and self-determination for others. In either case, assessment quickly moves beyond lethality to the problems which bring people to that point. Instead of saying, "Don't kill yourself," we say, "Wait—gives us some time to understand this and to see if some problems can be solved."

Risk Factors

Immediate risk factors which are related to *lethality*—or the likelihood that self-inflicted death will occur in the immediate future—are age, sex, the suicide plan, and the availability of means to carry out the plan.[15]

Mortality data indicate that adolescents be-tween the ages of 15 and 24 and people over 50 have higher suicide rates than other age groups. An adolescent, for example, is at higher risk than a 30-year-old in similar circumstances.

The *suicide plan* is an important criterion because it is an index of danger. It may also suggest something about the mental state of the client. Any plan that is straightforward, easy to carry out, and has a narrow or no margin for error is highly lethal. The difference between a plan to put a gun to one's head and pull the trigger and a plan to take pills is obvious. There is little margin for error with the gun, one gun being about as lethal as another. The margin for error with the pills can be expanded or contracted by the type of pill, the number of pills, and the possibility of reflex vomiting while the pills are being swallowed. In complex plans, the outcome may depend on a small detail. Bizarre plans may be evidence of psychosis. Conversely, many simple, highly lethal plans are dictated by hallucinated voices, as in the case of a young man who was rescued from the edge of a high roof. He had been instructed by an "angel of the Lord" to "rise up to meet God." Plans that are ceremonious may be the product of psychosis. Psychotic clients in general are a high-risk group because of their impulsivity and distorted thought processes. (See Chap. 14.) The plan may have a special significance or may have been decided upon because the alternative seems repulsive, as in the case of people who, because they can't stand the sight of blood, decide to take pills rather than cut their throats.

The availability of means is crucial to complete the simplest of plans. The person who has a gun but not bullets still has an important barrier standing between life and death. Another person who lives in New York and plans to commit suicide in Chicago has both time and space as intervening variables. These variables may not decrease the lethality of the actual plan, but they increase the possibility that the client will be rescued before the plan is carried out.

In the process of the first contact and immediate assessment, the nurse's goal is to diminish the lethality of the client's plan in any way that is necessary. It is not a situation for heroics but for cautious, deliberate action in calling on appropriate resources to protect the safety of the patient and others in his or her presence. Evidence of lethality and high intention indicates a need for continued observation in a safe setting.

Stress

Early in the assessment process, the nurse should let the client know that information is needed about what has happened. Clients in extreme anxiety states may be unable to identify precipitating factors. With such people it is helpful for the nurse to structure the interview by asking, "Why are you seeking help now?" or "What has happened in the last 24 hours (or week)?" Observing the client's age, the nurse may seek information about possible maturational crises such as separation from loved ones, particularly the death of a parent or spouse. Situational factors such as loss of job, change in social or economic status, marital difficulties, and so on should be explored. Loss of a loved one is a frequent cause of acute grief reactions in which people feel like taking their own lives.

Medical history is important; the client may have a chronic, painful illness from which he or she seeks relief by suicide. Detoxified alcoholics, who have lost their old defenses against anxiety, have to confront themselves without the help of new, healthier defenses.

Symptoms

Clients may display a variety of behaviors, but among the most common are depression, psychosis, and extreme irritability and agitation. Characteristics such as guilt and hopelessness, which were described earlier, are extremely common.

An important dimension of assessment is to determine how and how much the client's life-style and relationships have recently changed. Changes in activities of daily living—as in sleeping, eating, and working habits—may be indicative of severe personality disturbances. The severity of the symptoms usually has some relationship to the severity of the stress.[15]

Clients who tell of precipitating factors that sound like mild to moderate stresses but who yet show extreme symptoms may either be severely disturbed, be unable to focus on the serious problems, or be fearful of trouble with legal authorities.

Identification and Clarification of Problems—Nursing Diagnosis

One of the difficulties in talking about problems is that so many have to do with self-esteem, with outright violations of a person's "should" system. For example, many young people migrate to metropolitan areas each year to start their careers or to large colleges and universities to study. Starting a career sounds bland enough, but what sometimes happens is that John Doe gets a big sendoff from his family and friends to "make it big" in the city. After a few months of job hunting and rejections, John gets weary and depressed. A few more months pass and John has to face the reality that he is competing in a difficult job market and that menial jobs are the best he can hope for. A great deal of self-esteem depends on how the folks at home see him, and problems begin to mount as John's self-esteem diminishes and his self-image as a capable, competitive adventurer is shattered. He believes he should be able to get a good job; he should be sending money home; and he should be looking for a wife. The problems John relates to the nurse are (1) that he cannot get a job in his field and (2) the he hates living in the city. Exploration of what the "right" job would mean to him and the possibility that he may also be suffering from loneliness may help identify the most serious problem: John has broken off communication with family and friends because of his perceived failure.

On the basis of data gathered, the nurse proceeds to establish a list of problems, arranged in order of stressfulness. This list serves as a focal point for the nurse and client to consensually validate what they understand to be problems.

Communication problems, problems in relationships with significant others, and diminution of personal resources are frequently the common denominators of a long list of smaller problems. Some typical communication problems are (1) that people stop talking to each other about things and feelings that are important to them, (2) that people begin to assume that significant others automatically "know" what is going on inside them, and/or (3) that some people begin to interpret the attitudes of others as being hostile and rejecting because of their own feelings of worthlessness.

Once a problem list has been established, a therapeutic plan can be developed and essential resources can be mobilized.

Formulation of the Therapeutic Plan

Farberow characterizes suicidal crisis therapy by: (1) authority, (2) activity, and (3) involvement of others.[5] Rapaport, Hill, and others describe crisis therapy as ego work based on conscious reality (as opposed to probing of the unconscious and reconstructive work).[11] Undoubtedly both clients and therapists touch on unconscious feelings and develop insight in the process of the work, but these are side effects of the process.

Authoritativeness has already been described in the context of first-contact assessment. The helping person needs to communicate that he or she knows something about what the patient is experiencing. For this reason a young nurse's age can sometimes work against a relationship with a middle-aged client. The nurse must be sensitive to the difference between "authoritative" and "authoritarian." An authoritative person is one who is knowledgeable about a subject and can share that knowledge in a helping way in assisting clients to make better decisions based on new information and insights. An authoritarian person gives orders based on his or her knowledge, and the clients are expected to do as they are told if they hope to be helped. A helping person who appears knowledgeable and capable is reassuring, while a brassy know-it-all is an irritating menace.

Activity in intervention means that something is *done*. The client needs to know that the nurse will do whatever is possible and that the client will be expected to do something as well. The structuring of activity in time is an important supportive strategy. The time frame for crisis intervention may range from one contact of an hour or so to frequent contacts over a period of weeks. If the state of crisis lasts from 1 to 6 weeks, it is inappropriate to think of crisis intervention as extending beyond that. However, the client may begin short-term therapy in addition. The structuring of activity conveys the idea that certain outcomes are expected within an appropriate time period.

The activities are related to the problems on the problem list and are decided upon through problem solving with the client. The most pressing problem of John Doe, the young man who came to the city with great expectations, was his lack of communication with his family, who were important resources. The solution to his problem, however, was not a simple telephone call or letter. John had thought of that and, in fact, longed to talk with them, but the self-esteem issue was prohibiting contact. In problem solving with John, the nurse must help him expose his worst fears about making the call. For example, the nurse might ask John, "What is the worst you would expect to happen if you called home?" John may be afraid that the family will be ashamed of him in his failure, or he may be afraid that one of them has died since he last communicated with them 6 months ago. Any or all of his worst fears may come true or have already done so, but what is the likelihood of this? What has John's relationship been with his family? If it has been caring and mutually supportive, chances are they will be so happy to hear from him that they will consider his simply being alive and well to be wonderful news. Working through the worst fears to at least rational proportions is reality testing. Next, the nurse might ask John, "What is the best you would hope for if you called home?" John may want them to tell him they would like him to come home. Having established the worst-best outcomes, the nurse might now digress to worst again and explore with John how he would cope with any of the worst outcomes, using the nurse's support and any other resources. Then it would be logical to proceed to John's response to the best possible outcome. If he is given an invitation to return home, John must be helped to perceive this not as a pleasant escape but as an opportunity to make a decision. Should the family welcome John back home, this may be enough to relieve him of feeling trapped in the city. Being relieved of that stress and having reestablished communications with his family, he may decide to stay.

At the end of the initial contact with John Doe, our hypothetical client, plans must be made and goals established. The client should be informed that the services of the facility will be available to him for a definite, limited time. During that time the goals will be to (1) diminish his anxiety, (2) increase his ability to cope with his stresses, and (3) make changes in his life that will diminish the stresses. This particular client might be given 24 hours in which to make the conflict-provoking phone call to his family. Immediately after the phone call, he will call the therapist to discuss the outcomes and his feelings about them. This activity is within the capability of the client and is his responsibility. In the meantime the nurse may contact appropriate resources related to employment counseling and socialization. That activity is within the capability of the nurse and can be the nurse's share of responsibility in helping the client. Further sessions throughout the agreed-upon time period will keep the problems in focus in a deliberate effort to do something about them. Toward the end of the period of intervention, the client will be helped to focus on evaluating the events and activities and their significance for future experience. If further resources or treatment are necessary, the client will be referred appropriately. To summarize the intervention process, the nurse will initiate or participate in:

1 Assessment
  a Suicidal risk
  b Stress
  c Symptoms
2 Identification and clarification of problems
3 Formulation of the therapeutic plan
4 Follow-up

Hospitalization of Clients

At some point in the intervention process, it may be necessary for the client to be hospitalized. This decision is usually reached by a professional who determines that the client cannot control his or her destructive impulses without assistance. The suicidal client's safety is the primary reason for hospitalization, yet this rationale may be a source of conflict for nurses who participate in the client's care and treatment.

Typically, when a suicidal client is admitted to the hospital, his chart, or clinical record, is clearly labeled "suicide precautions"; included in the treatment orders are some that are designed to assure physical safety, such as these:

1 Search personal effects for toxic agents (such as drugs or alcohol).
2 Remove sharp instruments (razor blades, knives, letter openers, glass bottles which could be broken, etc.).
3 Remove straps from clothing (belts, neckties, stockings or pantyhose, etc.).
4 Place on one-to-one observation.

Such measures are intended to reduce obvious opportunities for clients to commit suicide. These physical safety precautions, however, have negative implications for nurse-patient relationships. The nurse sees a client admitted who is disconsolate—feeling worthless, hopeless, and guilty. The search of personal effects is an invasion of privacy such as would rarely be perpetrated on a client with a gallbladder problem. The removal of "sharps and straps" carries the message that the client cannot be trusted not to use them destructively. One-to-one observation may communicate that the client is being kept prisoner. The nurse may see the cumulative effects of hospitalization as the humiliation and depersonalization of someone who already has such diminished self-esteem that self-destruction is an imminent possiblity.

Although the criticism of safety precautions as potentially depersonalizing and offensive is realistic, the rationale for their implementation is based on the following:

1 The client would not need to be in the hospital if no danger were apparent.
2 The hospital accepts a legal obligation to provide protection for a client diagnosed as a suicide risk.
3 The nurse has a legal and professional responsibility to provide care which is life- and health-directed.

Until better strategies of protection and intervention are developed, these primitive measures are required. However, the manner in which they are implemented can do much to lessen their negative impact. The client deserves an explanation of why personal articles are searched and removed and should be told when, in relation to the client's progress, they will probably be returned.

Once the client is established on a service unit, the client's identity as a person, rather than a suicide risk, should be emphasized in introductions to others.

The client's self-destructive behavior should be treated as matter-of-factly as other clients' symptoms or problems. Even the marginally oriented psychiatric client knows that one-to-one observation means suicide precautions. No attempt should be made to keep the matter confidential; otherwise the client's interaction with other clients will be inhibited and isolation will become a barrier to intervention.

In-Hospital Suicide

Not all suicidal clients send messages, either overt or covert. Nurses should help clients talk about their feelings when suicidal thoughts arise. Some suicidal clients kill themselves in the hospital regardless of preventive measures. Other clients may appear to progress rapidly out of a high-risk suicidal condition and seek discharge or temporary leave from the hospital, and it is then that they kill themselves. After a client's suicide, either in the hospital or after discharge, other clients and staff have an intense reaction which includes anger, guilt, helplessness, and hopelessness. Clients on the unit may also demonstrate self-destructive behavior or even carry out their own suicides. Staff tend to go through a process of grief in addition to experiencing feelings of failure, guilt, and helplessness. It is usually helpful to assemble staff and patients together to share feelings of loss and to assist in their expression. Such feelings may include the clients' anger and fear for their own safety. As in the case of family members, surviving clients may identify with the person who committed suicide and be afraid that they will succumb to their own self-destructive feelings. The professional has the responsibilities of being supportive to and protective toward clients as well as working through his or her own feelings. The knowledge that the professionals were unable to prevent a suicide makes clients feel afraid that staff will be unable to prevent them from doing the same thing.

Evaluation
Intervention after Suicide

Grief following the loss of a loved one by natural death is a time-limited healing process of an emotional wound. Grief following the loss of a loved one by suicide is a self-perpetuating agony of loss from death, rejection, and disillusionment.[16]

Society provides rituals and conventional amenities through which bereaved families can receive support from friends who share their loss—provided the deceased died of natural causes. If the death was self-inflicted, the friends sometimes blame the family and are puzzled and perplexed as to what to do for the family; frequently they do nothing. The resulting isolation of the family confirms their sense of guilt. Families tend to respond to the loss by suicide as a rejection due to lack of trust, love, or even because of hatred. The family sinks into a morass of self-recrimination and guilt for having been inadequate or blind to the needs of the deceased. A family scapegoat may be identified as the destructive force which "caused" the suicide.

Children are particularly vulnerable to the death of a parent by suicide. Dorpat identified the following prominent psychopathological findings relating to parental suicide in a group of seventeen patients: (1) guilt feelings for having "caused" the parent's death, (2) depression, (3) preoccupation with suicide, (4) self-destructive behavior, (5) absence of grief, (6) arrests of some aspects of personality development.[17] Apparently suicidal behavior can be a learned pattern for coping with overwhelming stress; this may explain its frequency across generations and families.

The developmental arrest in surviving children's personalities is sometimes related to the families' tendency to try to keep from the child the facts of the parent's death. This is generally done by developing a mythical explanation which is supposedly less traumatic.[18] The child, however, frequently knows the truth anyway or is told by someone but is not permitted to deal with the fact of suicide because apparently the family is too fragile to allow this.

Because suicide is such an overwhelming trauma to loved ones, their tendency is to relive over and over the events surrounding the suicide. Occasionally, another family member will commit suicide later, near the date of the previous suicide; thus the term "anniversary suicide" has arisen. Some family members live for years expecting to die by suicide.

Many families will not permit the intrusion of a helping person following a suicide, but those who do allow this have a greater opportunity to grieve and to lessen the long-term effects of the loss. Very little clinical expertise has been developed for such intervention strategies, but experience has taught those who have tried to help *never* to attempt this alone. The family members are bombarding each other with hostile, destructive stimuli, and a stranger is an easy target.

Clients who Reject Treatment

Health professionals spend a great deal of time and use many resources in learning how to maintain health, intervene in illness, and support rehabilitation in terms of clients' needs. Clients, on the other hand, are expected to submit to the directions of a confusing variety of health-care providers in order to get their health needs met. Some people are comfortable with submission as the condition of their relationship to the "superior" knowledge of the physician or nurse about their health. Other people perceive themselves as consumers in that they seek out and pay for services from someone trained in one of the health professions. These people tend to negotiate egalitarian relationships with the providers of care and expect to participate in their own treatment as well as to evaluate it. When the provider is not approved of, or the treatment is not understandable or affordable—or when it is perceived as inappropriate—clients literally take their business elsewhere.

Another population of clients may recognize a health problem, seek assistance from a physician or a nurse, and then fail to carry out a plan of intervention which would be ameliorative, curative, or rehabilitative. No amount of follow-up, explanations, threats, coercion, support, or anything else will convince these clients that intervention is needed.

What does it mean when a diabetic does not take insulin and control his or her diet? Or when a woman with a breast lesion refuses surgery? Or when a patient with severe heart trouble goes on smoking? Or when a suicidal person refuses to be counseled? Such refusal of treatment strongly suggests self-destructiveness. Yet such clients may, by denying the possibility of their death and by continuing as if nothing were wrong, fantasize that their ailment will go away. Some clients may fear invalidism or disfigurement more than death and reject treatment on that basis. Still others may be afraid that changes in relationships with others might result from either the illness or its treatment. A few people may fear losing control of themselves or their fate and express the "I'll live as I please and die as I please" philosophy.

Nurses who come to know clients who reject treatment may experience frustration and anger at their lack of cooperation. These nurses may feel guilty for not having taken the "right approach" to convince their clients, or they may feel rejected if a client does not respond to their mutual "humanistic concern."

When clients do not improve and respond to the therapeutic plan within a given time, they are often transferred to other facilities such as the regional state hospital. These facilities frequently carry a connotation of hopelessness. Staff respond to the departure of these clients with feelings of guilt and failure. They may also avoid and reject the client once a decision to transfer has been made. The client is living proof of their inability to "cure." This is a threat to the self-image of mental health professionals.

Some clients will seek help but then become threatened or frightened by their self-exposure and refuse to follow through. For example, one man contacted a therapist and asked for help with some severe neurotic problems. On his second contact with the therapist he announced that he would terminate the relationship. However, the therapist set up another appointment and let the man decide whether to keep it or not. The client did keep the appointment and each additional one set up during 3 weeks, although he was angry and uncooperative. In the fourth week he contacted the therapist in a state of intoxication. His story revealed that he was trying to ask for help for alcoholism but could not deal with the loss of self-esteem involved in admitting this to anyone. Although he appeared to be rejecting the efforts of the therapist to conduct reasonable history gathering and interviews, he did not reject the contact. Thus the client's ambivalence eventually worked in his behalf.

When clients will permit nurses to discuss their refusal of treatment, it may be helpful for the nurse to explore the client's reasons without making judgments about them in any way. The client may be more willing to discuss his or her reasoning if the nurse asks to be helped to understand the decision. As long as the discussion stays open, there is a greater possibility that the client will eventually decide to accept treatment. Finally, the nurse needs to assure the client that people will be available to help should he or she make a different decision. If the nurse can manage feelings of anger, guilt, and rejection so that the client is not discarded as a hopeless case, some clients will eventually change their minds, although many do not.

References

1 Edwin Shneidman: in Albert C. Cain (ed.), *Survivors of Suicide,* Charles C Thomas, Springfield, Ill., 1972.

2 George P. Mudge: "The Mendelian Collection of Human Pedigrees," in Albert C. Cain (ed.), *Survivors of Suicide,* Charles C Thomas, Springfield, Ill., 1972.

3 Louis Shapiro: "Suicide: Psychology and Family Tendency," in Albert C. Cain (ed.), *Survivors of Suicide,* Charles C Thomas, Springfield, Ill., 1972.

4 Ronald Maris: *Social Forces and Urban Suicide,* Davey Press, Homewood, Ill., 1969.

5 Norman L. Farberow: "Crisis, Disaster, and Suicide: Theory and Therapy," in Edwin S. Shneidman (ed.), *Essays in Self-Destruction,* Science House, New York, 1967.

6 David Lester: *Why People Kill Themselves,* Charles C Thomas, Springfield, Ill., 1972.

7 Karl Menninger: *Man Against Himself,* Harcourt, Brace, New York, 1938.

8 Kresten Bjerg: "The Suicidal Life Space: Attempts at a Reconstruction from Suicide Notes," in Edwin S. Shneidman (ed.), *Essays in Self-Destruction,* Science House, New York, 1967.

9 Norman L. Farberow and Edwin Shneidman: *Cry for Help,* McGraw-Hill, New York, 1961.

10 Edwin Shneidman: "Sleep and Self-Destruction: A Phenomenological Approach," in Edwin S. Shneidman (ed.), *Essays in Self-Destruction,* Science House, New York, 1967.

11 Lydia Rappoport: "The State of Crisis: Some Theoretical Considerations," in Howard J. Parad (ed.), *Crisis Intervention: Selected Readings,* Family Service Association of America, New York, 1965.

12 Joseph Richman: "Family Determinants of Suicide Potential," in Dorothy B. Anderson and Leonora J. McLean (eds.), *Identifying Suicide Potential,* Behavioral Publications, New York, 1971.

*13 Florence Williams: "Intervention in Maturational

*Recommended reference by a nurse author.

Crises," *Perspectives in Psychiatric Care,* vol. 9, no. 6, 1971.

14 Jerome Motto: "Treatment and Management of Suicidal Adolescents," *Psychiatric Opinion,* vol. 12, no. 6, July 1975.

15 Norman L. Farberow, Samuel M. Heilig, and Robert Litman: *Techniques in Crisis Intervention: A Training Manual,* Suicide Prevention, Inc., Los Angeles, 1968.

16 Erich Lindeman and Ina May Greer: "A Study of Grief: Emotional Responses to Suicide," in Albert C. Cain (ed.), *Survivors of Suicide,* Charles C Thomas, Springfield, Ill., 1972.

17 T. L. Dorpat: "Psychological Effects of Parental Suicide on Surviving Children," in Albert C. Cain (ed.), *Survivors of Suicide,* Charles C Thomas, Springfield, Ill., 1972.

18 Max Warren: "Some Psychological Sequelae of Parental Suicide in Surviving Children," in Albert C. Cain (ed.), *Survivors of Suicide,* Charles C Thomas, Springfield, Ill., 1972.

Chapter

21

The Client Who Arouses Feelings about Sexual Identity

Anita M. Leach

Learning Objectives

After studying this chapter, the student should be able to:

1 Identify the causes of sexual dysfunction
2 Describe the ways in which pelvic surgery may affect sexual functioning
3 List the sexual concerns of clients who have had ostomy surgery
4 Name and describe the emotional impact of surgical procedures which cause sterility
5 Understand the effects of vascular disease and spinal cord injury on sexual functioning
6 Be aware of the nurses' response to clients with anxieties about sexual functioning
7 List self-assessment items for the nurse and for dealing with clients whose sexuality is threatened
8 Apply the nursing process to clients who experience disruption in their sexual functioning

The sexual functioning of clients is altered when they experience vascular disease, psychogenic stress, physical illness, and diseases affecting the nervous system. Sexual dysfunction is not limited to these categories but rather is experienced at one time or another by clients across the age span. Sexual dysfunction includes impotence as well as premature and retarded ejaculation in the male and frigidity, orgasmic dysfunction, and vaginismus in the female (see Chap. 12).

Sexual identity is part of the total self and is used therapeutically each time nurses lay on hands or counsel clients concerned with their sexual functioning. Nurses encounter clients who have different sexual values than their own as well as those whose sexual functioning has been limited or changed by illness. Education must deal not only with physical and emotional aspects of illness but with psychosexual development as well. Scientific data dealing with human sexual response and the effects of illness on sexuality need to be studied by all nurses if they are to acquire an open and healthy attitude toward their own sexuality and the sexuality of clients.

Diseases affect sexual functioning because they injure or impair sex organs, the nervous system, or the vascular system. Clients may also respond with diminished sexual activity for psychogenic reasons. They avoid fulfillment of sexual needs as they adjust to body-image changes (see Chap. 23), experience grief and mourning (see Chaps. 23 and 28), or simply respond to the impact of hospitalization and change in functional patterns (see Chap. 24).

Psychophysiological Sexual Dysfunction

Fatigue, stress, depression, and tension states are often the cause of sexual dysfunction. When clients are experiencing an emotional crisis or are depressed, sexual functioning assumes lesser importance in the hierarchy of needs.

Why stressful emotional states impair sexuality is not clearly understood. Some believe that the causes are purely psychogenic, while others hold that, in times of stress, energies are concentrated on resolving the crisis, thus making it difficult to concentrate on anything else. It is also possible that the physiologic and endocrine changes which accompany severe depression, stress, and fatigue may affect the central nervous system. A psychosomatic concept involving androgen is supported by recent findings. This theory states that in men, testosterone levels fluctuate in direct relation to chronic stress. Testosterone levels have also been shown to fall when men assume submissive roles.[1] Decrease in blood testosterone levels can precipitate a slowing of sex centers in the brain, causing lowered libido and a diminished sexual response. Stress may also adversely affect sexuality because of increased cortisone levels. In turn, the male's sexual interest decreases in response to the antiandrogen effects of the cortical steroids.[1] Serotonin is known to depress sexual activity and epinephrine to increase it. These substances are directly affected by emotional states (see Chap. 26).

Physical Illness and Sexual Dysfunction

Many organic conditions have general and nonspecific effects on sexual behavior. Common sense implies that clients who feel ill or are in pain will not usually be interested in pursuing sexual pleasure. For example, loss of libido occurs early in the course of a disease such as hepatitis. Likewise, diabetes often affects the male's ability to have an erection before there are other signs of the disease. Neuropathology, vascular damage, and the general debility and depression accompanying diabetes decrease libido and impair sexual response, particularly in the advanced stages of the disease. Problems of impotence and premature ejaculation are often the presenting symptoms in multiple sclerosis. Mutilative and lifesaving surgery also results in sexual dysfunction.[1]

Surgery and Sexual Dysfunction

Altered Body Image

Surgery as a lifesaving measure or as treatment for disease can temporarily or permanently alter a client's physical state and directly or indirectly affect sexual functioning. Clients who undergo a *mastectomy* (removal of a breast) have an *ostomy* (opening of bowel or bladder onto the abdomen) to treat carcinoma or ulcerative colitis will need to adjust to an *altered body image* before sexual activity can again take place.

Castration—either *oophorectomy* (removal of the ovaries in the female) or *orchidectomy* (removal of the testes in the male)—*prostatectomy, vasectomy, tubal ligation,* and *hysterectomy* (removal of the uterus in the female) affect the reproductive function of the sexual act by causing *sterility*. Surgery directly involving the genitalia and *pelvic exenteration* (removal of all pelvic organs) require the clients to adjust to physically altered excretory and sexual functioning, changed body image, and often sterility.[2]

Ostomy Surgery

Following an ileostomy, colostomy, or urostomy, 30 percent of males lose the *physical* capacity for erection, ejaculation, and orgasm. Most women can continue full sexual functioning. An ostomy performed as treatment for ulcerative colitis as opposed to carcinoma will have much less effect on the physiological ability of clients to function sexually.[3,4]

Sterility may result because of failure to ejaculate, although ostomy clients do reach orgasm. In a client with diagnosed carcinoma, the pelvic autonomic nerves are sometimes of necessity affected by surgery. The nervi erigentes from the sacral parasympathetic nerves conduct the impulses causing erection, and the hypogastric plexus conducts the impulses for ejaculation. Once these nerves are interrupted, there is little that can be done to restore physical sexual function in the male. In the female there is less likelihood that sexual functioning will be diminished, although the ability to have a vaginal or clitoral orgasm may be limited.

Five major emotional concerns of clients contribute to sexual dysfunction following ostomy surgery:

- Concern about body image and self-esteem
- Concern that an appliance or ostomy will interfere with coitus
- Concern about conception, pregnancy, and childbirth
- Concern about the perineal wound and scarring in women
- Concern about impotence and failure to ejaculate in men

Body image and self-esteem improve for some clients. The previously passive, conforming, and dependent behavior patterns of ulcerative colitis victims often change. These clients become less sensitive to rejection and more aggressive. Most ulcerative colitis victims who have surgery are between the ages of 20 and 30. Only 7 percent of these male clients experience impotence. The majority readily reestablish their sexual activity patterns and, after a period of adjustment, are known to enjoy sex more because of decreased concern over bowel function.

Those who have had the surgery because of chronic and medically incurable ulcerative colitis will sometimes feel a *sense of relief* after surgery. One man, expressing this relief, said, "At last I will be able to lead a normal life. I can go to business, socialize, and enjoy my sex life without having to worry about running to the bathroom."

On the other hand, feelings of revulsion, worthlessness, and altered body image may occur. Clients may see themselves as repulsive and unattractive. Still others fear their partners' reaction to their appliance. They experience frustration and impatience as they learn to cope with what they may perceive as a negative body image. They may be reluctant to resume sexual activity because of fears that their appliance will leak. Many express themselves by saying, "I'm finished," or "I'm half a person . . ." Once an ostomy is regulated and postoperative wound healing has occurred, clients should be encouraged to return to former sexual activity patterns. The client's spouse, when supportive, is the single most important factor in assisting the client to recover self-esteem and adjust to altered body image. A neat bandage can be placed over the stoma during coitus. When an appliance must be worn, it can be taped securely in place and out of the way of the genitals. Fear of impotency contributes to sexual dysfunctions. This fear is often linked to the man's self-esteem. Clients must be reassured that when potency returns, it does so within a year of the date of surgery.[5]

Women will often express concerns about conception, pregnancy, and childbirth. A male with an ostomy can father a child and a woman with an ostomy—once wound healing has occurred—can conceive and bear a child. However, when such surgery is elective and can be delayed, it is the practice to try to have a family prior to surgery. This is particularly true for the male, since there is a slight risk of failure to ejaculate after surgery.

Perineal wounds heal slowly, but scarring is generally minimal after ostomy surgery. Coitus should not take place until wound healing has occurred. Clients will need reassurance about their altered body image and will need to be encouraged to accept the fact that beauty and self-esteem are not skin deep.

Clients who have had ostomy surgery for carcinoma often experience problematic feelings that are not directly related to the surgery. Fears of death are expressed by many. It is people in this group who have difficulty accepting their ostomies, often choosing to think of them as temporary (denial). Displaced anger and depression are other feelings experienced by these clients. When the surgery is perceived by clients and their spouses as life-threatening, decreased communication may occur, with subsequent mutual withdrawal. The client is usually fearful of expressing

sexual concerns, feeling something like, "If I am dying, should I be sexual?" Clients and their spouses may be afraid of expressing sexual feelings, thinking them unimportant in the face of an apparent threat to life itself.

Clients who have had an ostomy for carcinoma are usually labeled "good" clients, undemanding, easy to please, and self-sacrificing. Their expressed concerns are not for themselves but for their families. This behavior is a subtle manifestation of their denial of the disease. The nurse should be prepared to confront these feelings in clients, serving as a guide as they cope with acceptance of their changed body image.

Mastectomy

Mastectomy—removal of a breast for a benign or malignant growth process—is a surgical procedure which affects the sexual identity of women. Although the breast is an organ of sexual arousal, the client who has a mastectomy can continue to live a full and rich sexual life. There is no interference with the physical ability to have intercourse and experience orgasm. However, because the female breast is laden with cultural and social significance and is intimately associated with female body image, psychological stress consequent to mastectomy will often precipitate a sexual identity crisis.

Fear and anxiety about the outcome of surgery are common emotions of the woman facing breast surgery. Grief and a period of mourning due to loss of a body part is a normal postoperative reaction. Clients experience an altered body image which can directly affect self-esteem. They may feel ugly, unattractive, and unable to accept the scarring that results from surgery. Fears concerning acceptance of scarring by the spouse are often present.

Most women do not confront the scarring and body-image issue until after the dressings are completely removed and they have returned to their homes. Often their spouses, who have not seen the wound, are concerned and shocked at first. Women sometimes interpret this reaction as rejection and withdraw from further contact. The support of the client's spouse, friends, and health professionals in the pre- and postoperative period will determine the woman's future sense of femininity and self-esteem. The outcome is directly dependent on the client's feelings of security and sense of self prior to the surgery.

Sterility

Many surgical procedures—both elective and those performed because of diseased organs—cause sterility. However, physical sexual function continues. The pleasure derived is often directly dependent on clients' acceptance and understanding of the surgery and their ability to look honestly at their feelings and those of their spouses.

Castration

Bilateral oophorectomy will result in a woman's inability to become pregnant. Surgical menopause results, and sometimes there are changes in vaginal secretions. Sexual activity, including the ability to reach orgasm, is not physically affected. The scarring caused by the surgery or a sense of loss of femininity may result in a change of body image, with subsequent psychogenic inability to reach orgasm.

Bilateral orchidectomy will result in an inability to ejaculate and, therefore, will render the client sterile. However, erection and orgasm remain possible. If the orchidectomy is performed prior to onset of puberty, it will halt the development of secondary sex characteristics (growth of beard, deepening of voice, growth of pubic and axillary hair, etc.) unless there is hormonal replacement. Lack of these male characteristics and the inability to father children may sufficiently affect body image and self-esteem that impotency and the inability to experience orgasm result.

Hysterectomy

The removal of a woman's uterus is known as hysterectomy. Once the uterus is removed, a woman is unable to bear children but can continue to enjoy intercourse and orgasm when wound healing has occurred. Because the surgery may result in tightening of the vaginal walls, initial coitus following hysterectomy should be approached gently. There may be need for the woman to perform exercises to stretch the vaginal vault before she returns to full sexual functioning. Some women have unrealistic fears of disturbing a suture line and consequently postpone or limit intercourse.

Because of the role the uterus plays in menstruation, pregnancy, and childbirth, it is central to perceptions and attitudes about female body image and self-esteem. Reactions to hysterectomy will vary depending on age, marital experience, children, and the client's security and comfort with sexual identity. Depression is the most common reaction. The degree of depression depends on the client's personality structure, family support, and the interventions of health professionals.[6] Some women experience defeminization as a result of the surgery. Some men also suffer threat to *their* sexual identity. They raise questions such as "A woman who does not have a uterus is really not a woman. If she isn't a woman, what am I if I have intercourse with her?" False beliefs about decrease in sexual desire will often lead women to decrease or eliminate sexual activity following hysterectomy. They may also become orgasmically dysfunctional because of stress (see Chap. 12).

In the immediate postoperative period, perineal care and dressing changes are necessary. Embarrassment due to perineal exposure is experienced by some clients. Anxiety regarding menstruation, intercourse, hormonal changes, and sexuality following surgery is also experienced. This is often allayed with accurate information and education by the nurse.

If the surgery has been performed for carcinoma of the cervix, the spouse may experience fear of "catching" cancer. Obviously, the client's spouse must be included in the educational process.

Prostatectomy

Prostatectomy or removal of the prostate gland in the male may cause concern about sexual functioning. The man who has had a prostatectomy will usually be sterile but can achieve erection, ejaculation (usually retrograde, into the bladder), and orgasm. When the suprapubic and transurethral surgical approaches are used, there is no interference with the physical ability to engage in intercourse; however, psychogenic impotence may result.[7] The perineal approach, on the other hand, may damage nerves and result in loss of the ability to have an erection, ejaculate, or reach orgasm. The feelings and concerns of the man who has had a prostatectomy generally parallel those of the woman who has had a hysterectomy.

Vasectomy and Tubal Ligation

Elective sterilization by surgical vasectomy or tubal ligation is becoming increasingly common as a method of limiting family size (see Chap. 32). Vasectomy in the male is performed by removing a section of the vas deferens. Tubal ligation in the female involves cutting and tying the fallopian tubes. Men and women who have had sexual difficulties prior to surgery continue to have them postoperatively. About 3 percent experience a decrease in their former sexual dysfunction when it was due in part to fear of impregnation. Arousal, erection, and ejaculation continue to be possible, although the man is sperm-free and infertile. Women continue to produce ova, but since these are blocked from reaching the sperm, they cannot be fertilized. Therefore these women cannot conceive.

Both vasectomy and tubal ligation are practically irreversible; therefore an in-depth interview prior to these procedures is essential. The decision-making process of the couple must be explored. Guilt in the individual having the procedure and anger toward the spouse are not uncommon. The relative risks of the surgery should be explained. Males who have had vasectomies should continue to use alternate methods of birth control until a sperm-free specimen of ejaculate is obtained. Women should have at least one normal period after tubal ligation before giving up other contraception. Follow-up counseling should continue until total adjustment occurs (see Chap. 32).

Altered Genitalia and Sterility

Pelvic Exenteration

The removal of all pelvic organs results in total change of body excretory and sexual function. A colostomy and urostomy are formed. In the female, the appearance of the genitalia is often disturbed. Sterility and the inability to achieve orgasm result from surgical interference with the nerves which carry erotic impulses, while erection and ejaculation are lost to the male. Such massive surgery is performed only as a lifesaving measure.[3,4]

Clients who have had a partial (vaginectomy or vulvectomy) or total pelvic exenteration must learn alternate means of sexual functioning. An artificial vagina is sometimes constructed for the female several months after the original surgery. This allows penetration and closeness, although orgasm rarely occurs. Some men elect to have a penile implant, which creates a permanent erection. As in the case of the female, orgasm rarely occurs. Closeness and pleasure for the partner does result. Sterility is inevitable.

These clients must cope with altered body image in its extreme. Grief and mourning are expected and depression is frequently seen long after the initial postoperative stage. Many clients express hopelessness, making statements like "You saved my life and now I'm half a man," or "You saved my life but what good am I if I can't have sex."

Patience and understanding from the spouse and supportive intervention of nurses is essential.

Vascular Disease and Sexual Dysfunction

Vascular disease impairs the vascular engorgement and muscular contractions which are part of the normal sexual response. While hypertension does not directly impair sexual functioning, many antihypertensive drugs do cause impotence by impairing neurovascular reflexes. Thrombotic obstruction, leukemia, sickle cell disorders, and penile trauma, because they interfere with penile blood supply, will impair the ability to have an erection; however, ejaculation and libido will remain intact.[1] Clients who have had an acute myocardial infarction may suffer decreased libido and impaired erection because of general debility and pain, but they do not lose their ability to reach orgasm.

Sexuality and the Client with Heart Disease

Clients who have had a myocardial infarction are usually 35 to 50 years of age, male, and have experienced good health prior to the heart attack. Illness strikes suddenly without warning, producing a crisis for clients and their families (see Chap. 5). Initially, the disruption to the lives of clients and their families is a major concern. After a few days, fears of dying as well as subsequent anger, denial, and depression usually emerge. As clients begin to recover, they experience fears and concerns about their future, not the least of these being related to sexual functioning. When these concerns are not addressed directly, problematic behavior occurs. It includes obsessive-compulsive intellectualization of the illness and treatment, regression, overdependency, and depression (see Chap. 26).

These clients, the majority of whom are male, often cover their fears and concerns with sexually provocative behavior. Banter with sexual overtones is common. Some nurses experience threat to their sexuality and embarrassment when faced with such situations. Limit setting and honest discussion wiht clients will assist in changing their behavior.

Depression is normal and common following a coronary. Clients and their spouses may believe that sexual arousal and fulfillment are harmful, making intercourse a tension-filled situation that results in little or no sexual gratification. If this process is not interrupted, subsequent abstinence

is followed by depression. Fears and depression sometimes result in reaction formation so that clients behave in ways directly contrary to what they are feeling. Spouses may become overprotective and parental toward the client while simultaneously feeling fearful and angry. Mutual withdrawal results if there is no intervention in the process.

Ignorance and misinformation prevent many clients who have recovered from heart disease from continuing an active sexual existence. Clients should be informed that some frequently prescribed drugs directly affect sexual functioning. *Reserpine* decreases libido and may cause impotence, while *aldomet* interferes with ejaculation. Most *tranquilizers* and *antidepressants* affect libido, ejaculation, and the ability to maintain an erection (see Chap. 8).

Many victims of coronary artery disease believe that sexual gratification is dangerous. Research has shown that sexual arousal and gratification have a stressful effect on the cardiovascular system (see Chap. 12) and that many sudden deaths have occurred during or immediately following coitus as a result of this stress. Rather than adopting total abstinence, clients should learn that exercise tolerance is the measure of whether or not sexual activity is safe for them. If clients with heart disease are able to walk a treadmill at 3 to 4 miles per hour and climb two flights of stairs without any increase in target pulse rate or elevation of blood pressure, their hearts can tolerate the energy demands of sexual intercourse.[8] After the onset of heart disease, the approach to this level of stress should be gradual; that is, sexual activity should not be resumed sooner than 30 to 40 days after bed rest has been discontinued. Clients with marginal stress tolerances can be helped by a regular progressive program of physical fitness aimed at increasing exercise tolerance.

Stressful and anxiety-provoking occurrences can have direct effects on cardiovascular functioning and should be avoided during, before and after sexual activity (see Chap. 14). In particular, extramarital sexual relations should be limited because they usually occur in unfamiliar surroundings with an unfamiliar partner and often add anxiety about discovery to the stress of coitus. Heavy meals and excessive drinking should be eliminated entirely. Sexual activity should be planned to occur several hours after meals, usually after a period of rest. Activity should remain within a client's exercise tolerance. Some coital positions, particularly those which avoid prolonged use of arms and legs for body support, are less strenuous than others and should be encouraged (see Chap. 12). Knowledge of stress tolerance and how drugs affect sexual performance beneficially is essential. *Nitroglycerin* prior to intercourse may prevent angina. *Propranolol* taken prophylactically decreases heart rate and blood pressure, thus decreasing cardiac labor during sexual arousal.

While the client with acute coronary disease is discussed here, the principle that sexual functioning is possible within the limits of exercise tolerance can be applied to any client who suffers from vascular or other physical diseases.

Disease of the Nervous System and Sexual Dysfunction

Disease or trauma which interferes with the nerve supply to reproductive organs will affect sexual functioning. Any injury or disorder (including surgery, as mentioned above) which affects the peripheral sensory nerves; visceral sensory nerves; the sympathetic, parasympathetic, or somatic motor nerves to the genitals; or the spinal cord reflex centers controlling vasocongestion and orgasm will impair sexual functioning.[1]

For example, multiple sclerosis, which causes degeneration of the spinal cord, can cause erectile or orgasmic dysfunction. Spinal cord injury as a result of trauma can affect control of erection and ejaculation. The woman with spinal cord injury may become unable to have orgasm.

Sexuality and Spinal Cord Injury

Paraplegics and quadriplegics are limited in the methods by which they can achieve sexual gratification. Once spinal cord nerves are severed, sexual gratification has to originate at levels other than the genital level.

In the period of time immediately following injury, fears of the unknown, about the inability to move unassisted, and about the loss of sensation are paramount. Grief and mourning for loss of body function occur (see Chap. 28). Restlessness and agitation secondary to pain are also seen. Concerns for sexual functioning usually begin after the acute trauma has subsided.[9]

The married injured are concerned about the understanding of the sexual partner, and for those who are not married, there is fear of rejection by potential partners. For both, these concerns have more importance than the lack of sexual functioning itself.[10] Those who are already married at the time of injury report increased marital and social conflict.[9] Depression and suicidal thoughts occur for many clients during the adjustment phase immediately following injury. Learning to be dependent creates conflict within the client and with caretakers. Self-pity and feelings of helplessness and hopelessness exist. If rehabilitation is successful, the client becomes aware of the need to restructure an entire life-style physically, emotionally, and socially. Sexual activity must also be totally restructured.

Clients with traumatic spinal cord injury usually suffer damage which affects the four phases of the sexual cycle (see Chap. 12). The autonomic nervous system controls tumescence during the excitement phase and detumescence during resolution. Innervation stems primarily from the sacral portion of the cauda equina and may run through an ancillary pathway from the thoracic regions. The plateau phase and orgasm itself are controlled by nerves originating in the lumbar area.[10]

The person who has suffered injury—once the rehabilitative stage of recovery begins—should be encouraged to engage in any types of sexual activity that are physiologically possible, pleasing, esthetically appealing, gratifying, and acceptable to them. It should be assumed that sexual intercourse is possible until experience, time, and complete neurological determinations indicate the contrary.[10] There are some alternative means of sexual gratification for the client who has suffered permanent damage to spinal cord nerves. Feelings of closeness with an understanding partner help to sublimate sexual needs. Learning to utilize alternate erotic zones (i.e., breasts) to derive sexual pleasure, taking advantage of spontaneous erections to gratify a partner, and utilizing fantasy and recall are other methods of deriving sexual pleasure. Oral sex and petting may also be used to gratify partners and derive self-pleasure. Some male clients may elect to have a penile implant. A permanent erection is thus created, enabling coitus to occur.

The positive or negative response of the sexual partner, the family, and health professionals will directly affect clients' return to their maximum level of function.

The Nurses' Response to Client Behavior

Sexuality is an integral part of the total person's self-concept and as such is involved in the individual's concept of body image and self-esteem. It is characteristic of being human. Any threat to sexual identity will have a marked effect on the totality of the self (see Chaps. 12, 13, and 19).

Before nurses can approach clients about sexuality, they must first approach themselves. Nurses, like clients, have beliefs and values about sexuality. These are the result of their cultural environment and must be confronted honestly (see Chap. 12). Once nurses have formed *adult* values about sexuality, they will be better able to counsel clients therapeutically. They must likewise accept or reject the limitations of the clients' sexual functioning.

Nursing as a profession has been given societal sanction to touch bodies and to be concerned about intimate and personal care. Initially, nurses may experience discomfort and even revulsion when asked to carry out these functions. Later, these feelings may be identified as shyness and insecurity. For many, the experience of bathing the genitalia of a person of the opposite sex may represent the first time they have seen a naked adult of that sex. Sex education and allowing

nurses to express their fears and concerns will help them deal therapeutically with this task. A nurse's self-composure and comfort combined with a direct, matter-of-fact approach will put clients at ease and help them overcome whatever discomfort or reluctance they may experience from the invasion of privacy.

Some nurses may deny sexuality either verbally or behaviorally. Avoidance of the subject of sex and vague or nonspecific responses to clients' concerns are some of the ways in which denial is expressed. Expressions such as "private parts" and "down below" are used by some when referring to the genitalia and are indicative of avoidance by the nurse. In some hospitals, rules exist that require that male professionals care for male clients and that female clients be cared for by females. Client comfort, not nursing avoidance, should be the motivation for such rules.

Insecurity and inhibition are other responses often experienced by nurses when confronted with a client's sexual concerns. Such responses interfere with therapeutic intervention with clients, causing decreased sensitivity and lack of objectivity. Nurses need to be aware of their own sexuality and to be secure enough to encourage verbalization of the client's underlying sexual concerns. The beliefs, attitudes, and values of the nurse cannot be imposed on the client. Fear of offending a client or embarrassment are responses which interfere with an objective approach to clients about their sexuality. Nurses' comfort with their own sexuality is essential.

Nurses sometimes reflect their own feelings and fears rather than empathizing with the feelings of clients about their sexuality. If the client is evasive, so is the nurse. If clients do not express concerns about sexuality, some nurses, because of their own feelings, are reluctant to approach the subject openly. Empathy is the ability to put oneself in another's place and to understand another's feelings and behaviors objectively (see Chap. 6). It is the key to a therapeutic approach. On the other hand, overidentification with the client is antitherapeutic and can sometimes be destructive.

Clients may become emotionally involved

with nurses who show interest and concern for their sexual well-being. It is the nurses' responsibility to maintain open and professional relationships characterized by empathy and shared problem solving. Authenticity in the relationship with clients and their spouses is learned and is a joint project. Any relationship with nurses should not threaten the client's spouse.

Sometimes nurses experience feelings of revulsion or pity when confronted by a client's sexual concerns. Nurses should not be forced to discuss sexual concerns or to care for a client with whom they are physically uncomfortable. Their discomfort can be transmitted to clients and it can thereby have a nontherapeutic effect. They should seek guidance from a peer, supervisor, or instructor to explore this aspect of the clients' and their totality.

Nurses' expectations of their clients may be unrealistic, thus threatening and angering them rather than helping them. For example, the nurse may explain various coital positions or discuss oral sex with clients whose culture or experience does not include these alternatives. Gentle encouragement and exploration of sexual adaptation with clients is more therapeutic than overenthusiasm. The moral, religious, and esthetic convictions of clients may differ from those of the nurse. Respect and a nonjudgmental manner are acceptable nursing responses.[9]

Assessment

Primary in the care of clients faced with conditions that threaten their sexuality—as well as the sexuality of the nurse—is an accurate and complete nursing assessment. This begins with the nurse's self-assessment. It is followed by assessment of clients and their families. Nurses must be fully aware of themselves as sexual beings if they are to intervene therapeutically (see Chaps. 12 and 13).

Self-Assessment

Because perceptions often color objective data, alertness to what is happening within themselves will offer nurses valuable data about their clients. The *process* occurring between nurses and clients when sexuality is discussed gives clues to appropriate and therapeutic intervention. In assessing themselves, nurses should ask the following questions:

1 What general feeling do I have in response to this client?

2 How is the client responding to me? Is my sex a factor in this response?

3 What personal experiences am I reminded of as I relate to this client?

4 Do my values about sexuality differ from those of the client?

5 Is my cultural outlook on sexuality different from or similar to that of the client?

6 How do I feel when I discuss sexual functioning with this client?

7 Am I more comfortable when the clients and I are the same sex or when their sex differs from mine?

8 How comfortable am I when I have to approach clients about bathing or caring for their genitals?

9 What is my feeling response to the client's sexual partner?

Honest answers to these questions will give nurses valuable information about their own sexuality. Exploration should follow with an informed person who can be objective and supportive in helping the nurse formulate a comfortable sexual self. Once nurses have confronted themselves, they are able to review the clients' situation objectively for the purpose of diagnosing sexual problems.

Client Assessment

Three primary concerns should be the focus of the initial assessment of a client's sexual functioning:

1 Has sexual functioning been disrupted because of a permanent, irreversible physical condition?

2 Has sexual functioning been disrupted because of psychogenic maladaptations to illness?

3 Has sexual functioning been interrupted temporarily or modified as a result of the illness?

Once nurses, in concert with other professionals, make assessments of a client's present and future physical state of sexual functioning, they can proceed to further information gathering and formulation of nursing diagnoses. Table 21-1 lists nursing assessments and diagnoses which may be applied to any client with sexual dysfunction. Table 21-2 deals specifically with the assessment of those clients whose sexual functioning is directly affected by surgery or by diseases of the vascular or nervous systems.

Goals

Realistic goals are based on the client's rehabilitive potential. The following goals can be set for all clients, regardless of their illness or health:

- Assist clients to recognize sexuality as an integral part of their personality, determined biologically at conception, influenced by the environment, sustained by health, threatened by disease, and changed by choice.
- Encourage clients to express themselves as sexual beings.
- Increase clients' knowledge of sexual psychology, physiology, and functioning.
- Teach the client how the disease process may or may not affect sexual performance.

Nurses can also formulate goals to guide their relationships with clients. These can include the following:

- Be aware of the influence one's sexuality can have on others.
- Use sexuality in a constructive and therapeutic manner.

- Be tolerant of the sexual attitudes and preferences of others (peers and clients).
- Develop an ability to assess clients' perceptions about their sexuality.
- Create an atmosphere conducive to discussion of sexual concerns.

Intervention

Based on their assessments, nurses initiate and complete the actions necessary to accomplish the defined goals of a client's care.[11] Intervention should follow from client assessment and diagnosis (see Tables 21-1 and 21-2). Planning for a client's return to the community at an optimum level of functioning begins when the client enters the hospital. Nurses need to involve professionals from other health-care disciplines in the care of clients whose sexuality has been disrupted.

Members of self-help groups such as ostomy clubs are invaluable in assisting with the rehabilitation of ostomates. One young male paraplegic stated that the turning point in his rehabilitation came when a nurse arranged for him to speak to another paraplegic who had adjusted to his limitations. Clients who have had an acute coronary thrombosis and their spouses are often most helped by those who have lived through similar experiences.

Evaluation

Periodic assessment of clients as they are in the here and now and alteration in planning as necessary is essential to the nursing process. The nurse intervening with clients about sexuality must evaluate plans frequently. Conclusive knowledge about sexual functioning is often not available when the plan is first initiated. Every change in physical or psychogenic state will necessitate a change in the plan. For example, needs for sexual fulfillment take on lesser importance in the immediate postoperative phase of illness but acquire

Table 21-1 Sexual Dysfunction — General Client Assessment, Diagnoses, and Interventions

Assessment	Diagnoses	Interventions
What was client's previous level of sexual functioning?	Comfortable sexual functioning; good relationship with spouse. Maladaptation in sexual functioning prior to illness. Conflictual relationship with spouse.	Use data from sexual history to assess client functioning. Teach client alternate sexual behaviors to obtain sexual fulfillment. Initiate couple counseling. Support spouse of client during adjustment to present state of sexual functioning.
What meaning does sexual activity have for client?	Client views sexual activity as (1) pleasure source for self, (2) pleasure source for self and partner, (3) tensions release, (4) means of procreation, (5) means of control.	Encourage verbalization of meaning of sexual activity. Take objective, nonjudgmental attitude in interactions.
What is client's cultural environment? What significance does physical wholeness have for client?	Client strongly identifies with ethnic group. Client's body image is culturally determined.	Explore client's adherence to behavior and standards of ethnic group. Explore client's acceptance of masturbation for tension release. Propose means of sublimation of sexual drive that are culturally acceptable to client.
Has client accepted or rejected current illness or surgical alteration?	Client acceptance. Client maladaptation.	Listen for client's nonverbal cues about sexual concern. Elicit verbalization of underlying concerns from client. Support client in adjustment process by encouraging verbalization about present physical state and client's perception of changes in sexuality.
What is client's support system?	Supportive partner. Support from job. Alone; no support. Support from other family members.	Conduct family conferences. Teach partner how to care for client's physical needs. Foster independence in clients who are alone by teaching self-help skills. Encourage clients to return to former social functioning by referral to and participation in community activities. Include employer in discharge planning.
What is client's sense of body image and self-esteem?	Well-adjusted adult. Maladjusted client with feelings of inadequacy, inferiority, shame, self-consciousness, worthlessness, pessimism, hopelessness.	Assist in identification of genital assets of client's sexuality. Provide opportunity for growth and self-actualization. Increase client's ability to cope with life stress. Help client with adjustment to any body-image change.
What is client's outlook for future?	Anxiety about discharge. Anxiety about future sexual functioning.	Provide opportunities for client to work and engage in constructive activity. Provide opportunity for social adaptation and involvement in community. Teach modification of environment that will be therapeutically useful. Investigate alternative methods of sexual functioning. Schedule discharge-planning interview with client and family.

Table 21-2 Physiological Sexual Dysfunctions

Assessment	Diagnoses	Interventions
	Surgery and sexuality	
Is there physical cause for client's sexual dysfunction?	Pelvic nerves disrupted. Client able or not able to experience orgasm. Erection possible or impossible. Ejaculation possible or impossible.	Collaborate with client's physician about extent of pelvic nerve disruption. Clarify degree of disruption.
What is client's perception of postsurgical sexual status?	Accepts or rejects limits placed on sexual function by surgery.	Reassure clients about feelings of femininity and masculinity. Clarify postsurgical function as it is known. Encourage client to attempt sexual activity until limitations are firmly established.
How much knowledge does client have about sexual alteration?	Knows what physician has explained. Knowledgeable. Has no knowledge.	Explore with clients the pros and cons of surgical intervention, such as creation of artificial vagina or penile implant. Give accurate information. Clarify and explore myths. Teach use of touch for sexual arousal.
Does client use appliance? Is client aware of prosthetic devices?	Needs to use appliance. Needs instruction on availability of prosthetic devices.	Teach use and care of stoma appliances and availability of prosthetic devices.
What devices are used by client for bowel and bladder function?	Ostomy appliance interferes with client's willingness to have intercourse. Indwelling catheter requires adjustment.	Suggest emptying appliance before intercourse; tape away from genital area. Stress cleanliness and preparedness. Teach techniques to accommodate. *Male:* bend catheter back along penis and apply condom; remove and clamp collecting device. *Female:* clamp catheter and tape away from vaginal opening.
What are psychogenic causes of client's fatigue or pain?	Incapacity. Pain. Job. Marital conflict.	Encourage clients to determine causes of stress and pain and ways of reducing it. Sensitize clients to partners' stress signals.
	Heart disease and sexuality	
What are perceptions of the client and spouse about the limitations cardiac illness places on sexual function?	Fearful of sexual function. Perceives marked change in sexual function. Overprotective spouse.	Explain client's exercise limits. Encourage verbalization of fears and concerns. Have spouse verbalize concerns and fears. Clarify realities of illness.
What is client's exercise tolerance?	Able to climb two flights of stairs without exceeding target pulse rate.	Outline graduated exercise program. Inform client of stresses to be avoided. Teach client to alternate rest with activity.
What activities, alone or in combination, cause fatigue?	Daily routine is	Help clients to plan for sexual activity after period of rest. Have clients identify most suitable times for sexual activity.
What coital positions induce feelings of relaxation and repose?	Side by side (face to face), woman on top (see Chap. 12).	Encourage clients to experiment with various sexual positions and approaches.

Table 21-2 Physiological Sexual Dysfunctions *(continued)*

Assessment	Diagnoses	Interventions
	Spinal Cord Injury and Sexuality	
What is the extent of physical disruption of client's sexual functions? Were pelvic nerves severed? What is the level of injury? Is there reflex response?	Neurological deficit: present or absent, degrees.	Assist client to understand the effect of neurological dysfunction. Explain present sexual functional capabilities to client.
What is client's sensory status?	Client responds to touch, pin prick, pressure, genital-area stimulation.	Assist client to identify hyper- and hyposensitive areas of body. Teach clients use of touch for sexual arousal and gratification. Assist client and partner to discover areas of erotic sensitivity (breasts, etc.).
What are alterations in client's perception and sensitivity to touch?	Is more responsive. Is less responsive.	Encourage openness and communication about what is helpful, pleasing, or hindering to sexual function. Teach awareness of alternate means of stimulation by stroking, oral and rectal stimulation, vibration.
What is client's capacity for mobility?	Client is dependent. Client is independent. Client can maintain position for a specified period of time. Client has full or partial range of motion.	Relate present mobility to former methods of sexual interaction. Teach alternate positioning for sexual intercourse (partner on top, side by side, etc.). Teach use of positioning aids such as pillow and use of water bed.
What degree of assistance does client need to fulfill sexual needs?	Client needs total assistance. Client is partially dependent. Client is independent.	Discuss need for assistance with client's sexual partner. Explore partner's concerns and feelings. Clarify potential for role conflict and stress when partner is care-giver.

more importance as clients prepare to return to their homes and former lives, often with an altered body image and lowered sense of self-esteem.

References

1 Helen Singer Kaplan: *The New Sex Therapy*, Brunner Mazel, New York, 1974.

*2 Linbania Jacobson: "Illness and Human Sexuality," *Nursing Outlook*, vol. 22, January 1974, pp. 50–53.

3 Linda Gross: *Ileostomy: An Introduction*, United Ostomy Association, 1976, pamphlet.

4 Linda Gross: *Urostomy: An Introduction*, United Ostomy Association, 1976, pamphlet.

*5 J. E. Mullens: "Sexuality in Ostomates," *ET Journal*, vol. 2, no. 2, pp. 1112–1113, Winter 1975–76.

*Recommended reference by a nurse author.

6 M. H. Hollender: "Hysterectomy and Feelings of Femininity," *Medical Aspects of Human Sexuality*, vol. 3, no. 6, 1969.

*7 Phyllis Carey: "Temporary Sexual Dysfunction in Reversible Health Situations," *Nursing Clinics of North America*, vol. 10, no. 3, pp. 575–586, September 1975.

8 Robert S. Eliot and Richard Miles: "What to Tell the Cardiac Patient about Sexual Intercourse," *Consultant*, September 1973, pp. 23–25.

*9 Isabel MacRae and Gloria Henderson: "Sexuality and Irreversible Health Limitations," *Nursing Clinics of North America*, vol. 10, no. 3, pp. 587–597, September 1975.

*10 Jim Smith and Bonnie Bullough: "Sexuality and the Severely Disabled," *American Journal of Nursing*, vol. 75, no. 12, pp. 2194–2197, September 1975.

11 Ray Buridge: "A Paraplegic Reflects," *American Journal of Nursing*, vol. 75, no. 4, pp. 643–644, April 1975.

Chapter

22
The Client Who Generates Identification Problems

Mary Teague

Learning Objectives

After studying this chapter, the student should be able to:

1 Discuss the dynamics of the identification process
2 Identify clients who generate identification problems
3 Discuss nurse responses to clients who generate identification problems
4 Identify assessment factors for staff and clients who are vulnerable to identification problems
5 Formulate nursing diagnoses and goals for clients who generate identification problems
6 Construct a plan of nursing intervention for clients who generate identification problems based on the client's individual needs
7 Evaluate the effectiveness of the nursing intervention

The intimate nature of the nurse-client relationship provides an atmosphere in which identification problems are likely to occur. An *identification problem* exists when the staff reacts to a client with emotions that are appropriate to persons or situations in the past but not the situation at hand. Freud described this phenomenon as *transference.* At first, Freud thought that it was unique to the doctor-patient relationship in psychoanalysis; however, he later found that it occurred in many everyday relationships as well. Sullivan called this same phenomenon *parataxic distortion.* Sullivan felt that if such distortions were not expected in the therapeutic relationship or were ignored, some of the most important information about the client would be missed. In the health-care setting, the authoritative role of the physician and the nurturant role of the nurse coupled with the regressive-dependent role of the client create an atmosphere reminiscent of the parent-child relationship and therefore one which fosters the development of identification problems.

There are two types of identification, *positive* and *negative.* Positive identifications are those in which individuals unconsciously attach to themselves certain qualities associated with others because they wish to be like the others. Negative identifications are those in which the painful or unpleasant emotions associated with people in the past are evoked by surrogate people in the present.[1] Both identifications are especially likely to occur in the nurse-client relationship because of its intimate nature, particularly when clients are endowed by the staff with special emotional significance because of their position, status, role, or age. The professional, the religious, the relative of staff, the client who is special because of age, and the "nice guy" are especially likely to precipitate such problems.

Since the identification phenomenon is the basis for serious misunderstandings and misconceptions in the nurse-client relationship, it is important that the nursing staff become aware of its development. Such awareness requires that the nursing staff pay attention to the behavior and responses that are present in both the client and the nurse. In each nurse-client relationship, the nursing process should focus not only on the dynamic issues presented by the client but also on (1) what the nurse and client say, (2) how each behaves, (3) the feelings experienced in the relationship, and (4) how the relationship is affecting nursing intervention.

Identification in Childhood

Identifications with significant persons are a normal and necessary part of personality development. The imitation of characteristics of parents and others to whom a child is emotionally attached shapes the child's personality. By identifying with parents, children learn how to behave in a variety of situations. For instance, children mimic both mother and father in work situations, in their manner of relating to one another, and in facial expressions and other idiosyncrasies. The childhood game of playing house shows how closely children identify with their parents' mannerisms.

Children not only identify with their parents' obvious habits and mannerisms but also incorporate parental attitudes and values. Marianne Jones, age 4, was scolded by her mother for taking her brother's candy without asking. Later in the day, Mrs. Jones chuckled as she observed Marianne, dressed in mother's hat and shoes, scolding a doll for eating candy that did not belong to it. Mrs. Jones saw that Marianne's tone of voice, facial expression, and hand gestures were remarkably similar to her own.

Between the ages of 2 and 5, children use identification to reduce the tension and relieve the anxiety induced by the clash between their desire for immediate gratification of needs and their awareness that sometimes, in order to be loved, the gratification of needs must be postponed. The classic example of the use of identification in the service of tension reduction is seen in the dynamics of the Oedipus complex (see Chaps. 4 and 5).

The situation known as the *Oedipus complex* was first described by Freud. He reported that, at about the age of 4 or 5, the little boy begins to want to take over his father's role with his mother. The little boy is jealous of their relationship but realizes that while the father is around, he has no chance with the mother. Therefore the little boy has fantasies of killing the father in order to get rid of the competition for his mother's love. However, due to the magical thinking typical of childhood, the little boy believes that the father knows about his murderous thoughts and that the father will punish him by castration. The little boy experiences acute anxiety over this imagined fate. In order to rid himself of the acute anxiety, the little boy represses his feelings toward his mother and, instead, identifies with the father's strength and power. Through this process of identification, which is unconscious, the little boy comes to believe that he too is strong and powerful and therefore need not fear his father.

In addition to identifying with the father's strength and power, the child also assimilates the father's values and attitudes. This identification with the moral, ethical, and social attitudes and values of the parent forms a rudimentary conscience or superego. Another important aspect of this process of identification is the acquisition of behavior consistent with our society's view of sex-appropriate roles. The situation with the little girl and her father is similar; however, the punishment that she fears is abandonment by the mother. She resolves the dilemma by repressing her feelings toward her father and identifying with her mother.

As the thought process becomes more logical in adulthood, identification is used less often as a method of reducing tension. However, this prelogical type of thinking is not completely lost with maturity. It may recur whenever situations arise in which emotions prevail over logical thought (see Chap. 13).

Identification in Adulthood

Most people reach adulthood with some unresolved conflicts and emotions. These feelings remain unresolved because, when originally experienced, they generated such a high level of anxiety that they were repressed before they could be worked out. Repression enables the individual to go on coping with life, but it also blocks further growth. A very simplified explanation of how emotions are usually resolved or worked out is as follows: (1) an emotional reaction is triggered by a person or an event; (2) the emotion is recognized or brought into awareness; (3) the precipitating event is recognized and the emotion is expressed—for example, through yelling, screaming, talking, or crying; and (4) tension is decreased and the emotion resolved. When this sequence is interrupted—for example, when awareness of the feeling or its source provokes too much anxiety—the emotion is repressed or pushed into the unconscious (See Chaps. 4 and 14).

Once disturbing emotions have been resolved, people are free to use all their emotional or psychic energy to deal with current matters. Repressed or unresolved emotions drain off some psychic energy, which is needed to keep the feelings repressed. In addition, these feelings continue to pose a threat because, when a situation occurs which endangers the person's emotional equilibrium, the repressed feelings may rise up into awareness or consciousness. One defense against this threat is the process of identification. The feelings which are often still too threatening to acknowledge, even in adulthood, are attached to a surrogate person in the present situation—often a nurse or physician. The dynamics of certain groups of clients enables us to predict that they will be likely to generate identification problems in the staff.

Selected Client Behaviors
The Professional Client

Denial of illness and fear of losing control are predominant issues when the clients are physicians or nurses. Denial is related to several factors. First, there is reluctance on the part of clients to assume the dependent role when they have been accustomed to being in charge. Second, the inability to prevent illness or to cure themselves poses a serious threat to their professional identity. Third, these clients fear loss of control. The loss of control includes three components: (1) loss of control over body functions, (2) loss of emotional control, and (3) loss of control over the day-to-day regulation of their lives.

When the client is a nurse or a physician, the staff's anxiety level increases. Illness in a colleague reminds the staff of their own vulnerability, and this is frightening. Therefore, the staff may identify with the client's denial and minimize the seriousness of the illness. If the staff is in a subordinate professional role to the client, the role reversal may increase the anxiety even more. For example, Miss Peters, a senior student nurse, awoke with a headache on the day she was scheduled to give preoperative care to Mrs. Rogers, one of her instructors who was a patient. After discussion with another instructor, Miss Peters became aware of her anxiety and her headache went away.

Another indication of the staff's identification problems is the tendency to treat these individuals as colleagues rather than as clients. Conflict in this situation revolves around two issues: telling the client too much or giving him or her too little information. Either course of action deprives such people of their need to be treated as clients. For example, the staff in the psychiatric setting may project their own characteristics of introspection and self-awareness onto a client who is a physician or a nurse, equating the client's *assumed* theoretical knowledge with insight into personal problems. However, nurses and physicians are not necessarily any more self-aware than anyone else.

Similar presumptions may be made about physician and nurse clients on the medical-surgical unit. For example, a patient who is a retired nursing supervisor and who was scheduled for a colostomy was given no preoperative instruction, despite the fact that she knew very little about what to expect postoperatively.

On the other hand, staff may feel that clients who are professionals will be able to deal effectively with all information available concerning their treatment. This thinking may lead the staff to overload these clients with too *much* information.[2] For example, information about tests, medication choices and dosages, and other decisions is not usually shared with clients. However, it may mistakenly be shared with *these* clients in ignorance of the fact that they may not be ready or able to assume the responsibility for decision making and may therefore suffer unnecessary anxiety. The result may be to deny the hospitalized physician or nurse the use of important coping mechanisms such as regression and withdrawal.

The nursing staff must be alert to signs of identification problems with clients who are nurses or physicians. An effective therapeutic relationship may never be established unless the staff deals with the issues of status and role very early in treatment.[3] It is important for staff to accept the fact that such clients do have needs that require gratification and that they should, while in treatment, be given the same consideration as any other client.

The "Nice-Guy" Client

Identification with the compliant, accepting attitude of the "nice guy" may cause the staff to discourage such a client from expressing their true feelings. The apparent compliance and acceptance is often a facade for denial, fear of rejection for failure to be "good," or a desire to manipulate the authority figures that the physician and nurse represent. The preoperative client who exhibits an unusually low degree of anxiety may be denying the dangers involved in the surgery. A common but often unexpressed fear of clients is that the staff will reject or neglect them if they are not "nice." Some clients refrain from asking the nursing staff to help them, so that when they "really" need someone, help will come quickly.

The clients on the psychiatric unit must conform to the staff's definition of mental health before they can be discharged. If such a client is not "good," there is the risk of loss of privileges, forcible restraint, or commitment. A compliant and accepting attitude may also be a facade for passive manipulation. Unwillingness to ask questions, share feelings, and verbalize needs can effectively thwart the efforts of the physician and the nursing staff to provide care to clients and to move them toward understanding problems, communicating openly, and coping effectively.

Consistent identification with the emotional tone of the client who is a nice guy may cause the staff to subtly influence the client away from the expression of real concerns.[4] Interactions with these clients may remain superficial, and the staff will then begin to realize that their relationship with the client lacks depth and trust. Often, after an adequate amount of contact, the staff realize that they have inadequate assessment data and do not have a clear understanding of the client. Equally common is a major difference of opinion among the staff about the approach to be taken with these clients. This may be due to the fact that some staff members have recognized covert feelings of fear, anger, or hopelessness in these clients even though their overt expressions are those of the nice guy. Unless the staff gently but persistently question this emotional facade, very little help will be provided to these clients.

Relatives of Staff

Problems of identification with clients who are relatives of staff often stem from the staff's feelings toward the client's relative rather than toward the client. If the relatives are powerful or influential, they may try to use their power or influence to obtain special privileges for themselves or for the client. For example, although it was the policy of the psychiatric unit that each client participate in group therapy, Ms. Lincoln, a nursing instructor, called the medical director of the unit and requested that her husband, a client on the unit, be excused from the group. Such behavior enhances the relatives' feelings of control and security, but it also undermines the staff, making them feel insecure and powerless. If limits are not clearly defined and enforceable, anxiety will rise and may be defensively exhibited as anger. The staff may then react to their anger with the *relative* by acting out against the *client*, rigidly enforcing policies and procedures.

When the client is a relative of staff, there is usually concern on the part of the staff that the client or the relative will try to manipulate the treatment situation. Sometimes this does happen, and it generally causes problems. For example, after Mark, the son of a prominent attorney, called his father to report that the staff would not give him medication for pain after his surgery, the staff found many reasons to restrict his teen-age friends from visiting and to report his "uncooperative" behavior to his doctor. Staff may also react by withdrawing. Both these behaviors protect the staff's credibility and self-esteem.

Although it may appear that the client who is a relative of staff gets special treatment—for example, visits and inquiries from the hospital hierarchy—in fact, these clients are often deprived of the care that they need. This deprivation may occur because the staff avoid the client or they avoid dealing with sensitive issues that are crucial to the client's care. Avoidance of the client often relates to the staff's fears that the client will find the care that they give deficient, that the client will reveal this to the relative, and that the dissatisfied family will, in turn, complain to superiors. The second type of avoidance is of sensitive issues in the care of the client. An example of such avoidance occurred when Joan, the 16-year-old daughter of a prominent physician, was admitted to the hospital because of an "accidental" overdose of tranquilizers. Joan was withdrawn and hostile toward the nursing staff, and visits between the father and daughter were charged with hostility. Although these observations were charted, Joan's physician refused to suggest psychiatric treatment, and the nursing staff did not pursue their observations by confronting the pair.

The Religious Client

Identification problems generated by nuns, priests, ministers, and rabbis are usually related to issues with which these clients have problems— identity and intimacy[5]—and to the staff's own stereotyped picture of such clients. The identity issue is exemplified by role expectations which carry connotations of status and altruism. The religious person is viewed as being strong, wise, and able to give to others. Clerical garb, if worn, seems to endow this person with special qualities. Religious articles around the hospital room also serve as reminders to the staff that this person is special. When the religious become clients, these factors may set them apart from other clients and from staff. They may be deprived of interpersonal support, adequate client teaching, and total nursing care. Most hospitals extend the courtesy of private rooms to the religious, thus only increasing their isolation. These clients may go to great lengths to minimize their special status.

For some of these clients, the issue of intimacy is of more significance than for others. Those whose education, training, and day-to-day living arrangements discourage the development of intimate relationships may find the intimate nature of the client role more difficult to cope with than do people whose backgrounds do not impose such limitations. Their education and training has often encouraged them to help others but discouraged identification and acknowledgement of their own needs. When acknowledgement of a problem does finally take place, radical intervention is often necessary. For example, Sister Helen, a schoolteacher, had an excoriation on her hip which was irritated by her undergarments. She said that she ignored it, thinking it would disappear. As it got bigger and began to ulcerate, she continued to neglect it, saying, "I couldn't miss school, the children need me." The ulcer became infected and foul-smelling. She was admitted to the hospital for debridement and skin grafts and had to remain in the hospital for 1 month.

While clients who are religious may set unusually high standards for themselves, these standards are often introjects of society's expectations of humility, obedience, stoicism, patience, wisdom, and kindness. Even though they know that they are maintaining a facade, the clients may be committed to this image. The nursing staff usually holds the same stereotyped ideas about the religious as does the rest of society. In short, the identification problems generated by these clients are based chiefly on social stereotypes and myths.

These stereotypes usually inhibit the staff's interaction with these clients. For example, the

staff may be reluctant to lay hands on them or to perform procedures that may cause embarrassment, such as catheterization. In addition, the staff may be reluctant to confront the behavior of these clients because of their special status. For example, although the staff was sure that Reverend Carter was eating more than his allotted calories on his diabetic diet, they were reluctant to discuss this with him because of his special status. After a discussion at a team meeting, the team leader decided she would talk with the Reverend about the matter. Reverend Carter readily admitted that he had a very difficult time staying within the allotted calories. He reported, in fact, that his "cheating" at home had necessitated his admission to the hospital. The team leader told him that she would have the dietician speak with him about some acceptable snacks and recommended that when he felt compelled to eat something, he call her or another member of the nursing staff to talk with him about his feelings.

Another consequence of the staff's stereotyping of these clients is that the staff may deny the impact of serious surgical procedures on them. The staff may think that these clients are uninterested in their personal appearance or sexual identity. Identification with the myth of stoicism may lead the staff to believe that the client will cope with any problem or diagnosis with equanimity. When one of these clients does not live up to the staff's expectations—that is, when the clients react in a way that is out of keeping with the stereotyped role in which the staff has cast them—the staff may feel inadequate, angry, betrayed, or cheated.

For example, Sister Mary Frances had just had a radical mastectomy. The staff was very involved with meeting her physical needs but avoided exploration of feelings and reactions regarding the diagnosis of cancer, change in feminine body image, and loss of a significant body part. Ms. Smith came in to give the client a bath and found her crying. She said, "Sister, you're crying! You look so upset." The Sister replied, "Upset? Of course I'm upset. Wouldn't you be if you found out you had cancer?" Ms. Smith said, "I know I would have many feelings. But you always seem so strong and composed, I guess it never occurred to me that you would be upset and need to talk about it." Sister and Ms. Smith spent some time talking about her loss. As Ms. Smith left, she said, "Let's spend some time talking again tomorrow." The religious want to be treated as human beings. The avoidance of issues and conferring of special status interferes with meeting their total needs.

The Client of a Special Age

Although there are many different staff-client age relationships which may trigger identification problems, three types are most common: (1) the younger client with the older staff member, (2) the older client with the younger staff member, and (3) the staff member with the client of approximately the same age.

Erik Erikson's model of age-related psychosocial developmental tasks and Sigmund Freud's model of psychosexual development provide a framework by which the dynamics that generate age-related identification problems may be understood. These theories propose that, from birth onward, the life cycle may be divided into developmental periods. During these periods, according to Erikson and Freud, certain critical tasks need to be accomplished if the individual is to function at an optimal level. A person's behavior during these developmental periods is characteristic of the struggle and conflict required to accomplish the tasks of the period and to progress to a more mature mode of functioning. A person's achievement of the tasks of some of the developmental periods may lead to antagonism toward others, especially those who are in close contact with the individual in times of stress. Some examples are authority relationships such as the parent-child relationship, teacher-student relationship, supervisor–staff nurse relationship, and staff-client relationship.

When the client is younger and the staff member older, the stage is set for the reenactment of parent-child conflicts. In this circumstance the staff members become the symbolic parents, since they are the enforcers of hospital rules and regulations. Adolescent clients, for example, are struggling for independence and emancipation from their families. The forced dependence and regression associated with hospitalization can be very threatening to the emerging and tenuously held independence of the adolescent client. Consequently, adolescent clients may, in order to hold onto their independence, refuse to follow hospital rules or treatment programs. Adolescent clients are also coping with sexual development and psychosexual drives. The intimacy of the staff-client relationship may be threatening to clients whose impulse control is tenuous. Identification problems may cause the older staff member to become rigid, restrictive, and even punitive with these clients. In contrast, some older staff members may subtly encourage the rebelliousness of adolescent clients who have rekindled the staff members' own unresolved adolescent rebellion.

In a situation where the staff members are younger than the client, the client may feel anger and resentment because younger people are in positions of authority. These clients may react to younger staff as they would toward their own children. Conversely, since hospitalization usually precipitates some regression in all clients, older clients may, because of the authority role of the young staff, react to them as they would toward their own parents. For example, Mrs. Gordon, a 45-year-old client, was very angry and uncooperative toward the staff, most of whom were in their twenties. Ms. Smith, the psychiatric liaison nurse, was asked to speak with the client because of her "uncooperative attitude." Mrs. Gordon told Ms. Smith that she thought that the nursing staff treated her "like a child." She felt that the nurses did not care about her, since they made her get out of bed when she had pain. She went on to tell Ms. Smith that, as a teen-ager, she had been bedridden at home for a year. Her mother had taken care of her in a very protective, nearly smothering manner. Mrs. Gordon expressed her ambivalent feelings about this period and about her mother. She said that she felt that her mother had probably prolonged her convalescence because of her own fears. Mrs. Gordon said that she had never expressed these feelings to her mother because she knew that her mother would be too hurt.

The present illness put Mrs. Gordon into a

dependent role which encouraged the development of an identification problem. This enforced dependence rekindled unresolved angry feelings toward her mother. Her anger at her mother was inappropriately focused on the nursing staff because they were fulfilling the same role that her mother had during the childhood illness. Mrs. Gordon was encouraged to express her angry feelings. She was also encouraged to help plan a schedule for getting out of bed when she felt stronger. The care plan encouraged increasing independence for Mrs. Gordon.

A third situation which may generate identification problems occurs when the staff member and the client are the same age. Since the developmental tasks that each is working through are similar, identification problems can easily arise. Ann, a 21-year-old member of the nursing staff, had been working with Peter, a 20-year-old college student, since his admission. Peter was in an automobile accident which caused a concussion and a fractured pelvis. Peter told Ann and several other staff members about the weekend parties at his dormitory. He said that he could hardly wait to return so that he could attend all the parties. At a team meeting, a discussion ensued regarding Peter's apparent lack of insight about his drinking and the dangers involved. Several staff members suggested that Peter should be referred for counseling. Ann, the staff nurse who had been working closely with Peter, became very indignant. She said that the staff were "squares," that Peter was not "crazy," and that he did not need counseling. She said that Peter had invited her to one of the parties, and she could see nothing wrong with going. Ann was identifying with Peter's rebellious attitude. Both client and nurse were still trying to establish their own identities, a crucial developmental task of people in their late teens and early twenties.

The nursing care of clients who generate identification problems in others requires an understanding of the clients, but equally important is self-understanding on the part of the staff. Identification problems do not exist in isolation; they are always interpersonal and at least two people are always involved. Therefore the nursing process must focus on the nurse, the client, and the interaction between them in order to deal successfully with such problems.

Nursing Assessment

Every nursing assessment should include a consideration of the possibility that identification problems may develop. The client's age, sex, role, status, understanding of the illness, expectations of treatment, and manner of relating to the interviewer may provide clues to potential identification problems. The staff should also be aware that they may be more vulnerable to such problems when there are changes in staff makeup or staff relationships. For example, the addition or loss of staff members, especially those who are of special emotional significance, may provoke such difficulties. The following signs may alert the staff to the possibility that an identification problem may be developing.

The Staff

1 An uneasy feeling during interactions with the client
2 Repeatedly feeling excessive sympathy or anger toward the client
3 Permitting or encouraging acting-out behavior
4 Deviations from the previously agreed upon team-treatment approach
5 Permitting deviations from ward rules and regulations
6 A repeated tendency to engage in gossip about the client
7 Repeated, lengthy, nonproductive discussions about the client
8 Avoidance of discussion of emotionally charged issues with the client
9 Consistently excusing inappropriate behavior or consistently finding fault with the client's behavior

10 Getting conscious satisfaction out of a client's praise or acting in ways to elicit praise

11 Being unduly disturbed by the client's unfounded reproaches[6]

The Client

1 Endowing the staff with magical powers to cure or heal

2 Having unrealistic expectations to be cared for, reassured, gratified, comforted, given more beauty, brains, power, health, a job, etc.

3 Exhibiting unjustified anger toward the staff

4 Expressing a desire to continue the relationship beyond the time that is appropriate

5 Expressing jealousy at the staff's relationships with other clients

6 Taking on the characteristics of staff in dress, speech, attitudes

7 Expressing unjustified hostile, angry, sexual, or aggressive feelings and/or behavior toward staff

8 Inability to express negative feelings toward the staff

First, the client who may generate identification problems must be recognized. Once this has been done, nursing diagnoses, goals, and approaches which will prevent the development of such problems can be established. The goals and approaches should focus on both the client and the staff, since identification problems are the result of the nurse-client interaction (see Tables 22-1, 22-2, 22-3, and 22-4).

Table 22–1 The "Nice-Guy" Client

Nursing diagnoses	Goals	Approaches
An excessively compliant attitude toward illness and treatment.	The client questions the staff about tests and procedures.	Spend extra time with the client.
		Give complete explanations about all procedures, even though the client may not appear to want or need such explanations.
Denial of the seriousness of the illness.	The client verbalizes understanding of the nature of the illness.	Cast doubt or indicate disbelief at the client's denial of anxiety. Example: "You do not seem *at all* concerned about your surgery. Most people are apprehensive."
	The client acknowledges appropriate feelings in response to procedures or treatment, for example, anger, fear, pain.	Reassure client that pain, fear, anger, and other "negative" feelings are acceptable and expression of them will not cause the nursing staff to abandon the client.
Staff discourages the expression of real concern and feelings by fostering compliant attitude.	Staff verbalizes doubts that the client's compliant or happy-go-lucky attitude is a genuine expression of feelings.	Staff discusses the following topics: Why the client is presenting the nice-guy facade. What the staff is doing to encourage this. Staff's feeling toward clients who express negative feelings about their care.

Table 22-2 The Religious Client

Nursing diagnoses	Goals	Approaches
Discomfort with the intimate nature of the staff-client relationship as exemplified by intrusive procedures such as enemas, catheterizations, seeking of personal information, etc.	The client verbalizes feelings about intrusive procedures and examinations, expresses desire for privacy.	Staff acknowledge awareness of possible embarrassment to client because of certain procedures. Assure client of confidentiality of records, etc. Ensure client's privacy during any procedures.
Identity as a religious threatened by requirements of hospitalization, i.e., anonymity of hospital gown, etc.	The client compensates for threat by keeping accoutrements of identity readily available. Discusses feelings about anonymity of client role.	Address client by proper title. Encourage client to wear any part of religious garb which will not interfere with treatment.
Reluctance to express feelings because of need to maintain stoical image.	Client expresses feelings—both positive and negative—about illness, procedures, care.	Deliberately bring up the topic for discussion.
Staff's own stereotyped image of the religious impairs their ability to care for clients.	Staff acknowledge feelings when assigned to care for clients who are nuns, priests, ministers, or rabbis.	Discuss own past experiences with clergy. Explore own stereotypes of these clients.

Evaluation

The purpose of evaluation in the nursing process is to assess the client's progress and to identify the degree to which the nursing approaches have contributed to the resolution of the identified nursing problems or nursing diagnoses. The evaluation process should begin at the time that the nursing-care plan is put into effect. The nursing team should reevaluate the plan daily, taking into ac-

Table 22-3 The Professional Client

Nursing diagnoses	Goals	Approaches
Professional identity threatened by client role, therefore does not relinquish professional role and is unable to become engaged in the therapeutic alliance.	Client discusses feelings about change in status (from professional to client), is receptive to the treatment regime.	Deliberately bring up the topic for discussion. Example: "Sometimes it is difficult to be the client after being the nurse (doctor)."
Fears of loss of control over emotions, body functions, day-to-day regulation of life.	Client expresses fears.	Emphasize client's right to have ordinary needs and feelings. Encourage activities which are of interest and meet client's needs for control.
Staff feel that their professional integrity is threatened by an ill colleague.	Staff identify and verbalize own feelings of vulnerability, anger, etc., toward ill colleague.	Discuss: Own experiences as a client. Meaning of illness (i.e., failure). Career choice (i.e., physician or nurse as healer).
Staff feel threatened when providing care to a peer, i.e., that peer will be evaluating them and will be critical.	Staff identify and verbalize fear of failure and inadequacy precipitated by these clients.	Feelings relating to caring for a professional peer.

Table 22-4 The Client of a Special Age

Nursing diagnoses	Goals	Approaches
Client has difficulty relating to staff because of age difference.	Staff and client discuss feelings about how client's age may influence care. Client shares feelings, etc., with staff members regardless of age.	Deliberately raise the topic for discussion with the client. Example: "Sometimes people your age worry about whether someone my age will understand how they feel."
Client's developmental tasks are interrupted by the requirements of hospitalization, i.e., rules, regulations, traditions, etc.	Client adapts to hospitalization, so that the work toward accomplishments of developmental tasks continues. Staff adapts hospital situation to the needs of the client as much as possible.	Provide experiences that encourage the client's development. Example: Ask adolescent clients to make decisions about reasonable bedtime, number of visitors, etc.
Staff has difficulty relating to client because of age	Enhance understanding of the relationship between the client's age and behavior. See to it that the hospital experience affects the client's development positively.	Identify how client's behavior reflects the developmental tasks of client's age. Enumerate ways that clients may continue to work on their developmental tasks while hospitalized.

count the client's progress and any new information obtained since the last discussion. Based on additional information, the nursing-care plan may be reinforced, changed, or modified.

Since identification problems are interactional, the behavior of both the clients and the staff must be evaluated. The accomplishment of the short-term goals should bring about obvious behavior changes in both the client and the nursing staff. For example, professionals who are clients should behave less like colleagues and more like clients. If the nursing diagnosis, goals, and approaches are correct, the staff should treat them more like clients and less like colleagues. If the nursing-care plan for the nice guy, for example, is effective, such a client will exhibit and express more appropriate reactions, including some negative reactions, to certain procedures. Also, the staff will encourage the expression of both positive and negative feelings by clients. If, after a reasonable

period of time, the behavior of clients and staff does not change, then the nursing goals and approaches should be reconsidered.

References

1 Phillip Polatin: *A Guide to Treatment in Psychiatry,* Lippincott, Philadelphia, 1966.

*2 Lisa Robinson: "Sick Doctors and Sick Nurses Are Sick Human Beings," *American Journal of Nursing,* September 1971, pp. 1728–1729.

3 E. M. Waring: *Today in Psychiatry,* Abbott Laboratories, 1975, tape, side 1.

4 Rosemary Marshall Balsam and Alan Balsam: *Becoming a Psychotherapist. A Clinical Primer,* Little, Brown, Boston, 1974.

5 Brian B. Doyle and Walter J. Smith: "Using Short Term Intervention with Priests," *Hospital and Community Psychiatry,* January 1975, pp. 30–32.

6 Karl Menninger: *Theory of Psychoanalytic Technique,* Harper & Row, New York, 1958.

*Recommended reading by a nurse author.

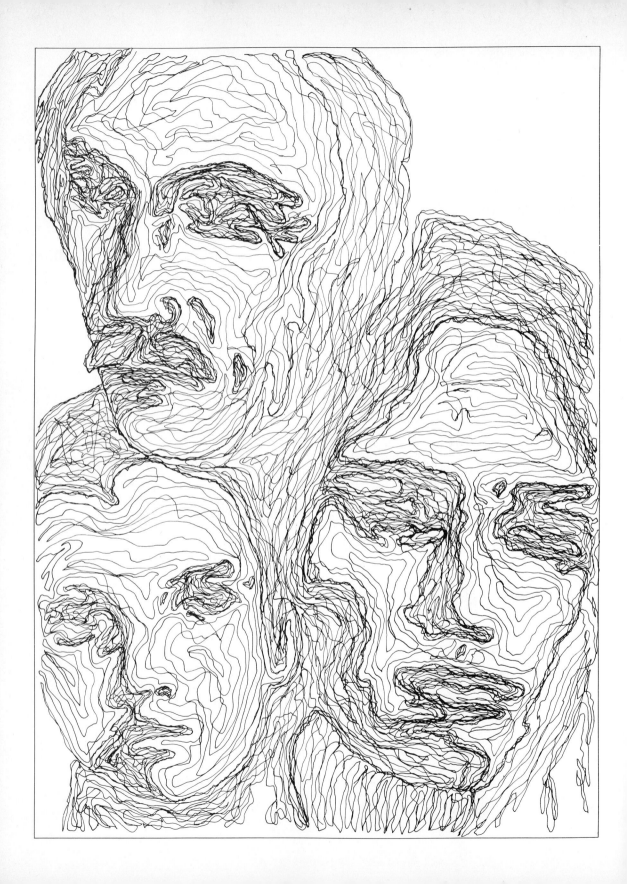

Four

Nursing Management of Family Systems without Manifest Psychiatric Disorders

Chapter

23
Psychodynamic Concepts Relating to Health

Roberta Mattheis

Learning Objectives

After studying this chapter, the student should be able to:

1 Define the concepts of identity, self- and body image, territory, rhythms, touch, sensory deprivation, and grief in relation to nursing practice

2 Use these concepts as a guide in the assessment of clients

3 Use these concepts in the formulation of nursing diagnoses

4 Use knowledge related to these concepts in determining and implementing nursing interventions

5 Use current self-knowledge as an effective tool in nursing care

Nursing science is moving toward maturity by developing, through research, a solid and valid foundation for nursing theory. Nursing practice is based on logically consistent concepts that are interrelated to form a theory; that becomes an explanatory system which describes and interprets phenomena observed in nursing practice. The selected concepts are a form of scientific language and a tool of science.[1] At this stage of theory construction, nursing is identifying, defining, and relating concepts derived from practice and from other disciplines. Selected concepts which have relevance to the care of clients and their psychosocial needs are examined in this chapter. Other central concepts—such as *stress, culture, values,* and *the nuclear family*—are defined and explained in Chapters 2, 3, 11, 25, 26, and 32.

Identity

"Identity" has become a word of the people. Identity is not a static, palpable thing but an ever-changing self-image that combines life experiences and perceptions with interpersonal relationships and emotions. Erikson states that identity formation involves simultaneous reflection and observation on all levels of mental functioning. Individuals use this process to judge the self in light of the apparent judgment of others in comparison to themselves.[2] One's identity is made up of experiences, memories, perceptions, emotions, and a mass of sensory inputs which somehow interact to form a gestalt of self-awareness.

The Body is Where the Self Resides

Self- and body image is what you think you are. But what determines what you think? Before you read this section, write down a description of yourself: fat, skinny, svelte, tall, short, dumpy, pear-shaped, intelligent, kind, efficient, disorganized, outgoing, motherly, informed, etc. Now look in the mirror. Does the written description match what you see? What are the discrepancies, if any? Most people carry around a mental image of themselves that includes the person they would like to be and the person they think they really are. Sometimes these images go out of date; a person who gains 15 pounds may have problems with splitting seams but even more difficulty adjusting his or her self- and body image to a larger size of clothing. Likewise, people who lose a great deal of weight may continue to think of themselves as fat when this is no longer true.

Generally, one's mental image is not completely up to date. Possibly that is because it is difficult to look objectively at oneself. Everyone is familiar with the various taboos of American culture regarding the body exploration games of young children; masturbation at any age has also been frowned upon for a long time. Both these instances carry overt associations of sexuality. The question is, then, when is any kind of body exploration permitted, let alone encouraged? Most natural opportunities for looking at and touching one's own body are linked with sexual play and are highly discouraged from childhood on. Fisher maintains that it is difficult to know one's own body because that involves *intimations of mortality.*[3] This conceptual framework serves as a boundary around the self, "the edge of me."[3]

These are powerful reasons for *not* knowing much about one's body. However, there are reasons just as powerful for acquiring accurate and specific knowledge about it. The most obvious is that a basic knowledge of a healthy body helps one to maintain health and increases one's level of response to a signal of disturbance in normal function. Self-knowledge is also important from a mental health standpoint. Fisher points out that those who are uncertain of their body boundaries tend to feel open and vulnerable to the world, with no secure, defensible border. People who are unsure of their boundaries—their *defensible borders*—will likely spend more and more time trying to check on those boundaries. They will be uncomfortable in group situations and generally will require more distance from other people. Having to continually shore up a shaky boundary obviously takes time and energy that might ordinarily be directed into more constructive behavior.[3]

If one lacks an accurate self- and body image, it becomes increasingly difficult to understand and interpret correctly the reactions of the rest of the world. People who cannot adjust their self- and body image to changes such as weight gain, amputation, or aging will experience increasing anxiety from the discrepancy and find it increasingly difficult to understand and react appropriately to the new way people are behaving toward them.

Each of the developmental tasks identified by Erikson contributes to identity formation. The physical, psychological, and social mastery of change in these areas of functioning provides a sound foundation and framework for a healthy identity, self-esteem, and self-acceptance. However, the identity, self-image, and body image do not become fixed with the attainment of adulthood. They continue to be challenged with the need to master developmental tasks throughout the life-span.

Identity Formation
Infancy
The self- and body image is essentially formed by the experience of *getting* things, of passively receiving nourishment, physical care, and love. Through this experience of receiving love and respect from a consistent mothering figure, *a sense of basic trust* in the self as well as the mother develops. This basic level of trust is the beginning of identity.[2]

Toddler
Possessing the sense of being a separate person and having developed motor skills and beginning language skills with which to engage the environment, toddlers are capable of controlling parts of the environment and parts of their bodies. The child intrudes on the world and a sense of initiative develops. Noticing physical differences and differing cultural expectations for the sexes, the child develops sexual orientations and role identifications. Children begin to interpret data from their environment regarding personal, physical, and intellectual characteristics; these influence self- and body-image formation.[2]

Childhood
At this stage of development there is a desire to increase knowledge and perfect skills; Erikson calls it a sense of industry. Self- and body image are influenced by the way in which the individual handles various tasks and assimilates new skills. Inability to deal with structured learning situations, which may be due to any of a multitude of reasons, can lead to a sense of inferiority. Self- and body image changes constantly throughout childhood. Bodily growth is phenomenal. As new tasks are encountered and mastered, new data for changes in self- and body image become available.[2]

Adolescence
Adolescence is often regarded as the stage of identity crisis; it is during this stage that all the accomplishments of preceding developmental stages come together to form an integrated identity. For some, this is a time of crisis, especially when some earlier task has not been satisfactorily completed. The last great spurt in bodily growth occurs, along with sexual maturation, adding new dimensions to self- and body image. The problem of autonomy arises again as the individual seeks emancipation from parents and childhood. Adolescents continually seek refinement and verification of their self- and body image through clothing styles, manner, music, social groupings, friendships, and first loves.[2]

Adulthood
During this period individuals develop their own resources; they are better able to postpone gratification and to give to others without necessarily expecting a return. Psychosexual adjustment and reinforcement of gender identity occurs in the process of selecting a mate and establishing and raising a family. There is a readiness for intimacy, the capacity to commit oneself to an affectional tie with a partner and to the care and nurture of a

child. Vocational identity is actualized and enhanced, providing satisfaction and opportunities for the further development of self-respect.[2] (See Chap. 32.)

Old Age
The realities of aging—changes in physical capacity, role definitions, and financial status—require an ongoing reassessment of identity in the elderly. Fears of chronic illness, loneliness, and dependency—as well as confrontation with the inevitability of death—challenge older people to examine their lives, present condition, and probable future. There is a need to see order and meaning in one's life and to accept the way one has lived. When there is integrity, the person defends the dignity of the life he or she has lived and accepts death as part of life and the history of humankind. Despair can be signified by a fear of death—a feeling that time is short and the life-cycle not yet complete.[2]

Periods of maturational crisis—such as marriage, parenthood, the "empty nest" stage, and retirement—require reassessment and revision of identity, of both self- and body image (see Chap. 5). Each maturational crisis is a time of both *increased vulnerability and heightened potential.* These crisis points in development are opportunities for a constructive reorientation and renewal in self- and body image.

There are also many other occurrences across the life-span that require adjustments in self- and body image, such as weight change, either loss or gain; chronic debilitating disease; mutilative surgery, disfigurement, or trauma; and changes in body function, such as impotence and menopause. Such changes may occur slowly or suddenly, as in the case of surgery or trauma. When a body part is amputated, most people retain a sense of feeling or phantom pain in the part that is no longer there. Nurses must prepare clients for this phenomenon prior to surgery, assist clients to deal with the grieving process for the lost part, and finally encourage the client in his or her reconstruction of self- and body image during the rehabilitation process.

After a psychotic episode in which self- and body image are disorganized and depleted, reintegration and reconstructive boundary building are required.[3] In psychosis, the body image becomes distorted; often one body part is perceived as being of greater or less than normal size or as having some gross structural or functional defect. Boundary perception is extremely unreliable. A psychotic person may not be able to tell where his or her body ends and the rest of the world begins and is often supersensitive to environmental stimuli such as light, noise, and the presence of others. Wearing bright clothing, touching the body, and even mutilating it serve to delineate a defensible border.[3] One of the now out-of-date treatments for psychotic episodes was the "wet-sheet wrap." This procedure was remarkably effective and may have provided the individual with a substitute body boundary.

Territory
Where the edge of one entity meets the edge of another there is a boundary. The concept of boundaries is applicable to objects large and small; living creatures, human and otherwise; and intangibles such as feelings, thoughts, and ideas. The most traditional application of the boundary concept is probably to physical spaces, as in the territorial boundaries of pieces of land. Boundary intersections are carefully surveyed and markers are established all the way from housing lots to international borders.

The initial boundary each individual is concerned with is the boundary of self. Many layers of fat can function as a reinforcement of the boundary of the self. Jewelry, styles of clothing, loud colors, cosmetics, tattoos, and perfumes are also used to define and reinforce one's self-boundary.[3] Self-touching or stroking, flexing one's muscles, clenching the teeth, and tapping one's feet or fingers are maneuvers that serve to reassure a person of the intactness of his or her boundaries, especially in stressful situations (see Chap. 15).

Mothers of small children are familiar with the magical powers of a kiss and Band-Aid to soothe the great distress that often accompanies small scrapes and cuts. All children know that when a balloon or stuffed toy is cut, the insides come out and the damage is severe. They reason quite properly that their own insides will spill out of a cut in the same way. The Band-Aid "closes up" the hole, making sure that no insides can spill out. What sort of psychological Band-Aids do *you* apply when something threatens the boundary of your self?

However, the self-boundary is flexible and there is a relationship between this boundary's integrity and the amount of physical space an individual requires to feel comfortable. "Shaky," insecure boundaries require more personal space; well-defined, secure boundaries require less.[3] In order to develop a secure boundary, an individual must first have a private space to work from.[3,4]

Personal space can be thought of as a semipermeable membrane which extends outward from the body. It is a portable territory which defines the space required between the self and another. This space requirement varies with the quality of the relationship. When the relationship is intimate, one loses part of the distinction between one's own body and that of another, and this entails some boundary loss. Interpersonal relationships have the potential for some degree of boundary disruption or, in intimacy, fusion with the boundary of another.[3]

The concept of boundaries can be further extended to include territory, which is a defined space or area an individual stakes out as his or her own. Territoriality has been well documented in animal behavior, and infringement gives rise to a fight-flight response. Humans share this need with the animal kingdom, and the invasion of territory is not dealt with rationally. Intrusion causes stress, which may be dealt with aggressively, passively, or by the displacement of feelings onto another person or the environment.

Surveyors' stakes and fences, uniforms, and defined work spaces all contribute external reassurances of territorial boundaries. White uniforms, caps in the general hospital, and keys in the psychiatric setting define professional boundaries. When these badges of power are not visible and the nurse is no longer easily identified, boundaries are not readily recognized; both the client and nurse may then experience anxiety.

Job situations also give rise to intangible territorial issues. Jobs with specific descriptions and those governed by rules and regulations obviously involve specific territorial responsibilities. Jobs with less specific boundaries require the individual to define the working territorial responsibility. It is easy to see that a less specific job description stresses the worker's personal boundaries more than a well-regulated position. Another territorial issue in work situations involves overlapping boundaries. Since two individuals cannot occupy the same space or "turf," overlapping job boundaries require some negotiation and compromise. When one is already insecure about a boundary, it can be very difficult to share a portion of territory with another, especially if the other is viewed as a competitor. This is an important concept for nurses to be familiar with since it is a rare situation, particularly in mental health work, that does not include some interdisciplinary mixing of personnel, with many fuzzy lines of responsibility and overlapping boundaries.

In health-care settings, caretakers and clients alike define their turf in terms of both physical space and responsibility. Perceived encroachment on this turf elicits defensive reactions.

Nurses must be both sensitive to the special needs of their clients and colleagues and aware of cultural influences. Hospitalization and the intimacy of nursing care disrupt client boundaries. These invasions are potentially stressful, arousing physiological and psychological responses such as increased grooming behaviors. Awareness of these boundary disruptions and their effect is the first step toward identifying ways to protect clients from loss of security, depersonalization, and powerlessness. Boundaries are an important consideration in communication, which is the essence of the nurse-client relationship.[5] (See Chap. 6.)

Aspects of Spatial Orientation

Rhythm

One of the key elements in the interaction of a living system with its environment is *rhythm*. A rhythm is a regularly recurring flow or movement, and each rhythm has specific features. Complex biological rhythms fall into two major categories: *exogenous* and *endogenous*.[6] "Exogenous" refers to those rhythms that are external, including the movements of stars and planets as well as gravitational and magnetic forces. "Endogenous" refers to internal biological rhythms, such as various biochemical processes, steroid and electrolyte excretion, cycles of temperature, heart rate, breathing rate, and levels of EEG (electroencephalogram) activity. The term *circadian* refers to daily rhythms of about 24 hours. A precise solar day is 24.0 hours, and a precise lunar cycle is 24.8 hours.[7] Rhythms of less than 24-hour or circadian cycles are called *ultradian*. Those with longer cycles, such as weeks or months, are called *infradian*. The term *cycle* refers to a circular process that starts from a specific point of origin and returns to it. *Period* is the time required to complete the cycle. *Frequency* is the reciprocal of the period; for example, sleep frequency in humans is 1:24 (i.e., one period of sleep every 24 hours). The *amplitude* of a rhythm is the amount or extent of change within a period. *Phase* refers to the time location of some part of a cycle, usually identified as *peak* or *trough* with reference to some external point such as clock time. Phases are the parameters of biological rhythms; for example, the diurnal portion of the circadian period is one phase, the nocturnal is another.[7,8]

In most organisms, biological rhythms are remarkably stable and accurate. Circadian cycles, as indicated by the feeding and activity phases, persist even when customary environmental cues such as changes in light and temperature are removed. Many creatures, including human beings, develop a *free-running* circadian cycle that typically fluctuates between 23- and 25-hour days when there are no environmental cues of any sort. When accustomed cues are restored, the cycle returns to a 24-hour day.[7]

When changes in the light-dark sequence or other parameters occur, the biological clock may get out of phase or synchronization with the exogenous cues of sunrise and sunset, etc. The creature then experiences *phase shifting* in order to conform with exogenous data.

Phase shifting is a stress which makes the individual more vulnerable. When rhythms are disrupted, demands are made on the person's adaptational system. Anyone who has experienced jet lag from crossing time zones by air travel can appreciate the process of phase shifting.[7,8]

In health, many body rhythms are not consciously perceived. When rhythms such as mood swings or hormone or electrolyte levels are phase-shifted or accentuated, the person senses dysfunction.

The human infant is widely considered to be erratic in terms of biological rhythms, but recent data indicate that even the fetus has intrinsic activity rhythms.[7] Two fetal rhythms have been detected by instruments in sleep research laboratories. One ranges from 30 to 50 minutes; the other, ranging from 80 to 100 minutes, is apparently related to the mother's REM (rapid eye movement) sleep cycle. Infants show a basic 60-minute rest and activity cycle, as demonstrated by quiescent and active sleep.[7]

At birth, there is only one truly circadian rhythm that has been identified: electric skin resistance, which is higher in the morning and lower at night.[7] By the second or third week, urine flow is greater by day regardless of fluid intake. At 4 to 6 weeks, heart rate becomes circadian. Between 5 and 9 months, higher diurnal body temperatures appear, along with circadian periodicities in blood-sugar levels and urine constituents.[7] A wide range of rhythms continue to stabilize throughout childhood, reaching the greatest level of stability in young adulthood. There is increasing evidence that some physiological rhythms may get out of phase in old age. The effect of social schedules on this dissociation has not been established, but certainly the circadian rhythms of old age more often resemble those of infancy than those of adulthood.

Sleep is one of the most tangible circadian rhythms. The sleep-wake cycle appears to synchronize other circadian rhythms such as temperature levels, hormone concentrations in blood and urine, deposition of carbohydrates in the liver, and urine production. Sleep itself is a series of cycles that are traceable by EEG. A normal adult sleep cycle occurs 4 to 5 times per night and lasts 85 to 110 minutes, usually averaging about 90 minutes. This basic ultradian rhythm period has also been demonstrated in waking activity cycles.

Sleep researchers have demonstrated four stages in the ultradian cycle: stage I or REM sleep is the lightest level of anesthesia. It is during this stage that most remembered dreams occur, as well as irregular pulse and respiration, increases in body temperature, changes in the conductivity of the skin, dilatation of peripheral blood vessels, production of corticosteroids, and—in males—erections. Stages II and III represent progressively deeper levels of anesthesia, with larger, more even EEG waves. In stage IV, the sleeper is difficult to arouse and exhibits slow, even EEG waves along with peak levels of growth hormone. Stage IV is also the point where most sleepwalking and bed wetting occurs.[7] It appears to be enhanced by exercise. The distribution of stages varies through the night, with stage IV predominating early in the night and stage I occurring mostly during the last third of the sleep period.[8]

Disturbed sleep patterns are common in the depressed. People who complain of poor sleep and various forms of insomnia usually demonstrate very disorganized sleep rhythms. They shift quickly from stage to stage, often awakening from REM sleep. A depressed person may fall directly into REM sleep instead of experiencing the usually complete cycle prior to the initial REM episode for the night. The depressed often invert the usual stage distribution, with REM predominating early

in the night and stage IV occurring toward morning if at all; they are thus clearly out of phase. Some people experience eight to ten cycles per night instead of the usual four to five, and there is an accompanying disorganization in hormonal rhythms. As other symptoms improve, sleep rhythm usually improves as well. Although the precise relationship between sleep and depression is not clear, tricyclic antidepressants seem to affect sleep patterns by increasing the amount of stage IV sleep, slightly decreasing REM sleep, and lengthening the entire cycle from about 90 to about 120 minutes.[7] Drugs such as phenelzine shorten the sleep cycle. Alcohol, amphetamines, and barbiturates also depress the REM cycle and the dreaming that accompanies it.

Sleep deprivation, especially deprivation of REM sleep, produces signs of emotional disturbance. If prolonged, it results in psychotic-like disturbances including delusions—often of a paranoid nature—confused sense of identity, and even hallucinations. Deprivation of stage IV sleep results in bodily malaise, apathy, and depression. Recovery from sleep deprivation seems to occur more readily in young, healthy personalities.[8]

Recent studies have indicated the importance of circadian rhythms in two significant areas of health care. There is increasing evidence that the susceptibility to infection is greater during periods of isolation from environmental cues and disruption of work-rest cycles. There is also significant variance in response to x-ray and chemical therapies at different points in the circadian cycle.[8]

Animal studies have shown that the same dose of bacteria is fatal given at the end of a rest period but nonlethal if given during the middle of an activity period.[7] Studies of large numbers of epileptics have shown that most seizure activity occurs during the same general time of day. Cardiac illnesses and diabetes show circadian symptom rhythms; asthma attacks and the peak levels of histamine response cluster in the early part of the night; and the effects of cortisone derivatives for asthma and antihistamines for allergic reactions are greater and longer-lasting when administered prior to 8 A.M. Salicylates remain in the body much longer when taken in the early morning than in the evening. Hormones used in treating Addison's disease—as well as insulin in diabetes—appear to be more beneficial early in the day. Some barbiturates, antibiotics, and hormones cause phase shifting after the drug is discontinued. Alcohol and various anesthetics appear to exert their greatest effect at the beginning of an activity cycle. Births and deaths cluster at night and early morning. Even protein is utilized most efficiently in the morning hours.[8]

Periodic illness such as manic-depressive disease and periodic catatonia have been documented for a long time. Premenstrual syndrome follows a roughly lunar cycle, as do emotional cycles in men, although male cycles are more subtle. During the premenstrual syndrome, women experience more infections, higher rates of psychiatric admission, higher accident and suicide rates, activation of chronic illnesses such as arthritis and ulcers, and notable changes in blood-sugar levels. Men also show marked mood changes with irritability, loss of energy, and depression occurring on a cyclic schedule.[8]

Statistics indicate that ulcers, allergies, and some psychoses are more symptomatic in spring, and that suicides peak in May.[7] Accidental deaths are much more prevalent during the summer months.

It is significant that hospitals maintain rigid schedules for patient care, meals, treatments, etc., and that patients incur the additional stress of having to adapt, or phase-shift, their own circadian rhythms to that of the institution, often without benefit of a wall clock or wristwatch (which is often put in the valuables locker for safety).[9] There is also evidence[8] that changes in the parameters of circadian rhythm due to illness can effect the functioning of the biological clock, making the patient's orientation to time and space that much more difficult and yielding an obvious clue to nursing care about the importance of supplying correct temporal and spatial cues. Temperature, in particular, has a demonstrable effect on the perception of time. As a person's body temperature increases, so does his or her perception of the passage of time; hence, when clients have elevated temperatures, they may feel that time is passing much more rapidly than the clock suggests. Those complaints about the long intervals between episodes of nursing care may not be at all unreasonable from the client's warmer point of view. The same logic applies for people experiencing severe pain.[10]

Another area of concern for nursing lies in the problems of shift work or personal work-rest cycles. Switching from one shift to another, particularly from day to night or the reverse, involves extensive phase shifting. Without complete phase-shifting efficiency levels are probably lower and the quality of work is in question, as well as the quality of sleep during the reversed work-rest cycle.[9] Some investigators[9] feel that the possibility of sleep-deprivation problems should be a real concern during shift rotations, since a considerable length of time is required for phase shifting of the circadian rhythms. Endogenous circadian rhythms —such as hormone production and temperature cycles—may take up to 3 weeks to shift. In the meantime, an individual may be attempting to work with a body primed for sleep and to sleep with a body primed for work. One must also be concerned with the rate of readaptation at the end of the reversed cycle, although that generally is much more rapid.

Another view of rhythm as a sensory input involves a more common concept: the rhythm of movement. Rhythm and music would seem to be inseparable components. Music and rhythmic dance movements are universal in the human experience, ranging from primitive tribal dancing to highly formalized Viennese waltzes to twentieth-century acid rock and the hustle. Music and its accompanying rhythmic dancing are expressions of a wide range of emotion; they can produce, in turn, just as wide a range of feelings. The tribal war dance stimulates feelings of aggression, the lullaby induces sleep. It would appear that much of the power of music can be attributed to its rhythm and the similarities of that rhythm to various biological rhythms.

The soothing rhythms of rocking and lullabies are being connected to the intrauterine experiences of the fetus.[11] Montagu points out that the fetal heart rate of 140 beats per minute combines with the mother's heart rate of 70 to produce a syncopated sound. It is not surprising, then—since the fetus experiences a rhythmic environment—that most children derive comfort from various methods of rocking, head rolling, crib rocking, and, as physiological development permits, dancing. Attempts to derive comfort from rocking and swaying movements are also easily observed among long-term residents of state hospitals, the retarded, and geriatric populations.

Touch

Montagu speaks eloquently of the soothing effects of rhythm combined with the tactual stimulation of touching. "To put one's arms around another is to communicate love to the other for which another word is security. To rhythmically rock the body when emotionally disturbed is comforting."[11] While the skin forms an obvious physical boundary to the body, it serves many vital functions, as Montagu points out, in terms of a communicator of sensory input. At almost any age, touching yields tremendous amounts of information concerning temperature, texture, shape, density, size, etc., of objects making up the organism's environment, making the skin a primary contributor to spatial orientation, along with eyes, ears, olfactory organs, taste buds, and inner-ear (balance) structures.[11]

This sort of physiological information is not the only datum available to the skin. A great deal of emotional information is also transmitted, as in the comforting gesture to which Montagu refers. The simple act of shaking hands transmits information from one person to another; the handshake is described as either forceful, crushing, strong, gentle, weak, limp, and so on. Speaking of American culture, Montagu notes that "One touches others largely in a sexual context."[11] This sort of interpersonal touching refers to postpubertal age groups and, of course, varies from culture to culture.

Krieger[12] has been engaged in research on "the laying on of hands" in nursing. She believes that the laying on of hands is a natural potential in

people, given at least two intervening variables: (1) the intent to help or heal another and (2) a fairly healthy body which would indicate an overflow of *prana* (vitality or vigor).[12] Beyond the therapeutic, comforting effects of touch, the force of *prana*, if it is possessed by the nurse, may be transmitted to the client, whose energy is deficient. Further research in this area and advances in the technological assessment of changes in health may yield theoretical implications for nursing practice.[13] Some research findings suggest that touching can be a positive communicator in work with patients suffering from chronic brain syndrome.[13] Bakker states that not all people can tolerate the same amount of closeness, pointing out the necessity, especially in psychiatry, of using touch discriminately.[4] The schizophrenic, whose boundaries are not well defined and whose identity is amorphous, may experience a loss of or invasion of self when touched.

Sensory Deprivation

Human beings are in constant interaction with their environment, exchanging a wide variety of sensory information. Sensory deprivation, especially of exogenous rhythmic input, creates stress, both psychological and physiological. The major symptoms of sensory deprivation are anxiety, tension, inability to concentrate or organize one's thoughts, increased suggestibility; vivid sensory imagery, usually visual and sometimes hallucinatory, with a delusionary quality; body illusions; somatic complaints; and intense subjective emotions.[14]

The two most popular theories for the phenomena of sensory deprivation are psychological and physiological.[14] Freud stated that sensory deprivation results in the suppression of secondary-process functioning, allowing primary-process functioning to emerge: "regression, confusion, disorientation, fantasy formation, primitive emotional responses, hallucinatory activity, and pseudopathological mental reactions."[14] The physiological theory states that optimal conscious awareness and accurate reality testing depend on a constant stream of environmental stimuli. The absence of such information promotes an increased prominence of various internal stimuli, rehearsals of memory, body-image awareness, and meditative thought. In the absence of environmental stimuli, repressed material tends to become conscious. Schultz's model of the nervous system, in which the reticular activating system functions as a homeostat, calls for more stimulation from the only available sources (repressed and unconscious material) during periods of sensory deprivation.[14]

A wide variety of clients are vulnerable to sensory deprivation: clients in ICUs (intensive care units), CCUs (coronary care units), the burn "bubble," and hyperbaric chambers; clients on respirators, medical or surgical clients subjected to decreased sensory stimulation, such as those recuperating from eye surgery or undergoing orthopedic treatment; the blind; the retarded; the chronically ill, the aged; and the infant. These clients must be assessed carefully for evidence of sensory deprivation and provided with sensory stimulation.

Increased sensory input is characterized by increased intensity, frequency, and/or rhythm. Manifestations of sensory overload approximate those of sensory deprivation.

Psychiatric clients are particularly vulnerable to sensory-input dysfunction. The basic factor in both deprivation and overload in all clients is the absence of meaningful contact with the environment. Clearly, optimum human functioning depends, at least in part, on continuous and varied environmental stimuli.

Grief

Grief is the normal process of resolving the loss of a highly valued (cathected) object, place, or person.[15] It is the process of separation. One of the more obvious separations in current American culture is divorce. As nuclear families split, spouses, parents, and children experience long or permanent separations from each other. Another current form of separation involves the mobility trends in this country. Relocation, particularly a long-distance move, involves separation from a familiar house/home, friends, possibly extended family, and local environment. Even when the relocation is desired by all concerned, the separation process will occur. A change in jobs that does not require relocation still involves separation from colleagues, familiar responsibilities, and established routines. Urban renewal—requiring the dissolution of "old" neighborhoods and dispersion of residents throughout the city—involves separation and loss of familiar surroundings and familiar faces. Less obvious and less disruptive separations are trading in an old car for a newer model (recalling memories of experiences in the old car), or discarding old clothing, memorabilia, or pieces of furniture.

When faced with an "empty nest," the woman who has made a major time and energy commitment to child rearing grieves for her lost role and the meaning of her life. The maturation process involves many separations. For the child and the parents, gradual separation is a developmental task. These separations are often symbolized by the child's graduation, moving out of the family home, first job, marriage. The feelings of loss evoked by these separations result in a grieving process.

Surgery, severe physical trauma, and chronic disease may alter body image, cause role reversal or loss, and disrupt significant relationships. Clients who have had hysterectomies, mastectomies, amputations, kidney failure, or disfiguring accidents must experience the grieving process to resolve the loss of body function, part, or image.

The ultimate separation of death itself can be sudden and unexpected, often called tragic by those left to grieve. It can be predicted in cases where there is a long illness or constant exposure to extreme danger, as in war. It can also be an accepted consequence of a long life, whether the lost object is a beloved family pet or an aged friend or relative.

With death, not only the survivors grieve. If the dying process occurs over time, the dying person must also separate from loved ones as well as from his or her own life. Thus, the dying person mourns the loss of self and relationships with friends and family.

An essential part of the process of grieving is referred to as "working through." *Working through grief* involves looking at a store of memories and things associated with the lost object, and *letting go*. While it is painful to think of what is lost, it often seems impossible not to.

The symptoms of grieving include the following:[16]

Somatic Problems Tightness in the throat; difficulty in swallowing or choking sensation; perceptible shortness of breath; sharp chest pains, light-headedness; empty feeling in the pit of the stomach; various digestive complaints ranging from nausea and vomiting in acute grief to apathy and lack of appetite at a later point; weary and weak feelings; heavy sighing evoked by thoughts about the loss.

Sleep Disturbances Insomnia, DFA (difficulty falling asleep), EMA (early morning awakening), nightmares; sleep is not refreshing.

Psychic Problems Preoccupation with the image of the dead person, lost body part, or object (grievers may be convinced they have seen the dead person, even seeking out "old haunts"); feelings of guilt about fantasied or real negligence toward the dead person or toward the self for not seeking treatment sooner; hostility toward those concerned with one's care or those who cared for the dead person; anxiety; inability to concentrate on normal patterns of living; depression; anger with friends for *not understanding*.

Grieving Behavior Clinging to possessions of the lost person or a former life-style; crying; dependency on anyone who is willing to temporarily assume the business or social responsibility; assimilation of the behavior traits and attitudes of the deceased by the griever; general restlessness.

The griever feels abandoned and experiences anger toward the lost person, but angry feelings are not acceptable and hence are guilt-provoking. Consequently, they are repressed and suppressed. Freud[15] wrote that ambivalent feelings, once aroused by the lost object, are redirected toward the self, thus accounting for the depression and anger (and sometimes even suicide) of the survivor. When ambivalence is strong, evidence of grieving may be absent. Unexpressed, these feelings have potential for causing physical and emotional distress and interpersonal dysfunction. A delayed grieving process also creates an additional problem for the person in that, when it is eventually expressed, it may puzzle others who do not understand the basis of the feelings and behavior exhibited. Consequently, support and understanding are not readily available to the griever.

Denial of the loss, a marked absence of grieving, extension of the process with intensification of the feelings, or evidence of depression with absence of feeling and marked apathy must be considered pathological.

Situations where the relationship with the lost object was troubled or where the griever has difficulty handling stress are especially likely to give rise to pathology. Maladaptive responses may include hyperactivity and sense of well-being inappropriate to the reality of the loss, often resulting in social and economic chaos; severe psychosomatic disease such as ulcerative colitis, asthma, rheumatoid arthritis, coronary disease, or assumption of the deceased person's symptoms; hallucinatory psychosis in which the dead one lives on; and agitated depression which may result in suicide.[16,17]

During the early stages of the grieving process, many grievers are concerned for their own sanity as they experience the intensity and pervasiveness of the symptoms. These acute symptoms generally last from 4 to 8 weeks. However, new situations and the anniversary of the loss may reawaken the intense feelings and reactivate the physical symptoms.

The healthy resolution of grieving, then, involves the incorporation of some aspect of the lost object into the ego structure of the griever. The intensity of the grieving is directly related to the intensity of the attachment to the lost object. In due time, because of the working-through processes, emotional attachment to the lost object decreases, leaving usually pleasant, even idealized memories relatively free of the initial intense emotion. At this point, usually 6 to 12 months after the loss, the grieving process is completed and the regular patterns of living gradually resume.

One of the most helpful things any person can do in preparation for dealing with object loss and particularly death is to be aware of his or her own feelings. Religious beliefs, philosophical orientations, and childhood experiences all contribute to one's thinking on death. Being aware of those contributions and being comfortable with them is the best preparation for dealing with grief, either personally or professionally.

References

1 Gordon DiRenzo: *Concepts, Theory and Explanation in the Behavioral Sciences,* Random House, New York, 1966.

2 Erik H. Erikson: *Identity, Youth and Crisis*, Norton, New York, 1968.

3 Seymour Fisher: *Body Consciousness: You Are What You Feel,* Prentice-Hall, Englewood Cliffs, N.J., 1973.

4 Cornelius B. Bakker and Marianne K. Bakker-Rabdau: *No Trespassing! Explorations in Human Territoriality,* Chandler & Sharp, San Francisco, 1973.

5 *Nonverbal Communication in Nursing,* Concept Media, Costa Mesa, Calif., 1975, pp. 48–57.

*6 Betty Bergerson: in Juanita Murphy (ed.), *Theoretical Issues In Professional Nursing,* Appleton-Century-Crofts, New York, 1971, p. 48.

7 Gay Geer Luce: *Biological Rhythms in Human and Animal Physiology,* Dover, New York, 1971.

8 *Biological Rhythms in Psychiatry and Medicine,* U.S. Department of Health, Education, and Welfare, NIMH, Chevy Chase, Maryland, 1970 (Public Health Service Publication # 2088).

9 William Peter Colguhoun: *Biological Rhythms and Human Performance,* Academic, London, 1971, p. 101.

10 M. J. Alderson: Effect of Increased Body Temperature on the Perception of Time, *Nursing Research,* vol. 23, pp. 42–49, January–February 1974.

*11 Ashley Montagu: *Touching: The Human Significance of the Skin,* Columbia University Press, New York, 1971.

*12 Delores Kreiger: "Therapeutic Touch—The Imprimatur of Nursing," *American Journal of Nursing,* vol. 75, no. 5, pp. 784–787, March 1975.

*13 I. M. Burnside: "Caring for the Aged: Touching Is Talking," *American Journal of Nursing,* vol. 73, pp. 1060–1063, December 1973.

*14 Phili Solomon and Susan T. Kleeman: "Sensory Deprivation," in A. M. Freedman, H. I. Kaplan, and B. J. Sadock (eds.), *Comprehensive Textbook of Psychiatry/II,* 2d ed., Williams & Wilkins, Baltimore, 1975, vol. 1, pp. 455–458.

15 Sigmund Freud: "Mourning and Melancholia," in James Strachey (ed.), with Anna Freud, *The Complete Psychological Works of Sigmund Freud,* Hogarth, London, 1966.

16 Erich Lindemann: "Symptomatology and Management of Acute Grief," *American Journal of Psychiatry,* vol. 101, pp. 141–148, September 1944.

17 Paul Huston: "Psychotic Depressive Reaction," in A. M. Freedman, H. I. Kaplan, and B. J. Sadock (eds.), *Comprehensive Textbook of Psychiatry/II,* 2d ed., Williams & Wilkins, Baltimore, 1975, vol. 1, pp. 1043–1055.

*Recommended reference by a nurse author.

24

Impact of Illness and Hospitalization

Mary Jane Kennedy

Learning Objectives

After studying this chapter, the student should be able to:

1 Define illness
2 Discuss the issues related to the right to hospitalization
3 Assess the impact of hospitalization on the individual and the family
4 Assess their response and its impact on the client's reaction to illness and hospitalization
5 Intervene to assist clients and their families to cope effectively with illness and hospitalization
6 Evaluate the effectiveness of nursing care

Illness

Illness has been defined as absence of health, a disturbed rhythm of life, diminished coping, an unsuccessful adjustment to life, and a loss of the sense of well-being and vitality.[1-4] In the past, illness has been considered an autonomous evil force outside the individual which attacks, debilitates, and kills. The advent of the scientific era brought the perception of illness as a defect in structure or fault in function that could be diagnosed, modified, or cured. More recently, the basis for illness has been seen to encompass the mutual interaction between the victim and the environment and the role of stress.[5,6]

People view illness as something to be treated with dispatch, prevented, avoided, denied, or used to control others in the environment so as to meet needs which have not been gratified in health. Help-seeking behavior is based less on symptomatology than on the person's perception, analysis, and unconscious feelings about the situation. Shontz has identified five factors which influence whether the person will seek or avoid professional help:

The degree and extent of symptom distress

The expectation of return to health if treatment is instituted

Fear of diagnostic and treatment procedures

Fear of discovery of serious illness

The self-concept that one is always healthy

Not all members of our society are health conscious or able to confront the possibility that they are ill—at least not until they are overwhelmed by symptoms. These people may recognize signs and symptoms of bodily dysfunction, but they fail or refuse to seek medical assistance because they believe that as long as the problem is undiagnosed, it does not exist; that the treatment would be worse than the symptoms; or that the illness must be endured because it is the consequence of unresolvable emotional conflict, a hex, punishment for misdeeds, or demonic possession.[5]

When illness strikes, it affects one's sense of well-being and life-style. Most health problems are minor, causing only a brief disruption in the person's or family's life. However, illness of a more serious nature requires hospitalization, in which case the person must cope not only with the loss of well-being but also with separation from family as well as protracted confinement in a strange environment.

The Right to Hospitalization

People have the right to quality health care, but there are limitations in our society on their ability to exercise this right. If illness strikes suddenly and severely, private physicians and clinics may not be accessible. To gain admittance to a hospital for treatment, a person must (1) be recommended by a physician who has privileges to practice in that particular hospital and (2) demonstrate the ability to pay for expenses incurred. According to the American Civil Liberties Union, in some instances people must indicate this ability to pay even before emergency services can be rendered.[7]

Once a physician has been selected for either an elective or emergency hospitalization, the client has no choice of institutions. This decision is governed by where the selected physician has privileges.

Today, health care in our society is an industry, and hospitals have unique organizational structures. They are organized partly around management and economic principles and partly around the prerogatives of the medical professionals who practice within the structure but are not a part of it. The consumers of service seem to have little influence except indirectly.

Thus the consumer of health care who requires hospitalization is admitted to an industrial, bureaucratic organization which is very complex, highly technological, and largely compartmentalized. The client may have developed a good rapport with the physician; however, once he or she is hospitalized for a major health problem, this physician may become only a background figure. Meanwhile, the client is taken over and bombarded by a wide variety of strangers—professionals and paraprofessionals—who are concerned only with well-defined components of the client's care. Upon hospitalization, when clients are psychologically stressed by the perceived loss of health, they must adapt to a myriad of strange people and experiences.

Impact of Illness and Hospitalization

Illness and hospitalization for physical or emotional problems has an impact not only on the client but on the family system as well. It is a crisis which may be coped with maladaptively, thus further disorganizing the individual and family. Or hospitalization may be dealt with constructively, thus providing an opportunity for growth and attainment of a higher level of wellness than had existed previously.

When people are admitted to the hospital, they surrender their roles in their families, businesses, and social worlds and assume the *sick role.* Parsons defined this role as a set of *institutional expectations* that people who are ill must meet and which society—inclusive of caregivers—expects of them.[8]

According to Parsons, the sick role is characterized by passivity. Care-givers are permitted to make all the decisions and perform any and all procedures without question. The person who is now a client is expected to tolerate everything without complaint: invasion of body and privacy, procedures which are painful or inconvenient, and suspension of preferences concerning eating, sleeping, and bathing. Paradoxically, this sick-role sanction carries with it the expectation that it will be abandoned as soon as possible and that the client will cooperate with the treatment program and work toward getting well.

Client Behaviors
Grief
Multiple losses are inherent in hospitalization. Confinement means a degree of isolation from significant others, while relationships in the work and social spheres of life are also disrupted. The client has an altered self-concept, being no longer healthy, functional, productive, or independent. The body image may be altered as well. These losses generate a grieving process. The degree of sadness, depression, and anxiety experienced and exhibited will be modified by the client's personality structure, perception of the present situation and the illness and view of other demands that were made in the past or are currently being made.

Hospitalization imposes a loss of control over the environment which may extend to bodily functions as well. A sense of powerlessness is experienced. Some clients find this anxiety-producing and respond with expressions of helplessness. Others deal with this powerlessness and anxiety by defending against their feelings with anger, which is projected or displaced onto the system, the caretakers, or the family.

Dependency
Physical illness which requires hospitalization demands varying degrees of dependency on caretakers. When the client's physiological status and feelings of distress are great, physical needs are primary and the dependency associated with these needs is in less conflict with the self-concept that values independence. However, as the client's condition improves physiologically, energy and attention are focused beyond the issue of survival and there is a striving for greater independence. At this time, enforced dependence on others as well as the demands of the hospital routine generate feelings of frustration and anger. The client becomes more irritable and frustrated. Family and staff may comment that the person "must be getting better" when they observe this irritability.

Regression
If the client is to assume the sick role and accept the passivity and dependency that go with it, some degree of regression must occur. Regression is an effective energy-conservation operation which

facilitates investment of all available energy in the restorative and reparative needs of the body. These clients become egocentric. Their world shrinks to include only their needs and satisfaction; survival becomes the primary goal. Concerns about home, work, or significant others which would otherwise occupy them are pushed out of awareness. The more severe the illness and the greater the physiological instability, the greater the client's capacity to regress. The extent of regression is usually evidenced by how easily and willingly the client accepts dependency. As the client moves toward health, the regression should diminish; this should be accompanied by a movement toward a more mature and independent level of functioning.

Fear and Anxiety

The illness experience in and of itself is anxiety-provoking, but this anxiety is compounded by the need for hospitalization. The societal perception that any illness requiring hospitalization is serious increases the feeling of threat and escalates fear and anxiety. People are confronted with their vulnerability, and this is frightening. Fears and fantasies, traumatic childhood experiences, medical television shows, or books and articles on health care may all heighten this anxiety. Each individual has a personal way of dealing with it. Some may be very quiet and minimally responsive to caretakers or family, while others are very talkative. There will be those admitted for elective surgery or diagnostic tests who will glue their eyes to the television set, a book, or handiwork such as needlepoint. Sleep is an escape some can use to avoid feelings, while others are plagued by insomnia. Physical movement is an effective way of reducing tension and—for those who are able—pacing the hallway may be therapeutic. The immobilized person loses this outlet; anxiety may consequently be free-floating or manifested in verbal and nonverbal behavior. Hospitalization may be equated with death because of the client's past experiences with family members, thus increasing fear for survival.

Problematic Client Behaviors

The emergence of maladaptive behavior interferes with caretaking, the treatment regimen, and progress toward health or a dignified dying process. These behaviors develop because (1) the client has an unrealistic perception of his or her illness; (2) the prognosis is poor, and/or family and caretakers are not hopeful; (3) situational supports such as significant others or nurturing caretakers are inadequate; and/or (4) needs are not being communicated, identified by caretakers, or satisfied, possibly indicating a nonsupportive environment.

The losses incurred by illness and hospitalization are real, and a degree of grieving is therefore to be expected. However, the losses may be temporary and limited in extent, in which case increasing depression and expressions of helplessness, hopelessness, and despair would be unwarranted. On the other hand, if the client's health status is serious and the prognosis poor, euphoric behavior would be equally inappropriate. Very sick people will employ denial to defend against the anxiety-provoking reality of their condition, but they will at some time grieve for their own loss and the loss of significant others (see Chaps. 23 and 31).

When clients resist or reject the sick role, dependency and regression do not develop. These clients often counter fears of regression and dependency with anger and hostility, which they project or displace onto the environment, caretakers, and family. Their angry, negativistic behavior often interferes with care and conservation of energy, making the convalescence more difficult and perhaps prolonging it. Their sarcasm, verbal assaults, and petulant behavior interfere with their communications and relationships with others. Often isolated as a consequence of this behavior, they begin to feel abandoned and rejected. If their personality structure is such that anger is their primary way of coping with stress, then this isolation, which is anxiety-provoking in itself, only serves to escalate their anger and hostility. Another problem with regression and dependency is that these behaviors do not always correlate well with the client's physiological status. A person may have made considerable progress physically but proceed more slowly in relinquishing regressive behavior, or just the reverse may occur. A client may proceed to an emotional plane which rejects regression and dependency prematurely; that is, the physical condition of the client may not have improved sufficiently to support the desired degree of independence.

When one is ill, anxiety, which is the consequence of necessary worry, is a motivating force for cooperation in the program of care. However, when anxiety escalates to unmanageable proportions, the client's behavior will not support efforts toward health (see Chap. 14). The demanding client who calls the nurse frequently, and often for seemingly unimportant reasons, may be communicating a fear of being abandoned and a need to test the environment before trust can emerge. Increased anxiety makes simple caretaking procedures painful or distressing. When intrusive procedures or tests are carried out, a high level of anxiety heightens pain sensitivity and may precipitate uncooperative behavior, which could result in injury to the client.

Family Behaviors

Families behave in many ways in response to a member's illness and hospitalization. Their behaviors are rooted in anxiety, fear or anger. Some families *rally around* to support the client through the experience. They are nurturing, attentive, and characterized by *"thereness."* This behavioral response may facilitate the client's acceptance of dependency and regression as integral to the sick role. When carried to excess, however, the family's support may interfere with the client's movement toward health, especially if family members fail to foster efforts toward independence as the client improves physically.

Some families feel abandoned by the one who is sick and burdened beyond coping with the additional responsibilities incurred by the hospitalization. Their anger and frustration may be directed at the client and exhibited by infrequent visiting or minimal communication with the client. The family may excuse this behavior by telling the client how burdened they are as a result of the hospitalization. Such messages may make the client feel guilty and anxious. This anger may also be projected or displaced onto staff or the hospital and expressed in a critical stance toward care or excessive demandingness concerning care.

Nurses' Response

According to Parsons, the sick role is an institutional expectation; providers, including nurses, expect that the sick person will abandon the self to the illness, surrender the prerogatives of other roles, accept without question their interventions, and do the work of getting well as they define it.[8] When the client's behavior is characterized by dependency and passivity and this is matched by the nurse's nurturing behavior, then there is congruency of expectations and behaviors. With this congruency, the "good nurse" and "good client" images emerge.

When anger, hostility, noncompliance, or free-floating anxiety are observed in the hospitalized individual, feelings of anxiety also tend to surface among the care-givers. Their expectations of the client are not met, and this, in turn, diminishes their own self-concept. Feelings of inadequacy and incompetence are generated. Individuals deal with stress in a manner consistent with the way in which other life stresses are handled. The personality structure of one nurse who feels incompetent and inadequate may lead her to respond with feelings of depression and apathy; another nurse in the same situation might become openly hostile and angry; while still a third nurse might use these feelings as a guide in assessing the interpersonal dynamics of the relationship with the client.

Anger usually begets anger. Thus clients who respond to their illness and hospitalization with hostility may be dealt with punitively by staff if the client's difficulty with dependency and regression is not understood. Nurses will tend to avoid these clients and display less accommodating behavior.

All behavior is communication, and as such it carries with it a message about how the sender preceives and experiences what is happening. It also, of course, generates feelings and perceptions in the receiver. Nurses who use this theory as a guide in their practice will examine their relationships with clients as sources of data concerning the reciprocal effects of client and caretaker on one another. Examination of these feelings and increasing self-awareness, coupled with behavioral theory, help the nurse to develop a greater understanding of the client's predicament and to identify appropriate interventions.

Nursing Interventions

The nursing assessment, diagnosis, and goals guide the nurse in the selection of appropriate interventions. Using Maslow's hierarchy of needs and the client's primary concern as guides, the nurse sets priorities regarding which problems are dealt with immediately and which are temporarily postponed.

Nursing interventions focus primarily on helping the client verbalize fears, fantasies, and perceptions so that misperceptions may be remedied by reality-based feedback and appropriate reassurance. The nurse acknowledges feelings and facilitates their expression in appropriate ways. When the client is receiving secondary gains from the illness which interfere with active efforts toward recovery, the nurse explores with the client and family the expectations in their relationship. These families may also need assistance in identifying and articulating needs and expectations and thus facilitating communication among members. As newer and healthier ways of meeting needs are used and found satisfying, the need to use the illness lessens (see Chap. 5).

Intervention involves helping the client to come to grips with the fact of being in crisis and facilitating the expression of whatever feelings are associated with the illness in order to bring them into awareness. If the client's coping behaviors are not helpful, the nurse can encourage the client to try alternative behaviors which will help the client

to redefine the situation and, if necessary, make some accommodation to an inescapable event. Reality-based reassurances and the clearing up of misconceptions or unrealistic expectations are extremely useful interventions.

A return to a state of equilibrium and the learning and adoption of new and more useful coping strategies signals a resolution of the crisis. At this time the client usually is able to make realistic plans for the future.

Evaluation

Case Studies

The following case studies illustrate the relationship between the components of the nursing process—assessment, planning, intervention, and evaluation—and the impact of the nurse's response.

The Client Who Demands Control

Mr. Boyd, a ranking university official, entered University Hospital for treatment of a recurrent gastric ulcer. Although private rooms were usually reserved for the critically ill on the unit to which he was assigned, he requested and received private accommodations.

Despite the admission order of strict bed rest and in spite of a stringent visiting policy in this institution, Mr. Boyd received visitors, mostly university officials, from early morning until 9 P.M. each night. When not in conference, he would be on the telephone. Whenever the nursing staff attempted to enter his room to provide care, it was usually necessary to wait until Mr. Boyd had completed some business transaction. Although smoking was prohibited for all patients, Mr. Boyd continued to smoke in his room. One evening before dinner, the hospital administrator was observed smoking in Mr. Boyd's room.

After 3 days of this activity, Ms. Lerner, the head nurse, called her supervisor and demanded that something be done to force Mr. Boyd to abide by hospital regulations. In conference, Ms. Lerner stated that she was angry because her authority was being undercut by administration as well as by the client. She also expressed frustration over the fact that a prestigious figure within the university had brought his powerful and controlling role into the hospital, thus effectively undermining her plan of care. Furthermore, and by no means least importantly, Ms. Lerner believed that, as a lay person, the client was not qualified to make these decisions.

Data analysis Mr. Boyd's behavior reflects a need to retain control in as many areas of his life as possible to compensate for his powerlessness concerning his health and confinement to the hospital. His special status in the system supports this defensive behavior. Regression and dependency may be very anxiety-provoking for this man, who is a decision maker and a powerful person when well. Because the system is supportive of the client's compensatory behavior, it may not be creating an environment which would facilitate adoption of the sick role and a lessening of denial.

Ms. Lerner is involved in her need to control and consequently is blocked from looking for the meaning in the client's behavior. Exploration of the conflict with her supervisor reveals the possibility that Mr. Boyd's behavior may be a defense against confronting the impact of illness and hospitalization. Redefinition of the problem—from a power struggle to defensive client behavior—alters the nurse's perception and indicates the direction for planning care.

Nursing diagnosis The nursing diagnosis is that use of denial and controlling behavior is interfering with the nursing care plan.

Goal The nursing goal is to assist client to accept the sick role and to participate in the treatment regimen.

Nursing intervention With an understanding of the use of denial as a mechanism for warding off anxiety, the nurse's posture changed from defensiveness to problem solving. The priorities for care were redefined as follows:

1 Explain care requirements and their rationale to client.

2 Involve client in planning a work-rest schedule which is flexible but which also maximizes the client's energy conservation.

3 Explore with the client how the nurse can help him follow the work-rest schedule and deal with visitors who do not honor hospital policies

Evaluation Once established in the helping role, Ms. Lerner became quite successful at convincing Mr. Boyd that abiding by the medical regimen, including the rule against smoking, might shorten his illness and hospitalization and keep his ulcer under control in the future. She also succeeded in helping Mr. Boyd to verbalize a realistic fear that illness posed a threat to his position of power within the university. Exploration of this fear led to a more realistic perception of the situation and a reduction in anxiety.

Mismanagement of the Family

Mrs. Carmella Pontillio, a 72-year-old widow, was admitted in acute congestive heart failure. Her seven adult children, their spouses, and their children descended on her en masse every evening an hour or more before visiting hours. In spite of the hospital policy limiting visitors to two per client, they all managed to gain entrance, and the two-bed room became jammed with people every evening. Mrs. Pontillio's sisters, nieces, and nephews visited throughout the day, often disrupting scheduled care and affording the other client neither rest nor privacy. Family members also insisted on bringing highly seasoned food from home after being told by the nurses that it would not be good for Mrs. Pontillio to ignore the diet prescribed by the doctor.

Mrs. Pontillio's condition showed little improvement since admission. Ms. Connors, the evening charge nurse, was cornered nightly by the critical and demanding family members to complain about the care. Members would also summon the nurse to the room frequently to fix Mrs. Pontillio's pillow, straighten covers, provide fresh water, or monitor the oxygen. On several occasions Ms. Connors suggested that the family limit the number of visitors and time spent so that Mrs.

Pontillio could rest. She also informed them that they were violating hospital policy.

One evening the unit was particularly busy. Two codes had been called, there was a new client who was confused and noisy, and one nurse who called in sick was not replaced. The woman sharing Mrs. Pontillio's room had an acute asthmatic attack during visiting hours. The charge nurse was summoned by panicked Pontillio family members who demanded not only that she do something immediately for the woman in acute respiratory distress but also that she move their mother to another room.

Ms. Connors bristled at their accusatory and demanding attack. She dispatched another nurse to tend to the distressed client and notified the medical resident on call. Then she loudly and angrily ordered all the Pontillio family off the unit. A heated, noisy argument followed and no one made any effort to leave. Ms. Connors called the evening supervisor and security from the bedside phone. The situation became chaotic and Mrs. Pontillio began to show signs of anoxia and respiratory distress, presenting a medical emergency.

With much effort and persuasion, security officers and the evening supervisor managed to move the family to the lounge at the other end of the floor, so that the nurses and doctors could attend to both women.

Data analysis Nursing ignored the family's invasion in spite of the violation of hospital policy. Since the other client in the room suffered in silence and did not complain, the nurses were able to avoid confronting this overbearing family.

The demanding and critical behavior exhibited by the family angered and frustrated the nurses. They tended to avoid and distance the client and family. When they were summoned to the room, they performed the requested tasks mechanically and perfunctorily.

Nursing recognized the deleterious effects of the number of visitors and the prohibited food and did inform the family. However, the nurses did not follow through, partly because they were intimidat-ed by the size of the family and their overbearing and argumentative manner.

The unwillingness of the nurses to enforce the hospital visiting policies also reflected their belief that they would not have been supported by administration had they acted to limit visitors. Policy exceptions had been made frequently in the past and without evidence to support the rationale for special privileges. On previous occasions when nurses had enforced the policy, they had been chastised. This left the nurses in an untenable position. Enforcement meant problems with administration, while ignoring the situation was less personally threatening but bad for the clients. Although annoyed by the family demands and criticisms about care and concerned about Mrs. Pontillio's progress, their own need to be secure in their jobs and to avoid the anger of the hospital authorities outweighed these issues.

Ms. Connors, under the pressure of an understaffed and overburdened unit, allowed the crisis of the moment to undermine a thoughtful and considered approach to the problem. Anger derived from past annoyances and frustrations was compounded by guilt feelings which arose when she recognized that her failure to consider the clients' needs first and act as their advocate resulted in a medical emergency for both.

Several problems for nursing care are present in this situation. Nursing felt they were placed in a double bind with administration and were unwilling to act. Their own needs became primary and they allowed the situation to get out of hand. When the situation was first noted and the impact on the client's health assessed, nursing failed to bring the problem to the attention of administration and the attending physicians. Documentation of Mrs. Pontillio's failure to respond to treatment and the family's sabotage of the treatment regimen would have provided a sound and valid basis for enlisting the needed support. The unfortunate failure of nursing to intervene early and firmly resulted in chaos and serious physical problems for both clients.

Failure to assess the impact of the Pontillios

on the other client violated her right to privacy and maximum opportunity for restoration of health.

The nurses' distancing and avoidance of the client and family were interpreted by the anxious family as a lack of caring and concern for their loved one. The nursing staff failed to recognize how natural it was, in view of their culture, for this large Italian family to rally around a sick member. In doing so, the nurses missed an opportunity to help the family understand and support the hospital policy and the dietary restrictions.

When the crisis did occur, the nurse responded with hostility and a show of force which only served to escalate the problem. The increased tension in the situation and Mrs. Pontillio's feelings of helplessness upset her to the point where her physiological equilibrium was still further stressed and she was precipitated into a respiratory and circulatory crisis.

Nursing diagnosis   The nursing diagnosis is that the large, demanding family is disruptive to the unit and to the care of the client.

Goals   The nursing goals are to assist the family to recognize the client's needs and the importance of supporting the treatment regimen, and to assist the client to stabilize physiologically.

Nursing intervention   Consequent to the incident, staff nurses, attending physicians, and administration sat down and discussed how they might work with the family and who would be the best liaison between family and caretakers. One of the day nurses who would be assigned to Mrs. Pontillio as primary nurse was also to provide this liaison. The family leader was identified and involved in the planning. From then on, he was kept well informed and allowed to participate in the planning. This enabled him to inform and reassure other family members and help them to understand the situation.

Nursing, medicine, and administration also studied the issue of policy enforcement. This unfortunate crisis brought the problem to everyone's attention and illustrated the need for administration to support staff and for staff to be more aware of the impact of rule violations on clients. It was decided that in the future, if a situation arose where special privileges were an issue, representatives from nursing, medicine, and administration would jointly discuss the issue and establish specific guidelines for the particular situation.

Evaluation   When the full implications of the family's behavior and its impact were discussed at length and supportively with family representatives, their behavior became more collaborative than disruptive. The son came daily to discuss his mother's care and progress with the primary nurse. The nutritionist provided family members with help on making the meals they prepared and brought in conform to the prescribed diet. The son was able to enforce limited visiting by establishing a rotating schedule for family members.

The discussion among nursing, medicine, and administration proved very valuable and productive. Each developed insight into the others' problems. The primacy of client needs was agreed upon and became the guide for all decision making.

References

1   R. Wu: *Behavior and Illness,* Prentice-Hall, Englewood Cliffs, N.J., 1973.

2   H. Sigerist: "The Special Position of the Sick," in M. I. Roemer and J. M. Mackintosh (eds.), *On the Sociology of Medicine,* M.D. Publications, New York, 1960.

3   T. Parsons: "Definitions of Health and Illness in the Light of American Values and Social Structure," in E. G. Jaco (ed.), *Patients, Physicians and Illness,* Free Press, New York, 1958.

4   G. Engel: "Homeostasis, Behaviorial Adjustment and the Concept of Health and Disease," in R. Grinker (ed.), *Midcentury Psychiatry,* Charles C Thomas, Springfield, Ill., 1963.

5   F. Shontz: *The Psychological Aspects of Physical Illness and Disability,* Macmillan, New York, 1975.

6   F. Backus and D. Dudley: "Observations of Psychosocial Factors and Their Relationship to Organic Disease," *International Journal of Psychiatry in Medicine,* vol. 5, no. 4, pp. 499–515, 1974.

7   G. Annas: *The Rights of Hospital Patients,* Avon, New York, 1975, p. 47.

8   T. Parsons: *The Social System,* Free Press, New York, 1951.

25

Stress and the Mind-Body Interrelationship

Barbara Flynn Sideleau

Learning Objectives

After studying this chapter, the student should be able to:

1 Define the concept of stress
2 Identify potential stressors
3 Identify factors which mediate the impact of potential stressors
4 Describe the physiological dynamics of stress and their relationship to emotions

Stress is a paradoxical concept which both enables people to survive and causes them to be disabled to the point of death. Stress has been defined in many ways and by many people throughout the ages. Presently it is a major concept used by nursing and is being researched extensively by many disciplines.

Historical Perspective

The term "stress" was first used by Cannon[1] in 1925 in relation to the fight-flight reaction observed in subjects exposed to cold, oxygen deprivation, and blood loss in a laboratory experiment. He described the subjects as being *under stress* as a consequence of these exposures. Cannon also coined the word *homeostasis,* which he attached to the adaptive functions of adrenalin and the sympathetic nervous system. He stated that there is a continual tendency in the subject to return to a *steady state* after a disturbance within the system, based upon a remarkable, complex system of buffers and feedback mechanisms. This work provided an important basis for the development of the concept of stress.[1][3]

Much later, Schoenheimer[4] extended Cannon's concept of homeostasis. He defined it as a *dynamic steady state,* that is, a constant process of turnover, change, and replacement. The living organism's tissue is subject to growth, change, and degradation and to the replacement and turnover of its molecular components.[2,4]

In the 1930s and 1940s, Selye differentiated between the *state of stress* and the *stress syndrome.* He defined stress as a *nonspecific response* of the body to any demand made upon it and as a *specific syndrome.* To clarify this point, it is important to understand that a *nonspecifically* caused change is one that can be produced by any agent. The *specific syndrome,* which will be discussed at a later point, is a defined pattern of physiological change induced in all subjects in response to stressors, or agents capable of eliciting this response. Exposure of subjects to such varied stressors as heat, cold, oxygen deprivation, prolonged conflict, or fluid and electrolyte derangements will elicit the same stress syndrome according to Selye.[2,3,5]

Wolff,[6] in the 1950s, described diseases influenced by *life stress*. He spoke of bodily changes resulting from stress and stress-producing factors in society which generate a person's response to the noxious agents and threats. In his view, stress resulted from disruption in life-style and/or relationships, deprivation of human needs, and failure to express needs or act to eliminate what is causing the distress. His thesis was that the stress accruing from a situation is based to a large extent on the way the affected subject perceives it. The perception depends upon a multiplicity of factors including genetic endowment, basic individual needs and longings, earlier conditioning influences and a number of life experiences, and societal pressures. In his view, the etiology of disease is a function of precipitating incident, setting, and past experiences.[6]

Schrodinger[7] elaborated the concepts of stress and homestasis by positing that, in the nonliving world, the amount of *free energy* (energy available for doing work) diminishes steadily and the amount of disorder and disorganization increases steadily. In the living world, on the other hand, over the course of biological evolution, the total amount of order and organization has increased steadily. Biological life can maintain its own organization and even increase the complexity of its organization. Living organisms maintain their dynamic state by acquiring free energy and information from the environment. Thus the *dynamic steady state* is a *dynamic equilibrium* of constantly interacting and inherently unstable biochemical systems.[2,7]

Thus the concept of homeostasis has developed from the idea of an internal dynamic state to that of a dynamic, equilibrious exchange between the system and the environment. The maintenance of human life is dependent upon such exchanges as heat and water across the skin; water, oxygen, and carbon dioxide across the lung tissue; nutrients and waste products across tissue in the gastrointestinal tract; water, salts, and organic substances across kidney tissue; and information and energy across all tissues which interface with the environment. The nervous and musculoskeletal systems are the major organs of adaptation which interface with the environment, but it is the integrated holistic organism which influences and is influenced through interaction with the environment.[2]

The Stress Syndrome

Selye defined stress as essentially the rate of wear and tear in the body. It is a dynamic state which raises the body's resistance to threatening and dangerous agents. It is experienced as fatigue, uneasiness, or illness and is manifested by the *general adaptation syndrome* or GAS[5] (see Table 25-1).

According to Selye, the response to stress is a tripartite mechanism: an alarm reaction, which is the direct effect of the stressor on the body; followed by the internal responses which stimulate defenses to emerge, or the stage of resistance; and, if adaptation does not occur, the internal responses which stimulate tissue surrender by inhibiting defenses, or the stage of exhaustion occurs (see Table 25-1).

When a stressor is applied, chemical alarm signals are sent out directly by the stressed tissues to the central nervous system and endocrine glands, particularly the pituitary and the adrenals, which in turn produce adaptive hormones. These adaptive hormones are the anti-inflammatory hormones (ACTH, cortisone, and COL) which inhibit excessive defensive reactions and the proinflammatory hormones (STH, aldosterone, and DOC) which stimulate defenses. The effects of these hormones can be modified or conditioned by other hormones—such as adrenalin or thyroxine—nervous reactions, diet, heredity, and the tissue memory of previous exposures to stress.[5]

Resistance and adaptation depend upon the ability to reestablish a proper balance in the internal milieu. Stages I and II of the GAS are experienced repeatedly throughout a lifetime. For learning, growth, development, and survival to occur, the person must experience and cope effectively with stresses. Mental and physical activity, emotions, and relationships with others are in and of themselves stressful and unavoidable. The local adaptation syndrome (LAS) is an inflammatory localized reaction to injury. It is an active defense reaction which strikingly resembles the GAS. There is an alarm signal caused by the stressor which mobilizes defenses; this is followed by the stage of resistance, which is outlined in Table 25-2. When exhaustion occurs, it is limited to the circumscribed area. However, several such limited exhaustive states may occur simultaneously in various parts of the body and, in proportion to their extent or intensity, they can activate the GAS mechanism described in Table 25-1.[5,8]

The stage of exhaustion in the GAS occurs when multiple stressors are affecting the body simultaneously or the stressor is applied repeatedly and/or in overwhelming intensity. When the stage-of-resistance mechanisms are worn out, adaptation fails to occur and the body surrenders. Although the body is an open system capable of acquiring free energy and information, the ability

---

Table 25-1 General Adaptation Syndrome (GAS)

Stage I: Alarm reaction
Weight loss
Enlargement of the adrenal cortex
Enlargement of lymph glands
Increase in hormone levels

Stage II: Stage of resistance (adaptation)
Weight returns to normal
Adrenal cortex becomes smaller
Lymph glands return to normal
Hormone levels are constant

Stage III: Stage of exhaustion
Enlargement of adrenal glands
Adrenal-gland depletion
Weight loss
Enlargement of the lymph glands
Dysfunction of lymph system
Increase in hormone levels
Hormonal depletion

Table 25-2 Local Adaptation Syndrome (LAS)

Momentary vasoconstriction
Vasodilation with hyperemia (redness and heat)
Engorgement of the site
Leukocytes migrate to site
Capillary-wall permeability reduced
Leukocytes phagocytize foreign substance and cellular
  debris
Leukocytes form a limiting circle around the site
A ring of fibrin is laid down around the site
Massive collection of leukocytes forms within ring
Bone marrow is stimulated to produce more leukocytes,
  particularly polymorphonuclear leukocytes

---

to exchange and utilize input has limitations. According to Selye,[3] the ultimate consequence of unremitting stress is the stage of exhaustion, which indicates that adaptational energy is finite. This energy is not yet measurable or operationally defined, but evidence is convincing that it exists and that it can be depleted.

Exhaustion is not always irreversible and complete as long as it affects only parts of the body and vigorous efforts are made to eliminate or ameliorate the stressor. However, if the total body's defense systems are involved or there are no respites—even brief ones—from the stress, the body's capacity to defend will be exhausted, adaptational energy will be depleted, and survival will be at risk.

Stressors

As previously indicated, agents capable of eliciting the GAS or LAS are many and varied. Potential sources of stress can be classified into three major categories: (1) the external physical environment, which includes both natural and the artificial agents; (2) the individual's internal milieu; and (3) the psychosocial milieu.

The External Physical Environment
Nature is the first and primary stressor encountered by living organisms. The natural physical environment possesses a number of potential agents which place demands on people's coping capacity. Environmental stressors of this nature include heat, cold, humidity, light, atmospheric electricity, pressure, and altitude. Overexposure to cold causes frostbite; and overexposure to heat causes thermal skin burns. If there is inadequate oxygen, hypoxia occurs; and changes in atmospheric pressure will alter blood gases.

The pollutant by-products of our industrial society affect the artificial physical environment as numerous noxious physical and chemical agents are released into it. High levels of gases, airborne particles, and chemicals in our water and food have been identified as being causes of disease or—in other words—triggers of the GAS and LAS. The ionizing radiation produced by x-ray equipment has not only diagnostic and treatment properties but may—if there has been overexposure— have deadly side effects as well. Noise is yet another stressor in the artificial physical environment. People who work with machines which produce a continuous ear-shattering din and those who work or live in the presence of jet-engine noise are subject to neural damage to their auditory system.

The Internal Environment
The division of potential sources of stress into the external and internal environments is an artificial way of organizing and classifying stressors; this is clearly indicated by considering the stress produced by a deficiency state of the internal milieu. Such a state often exists because there has been an interference in the supply of essential elements that must be obtained from the external environment. Inadequate nutrition, an insecure environment, and distortion of sensory input (deprivation or overload) are stresses which illustrate the mutual interaction between the external and internal environments. Maslow's concept of physical needs serves as a guide for identifying stressors in this category.

The person's internal milieu may also be stressed into disequilibrium if there is interference with the production or utilization of essential substances formed in the body. Derangements involving thyroxine, insulin, enzymes, or blood components such as platelets or leukocytes are examples of such stressors. Usually these internal endocrine, organ, or system derangements reflect a sustained stage of resistance or limited exhaustion as a consequence of the body's efforts to cope with other stressors.

A person's interaction with the environment will help to determine whether stressors will be manageable or exhausting. Factors within the internal milieu which mediate the effect of stressors include the genetic pool, maturation, earlier conditioning, and perception.

The Genetic Pool

The genetic pool is the foundation of each person's inherited physiological strengths/weaknesses and potential. The prenatal environment as well as later life experiences influence the expression or inhibition of these inherited "givens." People are born with variables in these givens which predetermine which body system or organ will be most vulnerable to stress and hence be the first to become exhausted.[9]

Maturation

Experiences in infancy influence the maturation of basic neuroendocrine processes which in turn influence body organs and systems and the development of rhythms, such as the circadian rhythm in adrenal function. The development of these neuroendocrine processes also has lifelong effects on adrenocortical activity. Corticovisceral theorists postulate that psychophysiological disturbances may be caused by faulty enteroceptive signaling, that is, by defects in those mechanisms whereby cortical impulses transmitted to internal organs are either inhibited or overactivated. These dysfunctions become an established pattern when stressful experiential events occur repeatedly and are translated into the altered psychophysiological states. These early psychophysiological changes provide the background for further environmental

stimuli which are superimposed. The combined neural and endocrine regulatory mechanisms affected by stressors influence not only the development of disease but its progression and severity as well.[9,10]

These involuntary neuroendocrine reaction patterns which have been conditioned in the past may be elicited by social stimuli symbolic of previous experiences which influenced their development. Thus psychosocial stress mediated by these altered neuroendocrine reaction patterns can affect heart rate, blood pressure, the amounts of circulating free fatty acids (producing rapid changes), ovulation, renal water transport (causing changes that range from diuresis to suppression), insulin production and function, the growth rate of neoplasms, and the effectiveness of the autoimmune system.[2]

Throughout the life-span, individuals are exposed to a wide variety of experiences. In some instances, the demands of growth, development, expectations of others, and the environment are congruent and within the individual's capacity to cope. The stresses they experience are growth-promoting and life-enhancing; their exposure to the demands of life are on a manageable gradient, broadly diverse and supported. For others, life experiences are more intense and accelerated, either too numerous or too limited, unsupported and punctuated by crisis. When such experiences make demands that overtax the developing person's capacity to control, mediate, or manage, inherent strengths may not be enhanced and weaknesses may be accentuated. These people are more apt to have their adaptational energy depleted; consequently they are at risk even when coping with the stress of daily living (see Chap. 5).

Perception

Each person is unique. Individualized needs, expectations, and perceptions derived from conditioning experiences and inherited potential influence the impact of stressors. What may be seen as a threat by one person is a challenge to another. One's personality structure and ego integration affects the perceived degree of threat presented by a stressor and the number of stressors that can be adequately managed at one time. Environmental support or perceived security also affects the capacity to confront and manage stress. Environments characterized by high levels of interpersonal involvement are associated with increased psychoendocrine and cardiovascular response. However, high levels of support, cohesion, and/or affiliation seem to reduce susceptibility to physiologic stress provided that one does not deviate from group norms.[11]

According to Wolff,[6] people react not only to the direct application of stressors but also to threats and symbols of the past. Each person perceives, interprets, and responds in the light of past experiences. If throughout childhood a person is rejected or treated harshly and unjustly by parental figures, confrontations with authority figures in adulthood will reactivate these memories and elicit an expectation of similar treatment. Such a person will, in later life, approach authority figures with anxiety or hostility, which may be either overt or manifested by dysfunction in a body organ or system. A child living in an argumentative family that communicates by fighting may learn, through a series of accidental events, that when he becomes ill and complains of abdominal pain, nausea, and vomiting, the family will abandon their battling and become nurturing. When confronted by a similarly hostile situation in adulthood, such an individual may experience an unconscious reactivation of this response mechanism and develop abdominal distress because he unconsciously hopes to defuse the situation and produce a more secure climate.[6]

Psychosocial Milieu

Psychosocial factors which are stressors include social milieu, change, conflict, power balance, responsibility, vocational satisfaction, and communication.

Any situation which elicits the activating emotions of fear, anger, anxiety, or elation is stressful and generates a physiological response. However,

one of the most important mediating factors affecting a person's response to a social situation which is potentially stressful is his or her perception of the event. Two people in the same situation may perceive and respond differently because of their unique inherited genetic potential, individual needs and aspirations, and earlier conditioning experiences.[6,12]

Social Milieu

Crowding and population density have been considered potentially stressful factors contributing to the development of disease and emotional disturbance. Animal studies have revealed dramatic negative effects, particularly a breakdown in social behavior, when there was increased density of population in an enclosed area. However, crowding in human populations does not always seem to produce stress-related problems. What seems to make a difference is not the number of people living and working in a limited amount of space but other factors such as food supply, pollution, availability of needed resources, and the effects of having to interact with a large number of individuals. If people are protected from noxious environmental stressors, are able to meet their needs, and not placed in situations where they are forced to interact with large numbers of others, then the density of the population does not seem to have an adverse effect on their coping capacity or health.[13]

Change

Any event which interferes with existing adaptive patterns of meeting needs for love, belonging and self-esteem generates stress and demands coping efforts.

Loss of a significant person, role, or relationship is inherently stressful. The grieving process is a healing one and an appropriate way of coping, but it is stressful both psychologically and physiologically. The psychological and somatic symptomatology that accompanies grief work reflect the effects of the stress (see Chap. 23). Research has documented the relationship between loss and the development of psychological and physiological disorders.[2,9,14-19] Change of any type is one of the most important stressors and most common. Our society is characterized by accelerated change which affects people in their work as well as their recreational and living environments.[20]

Disruption is inherent in change and change is inherent in interpersonal relationships, consequently demands for adaptation are inevitable. From the moment of birth to the end of life, people experience separation and differentiation from others. No human relationship is static. Forces emerge from the external and internal environments to alter these relationships. The growth and development process and differing personal perceptions of events, all of which alter roles and relationships, occur across the life-span. The child moves away from the parents, and these steps in separation generate feelings of loss in both the child and parents. Failure to separate and denial of the need for autonomy is also stressful. The maturational crises one encounters across the life-span are infused with stressors. The changes that occur in adolescence, marriage, procreation, the launching of children, aging, retirement, and death include elements of loss, altered expectations, and changes in need-fulfillment patterns (see Chaps. 5, 11, and 23).

According to Hinkle,[2] the major biological challenges in our society most often stem from the requirements of social roles and interpersonal relationships. Stressors capable of causing negative physiological or behavioral responses are likely to be those that are symbolic of change in relationships with significant others in the environment. Social demands appear to take priority over people's attendance to homeostatic needs and their gratification. Thus interpersonal transactions may produce direct neuroendocrine responses as well as overt behavioral responses which may have major physiological consequences. Overload of information and environmental stimuli may have destructive effects on psychological and physiological health; these effects depend on how the data are perceived, which in turn depends on how they are mediated by personality variables, roles, status, relationships, and behavioral patterns.[21]

Individuals and environments are in constant flux. Consequently there is an ever-present need to adapt to internal and external changes. A degree of instability always exists. Massive and accelerated changes within a short span of time will stress neuroendocrine mechanisms and even alter them, precipitating dysfunction in whatever organs, tissues, or cells are most vulnerable in the person affected.

Vacations, going away to college, a promotion, or relocation into a more spacious and luxurious home are all life events which imply happiness or success. Yet each life change of this kind also creates stress in those who experience it. Vacations do not always mean relief from the pressures of work and relaxation. The "workaholics" are so pathologically involved and bound to their work life that taking time to relax or have fun challenges their ego integration and life-style. The drastic changes and reorientation are anxiety-provoking, and these vacationers may feel guilty about not being productive. Freedom and relaxation are stressors to these people.

A promotion is usually considered a pleasant and positive experience; nevertheless, it is a potential stressor. Job change can mean increased responsibility, the need to develop new skills, and the loss of established patterns of behaving and interacting. When people are promoted to positions for which they are ill prepared or for which they lack inherent ability, the stress they experience contributes to the development of a wide range of psychophysiological disorders. The stress generated in such situations derives in part from the striving and work overload and in part from the distress these people feel when they recognize that they are actively trying to work and wanting to do a good job but unable to do so because of their incompetence.[22]

Upward mobility means changes in social and work relationships. The established patterns of relating, living, finding recreation, and valuing are disconfirmed by the expectations of the new social milieu. Previous ways of predicting social interactions and expectations and fulfilling needs are no longer relevant, so that each new encounter or event involves an element of the unknown which elicits activating emotions such as anxiety, fear, and anger.

The sudden acquisition of a large sum of money or the loss of financial security due to layoff or retirement have an equal potential for stress. Changes in body image create tension regardless of whether the alteration is due to pregnancy, weight reduction, aging, radical and disfiguring surgery, or debilitating disease.

Holmes and Rahe[23] developed the Social Readjustment Rating Scale to measure changes in people's life circumstances which would predict the onset of general disease or disability. Their research indicates that somatic and psychological illness is associated with a high life-change score for the time period immediately prior to the illness. These findings suggest that demands for multiple changes in one's life deplete adaptational energy and increase susceptibility to health problems.

Conflict

An environment that is stressful triggers anxiety and depression, which in turn may lead to conflict. People strive for goals, acceptance, or rewards but sense and anticipate danger which will jeopardize their status, role, or relationship to others. Lipowski[21] claims that affluent societies provide an overabundance of attractive stimuli, decision-making alternatives, and accelerated change which generate conflict, particulary in the context of ambiguous societal values and norms.

When conflict is present, defenses are elicited to protect the self from the perceived danger. However, the action necessary to satisfy needs may be blocked, so that a conflict develops between the drive to satisfy needs and the drive for security.[24]

Conflict has many positive functions. It prevents stagnation, stimulates interest and curiosity, and is a mechanism by which disagreements can

be resolved. Conflict is the root of personal and social change and as such is inherently stressful. It exists whenever incompatible activities occur. A number of variables affect its course and determine whether it will be a manageable or a destructive experience for the participants. The variables which influence the participants in the conflict process includes:[25,27]

- The congruence or incongruence of values
- Motivations, aspirations, objectives of each
- The physical, intellectual, and social resources of both
- The beliefs each holds about the conflict, strategies, tactics, and the rightness of his or her position
- The nature of the issue; its scope, rigidity, and significance
- Previous experiences with each other
- Expectations of the other
- Beliefs about the other's perception of the situation
- The degree of polarization that has occurred
- The social context in which the conflict is taking place; whether it facilitates or deters
- Norms, the existence of institutional mechanisms for regulating the conflict
- The interest and influence of other parties and their relationships to the participants
- The strategies and tactics used by each party in the conflict
- The consequences of the conflict for each party

Each of these factors influences the way the people engage in the conflict, the strategies and tactics they select, and their hope that resolution will not affect them adversely.

Most important to the course of conflict is whether it occurs within the context of competitive or cooperative processes. The former more often lead to destructive effects on one or all participants; whereas with the latter, *authentic conflict* may provide the basis for growth and improved relations. Destructive conflict, be it interpersonal or intrapsychic, is characterized by escalation of intensity and scope, unreliable and impoverished communication, an inadequate data base, the belief that solutions are polarized with either a win or lose outcome, and suspicious and hostile attitudes which increase sensitivity to differences while minimizing similarities. If a cooperative context exists, resolution of the conflict can be growth-promoting and mutually beneficial to all concerned. The nature of this context is characterized by open information exchange, recognition of the legitimacy of other positions, a maximization of similarities, and a minimization of differences.[25]

Conflicts can occur interpersonally between parent and child or husband and wife; among siblings, peers, coworkers, and family members; and with authority figures. But conflict can also arise intrapsychically. When people feel that they are in an untenable position—that confronting the conflict would threaten their very survival and that no possible solution would benefit them—they are subject to severe stress. The perception that no satisfactory solution is possible generates feelings of helplessness and hopelessness; if this state extends over time, the stage of exhaustion will be inevitable.

Power Balance

Power to cope effectively with stress is a function of the person's past successes or failures in managing stressful events, present physiological status, belief that the threat is manageable, and perceived support from the environment if the threat should be confronted. Problems in any of these dimensions will weaken the person's position. Environmental power is also variable. Forces impinging from other systems and the introduction of new people or changes in circumstances may alter the intensity and number of stressors emanating from the milieu.

Responsibility

Responsibility—which is a complex socioenvironmental dimension—is associated with physiological change and is thus a significant stressor. Responsibility for avoidance of threat to oneself or others and for symbolic outcomes can produce a physiological stress response.[11]

Vocational Satisfaction

Vocational satisfaction is yet another socioenvironmental stress variable. The fit between an individual's personality and the work environment is important. A job fraught with conflict, rapid change, role blurring, and unrealistically high performance standards is potentially stressful. However, it must be noted that two people in such a situation may perceive the same milieu differently or, given the same perception, may differ in their affective and adaptational responses to these perceptions.[11]

Communication

Communication networks are potentially stressful when informational incongruities invalidate one's beliefs, ideals, and perceptions. If they are not resolved, these incongruities increase susceptibility to illness; the stress evoked alters physiological functioning and produces changes in the social network. If alienation and anomie persist, the subjective noninvolvement and withdrawal from social relations results in an impoverished data base which, in turn, contributes to misperception and increased stress.[28]

Adaptation

When people are confronted by a threatening stressor, according to Withey,[29] they make a series of thoughtful appraisals. They attempt to estimate:

- The nature of the impending danger and its expected unfavorable consequences

- The probability that the dangerous event will occur
- The severity of the loss to self if the event materializes
- The means available for coping with the potential danger
- The probability of success of alternative means
- The probable cost of using each of the alternative effective means
- The course of action that will most likely succeed at minimal cost

The individual's ability to follow this cognitive process to its end will depend on his or her mental set. If anxiety is pervasive, this cognitive, deliberate problem-solving process will be overwhelmed by the affective domain. Strong activating emotions interfere with the use of logic and the effectiveness of the perceptual system. When problem-solving ability is dysfunctional, the noxious effects of the stressor predominate, becoming intense and/or prolonged. Problem solving based on cognition enhances coping while predominantly affective reactions predispose to maladaptation.

Physiological Dynamics

The subjective indices that one is being stressed include nervousness, inertia, insomnia, heart palpitations, trembling hands, sweating, headaches, dizziness, fainting, and nightmares.[30] These symptoms, psychopathology, and organ and body-system dysfunction develop as a consequence of stress. The cerebral cortex, autonomic nervous system, endocrine system, and hypothalamus mediate this physiological response to stress.*

When people encounter stressors, the fight-flight response is activated. They either flee the

*The student is directed to a text dealing with anatomy and physiology for further discussion of the structure and function of these organs and systems.

situation or get ready for battle. Figure 25-1 illustrates the polarity of the responses as well as the behaviors and feelings which accompany both fight and flight.

The fight-flight response developed as a survival mechanism in the course of evolution. It is a primitive response which was necessary in the past for the survival of the species. The anxiety which is evoked in the face of danger activates the complex physiological response which enables the person to either fight or flee.[31]

When stressors impinge on people, their reactions are mediated by the perceptual system, which in turn notifies the central nervous system. The central nervous system can respond by initiating activity in any part of the body, since all vital organs are under its control. There may be gross motor activity, which enables the person to run from the situation, as well as alterations in the functioning of the autonomic nervous system and in the activation of the endocrine system.[2]

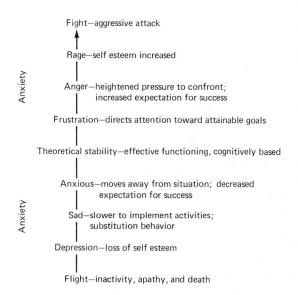

Figure 25-1 Anxiety is a basic human response to conflict, change, or unmet needs that may be manifested by flight behavior (a progressive distancing of self from the perceived source of anxiety) or fight behavior (a progressive confrontation).

The autonomic nervous system has two divisions, the sympathetic and parasympathetic. It has important short- and long-term effects upon the function of any muscular or glandular organ it innervates. Its two divisions convey impulses having opposite or antagonistic effects, depending on circumstances such as physiological requirements and the organ concerned. One division may override the other; however, there is generally a balance between impulses sent by both divisions, and this balance plays a major role in the maintenance of homeostasis.[32]

The autonomic nervous system contributes to the maintenance of dynamic equilibrium by acting on sweat glands, body-fluid balance (by controlling the excretion of sweat glands and kidneys), the heart (its rate and the force of its contractions), blood pressure, enzyme production, blood-sugar levels, hormone production, and digestion. The autonomic nervous system also influences such physiological processes as the secretion of sebum; the secretion of aqueous humor in the eye;

nasal and bronchial secretion; the motor and secretory activity of the esophagus, stomach, biliary tract, pancreas, and large and small intestines; and the engorgement and secretions of the genital tract.[32]

The endocrine system also plays an important role in a person's reaction to stress. This system, acting either directly or through a variety of complex interactions with the nervous system, may have a pervasive influence upon the enzyme system, metabolic processes, and membrane permeability at the molecular and intracellular levels. These, in turn, influence processes such as cell division, growth, maturation, energy metabolism, fluid and electrolyte metabolism, the inflammatory process, the immune system (specifically antibody production), and ovulation or spermatogenesis.[2]

The endocrine glands are interdependent to varying degrees. Their reciprocal relationships provide an important feedback mechanism. The endocrine mechanisms appear to be a signaling

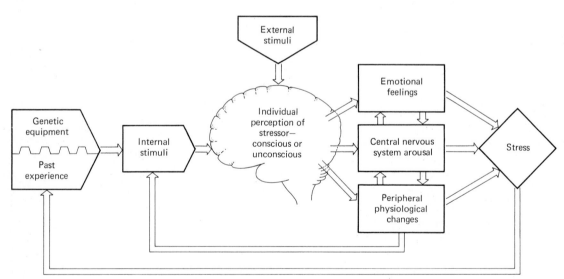

Figure 25-2 Stress may be derived from either the internal or external environment, is mediated by genetic endowment, past experience, and perception, and elicits emotional, physiological, and social responses in the individual. (Used with the permission of Alma Miller Ware, M.N., R.N.)

system between cells and the system itself constitutes a physiological mechanism of adaptation.

Neuron tracts extend from the cerebral cortex to the hypothalamus and thus influence the function of the latter. The hypothalamus directs much of the pituitary activity which, in turn, influences the other endocrine glands either directly or indirectly. The neurohumoral link between the hypothalamus and the pituitary appears to be important to the function of neuroendocrine mediating mechanisms. The linking of the emotions, the cerebral cortex, the autonomic nervous system, the endocrine system, and the hypothalamus illustrated in Fig. 25-2 is the foundation for somatopsychophysiologic theory.[2,32,33]

References

1 W. B. Cannon: "Stresses and Strains of Homeostasis," *American Journal of Medical Science,* vol. 189, p. 1, 1935.

2 L. E. Hinkle: "The Concept of Stress in the Biological and Social Sciences," *The International Journal of Psychiatry in Medicine,* vol. 5, no. 4, pp. 335–357, 1974.

3 H. Selye: *Stress Without Distress,* Lippincott, New York, 1974.

4 R. Schoenheimer: *Dynamic Steady State of Body Constituents,* Harvard University Press, Cambridge, Mass., 1942.

5 H. Selye: *The Stress of Life,* McGraw-Hill, New York, 1956.

6 H. Wolff: *Stress and Disease,* Charles C Thomas, Springfield, Ill., 1953.

7 E. Schrodinger: *What Is Life? The Physical Aspect of the Living Cell; & Mind and Matter,* Cambridge University Press, London, 1967.

8 M. Levine: *Introduction to Clinical Nursing,* Davis, Philadelphia, 1969.

9 R. Ader: "The Role of Developmental Factors in Susceptibility to Disease," *The International Journal of Psychiatry in Medicine,* vol. 5, no. 4, pp. 367–376, 1974.

10 E. Wittkower: "Historical Perspective of Contempory Psychosomatic Medicine," *The International Journal of Psychiatry in Medicine,* vol. 5, no. 4, 1974, p. 315.

11 R. Moos: "Determinants of Physiological Responses to Symbolic Stimuli: The Role of the Social Environment," *The International Journal of Psychiatry in Medicine,* vol. 5, no. 4, pp. 389–399, 1974.

12 I. Janis: *Psychological Stress,* Wiley, New York, 1958.

13 J. Freedman: "The Crowd May Not Be So Madding After All," *Psychology Today,* September 1971, p. 58.

14 Erich Lindemann: "Symptomatology and Management of Acute Grief," *American Journal of Psychiatry,* vol. 101, September 1944, pp. 141–148.

15 H. Parens, B. McConville, and S. Kaplan: "The Prediction of Frequency of Illness from the Response to Separation," *Psychosomatic Medicine,* vol. 28, March–April 1966, p. 2.

16 C. M. Parkes: "Broken Heart: A Statistical Study of Increased Mortality Among Widowers," *British Medical Journal,* March 1969, pp. 740–743.

17 A. H. Schmale: "Relationship of Separation and Depression to Disease," *Psychosomatic Medicine,* vol. 10, July–August 1958, p. 259.

18 A. Stenbeck: "Object Loss and Depression," *Archives of General Psychiatry,* vol. 12, February 1965, pp. 144–151.

19 John Thurlow: "General Susceptibility to Illness," *Canadian Medical Association Journal,* vol. 97, pp. 1397–1404, Dec. 2, 1967.

20 A. Toffler: *Future Shock,* Random House, New York, 1970.

21 Z. Lipowski: "Physical Illness and Psychopathology," *The International Journal of Psychiatry in Medicine,* vol. 5, no. 4, pp. 483–497, 1974.

22 L. Peter and R. Hull: *The Peter Principle,* Morrow, New York, 1969.

23 T. H. Holmes and R. H. Rahe: "The Social Readjustment Rating Scale," *Journal of Psychosomatic Research,* vol. 11, p. 213, 1967.

24 Charles Brenner: "Affects and Psychic Conflict," *The Psychoanalytic Quarterly,* vol. 44, no. 1, pp. 5–28, January 1975.

25 M. Deutsch: *The Resolution of Conflict,* Yale University Press, New Haven, 1973.

26 L. Coser: *The Function of Social Conflict,* Free Press, Chicago, 1956.

27 G. Simmel: *Conflict,* Free Press, Chicago, 1955.

28 G. Moss: "Biosocial Resonation: A Conceptual Model of the Links between Social Behavior and

Physical Illness," *The International Journal of Psychiatry in Medicine,* vol. 5, no. 4, 1974.

29 S. Withey: "Reaction to Uncertain Threat," in G. Baker, D. Chapman, and M. Wolfstein (eds.), *Society in Disaster,* Free Press, Glencoe, Ill., 1957.

30 U.S. Department of Health, Education, and Welfare and U.S. Public Health Service: *Selected Symptoms of Psychological Distress,* National Center for Health Statistics, series II, no. 37, Public Health Service Publication #1000, Washington, D.C., 1970.

31 K. Lamott: *Escape from Stress,* Putnam, New York, 1975.

32 W. Evans: *Anatomy and Physiology,* 2d ed., Prentice-Hall, Englewood Cliffs, N.J., 1976.

33 P. C. Whybrow and P. M. Silberfarb: "Neuroendocrine Mediating Mechanisms: From the Symbolic Stimulus to the Physiological Response," *The International Journal of Psychiatry in Medicine,* vol. 5, no. 4, pp. 531–539, 1974.

26

Physiological Maladaptation to Stress

Barbara Flynn Sideleau

Learning Objectives

After studying this chapter, the student should be able to:

1 Discuss the psychodynamics and environmental factors which predispose the individual to stress-induced illness
2 Discuss the family dynamics which predispose the individual to stress-induced illness
3 Discriminate between adaptive and maladaptive responses to acute coronary heart disease
4 Assess the factors affecting adaptation following an acute coronary episode
5 Discuss the family dynamics which affect adaptation following an acute coronary episode
6 Plan care for clients and families coping with an acute coronary episode
7 Intervene to assist clients and families to prevent stress-induced illness
8 Intervene to assist clients and families to cope with inevitable stressful events
9 Intervene to assist clients and families modify stressful life-styles
10 Discuss alternative stress-reducing activities

Psychosomatic Medicine

Early research in psychosomatic medicine focused on the development of specific diseases as a consequence of particular emotional states and the symbolic meaning of disease. Wolff's work focused on associations such as that between migraine and an obsessive personality structure characterized by striving for success and feelings of anger and resentment; respiratory disease and the symbolic shutting out and washing away of feelings of resentment, frustration, humiliation, and guilt; and problems of the lower gastrointestinal tract and the riddance pattern expressed by diarrhea or ulcerative colitis.[1]

The results of this research, rather than discovering specificity of relation between a specific emotion and a disease, supported multicausation. Emotional stress was a key factor, but other mediating factors influenced the noxious quality of the stressor and even its neutralization. More recently, psychosomatic medicine has directed its research toward developing a greater understanding of the physiological processes involved in disease, the psychological processes which make a person's encounters with the environment stressful, the self-regulatory or coping processes, and the steps in these processes that lead to bodily states that Levi and Kagen have called the *precursors of disease.*[23]

The mind-body dualism which has dominated the thinking in health care in our society has become obsolescent because it cannot adequately explain health-illness phenomena. The holistic view which encompasses multifaceted realities and the relationship of the person to the environment provides a more relevant framework for understanding disease causation. Research on specificity of stressors or single causation of diseases has only served to substantiate the position that the person is a holistic system mutually interacting with the environment (see Chap. 25).

Stress is a primary factor in the development of disease. Stressors elicit physiological responses in the autonomic nervous system, endocrine system, hypothalamus, and cerebral cortex, which in turn influence other body systems and organs.

There is no simple cause-and-effect relationship in the development of disease; rather, it is the complex interrelationship of multiple factors which determines whether one succumbs to the stress and becomes dysfunctional and how the body will manifest the inability to cope with the stress (see Chap. 25).

Psychodynamics

According to Thurlow, disease-producing stress occurs when an individual feels less able to cope. In such instances the person exhibits a withdrawal pattern, psychologically and physiologically, to conserve energy.[4] Although specific personality types have not been positively correlated with personality profiles, response patterns are evident in the various disease processes. Researchers have found a specific relationship between the way people feel and what they want to do about these feelings at the time they develop symptoms of disease. Their attitudes are not seen as being responsible for the development of the disease but as being part of the disease process. Backus gives the example that one does not have an *attitude* for hives; rather, the stress of the dilemma increases skin temperature, which increases the skin's susceptibility to this dermatological condition.[5] The reasons for the increase in temperature and the skin's susceptibility are probably related to inherited predisposition and/or early conditioning (see Chap. 25). According to Backus, the object relationships of psychosomatic clients are characterized by a poverty of fantasies and mental representations and a lack of affective involvement.[5] Interpersonal relationships with significant others which are impoverished, conflicted, and nonsupportive interfere with satisfying object relations.[6]

In the maturation process, undifferentiated infantile patterns of hypersecretion, hypermotility, and hyperemia move from involuntary control in the oral stage, to combined involuntary-voluntary control in the anal stage, and finally to the voluntary control in the genital stage. If people are confronted with stressors that tax them beyond their capacity, to master the event regression occurs. The earlier undifferentiated physiological responses are decontrolled and their unregulated activity becomes the basis for the development of psychosomatic disease[6] (see Chap. 25).

Ruesch maintains that people with psychosomatic ailments are immature and their disease is a consequence of their inability to manipulate symbolic processes in order to communicate. Instead, these people communicate at the preverbal level via the autonomic nervous system.[67]

The giving-up–given-up complex described by Engel encompasses the relationship between the person's internal and external milieu. It is a depressed psychological state characterized by expressions of helplessness, hopelessness, and worthlessness; it is compounded by impaired interpersonal relationships; a disruption in the sense of continuity between the past, present, and future; and a reactivation of memories connected with previous experiences that evoked similar feelings.[8] According to Thurlow, the overall pathology of this complex indicates an inability to seek out and implement new ways of dealing with the environment and the present state of affairs. There is overt and covert resistance to modification of old behavior patterns. The person's sense of impotence contributes to a state of psychobiological disequilibrium. When this complex is present, the person appears to have surrendered to the stress; vulnerability to exhaustion is then increased[7][9] (see Chap. 31).

Family Dynamics

The family is an emotional system, and the *resonancy phenomenon* links the impact of stress among members.[10] The influence of dynamic factors within the family has been associated with the psychogenesis of maladaptive emotional behavior and physiological dysfunction.[11-16] The interpersonal stress in family life is a factor in neuroendocrine dysfunctional adaptation.[11]

Dependency conflicts, psychosexual insecurity, the projection process, overadequate-inadequate reciprocity, and the multigenerational transmission process are significant factors in the development of psychosomatic disease. The affective system in these families seems to foster immaturity and to sabotage or fail to support the differentiation of members. Family disorganization and emotional disturbance interfere with the provision of appropriate support to members. Family disruption may be a temporary reaction to an emotionally significant event which disturbs the balance, or it may reflect a chronic situation. In the latter case, there is a greater potential for psychopathology or pathophysiology in one or several members (see Chaps. 11 and 25).

Psychosomatic Disease
Respiratory Disorders

The effects of psychosocial stress are easier to recognize in respiratory ailments than in other system disorders because of the rapidity with which symptoms are manifested.

Hay Fever

Backus points out that hay-fever sufferers react differently to the offending substances depending on their psychological state. When these people are stressed into feeling helpless, nasal secretions are increased, hypervascularity occurs, and the consequent membrane edema and obstruction occur. If they are feeling secure and have a sense of well-being, exposure to the offending substance does not elicit symptoms.[5]

Asthma

Several researchers point to conditioned visceral learning, mediated by the autonomic nervous system, as significant in the development and aggravation of asthma. However, the importance of psychosocial stressors lies in their influence in triggering diffuse pulmonic obstruction, hypersecretion, mucosal edema, and the consequent acute respiratory status. This physiological response resembles the regressive undifferentiated reaction of infancy. It is notable that such attacks often occur when the environment has generated feelings of helplessness and exclusion which have potential for reactivating memories of similar events in the past, thus escalating the impact of the stress.[5,17]

Although a wide variety of personality types have been identified among sufferers, the following psychodynamic themes have been noted: an exaggerated bond with the mother figure, an acute fear of separation from this significant person, and antecedent events—such as sexual encounters—which generate overwhelming feelings of hostility, anxiety, or competitiveness.[7,17]

Emphysema

The emphysemic resembles the asthmatic during a severe attack. Both types of episodes are precipitated by activating emotions such as anger, anxiety, or elation which require increased ventilation. Thus psychosocial stressors are significant in the development of the disability once the disease is present. These people tend to avoid any emotionally charged life experiences. They employ repression, denial, regression, and isolation to ensure their comfort and survival. People in their environment also tend to avoid conflict to prevent precipitating an attack. As a result of this avoidance of authentic conflict and emotional release, their frustration may be further increased.[5]

Autoimmune Disorders

Psychosocial stress has been associated with the onset and course of diseases of the autoimmune system. The dysfunction and hypofunction are mediated by neuroendocrine mechanisms. Rheumatoid arthritis, systemic lupus erythematosus, and ulcerative colitis seem to be associated with states of immunologic incompetence. This immune deficiency may be induced by unmanageable psychosocial stress. Research suggests that the onset of these diseases follows closely on emotional decompensation in predisposed individuals.[11,18]

Ulcerative Colitis

Ulcerative colitis has frequently been associated with anticolon antibodies. Confronted with unmanageable stress, the neuroendocrine mechanisms create disequilibrium in the immune system, thus allowing these destructive antibodies to proliferate. People with a predisposition for ulcerative colitis respond to activating emotions with a marked increase in bowel motility, hyperemia, increased fragility of the bowel wall, and a marked increase in lysozyme levels, producing effects similar to those caused by strong cholinergic stimulation. According to Backus, it is possible to observe the development of small ulcerations and petechial hemorrhages when these people are experiencing rage, resentment, and anger. Strong activating emotions appear to decrease bowel-wall defenses and increase the levels of proteolytic enzymes.[5,18,19]

The victims of ulcerative colitis have been portrayed in the literature as passive, conforming, dependent, conscientious, indecisive, and obstinate. However, when they have schizoid or paranoid tendencies, messiness and disorderliness predominate. People with ulcerative colitis tend to exhibit guarding of affectivity, overintellectualization, rigid attitudes toward morality, a defective sense of humor, and extreme sensitivity to rejection and hostility from others. They are also likely to expend considerable energy warding off potential rejections. Their outward manner—which is often energetic, ambitious, and efficient—may mask feelings of inferiority. They possess an acute sense of obligation and a close bond with one or two parent figures on whom they depend for guidance. They tend to act on the conscious or unconscious wishes of these figures and then to experience hostility, which cannot be discharged because of fears of rejection. These people perceive the mother figure as an overwhelming perfectionist. Love in this relationship is conditional, depending on the ability of the "child" to fulfill the parental figure's expectations. Male clients see their fathers as punitive and exceptionally masculine, while female clients see their fathers as passive and ineffective. The profile of these clients has been interpreted as showing a regressive seeking of dependency but with underlying oral aggressive and self-destructive tendencies, while the family dynamics are characterized by pseudomutuality.[19]

Arthritis

Stress plays an important part in the causation and exacerbation of arthritis. The psychophysiological mechanisms are complex. Hormones involved in the regulation of connective-tissue synthesis (the growth hormone, thyroxine, androgens, estrogens, and adrenal corticosteroids) interfere with the immune mechanisms and with the production of collagens. The neuroendocrine mechanisms also affect the network of capillaries and nerve fibers surrounding the synovium. Life changes are of major importance in generating the activating emotions and the level of stress capable of altering these neuroendocrine mechanisms.[18,20]

The arthritic has been described as being shy, socially inadequate, self-sacrificing, and having problems handling aggression. It would appear that, in the arthritic, pent-up rage and desire to strike out is blocked and expressed in the crippling manifestations of the disease. But not all "nice-guy" types develop arthritis, so that a predisposition and organ weakness must exist for the stress to be manifested by this disease process.[5,11]

Cancer

Similar personality factors have been linked to the pathogenesis of cancer, both clinically and experimentally.[18] These people have been described as selfless, undemanding, easy to please, unaggressive, self-sacrificing, and self-effacing.[11] Multiple life changes accompanied by feelings of helplessness, hopelessness, and despair have been associated with the immediate preneoplastic time period.[11] Complex immunologic factors are being studied extensively; as a result, there is increasing understanding of the role the immune system plays in surveillance against the mutant neoplastic cell that the system responds to as a foreign body. Emotional disruption affects hormone levels and increases corticosteroid levels, thus apparently undermining the effectiveness of the immune system's defenses. Hence failing psychological defenses have been correlated with the onset and accelerated course of autoimmune diseases and cancer.[18]

Allergic and Skin Disorders

The skin interfaces with the environment and is a somatic sounding board for emotions. It is a major component in the body's homeostatic system. It plays a major role in heat and fluid regulation; its sense receptors for pain, touch, and temperature affect development and survival. States of fear, rage, and tension can induce increased sweat production, and excessive sweating under prolonged stress leads to secondary skin changes. This anxiety phenomenon is mediated by the autonomic nervous system. Tension, anxiety, and anger predispose the person to itching and scratching. Anxious and tense people may be more conscious than others of itchy sensations. Given this possibility and the skin changes which occur under stress, self-inflicted excoriations, urticaria, and aggravations of psoriasis can be better understood.[21]

Other allergic conditions show a strong correlation to emotional disrupting events and suggest that they derive from a conditioned response.[21]

Endocrine Disorders

As with the systems previously discussed, recent studies correlate degree of life stress with the onset of endocrine problems; however, no pattern of endocrine functioning has been shown to be characteristic of particular emotions such as anger, fear, or affection. Adrenal secretions are increased with emotional arousal, and the role of the hypothalamus is significant in its effect on the endocrine system.[22–25]

Gonadal Dysfunction

Menstrual dysfunction, particularly amenorrhea, has been associated with psychogenic causes such as postpsychic trauma after rape and abortion and anorexia nervosa. Fertility and infertility have psychogenic bases resulting from psychologically based impotence or frigidity, premature ejaculation, and aberrant sexual behavior. Hypothalamic dysfunction, psychogenically or physically based, leads to infertility. In the woman, it can cause anovulation, an inhospitable viscous cervical mucus, or an improperly prepared uterus. In the man, hypothalamic dysfunction may cause oligospermia or inadequate motility of sperm.[25]

Thyroid

Paykel and Herman do not support earlier hypotheses regarding the role of specific personality and family patterns in the etiology of thyroid dysfunction. Research has not yet validated the role of stress; however, when the thyroid-stimulating hormone (TSH) and vasoconstrictor substances associated with increased tension are secreted, both act together to traumatize the thyroid and expose cell walls to the body's immune system. This immune system, in turn, may respond by causing long-acting stimulation of the thyroid and eventual exhaustion as seen in Hashimoto disease.[25-27]

Gastrointestinal Disorders

Organic bowel disorders such as regional enteritis, colitis, spastic colon, diarrhea, and malabsorption syndromes are somatopsychophysiological problems characterized by riddance and retention. The conflict between physiological functioning and the socializing demands for bowel control and cleanliness determines the role of the bowel in psychogenic disorders.[28,29]

Research suggests that gastric erosion and ulceration depend on factors which decrease the competence of the gastric mucosa. The normal hypersecretion and hypermotility patterns of infancy—which may be in part genetically determined and in part learned in the mother-child relationship—are significant factors in the development of gastrointestinal disturbances. Psychic tension ebbs and flows in the *hunger-crying-feeding-satiation-sleep* sequence of infancy. Tension reduction is regulated by the relationship with the nurturer and oral satisfaction. Incongruency in the mother-child relationship may interrupt the sequence, so that satiation and sleep are delayed or blocked. If this occurs, it may intensify and ingrain in the child strong oral-dependent wishes. Current psychosocial stresses may trigger these physiological changes and produce disease.[29]

People with gastrointestinal illness, particularly ulcer problems, exhibit oral character traits and conflict around dependence-independence. Some present as dependent, passive people, while others deny their needs and appear highly independent, self-reliant, aggressive, and continually overactive. In our society, the male victims are often supermasculine while the females show a strong male identification which is compatible with career success.[29]

As a group, these people are controlling and unconsciously have their needs met by this behavior. Some may mask this control by being outwardly compliant, ingratiating, and demanding in a passive-aggressive way, obtaining need satisfaction from the secondary gains of manifest illness. The sequence of events which culminates in illness has been described by Engel[29] as:

1 Intensification of psychological and social devices usually used in need satisfaction
2 Device failure with increasing anger, which is suppressed or denied if it threatens need satisfaction
3 Internalization of aggressive impulses
4 Perceived inability to cope, accompanied by feelings of helplessness and hopelessness

Anorexia Nervosa

Anorexia nervosa is characterized by drastic weight loss, a cachectic appearance, slow pulse, emaciation, amenorrhea, and a morbid fear of obesity. Psychogenic malnutrition may occur in clients with mania or schizophrenia because of agitation, overactivity, apathy, or because they have delusions that their food is poisoned and not edible. Depressed people may also lose weight, but their problem is based on apathy and retarded motor activity which interferes with appetite and the demands of feeding themselves. Anorexia differs from these psychogenically based cases of malnutrition.[30,31]

People who develop anorexia nervosa are usually females (90 to 95 percent) ranging in age from 16 to 23 years. They exhibit an obsessional preoccupation with the desire to be thin and a compulsive avoidance of food. As a group, they exhibit a remarkably high level of activity in spite of their frail appearance. Often these women are shy, timid, neat, and controlled adolescents who were obese and dieted. During the weight reduction process, they became counterphobic to avoid obesity. They also tend to be uninformed and fearful about sex. Fearing fantasied pregnancy, they starve themselves to prevent the development of any abdominal protrusion. They seem to hold a deep-seated wish to remain tiny and immature and to retain an intrauterine type of passive dependency on parental figures. Some spend time narcissistically admiring their emaciated bodies in the mirror. As the disease progresses, they develop hypotension, cyanosis of the extremities, pigmentation and hyperkeratosis of the skin, and increased lanugo hair over the body. The breasts atrophy; axillary and pubic hair is reduced. Leukopenia, lymphocytosis, anemias, hypoglycemia, hypocholesteremia, and hypoproteinemia develop. Generally there are no notable changes in hormone levels with the exception of the gonadotropins and ovarian hormones. Amenorrhea, which is characteristic of the disorder, occurs in 50 percent of these women before weight loss; the menstrual cycle may not return to normal for some time even when the nutritional status has returned to and been maintained at a normal level. These facts suggest psychogenic causation.[30,31]

Anorexia nervosa is usually precipitated by traumatic events which center around separation, the bodily changes of puberty, and sexual experiences and failures. Food comes to symbolize evil and self-indulgence, and severe dieting is used to control the body, its impulses, and sexuality. The cachexia is seen as a way of becoming inconspicuous, while the disease process enables the victim to avoid both responsibility and the need to deal with the emerging secondary sex characteristics and their implication. If there has been sexual activity, even masturbation, these women may feel guilty and use the strict dietary regimen for self-punishment. Misconceptions causing fear of pregnancy are not uncommon.[30]

As the disease progresses and the physiological status deteriorates, these clients come to represent psychiatric and medical emergencies. Somewhere between 3 to 15 percent die of malnutrition or intercurrent infections. No specific treatment is available to reverse the process. Psychotherapy, family therapy, and behavior modification are used with varying degrees of success.[30]

Food and its consumption becomes a control issue. These clients may starve themselves to dangerous levels but do not seem aware of the lethal implications of their behavior. In their hatred of food, these clients' internal signals of hunger are disrupted and signs of satiation are misinterpreted or lost. Some fluctuate between starvation and bulemia and pica occurs in others, while all employ a variety of strategies to eliminate food from their bodies. Initially, the anorexic client may stick a finger down her throat to induce vomiting if she is prevented from hiding or disposing of food by other means. With time, these clients learn to disgorge the contents of their stomachs at will. Those who do eat may consume large doses of cathartics or use self-administered enemas to rid their bodies of the unwanted food.[30]

Cardiovascular Disorders

Cardiovascular disorders are caused by the interaction between biological and psychological factors. The neuroendocrine mechanisms play an important role in their development. Activating emotions not only increase blood pressure, heart rate, and oxygen consumption but also cause sudden and marked increases in the serum cholesterol and decreases in clotting time and hemoconcentration. These responses predispose the individual to migraine headaches, hypertension, stroke, and coronary heart disease.

Psychogenic Headaches

Headaches are a common complaint most commonly resulting from painful dilation and distention of cranial arteries or sustained contraction of skeletal muscles around the face, scalp, and neck. They tend to occur in a life setting that engenders frustration, resentment, anxiety, emotional tension, and fatigue.[32] Anxiety has been found to be the predominant predisposing factor. No one specific personality type is associated with chronic recurring headaches; however, personality disorders such as passive aggressiveness, obsessive compulsiveness, and hysteria and their underlying conflicts seem to predispose the individual to such headaches.[33]

The migraine is a particularly painful and immobilizing paroxysmal headache. Although heredity is recognized as a primary predisposing factor, tension plays a role in triggering an attack. These people have been described as rigid, pent up, perfectionistic, overconscientious, ambitious, and obsessional.[33]

Prior to an attack, the migraine sufferer usually engages in a high level of activity and experiences increased tension, which is followed by a sudden and drastic change in life pace and pressure characterized by a feeling of relaxation. According to Backus,[5] during or immediately following this *letdown,* there is a contraction of cranial arteries, including the retinal artery, which produces prodromal symptoms such as an aura or visual disturbances (blurred vision, flashes of light, or diplopia). The pounding and throbbing pain is produced by the distorted vessels and increased fluid impinging on surrounding interstitial tissue.[33]

Repressed and suppressed hostile impulses seem to be the chief source of the neurotic conflicts that precipitate an attack. In some instances the headache may be partly caused by this rage and partly by hysteria.[33] According to Friedman and Brenner,[33] positive or negative identification with a parental figure and introjection of that figure also play a role when symptoms arise from the person's wish to gain affection or attention. The headache may reflect a need to be dependent.[33]

Hypertension

Hypertensive disease is a major health problem in our society. It is a significant contributing factor in the development of coronary heart disease and cerebrovascular accidents. Elevation of the blood pressure is a component of the fight-flight mechanism. A wide range of environmental stimuli generate the fear, anger, and frustration that elevate the arterial blood pressure (see Chap. 25). Hypertensives may learn—through conditioning and as an adaptive response—to screen out of awareness potentially noxious stimuli, but they continue to respond to these stimuli physiologically with their conditioned and/or inherited hyperreactive pressor systems.[5,34,35]

These people often suffer from chronic rage or guilt over their aggressive tendencies. However, they may appear as the "nice guy," repressing or suppressing angry and aggressive feelings but suffering the consequences of this tension physiologically, through sustained diastolic elevation.

When the chronically elevated blood pressure results in a stroke, the person has usually experienced a period of sustained and relatively severe emotional disturbance which was often intensified before the onset of illness. As a group, these people assume an unusual degree of personal responsibility for their situations. Prior to the stroke, they felt pressured to meet goals which they had set for themselves; but they often felt that they were not in control of either their lives or the environment and were failing to meet their own expectations.[35,36]

Coronary Heart Disease

The heart has symbolic meaning and may be used to communicate psychological conflicts and distress.[34] There is a higher correlation between personality type and disease manifestation in heart disease than is the case with other psychosomatic disorders. Individuals susceptible to heart attacks are described as type-A personalities by Friedman and Rosenman.[37] Table 26-1 lists those characteristic behaviors of type-A personalities which appear to go with a predisposition to coronary heart disease. As a group, these people are outwardly controlled and apt to be successful in repressing and denying anxiety, anger, and depression. Other psychological variables which also seem to play an important role are upward mobility, significant loss, multiple life changes, overwork, and job dissatisfaction. An unfamiliar social or work environment, increased responsibilities, and discrepancies between the expectations of the culture of origin and the current cultural situation place demands on the individual's capacity for psychosocial coping. Bereavement is a significant factor, particularly with regard to losses in relationships, roles, and status. Surviving spouses during the first year after the death of a husband or wife are particularly vulnerable.[34,38,39]

Table 26-1 Personality Type A

Aggressive, ambitious, unable to delegate authority
Possesses intense physical and emotional drives
Concentrates on career and has no hobbies
Experiences a chronic sense of time urgency
Preoccupied with deadlines
Exhibits excessive competitive drive
Exhibits easily aroused hostility under very diverse conditions
Meets challenges by expending extra effort
Takes little satisfaction from accomplishments
Obsessed with numbers
Obsessed with money
Presents as self-assured and self-confident
Measures self by number of achievements
Insecure about status
Restless during leisure time and guilty about relaxing

If the person is unable to master the stress of these situations, the fight-flight mechanism which was designed for short-term emergency situations is prolonged and becomes detrimental (see Chap. 25). The homeostatic mechanisms remain chronically mobilized, which eventually leads to exhaustion. Often the illness strikes not at the peak of the stressful experience but rather shortly after the pressures of the situation have diminished, when exhaustion begins to occur. It is during this *letdown* period that the viscosity of the blood increases, clotting time decreases, and there is a sudden drop in cardiac output and oxygen consumption, creating a period of maximal vulnerability consequent to the lowering of coronary blood flow.[34,40]

Myocardial Infarction

Myocardial infarction strikes its victims suddenly and without warning. These people are admitted to the coronary-care unit (CCU) and connected to monitoring equipment. Chapter 29 discusses the impact of the life-support systems and special-care unit on clients and staff.

The first day after admission, these people are in crisis and feel anxious. By day two they usually mobilize denial as defense. They may protest being in the CCU, insist they feel much better, and claim that their problem was only acute indigestion. By the third or fourth day awareness of the implications of the disease generates feelings of depression. Premorbid abrasive personality traits emerge to defend against depressive feelings. These clients often become demanding, hostile, and irritable toward staff.[41]

Anxiety

Anxiety is inevitable, but it is the most problematic emotion for these clients because it activates the sympathetic nervous system, causing the release of epinephrine, which increases the heart rate and blood pressure and speeds up metabolic processes. These neuroendocrine mechanisms jeopardize the integrity of the myocardium. Even more problematic are the clients who mask this anxiety and suffer silently with their fear of death, misconceptions, loss of control, and isolation.[41,42] Discrete social interactions can have an anxiety-producing effect on the heart activity of clients in the CCU. The rate, rhythm, and frequency of ectopic beats may be altered by socioenvironmental events. One study revealed that there was a significant increase in the number of sudden deaths in the CCU after or during ward rounds by the medical staff. These findings suggest that rounds increased the clients' anxiety concerning their health status, which triggered lethal arrhythmias. Assessing a client's pulse is a frequent nursing activity in a CCU. This simple assessment is potentially stressful, depending on the client's emotional interpretation of and cardiac reaction to being touched and perception of the purpose of the assessment.[43,44]

Regression

Regression, a component of the sick role, can help the client conserve energy and prevent lethal arrhythmias. It is a normal stage in the acceptance of the illness. For some coronary clients, regression generates anxiety and hostility. Others appear compliant and docile because they are masking their feelings. In both cases, failure to regress with ease increases the risk to lethal arrthymias or extension of the infarction[41] (see Chap. 25).

Denial

Denial is a major and necessary defense for these clients. Deniers have been classified as major, partial, and minimal. Major deniers negate the stress of the experience. Research findings reveal that people in this category did not die. This suggests that the ability to deny the implications of the illness and to cope with awareness a little at a time has value for immediate survival.[41,42]

Depression

Depression, like anxiety, is to a degree inevitable, but it introduces some risk for these clients. Re-search has revealed that all those who died in the population studied were judged to be depressed. Depressed clients cry, exhibit a sad face, and have slowed speech. The feeling is generated by the multiple losses which have occurred and those which are anticipated. Expressions of hopelessness are associated with mortality and are therefore a concern to caretakers.[4]

Clients in CCUs may be reassured by the speed, efficiency, and expertise of the staff in responding to emergencies. Nevertheless, they harbor a strong fear of dying. Exposure to others in the unit with the same diagnosis who are arresting or who have died is anxiety-producing. To defend against these realities and identification with the victims, clients tend to perceive themselves and/or their condition as different from that of the victims.[41,42]

When clients do arrest, they often exhibit symptoms of organic brain syndrome which may be either transient or permanent (see Chap. 30). Most of these people do not confront or explore the implications of their arrest, but they do report violent dreams with sudden-death scenarios. They also suffer from insomnia and exhibit cognitive impairment. They feel that their experience has made them unique, and they may have unspoken fears and fantasies about their "death" experience.

Problematic Behaviors

Some clients cannot accept their disease or its implications and defend maladaptively against awareness and the massive fear. The most lethal of these behaviors is signing out of the hospital against medical advice. Euphoric behavior need not be dangerous unless the client's activity level stresses the myocardium. Sexually provocative, openly hostile, and manipulative behavior communicates the client's fears but often generates problems when misinterpreted by caretakers[41] (see Chap. 17).

The maladaptive coping styles most frequently seen in the CCU are obsessive-compulsive, repressive, dependent, hyperindependent, paranoid, and depressive.[45]

Obsessive-Compulsive Reaction

Obsessive-compulsive people deal with stress by studying and structuring both the environment and events. They seek to subjugate everything that happens to intellectual mastery and present themselves as doubters, question raisers, and careful thinkers. In approaching problems from this position, they tend to intellectualize. Difficulties arise when these people are not able to get all the information and rationales they feel they need to occupy their thinking and structure what is happening[45] (see Chap. 16).

Repressive Reaction

Repressive individuals are the opposite of obsessive-compulsives. They operate on an impressionistic mode and do not want or need to examine situations closely. These people deal with stressful occurrences by pushing them out of awareness, and they want others to do the same. When confronted with an event which cannot be handled in this way, their impressionistic perceptual set leads to a global, intense, diffuse overreaction.[45]

Excessive Dependency

Dependency is necessary to the assumption of the sick role. It allows the person, through a childlike dependency on the caretakers, to receive care and empathy and to feel more secure. However, if intense or prolonged, this dependency interferes with the assumption of self-care and participation in the rehabilitation regimen[45] (see Chap. 24).

Hyperindependence

People who cannot accept dependency because they fear loss of control or are shy or intimidated will act totally independent and will put up barriers between themselves and the caretakers. They deny fears and feelings of helplessness. The reactivation of memories of past dependencies may be more anxiety-producing and frightening than the present situation (see Chap. 24).

Paranoid Reaction

Some clients react to the stress of their illness and confinement to the special-care unit with paranoia. They feel that the world is a dangerous place and that people are not to be trusted. They expect to be hurt, disappointed, or rejected, and the severe illness of a myocardial infarction confirms this belief. Suspicious and fearful, they tend to distance others as a defense[45] (see Chap. 16).

Depressive Reaction

Depression which becomes intensified and prolonged causes the person to feel overwhelmed and intensely guilty. There is a loss of self-esteem accompanied by disgust toward the self. These people feel a personal responsibility for the crisis, which to them is one more example of their failure in life. They feel that by becoming ill, *by their own doing,* they have adversely affected their families. Although there may be unconscious antagonism toward the family, they are aware only of the guilt[45] (see Chap. 18).

Transient Psychosis

Psychosis in these clients may be due partly to organic brain syndrome precipitated by the physiological derangements of the crisis, the client's psychological style, or sensory and psychomotor deprivation. Delirious psychotic reactions are not as common to CCUs as they are to other special-care units, but they do occur. Personality predisposition is characterized by a repressive style of coping. The psychosis is characterized by transient perceptual distortion, visual and auditory hallucinations, disorientation, and paranoid delusions[42,45] (see Chap. 15).

Family Dynamics

At the time of infarction, family members experience feelings of loss, depression, and guilt. As the client's physiological status stabilizes, the fear of death lessens but insomnia and appetite disturbances continue. The grief reaction is often greater in wives under 45 and those with a psychiatric history than in older wives.[46]

Many family members, particularly spouses, complain of symptoms such as headaches, chest pains, or shortness of breath. These symptoms may persist through the acute and convalescent periods. Some spouses tend to be overprotective, which often leads to marital discord and sexual problems (see Chap. 21). Spouses and children often avoid conflict, and the client, too, tends to avoid arousing activating emotions. Suppression of feelings and the failure to recognize and resolve conflict increase and escalate tension within the family.[46]

Research findings reveal that a year after the heart attack, spouses felt marital relations to be different from what they were during the premorbid period. When relations were markedly changed, the wife had assumed a managing role and tended to be overprotective, while the husband remained irritable and less independent.[46]

Families experience financial strains as a result of the costs of the hospitalization, which is compounded after discharge by layoffs, job changes which mean lower pay, forced retirement, dependence on disability pensions, or difficulty in finding employment. Socioeconomic problems often interfere with the resumption of the earlier life-style. Often these clients are unable to get auto or life insurance, keep their homes repaired or as clean as they had been, or maintain their premorbid standard of living. Role reversals in the marital dyad and a shift in parenting responsibilities further stresses the family's ability to cope. When this stress is experienced as intense or prolonged and solutions seem unavailable, the family may become disorganized and family members may become predisposed to psychophysiological disorders.[4,11,35,40,47,48]

Psychogenic Pain
Pain is both a torment to the sufferer and a vital warning signal that something is amiss. Many theories have been postulated regarding the pain response mechanism.* In addition to the physical stressors which elicit and sustain pain, there is also the psychological component.

To experience pain, the person must be conscious, attentive, and self-concerned. During the growth process, pain is perceived as a consequence of a variety of stimuli and is associated with feelings, ideas, actions, and people. Pain may become psychologically meaningful and influence adaptive behavior. Memories of painful experiences acquired in childhood may be reactivated, fantasied, or hallucinated later.[49] Symbolic stimuli are incorporated into the person's reward and punishment systems on the physiological level. Cognitive appraisal of a situation and the personal interpretation and meaning elicit a physiological and behavioral coping pattern[50] (see Chap. 25).

Punishment in childhood is often associated with a way of controlling bad behavior and is exaggerated in retrospect. As adults, these people may, on the basis of childhood experiences, suffer pain as a neurotic symbol to evade guilt feelings generated by an impulse or action that is judged bad.[49] This conditioning influences the development of pain behavior as a way of getting needed love and attention.

Psychogenic pain occurs in many clinical syndromes through several mechanisms. According to Kapp, it may be a secondary symptom of a psychophysiological disorder, or it may be a neurotic conversion symptom. In either case, the person is not aware of the underlying conflicts around dependency, hostility, and sexuality.[49]

When psychogenic pain is secondary to physiological dysfunction, it is induced by chronic activating emotions which trigger neuroendocrine mechanisms affecting various organs and systems.[50] A neurotic conversion pain originates in the mind but is experienced as if it were in the body. It is derived from reactivated memories of bodily functions that are used to represent unconscious conflicts in a symbolic manner. According

*The student is referred to Margo McCaffery, *Nursing Management of the Patient with Pain,* for further discussion of these theories.

to Kapp, conversion pain is a neurotic process whereby an unacceptable idea, wish, or fantasy is expressed as a bodily pain.[50] For further discussion of the conversion mechanism, see Chap. 16.

Nurses' Response

People with psychophysiological ailments exhibit a wide variety of personality types and coping patterns. However, if their disease is labeled as psychosomatic, the diagnosis is likely to be taken to mean that the problem exists only "in the person's head"; this perception, of course, influences nurses' perceptions and responses. As a society, we tend to feel that if our emotions are affecting our health, we must simply control or modify them. Nurses are not immune to this belief unless they develop a working knowledge about the perceptual, neuroendocrine, and defense systems. Without a sound understanding of these, nurses tend to take the position that individuals with psychosomatic ailments are willfully creating their own problems.

If nurses ascribe responsibility to the individual "to know" the underlying psychodynamics motivating the maladaptive behavior and "to know" how to change these behaviors, it becomes difficult for them to define their roles and to plan appropriate care. With this perception, nurses are apt to become frustrated and angry if clients do not "see" or "understand" the stresses they are experiencing and how their personality styles and defenses are creating problems (see Chaps. 5, 16, and 17). This frustration and anger may baffle clients, whose view of the situation may differ markedly. Many lack insight into their conflict or feel that they do not know how to change their ingrained personality style or the stressful forces in the environment contributing to their distress.

Anorectic clients are particularly frustrating to the nurse. Their cachectic state and life-threatening anorectic behavior challenges the nurse's professional self-concept as well as the professional goal of assisting clients to attain optimal health. When nurses find themselves acting like jailers toward these uncooperative people who, in spite of diligent supervision, manage to disgorge whatever nutrients they ingest, they experience a stressful conflict between their need to help improve the client's physiological and nutritional status and their wish to abandon a situation which is frustrating, unrewarding, and seemingly doomed to failure. If tube feedings are ordered, the nurse may unconsciously implement the procedure with a punitive vengeance.

The coronary client who fails to adopt the sick role and—in spite of life-threatening cardiac problems—continues to sabotage all interventions directed at conserving energy also frustrates nurses and challenges their self-perception as professionals (see Chap. 16).

Nurses working on busy and stressful units tend to organize and structure their work carefully so as to be certain of allotting adequate time to each person. This organization and the work schedule they develop may be efficient, but it is also rigid. If flexibility is lost or lacking and the nurse encounters clients who need to manage their illness by controlling the environment, a power struggle ensues. The nurse may feel threatened or disorganized if the client does not conform to the established care schedule. Controlling clients also ask the nurse many questions and request detailed explanations. The sick role in our society defines the client as a passive recipient of care, not an active participator. When clients question the rationale for nursing interventions, nurses may feel defensive and irritated that a client should question a professional decision. If nurses unnecessarily withhold information from these clients, the relationship becomes strained and unrewarding for both participants. The nurse in this situation may label the client as "difficult" and withdraw from all but the necessary encounters (see Chap. 29).

A discrepancy which can generate strong feelings also occurs when the nurse wishes to give clients information about their illness and its implications but the clients deal with stressful events by using denial and avoidance. These clients may screen out anxiety-provoking messages, and the nurses feel frustrated because—in spite of their efforts—the clients fail to learn or understand what is being communicated. If the nurse does manage to break down this barrier, the client may manifest a global, intense overreaction and anxiety which, in turn, generates anxiety and feelings of incompetence in the nurse who was unable to help the client cope more effectively.

When clients react to illness with depressive and paranoid reactions, this too generates feelings in nurses. Chapters 18 and 14 discuss these responses and their impact on care. Transient psychotic behavior in a special-care setting is usually seen as an organic disturbance, and within this medical model nurses respond to bizarre behavior differently than they do in other contexts (see Chap. 30). They feel less personally threatened or anxious. The responsibility for remediation of the psychosis is seen as a matter of medical management.

When a client is not responding to treatment and there is the possibility of a conversion reaction, the nurse may allow this diagnosis to skew perceptions during the assessment and evaluation phases. When this occurs, it may affect the nurse's sensitivity to data and analysis of findings; these may prove inaccurate because the nurse dismisses some observations as simply hysterical responses.

Identification problems may be a source of difficulty in caring for these clients. When this phenomenon occurs, it may distort observations and affect the nurse-client relationship. Chapter 22 explores this issue in depth.

Nurses have expectations of how a "good" family should behave. If they visit "too often" or "too little," ask "too many questions" or display anger, nurses may label them as "problems" and minimize communication and support. When nurses feel that the family is in some way responsible for the client's distress or see them as unwilling to support the client and the treatment, they may allow anger and frustration to interfere with the development of an effective working relationship with the family system. Rather than counseling and supporting, they may wield their authority in a directive, controlling, and punitive manner (see Chap. 24).

The CCU is a stressful environment in spite of its seemingly quiet climate and freedom from hustle and bustle. Working in a life-or-death environment stresses caretakers, even though they may carry out their tasks in a subdued, patient, and calm manner. The setting escalates feelings of tension and anxiety when the nurses feel that working conditions are not supportive of their needs. If they feel that help is unavailable, continuing education is lacking, and a team spirit is absent, they experience increasing tension and job dissatisfaction. Nurses in CCUs seem to have greater expectations and sensitivity to working conditions and to feel more vulnerable than do nurses in general-care units; this may reflect the greater responsibility they feel they bear in the life-and-death decision-making situations.[51] (see Chap. 29).

Planning Care

Assessment

Clients suffering from psychophysiological disorders exhibit a wide variety of disease processes and symptoms. The one thing they have in common is that all have coped maladaptively with stress and their disease is a manifestation of this failure. For their bodies to do the work of repair, energy must be diverted to this task. Thus nursing is primarily concerned with helping these people learn how to cope more effectively and managing the environment to modify the number and intensity of stimuli which would generate further stress. The assessment process focuses on identifying stressors and determining their impact on the client. The following is a guide for gathering data on these sources of stress:

The Environment

1 What stressful factors are present in the physical environment (light, temperature, noise, odors, technology)?
2 What is the level of sensory input?
3 What is the response of caretakers to the client?
4 What is the degree of flexibility?
5 Are caretakers sensitive to the clients' "need to know" and to participate in their care?
6 How do caretakers deal with feelings and their behavioral manifestations?
7 What are the caretakers' perceptions of the causes for the client's illness and distress?
8 Is the client's means of support threatened by this illness?

The Client

1 How does the client communicate needs and feelings?
2 What is the client's perception of the cause of the illness?
3 What is the client's perception of the implications of the disease process?
4 How does the client cope with change?
5 How is the client adapting to the sick role?
6 Which coping mechanisms is the client employing?
7 Are these coping mechanisms helping the client cope effectively and conserve energy?
8 How does the client cope with conflict?
9 What are the client's expectations of the caretaker?
10 What are the client's self-expectations?
11 What is the client's support system?
12 How does the client perceive this support system?
13 What is the system's impact on the client?
14 Is the client able to explore alternatives in his or her life-style?

15 Is the client exhibiting a mental set or behaviors that interfere with conservation of energy and effective coping?
16 How does the client solve problems and make decisions?
17 Does the client have financial burdens?
18 What changes in life-style has the illness imposed?

The Family

1 What behaviors does the family foster in the client?
2 Is the family relationship supportive or destructive of the client's coping?
3 How does the family handle conflict?
4 How does the family handle change?
5 How does the family handle feelings?
6 How are needs being met within the family?
7 How does the family relate to staff?
8 Does the family need information or support?
9 What is the family's perception of the illness and its implications?
10 How does the family make decisions?

Nursing Diagnosis
The nursing diagnosis is a process that involves interaction between the client and nurse. The nurse assists the client to verbalize needs, feelings, perceptions, and thoughts related to the illness episode and to the client's ability, past and present, to cope with stress. The nurse also assesses the client's nonverbal behavior and looks for discrepancies between words and actions. For example, the client may say, "I know I'm supposed to stay in bed, it would be dangerous to exert myself now." This statement, on the surface, would suggest that the client understands the bed-rest restriction and its rationale. However, the nurse may find this client using the bathroom rather than calling the nurse for the urinal.

Table 26-2 Nursing Diagnoses and Goals For Selected Behaviors

Client behavior	Nursing diagnoses	Nursing goals
Client shows global anxiety on admission to CCU.	Inability to use denial to defend against anxiety and fear of death.	Help client to conserve energy and use effective coping mechanisms.
Postmyocardial client on bed rest goes to bathroom and refuses to call the nurse for urinal.	Inability to adopt sick role is interfering with client's adherence to activity restrictions.	Help client to accept sick role and necessary dependency as well as to verbalize needs.
Client verbalizes helplessness and hopelessness concerning recovery.	Depressive mental set is interfering with client's mobilization of effective coping strategies.	Encourage client to use coping mechanisms compatible with movement toward health; foster realistic perception of events and prognosis.
Client refuses to feed or wash self in spite of physiological stability.	Excessive dependency is interfering with client's rehabilitative progress.	Help client to participate actively in care.
Client has asthmatic attacks when parents visit.	Respiratory distress is elicited by underlying conflict with parental figures.	Encourage differentiation from the family system; help client to engage in authentic conflict to resolve disagreements.
Client is preoccupied with work to the exclusion of other interests and activities; maintains unrealistic work schedule.	Client is unable to relax and follow a realistic work schedule.	Help client to: Develop interests outside of work arena Pace work schedule within realistic limitations Adopt realistic expectations Pursue recreational activities Explore ways to relax Limit assumption of responsibility
Client has peristaltic rushes manifested by diarrhea in stressful situations.	Client's bowel frequency is response to impaired ability to modify anxiety.	Encourage client to: Deal with activating emotions by labeling them Analyze anxiety-provoking situations Use effective problem-solving approaches
Client's wife is overprotective and managing; husband is irritable, demanding, and dependent.	Behavior reflects role reversal causing marital discord and impairing husband's rehabilitation.	Help couple examine changes in their relationship; encourage them to confront conflict.

Nursing diagnoses reflect the needs and problems clients exhibit in response to their illness episode which—if not resolved—will interfere with restoration of health. Table 26-2 includes samples of client behavior, the nursing diagnoses, and goals.

The number of potential or actual stresses and their intensity are examined to determine which can be prevented, modified, or eliminated to lessen the demands on the client and promote effective coping. The person's previous and present coping patterns provide data on how stress is managed and suggest areas that need modification. The roots of maladaptive neuroendocrine responses go deep into the client's past; therefore

changes may be small, slow, and almost imperceptible. Thus goals that are realistic and useful in evaluating care must reflect this very gradual step-by-step process of change.

In many instances the nurse only initiates the process of change. It is the client who must, over time, work on modifying life-style, perceptions, and the environment. Motivation to change is an important, complicated, and problematic issue. A first step toward resolving the issue of motivation is to determine the client's needs, the way in which they are satisfied, and what alternative, healthier ways of meeting them may be available. All behavior, adaptive and maladaptive, satisfies needs. The nurse's perception of the client's problems and the priority for need fulfillment may not agree with the client's perception. From the nurse's viewpoint, the emaciated anorectic adolescent has a primary need for adequate nutrition, but to the adolescent, the need to manage the fear of obesity or to be dependent has priority. Therefore the nurse must determine which needs take priority for the client, how they are being met, and what alternatives are available for the fulfillment of these needs. If these primary needs are satisfied, then the needs that the nurse sees as important to the restoration of health will emerge.

Nursing Interventions

People encounter stress from many sources across the life-span. Its inevitability is unquestioned. However, stress may be growth-promoting rather than destructive depending on the person's ability to cope effectively. Stress becomes destructive when exhaustion occurs and disease or psychopathology develop.

Dumas has classified nursing interventions directed toward the management of stress as prophylactic, mitigative, and remedial.[52]

Primary Prevention—Prophylactic Action

Primary prevention has great importance in the area of psychosomatic dysfunction. This level of intervention is directed primarily at the family, the growth and development of the individual, and the prevention of maladaptive neuroendocrine responses. Therefore the healthier the family, the better able it will be to provide a milieu that is conducive to the effective management of stress.

Prenatal care which maximizes maternal health and adaptation influences the child's neuroendocrine development and function (see Chap. 32). LeBoyer's concept of *birth without violence* may have a profound impact on how the person interacts with the environment throughout the life-span. Findings to date from longitudinal studies of babies delivered by LeBoyer's method indicate that these children's developmental quotient is higher than the norm, psychomotor development is more advanced, toilet training is less difficult, colic and respiratory difficulties common to the first months of life are absent, and the parents have a greater interest in their child.[53] Future findings may support the notion that mediation of stressful experiences must begin early to maximize healthy adaptation.

The attachment process and the ongoing relationship of the child to family members are basic to helping the child mediate the stresses that will be encountered across the life-span (see Chap. 32). A healthy family system helps the child develop a positive self-concept, effective coping patterns, and the ability to perceive and interact realistically with the environment.

Nursing interventions include teaching, counseling, role modeling, and supporting activities directed toward helping the family develop healthy patterns of functioning. The research findings of Lewis and his group identified the following significant factors in the development of effective relational patterns supportive of an emotionally healthy family system:[54]

1 Development of a climate which encourages members to reach out and to expect caring, support, and empathy.
2 Development of a climate in which it is safe and acceptable to talk about feelings.
3 Acceptance of conflict and differing views as a part of family life. Disagreements are resolved by authentic conflict resolution using cooperative processes (see Chap. 25).
4 Members assume responsibility for their own feelings, thoughts, and actions.
5 Gender and generation boundaries firmly established. Parental coalition and complementarity support these boundaries and defend against emotionally charged alliances with children, particularly those of the opposite sex.
6 Capacity to tolerate personal autonomy of members. Separation of the children from the family is gradual and appropriate to the

child's developmental age. Members differentiate (see Chap. 11).

7 The power is clear and used judiciously. Negotiation rather than authoritarianism predominates.

8 Problems are resolved by exploring options.

9 Complex motivation for behavior is acknowledged and accepted.

10 Family and individual members exhibit initiative. Members reach out to the community constructively and are involved. Members have many interests and relationships outside the family.

Primary prevention can also be directed toward helping the adult population become aware that multiple life changes predispose them to illness. By helping them explore options for stabilizing their lives, nurses may be able to assist clients to control their environment and the number of stressors they must cope with at any given time.

Secondary Prevention—Mitigative Action

Mitigative nursing actions include those taken to weaken the impact of an inevitable situation which is potentially or actually stressful.[56] A person's perception of an event is a significant mediating factor on the impact of the stressor.

Research indicates that when people are warned and prepared for stressful events such as pain, change, or conflict and given sufficient reassurances, fear levels are controlled and they are less likely to develop acute emotional disturbances than those who are not warned.[55-57] According to Janis,[57] for these interventions to effectively prepare the person, it is necessary to:

- Interfere with the person's spontaneous efforts to ward off awareness of the impending threat
- Provide information that gives a realistic picture
- Provide information in tritated doses to

elicit a cognitive problem-solving approach and lessen affective interference

When the person's knowledge base is inadequate and perceptions concerning an inevitable impending stressful event are distorted, anxiety and tension increase. By maximizing reality-based communications, the nurse can assess the person's perception of the event, provide the requisite information that helps the person structure (or give meaning to) the event and understand its ramifications, and help the person identify the most effective way of coping with the event.[52,55] For example, clients who must undergo surgery or a painful procedure are better able to handle the inherent anxiety if they know what the procedure will be like and how it will affect them.[52,55]

The nurse can also manage the environment so as to minimize external stressful stimuli such as noise, light, and numbers of interpersonal contacts. Reduction of environmental stressors conserves the person's energy and facilitates the coping process.

Tertiary Prevention—Remedial Action

Remedial actions are those directed toward relief from stress.[52] People in stressful situations are in a dilemma and may feel that no solution is available. They may blame themselves for the situation and thus not be motivated to act in their own behalf, believing that the distress they are experiencing is just punishment for past misdeeds. In some instances the solutions they are able to identify seem more threatening and devastating than the stress they are experiencing. In such instances the nurse can help these people examine the situation, identify alternative solutions, explore the consequences of these alternatives, and accept feelings without guilt or fear.

The coronary client who has followed a fast-paced work schedule with no time out for rest or relaxation may see the situation as one that cannot be changed. Exploration of alternatives may help such a client learn how to delegate tasks and responsibilities. For example, through discussion and analysis of his life with the nurse, Mr. Adgar was able to relinquish the landscaping work around the house and assign it to his adolescent sons. He wrote detailed instructions for them to follow and, with time, was able to sit and watch them perform the work without interfering or taking over.

When people have difficulty expressing their feelings and perceptions, nurses use a variety of communication techniques and actively listen to what is related in an accepting and empathic manner (see Chap. 6).

People suffering from psychophysiological disorders often need to alter their life-styles and ways of relating to others. In order to change the basic matrix of one's life, values, attitudes, and behavior, one must go through a change process which is demanding and time-consuming. These people often resist recognizing the need to change and to engage in the change process. In Table 26-3, Janis's[57] stages in decision making are used as a framework for nursing intervention.

Mastery of destructive stress requires more than a repertoire of patchwork activities. It is an active process which is responsive over time to ever-changing environmental demands. These demands are often ambiguous and intangible, since they arise out of the social fabric and climate.[58]

Alternatives to Relaxation

Many people suffering from stress-related diseases need to learn how to control their lives, their environment, and their autonomic nervous systems. They need to *let go* and to relax. Scientists are beginning to study a wide variety of alternatives which in the past would have been dismissed. To find out how to achieve a relaxation response in chronically tense people, scientists are examining not only biofeedback techniques and autogenic training but also meditation and hypnosis.

Biofeedback is an application of cybernetic theory. A bodily function such as blood pressure is measured and readings are reported to the individual by way of a visual or auditory feedback system. Through autogenic training, the person is taught to consciously control the body function and alter it at will. Research has revealed this method to be effective; however, the learning retention rate is now being questioned.[59]

Altered states of consciousness are attainable through the use of Yoga, Zen, or Transcendental Meditation. Mystics have employed these methods of letting go—of decreasing their heart rate, blood pressure, and other bodily functions—for centuries. These altered states of consciousness lie on a continuum of brain activity somewhere between sleep and wakefulness and are reflected in altered brain-wave patterns. Hypnosis is a type of altered consciousness which has had a controversial history and has still not been well defined by the scientific community. There have been reports of its effectiveness in pain relief, mobilization of the will to return to health, and inhibition of hemorrhage, but rigorous research is still needed.[59]

Biofeedback, meditation, and hypnosis have intense concentration in common. For each approach, the subject must exclude other thoughts from consciousness and concentrate exclusively on a specific word or information input.[59] This intense concentration on a subject that is not emotionally charged appears to facilitate letting go of bodily functioning. Learned physiological mechanisms which reflect tension seem to dissipate and physiological equilibrium is restored. Future research in this area may identify ways that will help people who are suffering from chronic stress in a world of accelerating change.

Evaluation

Evaluation is a necessary component of the nursing process. The effectiveness of nursing interventions must be determined to make sure that goals have been met. Purposeful assessment of effectiveness includes not only observations made by the caretaker but also assessment of documenta-

Table 26-3 Change Process

Client tasks	Nursing interventions
Step 1	
Recognize that the problem is serious enough to require a change.	Challenge the client's position that the problem is not serious.
Recognize that there are undesirable consequences in the present coping pattern that should be avoided.	Provide reality-based information on the severity of the consequences if no change is effected.
Consider the possibility that there are other, alternative ways of living, relating, and/or behaving.	Explore other alternatives and their consequences.
Step 2	
Experience doubt about the present coping pattern.	Point out the deleterious effects of present coping pattern.
Seek information about alternatives.	Provide data regarding alternatives.
Appraise alternatives from the standpoint of averting negative consequences.	Support examination of alternatives.
Discard alternatives which appear to be unsafe or too costly.	Assist client to examine consequences of alternatives — the risks and benefits.
Identify feasible alternatives.	
Step 3	
Examine pros and cons of feasible alternatives.	Assist client to identify the advantages and disadvantages.
Identify the alternative that meets realistic personal criteria.	Assist client to clarify how realistic his or her personal criteria are and the relevance and appropriateness of the selected alternative.
Examine utilitarian gains or losses to the self and to significant others.	
Examine the possibility of approval or disapproval of significant others.	Help client explore impact of change on the self and significant others.
Examine whether there will be self-approval or disapproval.	
Step 4	
Decide to adopt change.	Support decision to change.
Tell others that they are going to adopt the selected alternative way of living, relating, or behaving.	Reassure client that change is possible.
	Support telling others to maximize commitment.
Implement the alternative.	Give positive feedback when change is implemented.
	Emphathize regarding the difficulties expressed by client.
Step 5	
Confront whether persistence in change will be possible in face of problems encountered.	Assist client to employ a problem-solving approach when difficulties occur.
Examine negative social feedback, both covert and overt disapproval.	Explore perceptions that the change is not supported by significant others.
Examine expectations when they are not met.	Help client clarify the importance of negative social feedback.
	Assist client to examine expectations.

tion by others involved in the care and—most importantly—subjective validation by the client and family. Long- and short-term goals are examined in light of assessment data on the client's present status. Evidence that goals are not adequately met indicates that the situation must be reassessed, further planning initiated, and alternative interventions identified. The client and family are included in this process to increase the possibility that goals will be successfully met by the revised plan and identified interventions.

References

1 H. Wolff: *Stress and Disease,* Charles C Thomas, Springfield, Ill., 1953.

2 L. Levi and A. Kagan: "Adaptation of the Psychosocial Environment to Man's Abilities and Needs," in L. Levi (ed.), *Society, Stress and Disease,* Oxford University Press, London, 1971, vol. 1, pp. 399–404.

3 R. S. Lazarus: "Psychological Stress and Coping in Adaptation and Illness," *International Journal of Psychiatry in Medicine,* vol. 5, no. 4, pp. 321–333, 1974.

4 J. Thurlow: "General Susceptibility to Illness," *Canadian Medical Association Journal,* vol. 97, pp. 1397–1404, December 2, 1967.

5 F. Backus and D. Dudley: "Observations of Psychosocial Factors and Their Relationship to Organic Disease," *International Journal of Psychiatry In Medicine,* vol. 5, no. 4, pp. 499–515, 1974.

6 E. Wittkower: "Historical Perspective of Contemporary Psychosomatic Medicine," *International Journal of Psychiatry in Medicine,* vol. 5, no. 4, p. 315, 1974.

7 S. Ruesch: "The Infantile Personality—The Care Problem of Psychosomatic Medicine," *Psychosomatic Medicine,* vol. 10, pp. 134–144, 1948.

8 G. Engel: "A Life Setting Conducive to Illness—The Giving-up–Given-up Complex," *Annals of Internal Medicine,* vol. 69, pp. 293–300, August 1968.

9 Barbara Sideleau: "Response to Loss," unpublished thesis, Yale University, New Haven, Conn., 1970.

10 E. Andrews: *The Emotionally Disturbed Family,* Jason Aronson, New York, 1974.

11 W. Meissner: "Family Process and Psychosomatic Disease," *International Journal of Psychiatry in Medicine,* vol. 5, no. 4, pp. 411–430, 1974.

12 W. Meissner: "Thinking About the Family—Psychiatric Aspects," *Family Process,* vol. 3, pp. 1–4, 1964.

13 T. Lidz and S. Fleck: *Schizophrenia and the Family,* International Universities Press, New York, 1965.

14 H. Bruch and G. Touraine: "Obesity in Childhood: The Family Frame of Obese Children," *Psychosomatic Medicine,* vol. 2, pp. 141–206, 1940.

15 F. Honker: "Physical Illness in Disturbed Marriages," *Medical Times,* vol. 92, pp. 206–208, 1964.

16 E. M. Goldberg: *Family Influences and Psychosomatic Illness,* Tavistock Publications, London, 1958.

17 L. Vachan and E. Rich: "Visceral Learning in Asthma," *Psychosomatic Medicine,* vol. 38, no. 2, pp. 122–129, March–April 1976.

18 A. Amkraut and G. Solomon: "From the Symbolic Stimulus to the Pathophysiologic Response: Immune Mechanisms," *International Journal of Psychiatry in Medicine,* vol. 5, no. 1, pp. 541–563, 1974.

19 G. Engel: "Intestinal Disorders," in A. Freedman, H. Kaplan, and B. Sadock (eds.), *Comprehensive Textbook of Psychiatry,* 2d ed., Williams & Wilkins, Baltimore, 1975.

20 A. Silverman: "Rheumatoid Arthritis," in A. Freedman, H. Kaplan, and B. Sadock (eds.), *Comprehensive Textbook of Psychiatry,* 2d ed., Williams & Wilkins, Baltimore, 1975.

21 D. Engleds and E. Wittkower: "Psychophysiological Allergic and Skin Disorders," in A. Freedman, H. Kaplan, and B. Sadock (eds.), *Comprehensive Textbook of Psychiatry,* Williams & Wilkins, Baltimore, 1975.

22 R. Rahe et al.: "Prediction of Near-Future Health Change from Subjects' Preceding Life Changes," *Journal of Psychosomatic Research,* vol. 14, p. 401, 1970.

23 M. Frankenhaeuser: "Experimental Approaches to the Study of Human Behavior as Related to Neuroendocrine Functions," in L. Levi (ed.), *Society, Stress and Disease,* Oxford University Press, London, 1971, vol. 1.

24 J. Froberg et al.: "Physiological and Biochemical Stress Reactions Induced by Psychosocial Stimuli," in L. Levi (ed.), *Society, Stress and Disease,* Oxford University Press, London, 1971.

25 L. Koran and D. Hamburg: "Psychophysiological Endocrine Disorders," in A. Freedman, H. Kaplan,

and B. Sadock (eds.), *Comprehensive Textbook of Psychiatry,* 2d ed., Williams & Wilkins, Baltimore, 1975.

26 E. S. Paykel: "Abnormal Personality and Thyroid Toxicosis: A Follow-up Study," *Journal of Psychosomatic Research,* vol. 10, p. 143, 1966.

27 H. T. Hermann and G. C. Quarton: "Psychological Changes and Psychogenesis in Thyroid Hormone Disorders," *Journal of Clinical Endocrinology,* vol. 25, p. 327, 1965.

28 G. Engel: "Intestinal Disorders," in A. Freedman, H. Kaplan, and B. Sadock (eds.), *Comprehensive Textbook of Psychiatry,* 2d ed., Williams & Wilkins, Baltimore, 1975.

29 G. Engel: "Peptic Ulcers," in A. Freedman, H. Kaplan, and B. Sadock (eds.), *Comprehensive Textbook of Psychiatry,* 2d ed., Williams & Wilkins, Baltimore, 1975, vol. 2

30 E. Bliss: "Anorexia Nervosa," in A. Freedman, H. Kaplan, and B. Sadock (eds.), *Comprehensive Textbook of Psychiatry,* 2d ed., Williams & Wilkins, Baltimore, 1975.

31 L. Linn: "Other Psychiatric Emergencies," in A. Freedman, H. Kaplan, and B. Sadock (eds.), *Comprehensive Textbook of Psychiatry,* 2d ed., Williams & Wilkins, Baltimore, 1975.

32 F. Plum: "Headache," in P. Beeson and W. McDermott (eds.), *Cecil-Loeb Textbook of Medicine,* 13th ed., Saunders, Philadelphia, 1971.

33 A. Friedman and C. Brenner, "Psychological Mechanisms in Chronic Headache," *Proceedings of the Association of Research on Nervous Diseases,* vol. 19, p. 605, 1950.

34 Z. J. Lipowski: "Psychophysiological Cardiovascular Disorders," in A. Freedman, H. Kaplan, and B. Sadock (eds.), *Comprehensive Textbook of Psychiatry,* 2d ed., Williams & Wilkins, Baltimore, 1975.

35 R. Moos: "Determinants of Physiological Responses to Symbolic Stimuli: The Role of the Social Environment," *International Journal of Psychiatry in Medicine,* vol. 5, no. 4, pp. 389–399, 1974.

36 R. Adler et al.: "Psychological Process and Ischemic Stroke," *Psychosomatic Medicine,* vol. 33, pp. 1–29, 1971.

37 M. Friedman and R. Rosenman: *Type A Behavior and Your Heart,* Fawcett Publications, Greenwich, Conn., 1974.

38 C. M. Parkes: "Broken Heart: A Statistical Study of Increased Mortality Among Widowers," *British Medical Journal,* March 1969, pp. 740–743.

39 C. M. Parkes: *Bereavement,* International Universities Press, New York, 1972.

40 H. Russek and L. Russek: "Is Emotional Stress an Etiologic Factor in Coronary Heart Disease?" *Psychosomatics,* vol. 17, no. 2, pp. 63–67, April–May–June 1976.

41 Alma Wooley: "Excellence in Nursing in the Coronary Care Unit," *Heart and Lung,* vol. 1, no. 6, pp. 785–792, November–December 1972.

42 H. Cassem et al.: "Reactions of Coronary Patients to the Coronary Care Unit Nurse," *American Journal of Nursing,* vol. 70, no. 2, p. 319, February 1970.

43 J. Lynch et al.: "The Effects of Human Contact on Cardiac Arrhythmia in Coronary Care Patients," *Journal of Nervous and Mental Disease,* vol. 158, no. 2, pp. 88–99, February 1974.

44 K. A. J. Järvinen: "Can Ward Rounds Be a Danger to Patients with Myocardial Infarction?" *British Medical Journal,* vol. 1, pp. 318–320, 1955.

45 R. Lee and P. Ball: "Some Thoughts on the Psychology of the Coronary Care Unit Patient," *American Journal of Nursing,* vol. 75, no. 9, pp. 1498–1501, September 1975.

46 M. S. Dominian: "Psychological Stress in Wives of Patients with Myocardial Infarction," *British Medical Journal,* vol. 2, pp. 101–103, April 14, 1973.

47 P. Tyzenhouse: "Myocardial Infarction: Its Effect on the Family," *American Journal of Nursing,* vol. 73, no. 6, pp. 1012–1013, June 1973.

48 R. Ader: "The Role of Developmental Factors in Susceptibility to Disease," *International Journal of Psychiatry in Medicine,* vol. 5, no. 4, pp. 367–376, 1974.

49 F. Kapp: "Psychogenic Pain," in A. Freedman, H. Kaplan, and B. Sadock (eds.), *Comprehensive Textbook of Psychiatry,* 2d ed., Williams & Wilkins, Baltimore, 1975.

50 W. Kiely: "From the Symbolic Stimulus to the Pathophysiological Response: Neurophysiological Mechanism," *International Journal of Psychiatry in Medicine,* vol. 5, no. 4, pp. 517–529, 1974.

51 E. Friedman: "Stress and Intensive Care Nursing," *Heart and Lung,* vol. 1, no. 6, pp. 753–754, November–December 1972.

52 Rhetaugh Dumas: "Utilization of Concept of Stress as a Basis For Nursing Practice," unpublished paper, Yale University, New Haven, Conn., 1969.

53 Robert Trotter: "LeBoyer's Babies," *Science News,* vol. 3, January 22, 1977, p. 59.

54 J. Lewis et al.: *No Single Thread,* Brunner-Mazel, New York, 1976.

55 M. Meyers: "The Effect of Types of Communication on Patients' Reaction to Stress," *Nursing Research,* vol. 13, no. 2, pp. 126–132, Spring 1964.

56 R. Dumas and R. Leonard: "The Effect of Nursing on the Incidence of Postoperative Vomiting," *Nursing Research,* vol. 12, no. 1, pp. 12–15, Winter 1963.

57 Irving Janis: "Vigilance and Decision Making in a Personal Crisis," in G. Coehlo, D. Hamburg, J. Adams (eds.), *Coping and Adaptation,* Basic Books, New York, 1974.

58 D. Mechanic: "Social Structure and Personal Adaptation: Some Neglected Dimensions," in G. Coelho, D. Hamburg, and J. Adams (eds.), *Coping and Adaptation,* Basic Books, New York, 1974.

59 K. Lamott: *Escape From Stress,* Putnam, New York, 1975.

Chapter

27

The Rehabilitative Process

Phyllis E. Porter

Learning Objectives

After studying this chapter, the student should be able to:

1 Define "rehabilitation" as a philosophy, an objective, and a method
2 Describe the historical development of rehabilitation
3 List the events of historical significance in the development of rehabilitation
4 Describe the meaning of rehabilitation and its philosophical implications to the family, the professionals, the patient, and society
5 Describe the characteristics of the client population needing rehabilitation
6 Describe the characteristics of the client population needing rehabilitation
7 Distinguish between the rehabilitative needs of the chronically ill and those of the permanently disabled
8 List the responses of clients and their families to problems creating the need for the rehabilitative process
9 Identify problems for providers of care to clients requiring rehabilitation
10 Identify coping patterns of response
11 List members of the rehabilitation team and their functions and responsibilities
12 Identify the nursing role in planning and implementing care that is rehabilitative

In today's society, the term "rehabilitation" is frequently used in reference not only to individuals suffering from physical maladies but also to those affected by social and psychological patterns of disruption. "Rehabilitation" also often serves to describe the bringing of restorative and remedial processes to communities and their social problems.

"Rehabilitation," therefore, may be variously defined. To define may be to limit perspective, but an understanding of some of the more common definitions may serve as a focal point for discussion. One of the most widely known definitions is that of the National Council on Rehabilitation, issued in 1942, which states: "Rehabilitation is the restoration of the handicapped to the fullest physical, mental, social, vocational, and economic usefulness of which they are capable."[1] This definition illustrates two major components inherent in rehabilitation: the notion of restoration and its comprehensiveness. Whitehouse's definition of "rehabilitation" points to a third major component; the underlying philosophical base. Whitehouse states that "Rehabilitation is the logical fruit of a progressive concern for human welfare . . . engulfed by religious and ethical concepts."[2]

A review of the definitions of "rehabilitation" indicates that the concept must include: a philosophical basis, a concern for human welfare, recognition of the need for restoration, and a comprehensive perspective.

Dimensions of Rehabilitation

The philosophy of rehabilitation becomes the cornerstone for health-care practice and subsequently for nursing practice. Rehabilitation can be viewed from a tridimensional perspective: as a philosophy, as an objective, and as a method. The personnel and structures involved in rehabilitation serve these dimensions in various capacities and may sometimes focus more directly on one or more of the dimensions. An understanding of these dimensions of rehabilitative nursing is essential.

The tridimensional components of rehabilitation concepts are inextricably intertwined. The philosophy of rehabilitation held by the practitioner and the agency determines the objectives of care, and the objectives, in turn, clarify direction and methodology.

philosophy $\longrightarrow$ objectives $\longrightarrow$ method

Thus if there is confusion about a philosophy, the subsequent objectives and methodology will also be lacking in clarity. The result may be total confusion in the rehabilitative process.

Porter[3] states that a basic tenet in a rehabilitative philosophy of nursing is a firm belief in the worth and dignity of the individual. The problems posed by clients requiring rehabilitation are complex and not easily solvable; in many instances they are not solvable at all. It is therefore imperative that nurses involved with these clients have a firm commitment to their care—a commitment based on a firm belief in the worth and dignity of the individual.

The nurse who cares for clients needing rehabilitation must be able to view them and their problems positively. This optimism should not be unrealistic but should be based on an objective assessment of the client's abilities, potential capacities, and limitations. With such a philosophy and objective assessment, the nurse will be able to help the client to achieve the maximum benefits of rehabilitation. Clients and their families can derive the best results from the rehabilitation process only when they understand the realities of their situation. Nurses must be willing to share their knowledge and skills with clients and their families. They must be able to communicate this knowledge and skill in a nonthreatening therapeutic manner and at a level that is understandable to the clients and their families.

Philosophically, the nurse must foster independence in the client; except in those instances where dependence is necessary, the nurse must help the clients deal with their dependence. Clients should be encouraged to gain whatever measure of independence they can, no matter how small that gain may be. In rehabilitative care, the nurse, when necessary, does *for* the client; however in nursing, which is rehabilitative, the nurse works primarily *with* the client. This is often one of the most difficult approaches for the nurse to put into practice.

Finally, rehabilitation must be seen as the right of every client. Rehabilitation must be available for all: the rich and poor, young and old, civilian and military, advantaged and disadvantaged alike. A society that makes available a sophisticated system of medical care capable of saving lives is equally accountable and responsible for developing the rehabilitation services necessary to ensure that the lives saved are worth living.

Rehabilitation as an objective may be seen at two levels. The objective of rehabilitation from the broad societal point of view is in essence as follows: The major objective for the rehabilitation movement is the return of handicapped people to their maximum function in all areas of the human situation, physical, emotional, social, economic, and intellectual. The second level is the implementation of this broad objective in specific instances, applying it in terms of the individual client's and family's needs. This translation into specific objectives provides for an individualized rehabilitation program. Both levels of objectives serve to set directions and goals, one level for rehabilitation programs and one for the specific needs of clients.

The third dimension essential to the concept is that of rehabilitation as a method. This dimension clarifies the concept of *how*. The health-care delivery system must provide rehabilitation services to the consumer. This requires an organization of rehabilitation health-care services. These organizations at the national and community levels represent private and community agencies as well as hospitals and rehabilitation centers. In some instances, agencies are organized to provide special services for selected positions of the consumer population requiring rehabilitation, namely, for those suffering from cerebral palsy, mental retardation, alcoholism, and drug abuse. A broad range of both inpatient and outpatient rehabilitation services is provided by rehabilitation centers that serve clients with a variety of pathological problems representing a variety of age groups.

In addition to agencies, one of the essential components of rehabilitation methodology is the personnel required to provide these services.

The Consumer of Rehabilitation

Everyone requiring health-care service is a consumer of rehabilitation. The dimensions explored in the discussion of rehabilitation should be characteristic of all services in health care. Nursing, in particular, stresses that there is no difference between rehabilitation nursing and comprehensive nursing.

The emphasis in rehabilitation nursing can best be illustrated in the care of clients whose needs require an emphasis on the rehabilitative components of care. These clients are people with chronic diseases or permanent disabilities.

Chronic Illness

Any illness which extends over a prolonged period of time can be considered a chronic illness. The length of time may vary, but in chronic disease there is no hope of full recovery. The disease process may remain fairly stable, with the elements of dysfunction also remaining stable. In other instances, the chronicity is characterized by periods of remission and exacerbation, with concomitant fluctuation in the client's ability to function. Clients with multiple sclerosis often find themselves in this category. In still other instances of chronic disease, there is a steady degenerative disease, the rate of disease progression and the time lapsed is extremely variable. It is not usually possible to predict the rate at which the disease will progress. Many clients with neuromusculoskeletal diseases exhibit this pattern. It can be seen that the variability of the chronic disease pattern is one of its insidious problems.

Case finding may occur in the psychiatric setting because the psychodynamic and behavioral evidence and the feelings experienced by clients with multiple sclerosis or other neurological diseases cause them to to seek psychiatric help. In such instances, careful physical assessment and diagnosis in the psychiatric setting may reveal the underlying causes of the clients' behavior.

Clients with chronic diseases represent an increasing percentage of the general client population. As might be expected, chronic illness is more prevalent in the older age group, but it is also found in people of middle age and in children. In addition, any normal system affected by acute illness can also become heir to chronic disease. Such pathophysiological entities as Parkinson's disease, arthritis, multiple sclerosis, emphysema, circulatory deficiency, and cardiac disease are among the most prevalent chronic diseases today.

Permanent Disability

The term "permanent disability" represents one segment of the client population with chronic disease. Pragmatically, there is value in distinguishing between clients with chronic degenerative disease and clients with permanent disability. When there is permanent disability, the focal point is not the disease or injury but rather the kind and extent of function or dysfunction. Hirschburg[4] divides permanent disability into primary and secondary types. Primary disabilities result from pathological processes and may be caused by congenital disorder, disease, or trauma. Common examples of such primary disabilities would include cerebral palsy, spinal-cord injury, hemiplegia, and amputation. Secondary disabilities represent preventable problems. When they arise from inactivity, they are called *disuse syndromes;* those that stem from contraindicated activity are called *misuse syndromes.*[4]

There are some pragmatic differences between clients with chronic degenerative diseases and clients with permanent disabilities. The underlying rehabilitation approaches for both groups remain the same. However the prognoses for these groups are quite different. Therefore the specific rehabilitation programs may differ.

The client with a chronic degenerative problem represents to nursing and to the health-care delivery system a medical problem that is not solvable and which is predictably going to become worse and ultimately terminal. In general, the rehabilitation program for these clients is designed to prevent secondary disability, to prevent futher primary disability, and to maintain optimal function for as long as possible within the limits imposed by the pathological process. The implementation of such a program falls heavily on the nursing profession and represents one of its greatest challenges.

Clients with permanent disabilities which are not progressive in nature have an entirely different prognosis. The child with cerebral palsy, the young man with spinal-cord injury, or the middle-aged woman with a mastectomy have problems that are permanent and complex, but their conditions are not degenerative. Such clients need a dynamic rehabilitation program in order to return to society at their maximum potential. Although the problems of these clients are not readily or easily solved, a positive prognosis for rehabilitation can be expected within the limits of their disabilities.

The implications of chronic degenerative disease and permanent disability in an increasing segment of the population are enormous. The problems of these clients represent at best the ultimate challenge and at worst an overwhelming despair.

Clients and their families must learn to live with problems that are permanent and that, for some, may be degenerative. They must also deal with many additional stresses including changing family relationships, increased financial stress, and potential changes in employment.

An increasing client population with chronic degenerative disease and/or permanent disability adds many dimensions and stresses to the health-care delivery system and the work of the health professional. The current foci and emphases of many physicians and nurses are care, treatment, and *cure* of the client with acute illness. However, rehabilitation requires a different orientation and a redefinition of goals. The zeal that is brought to the treatment of acute illnesses is also needed in the area of chronic disease and rehabilitation. It is important to stress—to both physicians and nurses—the maximization of potential, the prevention of secondary disability, and the need to cope with the impact of change in function, identity, and body image.

The implications for the community of an increasing population requiring rehabilitation are equally challenging. What place will the disabled person have in the community? How will the community help the disabled to provide for housing, employment, and education/recreational needs? When will the architectural barriers come down? What rehabilitation services will the community provide? Will they come from the private or or public sector? How will programs be financed, organized, and implemented? How will the community find a way to reap the benefits and contributions that its disabled citizens can make?

The Rehabilitative Process

Response to Chronic Disease and Disability

It is in the actual rehabilitative process that the philosophy, objectives, and methodology of rehabilitation—as well as the clients and providers themselves—interact. The rehabilitative process is extremely variable for each client. It is difficult to predict the final outcome and the time that will be needed to reach it because the factors involved are complex. In most instances the process will not move in a straight line; rather, it will be typified by peaks and valleys of success and and frustration and will occasionally be sidetracked. Constant evaluation and reevaluation are therefore vital components.

The rehabilitative process should begin immediately at the onset of illness or injury. The early objectives and program will be set according to the health-care needs of the clients. The nurse and other members of the rehabilitation team may encounter the client initially in any one of several phases of treatment. The client's and family's responses vary at different phases of the rehabili-

tative process; also, this process may occur in a variety of settings. These two factors will influence the client's behavior. It is essential that these two components be remembered by nurses as they begin to implement the rehabilitative process.

It is helpful to divide the rehabilitative process into three periods, the early or acute stage, the middle phase or secondary period, and the third or final phase. In general, the client's and family's patterns of behavior will vary from phase to phase and will be quite characteristic in each of the phases.

Acute Stage

The early phase is characterized by the client's and family's responses to the crisis (see Chap. 5). All clients with disabilities have at some point gone through an acute phase. Their response at this point will be characteristic of the general reactions of clients to illness. It will be individualized according to the specific behavior pattern of the client. For some clients, particularly those with severe trauma, the acute stage is actually a life-threatening stage (see Chap. 29).

Although the rehabilitative process should begin at this stage, it must be remembered that the resources and energies of the client, family, and health team must often be focused on and limited to treatment of the acute injury or illness. This need not, however, preclude preventive rehabilitative measures as they relate to the *disuse* and *misuse* syndromes.

The professional nurse must be especially responsive to nursing diagnoses, goals, and care plans that encompass preventive measures; these are critical during the acute stage and determine the client's ultimate prognosis.

Nursing diagnoses, objectives, and care plans must take into account not only the physical problems and their treatment but also the client's emotional and behavioral responses. As indicated earlier, clients and their families will respond in the myriad of ways in which all clients respond to illness and life-threatening situations (see Chap. 24).

On the positive side, clients characteristically respond by trying to cope with the acute crisis situation. Similarly, families respond with a *rallying-around mechanism* and are usually very concerned and supportive. They demonstrate this, when possible, by frequent telephone calls and visits to the bedside.

The early stage is also marked by less positive behavior. It is critical to remember that the client's responses at this stage are normal and expected. The client is not showing signs of psychopathology when he or she displays fear, anxiety, anger, hostility, dependency, and overwhelming feelings of helplessness. The client's and family's patterns of response are confused and disorganized. During the period of emotional stress, nursing care should be supportive. According to the client's and family's individual responses, nursing care will have to be planned to incorporate a therapeutic response to the client's behavior. For example, if the behavior is hostile, then the nursing diagnosis, intervention, and evaluation should incorporate measures for coping with the hostile client (see Chaps. 17, 19, 13, and 28). The same would apply with regard to client behavior that is indicative of dependence, anxiety, fear, and denial. Again, it must be stressed that sensitivity to the timing of events is essential in the emotional care of clients and their families during this period.

Middle Phase

There are no specific guidelines for the client's transition from the early phase to the middle phase. There may be a clear physical demarcation, however; this is usually characterized by the stability of the client's physical condition. There may even be a physical transfer of the client from one setting to another. The emotional transition is less clear, but at some point all clients emerge into behavior patterns characteristic of the middle period.

The middle stage of the rehabilitative process represents a period of discouragement and uncertainty for the client and family. It is marked by a plateau and low ebb of psychic energy and motivation. Nevertheless, the physical process of rehabilitation should be continued. The plans for physical treatment and rehabilitation are reevaluated and revised in relation to the client's physical condition. It is critical that the client be an active partner with the rehabilitation team during this process.

Emotionally, this period represents a difficult time for client and family. It is early in this period that the client and family recognize the long-term implications of the illness or injury. The awareness that the disability is permanent or progressive constitutes a threat to the ego structure. The client's body image is disrupted and disturbed, resulting in damage to the entire self-concept. The pattern of emotional behavior changes to one that is characteristic of depression. Denial of the disability is a common mechanism for coping. As the disability becomes more real and apparent, however, it becomes more difficult for the client to deny the problem. Anxiety therefore increases and there is a change in the emotional response.

At this point, clients undergo a grieving and mourning process (see Chap. 23). They are mourning for the losses the disability represents. Emotionally, the client is not capable of evaluating the loss realistically; he or she will often perceive it as being greater than it really is. Wright[5] refers to this as *generalizing the disability effect*. These clients are so distraught that they may be overwhelmed by feelings of worthlessness and helplessness. The depression is sometimes also marked by withdrawal behavior.

This phase is particularly challenging to the nurse. The therapeutic relationship with the client and the family must be aimed at helping clients to work through their depression and mourning. The clients may express their grief overtly, or they may tend to keep it to themselves. It is frequently easier for clients to recognize their disability intellectually than emotionally. Some clients talk quite openly about how they feel, with an "I'm no good for anything anymore" response. Others are less open, sometimes hiding their feelings through intellectualization.

Whatever the client's response, nursing therapy must be directed toward maximum support of the client. The timing of therapeutic intervention is important too. The nurse must be alert to clues from clients that they are capable of receiving positive direction. Clients need help in looking into the future, beyond the immediacy of their depression. The sensitivity of the nurse is critical. If the nurse is premature in encouraging the client and too positive too soon, the patient will respond negatively.

On the other hand, prolonged mourning and depression may move from the normal, expected response to a pathological one (see Chaps. 23 and 28). If this occurs, additional psychological help may be called for. Another challenge for the nurse during this period is to help the client maintain motivation for participation in therapy in spite of the pervasive feelings of depression and withdrawal which may interfere with the program plan. Maintenance of the therapy program is important to the client's future. At some point the client will begin to terminate this negative phase. This will not be a sudden step but rather one that is marked by a gradual, positive response on the part of the client. The client experiences a satiation effect with depression and he or she also begins to become aware of the value of being alive.[5]

Final Phase

Following the middle phase, clients will move into the final phase of the rehabilitative process. At this stage, the client and family have begun the process of accepting and adjusting to the disability. The amount of time the client spends on the second phase is extremely variable. However, for clients to achieve the maximum benefits from the rehabilitative process, they must reach some degree of acceptance and adjustment to their disability.

There are a number of individual factors influencing the ability of clients and their families to cope. Of these, probably the single most critical one is the client's personality before illness occurred. If the client was not a well-adjusted, stable person at that time, then he or she will have great difficulty in coping with the disability. The same is true of the family relationship: if this was under stress prior to the disability, it will, in all likelihood, not be able to stand the strain of chronic illness and disability.

Additional client factors influencing acceptance and adjustment include the physical extent of the disability, the impact on life style, the meaning of the disability to the individual, and the client's preconceptions about the disability. The interaction of these components—along with the rehabilitation program and the client's involvement—determine in large measure the final outcomes of the rehabilitative process.

The psychodynamics of acceptance include the following: (1) clients are able to enlarge the scope of their values, making possible an emotional realization of values other than those lost and mourned; (2) the clients' responses to body-image changes become more realistic, less importance is ascribed to physical appearance; (3) clients are able to contain the disability effects, they no longer generalize the disability but are able to appraise realistically their abilities and their limitations; (4) clients are able to appreciate their personal assets just as they are rather than in relation to those of others, and they are able to achieve satisfaction from their accomplishments without comparing them to those of others.[5]

Because clients have begun to cope with the disability, it is at this stage that they are able to achieve the maximum benefits from the rehabilitative process. They are able to put all their energies into their rehabilitation programs. The nurse and other members of the rehabilitation team, along with the client, reevaluate program objectives and goals. Clients and their families continue to need support and reassurance. Final planning for discharge occurs during this phase. As discharge approaches, the clients and their families may feel insecure and may need additional support. At the termination of this stage, clients will have made major adjustments to their disabilities. They will have incorporated a new body image and a new value system. They will be able to accept the limits of their disability and will have established realistic goals for the future. Total acceptance and adjustment will remain a lifelong process, but when rehabilitation is complete, the client will have achieved the means for accomplishing this.

Maladaptive Responses

Not all clients and their families will be able to achieve maximum benefits from the rehabilitative program. As discussed previously, there are many factors which determine the response of the client and the family to the disability and subsequently to the rehabilitative process.

Maladaptive patterns present two inherent dangers. The first of these is too early a conclusion on the part of the rehabilitation staff that the client's response is indeed maladaptive. Clients and their families must be allowed time and given support to work through their emotional responses to their problems. Too early and too zealous an intervention in this process may enhance the confusion and disruption felt by clients and their families and thus may further deter psychological progress.

Conversely, if the staff does not recognize maladaptive behavior patterns until they are well ingrained, then therapeutic intervention becomes more difficult. Hence, rehabilitation personnel must be sensitive to the meaning of the client's behavior as it relates to the total rehabilitative process.

Behavior patterns which are truly maladaptive may take many forms. Most commonly they constitute an exaggeration of the client's premorbid behavior pattern. This exaggeration may be seen in the client's emotional response (e.g., the degree of anger or hostility). It may also be reflected in the time factor; for example, the period of mourning or depression may be prolonged and continue to interfere with the rehabilitative program. It is at the point when maladaptive behavior interrupts the rehabilitation program that these behaviors are usually recognized and/or labeled disruptive. Clients may refuse to dress, go to therapy, or to participate in the rehabilitation program in other ways. They may become more withdrawn, depressed, and dependent. Families, too, may ex-

hibit maladaptive response behavior. They may withdraw from the situation, fail to visit the client, refuse to allow the client home on weekends, encourage overdependence in the client, or refuse to learn the techniques needed to care for the client. In such instances, intensive therapeutic intervention by members of the rehabilitation team is needed and psychiatric consultation may be helpful.

Clients who refuse to participate in their rehabilitation programs often present particular difficulty to the rehabilitation team. Unless careful analysis is made and care is taken, the team's response to the client may become negative and nontherapeutic, thus further disrupting the rehabilitative process. Team members who are frustrated in their efforts may become angry and authoritative with the clients. Team members may also feel guilty and feel that they have failed to help the client. In such difficult situations, consultation may be of help to the staff in their analysis and treatment of the client's response to the rehabilitation program.

All clients and their families will not be able to achieve the ultimate goals in rehabilitation. However, with careful analysis and planning of the rehabilitation program, the number of those who fall short should be small, and even those with greater problems and fewer resources should be able to attain some measure of success.

References

1   W. Scott Allan: *Rehabilitation: A Community Challenge*, Wiley, New York, 1958, p. 2.
2   Frederick A. Whitehouse: "Rehabilitation as a Dimension of Human Welfare," *Journal of Rehabilitation*, July–August 1961, p. 11.
3   Phyllis E. Porter: "The Worth of Man as an Individual: A Philosophical Approach to Rehabilitative Nursing," *Journal of Rehabilitation*, September–October, 1962, p. 11.
4   Gerald Hirschberg, Leon Lewis, and Dorothy Thomas: *Rehabilitation*, Lippincott, Philadelphia, 1964, p. 12–14.
5   Beatrice A. Wright: *Physical Disability—A Psychological Approach*, Harper, New York, 1960, pp. 108–131.

28

Clients Dependent on Technology

Judith Gregorie D'Afflitti

Learning Objectives

After studying this chapter, the student should be able to:

1 Assess the psychodynamics of clients with chronic illness who are dependent on life-sustaining technology

2 Identify the losses and changes experienced by the client and family

3 Assess the impact of these losses and changes on the client and family

4 Assess their own response to the client and family and its effect on the delivery of care

5 Formulate nursing goals for the client and family

6 Formulate nursing diagnoses of the client's and family's responses to the chronic disease and dependency on technology

7 Intervene to assist the client and family cope effectively

8 Analyze the rationale, risk/benefit, and implications of transplantation

9 Evaluate the effectiveness of nursing interventions

When people become ill, the first concern is that for life itself. Nothing else matters until and unless these people are reassured that they will live. The next concern is *how* life? In what ways will the illness mandate changes in the person's life? What losses must be faced?

Many times the answer to this question involves the acceptance of a regular medication, a special diet, and/or a procedure which is essential to living with the disease. If the illness is *chronic,* with irreversible physical changes and usually no possibility of cure, the medications, diet, and life-essential procedures are also chronic.

Clients with renal failure, stroke, brittle diabetes, pacemaker implantation, and traumatic neurological deficits as well as those who are victims of degenerative and debilitating diseases are faced with adjustment to the disease and also to the treatment for the disease.

Psychodynamics

Emotional Response to Chronic Disease: Grief and Mourning

Nursing is the diagnosis and treatment of a client's response to disease. With chronic disease, the two major concerns are (1) the person's reaction and adjustment to change and loss in many areas of life and (2) the person's cooperation and responses to the necessary treatments. When clients have chronic diseases, nurses are primarily dealing with the emotional response of grief and the psychobiological process of mourning, Nurses must recognize how these clients are responding to their losses and help them to reach a resolution of those losses (see Chap. 23).

People's responses to loss are dependent on their personalities, the patterns they have developed in dealing with past losses, and the present situation in terms of environmental and interpersonal interactions and supports (see Fig. 28-1). Each of these factors must be evaluated on an individual basis through interviews and interac-

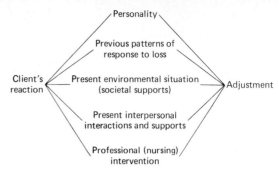

Figure 28-1 Factors in response to loss.

tions with client and family. The overall human response to loss however, has been well described by many authors[1-3] and can be reviewed in terms of three phases: (1) protest and denial, (2) depression and despair, and (3) detachment and reinvestment (see Chap. 23).

Protest and Denial

In the first stage people are very much involved with what has been lost and are constantly disappointed as they try to regain this. Anxiety, intense sadness, and anger are the prevalent feelings. Weeping is common. The person says and thinks such things as: "How could this happen to me?" "It can't be true." "I'm sure when I wake in the morning it will be gone." "I'm getting better every day, soon I'll be my old self." Some denial is an essential defense so that the person will not be overwhelmed with the feelings of loss. Reality is handled in tolerable doses, and eventually the protesting stops. Then these people can allow themselves to feel.

Depression and Despair

Depression and despair predominate when these persons stop putting energy into futile attempts to recover what has been lost and allow themselves to feel the empty spaces created by the loss. There is a painful disorganization, restlessness, and depression. The person thinks and says such things as: "Why did this happen to me?" "I've always led a good life." "How am I going to manage now?" "Nothing—no one—can help me." Since these people still see help in terms of regaining what has been lost, they feel hopeless. It is often a time for lashing out at family and hospital staff because they are unable to do the impossible—bring back what has been lost. People must begin to allow themselves to feel and express the agonies of the loss.

Detachment and Reinvestment
In this stage people are able to detach themselves sufficiently from the lost objects to have the energy for new investments and relationships. They begin to accept what they have and to work with that. They may think and act on such thoughts as: "I won't be able to travel the way I used to, but with good planning we could have an occasional trip." "I couldn't manage my old job, but my sister needs some help in her office, and I could handle that work now." There is growth in new directions with personal rewards.

Two points must be stressed about these phases of loss. The first is that the process is not really a sequence of steps but rather an intermingling of all the phases with a predominance of one. A person can experience the phases in any order and even all at once. The successful end of the process, however, should be detachment and reinvestment. The time it takes a person to successfully deal with a loss is highly variable and dependent on the nature of the loss, the individual's personality, and many environmental and interpersonal factors. Those who are not involved in the grieving often expect the person to resolve the loss too quickly. A year is *not* a long time in dealing with loss. And for people with chronic disease, the losses are often progressive, so it is difficult for them to stop grieving (see Chap. 23).

Types of Loss with Chronic Disease

Loss of Well-Being (Health)
Initially, the person experiences a physical crisis and responds realistically with great fear and anxiety for life itself. People around the ill person offer reassurance about what can be done. If treatment does indeed help the person's physical functioning, fear of extinction moves into the background as attempts are made to deal with many other changes. However, the fear of death is a backdrop for all the less catastrophic fears to follow.

Loss of Independence
From the moment of birth we struggle for an appropriate amount of personal independence in our environment and human relationships. Events throughout our lives, physical and emotional, help form our patterns of dependence-independence. If all goes well, there will, as we reach adulthood, be a balanced personality structure that allows for maximum creativity and integrity. When people become ill, they are forced back into patterns of dependence they had long since abandoned. They must often depend on others for assistance with bodily needs and functions, from help with personal hygiene and mobility to help with toileting. Other adults, from family members to stranger-professionals, often take over decision making for the ill person. It is at best frightening and conflicting for adults when they are suddenly forced to revert to patterns of dependence they may have abandoned in childhood.

The client with renal failure is dependent on a hospital and its personnel, a machine, a diet, medications, possibly a shunt, perhaps society for financial assistance, and many other things which comprise a "program" to maintain life. The client with a pacemaker and the brittle diabetic are also dependent on the health-care system for periodic care and emergency treatment. Not since infancy has such a person been so dependent on people and things outside the self for survival. At the same time that they have lost adult independence in so many areas, they are expected to maintain independent adult behavior in areas of work, finances, family, and other social relationships. This is a difficult task at best, requiring the development of new self-concepts and patterns of dependence-independence. Of course the degree to which these people were successful in working with the human condition of dependence-independence before the illness will directly affect the degree to which they can adjust creatively to the demands of chronic disease.

Loss of Familiar Surroundings

At a time when clients could most use the reassurances of the place and people they know best, they are forced to move to a hospital, which is a strange environment, and to relate in a dependent manner to many strangers who purport to help them. When the illness is chronic, the person faces repeated hospitalizations. In the case of chronic kidney failure, the treatment of hemodialysis is often done in the hospital setting. No matter how familiar a setting the hospital becomes, it is never a place where the person controls the environment.

Loss of Comfort

It is very distracting and frightening to be physically uncomfortable. The discomfort is an ever-present reminder of vulnerability and does not allow a person to focus well on other aspects of life. The more severe the discomfort, the more severe the disruption of activities, ranging from care of one's own body to interpersonal relationships. The person with chronic kidney disease suffers pain, itching, weakness, and some periodic mental slowness and confusion. The paraplegic must learn to live with frequent muscle spasms, and other clients with limited mobility must also cope with frequent discomfort.

Loss of Physical Function

Many people with chronic illnesses experience intermittent or permanent loss of various valued physical functions. People with kidney failure are no longer handling fluids and urination as they once did. They often complain of an overall weakness and malaise which prevents them from performing usual and desired activities. With many chronic illnesses, active participation in sports or jobs requiring physical strength or stamina must

be abandoned. The treatment of people with kidney failure and diabetes includes strict dietary requirements, so that they cannot eat and enjoy food and drink in the same way as before. Sexual functioning is often impaired or lost when there is chronic illness. In some instances, the problem is simply a result of low energy and interest because of preoccupation with one's physical problems. In other cases—as with long-term renal failure, diabetes, or the use of certain antihypertensive and diuretic medications—there is impotence and an inability to have an orgasm.

The treatment of hemodialysis—requiring physical connection to a machine two to three times a week for 6 to 8 hours at a time, the implanted pacemaker, and the daily insulin injection are ongoing reminders of the loss of physical function.

Loss of Mental Function

The emotional stress of trying to cope with the many losses of chronic disease results in states of anxiety and depression. People are often less able to concentrate and organize thoughts efficiently, so that they cannot think as clearly as they did before the illness. In addition, many illnesses result in organic changes which affect mental functioning. Fluid and electrolyte imbalances and the buildup of toxins or waste products caused by kidney or liver dysfunction can result in organic brain problems such as language or memory impairment. Medications such as diuretics and antihypertensives can also cause mental confusion. Brain-tissue damage caused by cerebrovascular accidents is also a chronic disease process that affects cognitive and affective functioning (see Chap. 30).

Loss of Familiar Appearance (Change in Body Image)

Loss of physical function is often related to changes in body image and self-concept. Changes in physical appearance may occur suddenly, sporadically, or continuously during chronic illness and result in a profound alteration in body image. Chronic kidney failure usually results in decreased body fat; periodic puffiness of tissue due to fluid retention; a change in skin color to a sallow, jaundiced look; and a slowing of body movement. As a result, these people often appear to be suffering from chronic disease. The treatment of hemodialysis causes bruises and punctures in arms and/or legs; sometimes a disfiguring plastic shunt is permanently inserted in an arm or leg; and peritoneal dialysis causes distortion of the abdomen. Renal transplantation is major surgery and brings with it all the bodily wounds and consequent scars associated with such surgery. Chronic illnesses which cause muscular wasting, paralysis, or disfigurement disrupt the body image and self-concept (see Chap. 23).

Loss of Roles in Society

People develop a life-style which includes participation in travel, the theater, church, community, work, sports, school, and social groups. Such activities may be disrupted temporarily or permanently by chronic illness. Our society stresses independence as a virtue, and the dependence forced on people by illness results in a loss of cultural as well as personal esteem.

Loss of Roles in Family

Change in family role can be in terms of concrete functions and interpersonal relationships. The sick person may no longer be able to maintain the household physically, feed the family, or bring in a salary for financial support. The client may have been the family member who mediated disputes or perhaps served as the family scapegoat. Chronic illness can force changes in these roles and relationships. Anger or impatience toward the sick member may evoke feelings of guilt in family members. The conflicts generated by the normal "sandpaper effect" of living together may not be openly and authentically resolved, causing increasing tensions. These tensions, if unresolved, may be acted out in ways which interfere with the treatment plan, isolate the client within the family, or cause behavioral or physical problems in other members.

A problem that is often mentioned when the client is male is that of *role reversal*. Our culture still infuses the male role with power and dominance and an expectation that the male will be the breadwinner. Chronic illness can make a man physically, financially, and emotionally dependent on his wife. He may perceive this position as feminine or childlike, as a loss of control and leadership to the wife. The wife, burdened with the chronically sick husband, may have to assume a major role in supporting the home and rearing the children, forcing her to revise her earlier definition and expectations of family life. Women with chronic illness, forced to relinquish their role as homemakers, may be equally distressed by the loss of their position as nurturers and caretakers in their families. It may frustrate and depress such a woman to see chores poorly done, not done at all, or constituting a burden to her spouse and children.

In our present culture, many women are struggling for a new emotional and financial independence. It can be a bitter and difficult adjustment for these women to face the dependence imposed by chronic disease. They may be forced to surrender hard-won positions in the business world and their own homes. They may be forced to return to their families of origin, only to be placed in a childlike role. All these concrete and emotional losses in family role mean change for the ill person and for the whole family as a system.

Loss of Self-Concept

The combined result of the physical, emotional, interpersonal, and social-system role changes just discussed is a change in self-concept for the individual. People with an illness feel differently about themselves in relation to their world, and they are viewed differently by that world. Since self-concept is a combination of internal and external opinion, adaptive and creative response to chronic disease must be a positive interaction between the person with the disease and the individuals and social structures around that person. Neither will succeed in isolation (see Chap. 23).

Nurse's Response

It has been observed that there are unique responses and problems for the medical and nursing staff caring for the chronically ill person, especially the client with chronic renal failure. The difficulty in working with the person with chronic disease is akin to the difficulty in working with the dying person. There is no "cure," and the client's problems cannot be eliminated. The medical and nursing task is to help people live as comfortably and fully as possible with their limitations. This involves the staff's ability to face disappointment and loss on a regular basis and to continue to give sensitive care. Abram[1,4] points out that staff use denial along with client and family to avoid facing painful facts, such as the client's deterioration or loss of will to continue living with the limitations imposed by the disease process. This denial often results in staff anger when some crisis forces reality on everyone. On the basis of a 2-year study of the emotional problems of a medical team, De-Nour and Czackes[5] report that guilt, possessiveness, overprotectiveness, and withdrawal from patients are the major responses. They attribute anxiety and guilt to frustration and anger around the fact that the staff recognize that they are not omnipotent. Hostility toward an ever-demanding client whose lack of improvement generates feelings of helplessness and incompetence in the caretakers is the underlying basis for both the overprotective and rejecting withdrawal reactions.

It is difficult for staff to feel that they are doing all they can and still, often, see an end result that amounts to physical and emotional misery. There is underlying doubt about the good of the treatment they are offering. This doubt makes staff very sensitive to any criticism or lack of cooperation on the part of the client. The "good" clients are those who do exactly as they are told and do not confront the staff with their denied frustrations and limitations. If clients act out their frustrations with treatment by not following the treatment regimen in some way, the staff become angry and withdraw from these people. This isolates clients and does not allow for the expression of negative feelings; it certainly interferes still further with the effectiveness of treatment. The same staff responses occur,

along with defensiveness, when clients do express their anger openly and direct it toward the caretakers, the agency, or the treatment program.

The first thing to remember is that clients need help with their *response* to disease. Nursing's responsibility is primarily to help clients cope with this response, even if it is not always possible to alleviate suffering. However, nurses can help clients to live with their suffering so that they can continue to create, grow, and relate in everyday life. Nursing's goal and reward cannot always be a happy, comfortable client.

Caring for a person with a chronic disease, like caring for the geriatric client in a home or the person who is terminally ill, necessitates extra support for the staff simply because they are all human. It is impossible to deal with physical and emotional suffering day after day in an open, sensitive, objective way without support from peers and authorities. Regular, at least weekly, conferences for staff to discuss together their clients and problems can nurture staff and provide more objective, effective management of the client. The conferences should be run by a *benevolent authority* on the problems of chronic illness who understands the stresses experienced by staff and provides direction and rewards for care given. This person can be an authority on the unit who does not have a direct personal relationship with the clients and the resulting emotional involvement; or the leader may be an outside consultant, such as a psychiatric liaison nurse. It is useful for these conferences to be interdisciplinary, as this facilitates collaboration among the team of professionals coordinating care for the client.

Death on a dialysis or chronic-care unit is a very difficult experience for clients and staff alike. It confronts everyone with a reality they are trying to avoid; the fact that chronic kidney failure or other such diseases are ultimately fatal. Past feelings of hostility and frustration toward the client now give rise to guilt and a feeling of failure. Everyone is quite naturally depressed by the loss and its implications. The principles for successful mourning apply in this situation also. There needs to be expression of feelings in order for depression to resolve into a reinvestment of energies. The staff must help clients express their grief, and it is equally important that staff express their feelings to each other. This is an important use for the regular conference previously described (see Chap. 31).

Assessment

The kidney client typifies the client with a chronic disease who is dependent on technology for survival but does not require continuous hospitalization. The client suffering from heart disease who has a pacemaker or the diabetic on insulin—neither of whom is greatly restricted by the disease or its treatment—have similar emotional responses and adjustments.

The overall framework for assessing, understanding, and dealing with a person's response to illness is that of loss and grief. Within that framework, however, there are other areas for assessment which stem from the specific illness and its treatment as well as the client's personality and interpersonal and environmental supports. In the following paragraphs, general issues will be addressed using the kidney client as the primary example.

There are many causes of chronic renal failure and the need for dialysis, including glomerular disease, vascular disease, infections, obstructions, collagen disease, and polycystic kidney disease. The person's initial response to renal failure will be influenced to some degree by whether the onset is sudden and catastrophic, as with obstruction, or gradual, as when failure results from chronic infection. The nurse may observe a person numb with shock, unable to believe what has happened, or someone in deepened depression who is trying to summon coping energy that has already been depleted by prolonged illness. If the etiology is polycystic disease, the issue of heredity further complicates the emotional response. There is increased guilt in the parents, who feel they are directly responsible for the illness; the family also experiences heightened anxieties and fears that the disease could vic-

timize any other member. The impact of hereditary diseases on family members is discussed in Chap. 37. Thus the cause and manner of onset of renal failure or any chronic disease are important factors in the way a person begins to deal with illness.

The kidney is the main organ which eliminates the end products of protein metabolism, and it maintains the water and electrolyte balance within the body. When the kidney fails, treatment includes a special diet to control protein, fluid, and electrolyte intake; medications mostly for the control of blood pressure and fluid balance; and hemodialysis—either at home or at a community facility or hospital unit—*or* peritoneal dialysis *or* kidney transplantation. Many factors are involved in the decision regarding the type of dialysis to be used or whether transplantation will be offered to the client. These factors include the client's medical situation; the facilities available; the financial situation of client and agency; and, at times, the psychological needs of a client and family. As yet there are no sound criteria for correlating these needs with type of treatment.

The artificial kidney machine used in hemodialysis was the first mechanical device to substitute for a body organ. Presently this is the most successful treatment for kidney failure, since people generally live longer on dialysis then they do following transplantation. The strong wishes of many patients for transplantation have less to do with life itself than with the *how* of life. Most people do not want to adjust to a chronic treatment for chronic disease. They want a cure, even if it involves a considerable risk to life itself.

Assessment of the client with a chronic illness that involves ongoing dependence on technology focuses on five major areas of concern: (1) the independence-dependence conflict, (2) the use of denial, (3) anxiety and depression, (4) anger, and (5) the family.

Independence-Dependence Conflict

The independence-dependence conflict is one of the most troublesome for the person with chronic illness, particularly renal failure.[4] Although this is an important conflict for any chronically ill person, it is perhaps more salient for a client who is involved with frequent, direct dependence on a machine and the person who is assisting with the use of that machine. It is most difficult to be dependent in the area of treatment of an illness and then to function independently in the rest of life. There are some people who are able to accomplish this well, but many clients exhibit either excessive dependence in all areas of their lives or a rebellious, adolescent-type of counterdependence which does not allow effective medical management of the illness.

Nurses tend to become exasperated with overdependence and counterdependence. The former makes them feel abused and burdened, and the latter makes them feel ineffective and helpless. Since both behaviors cause withdrawal by staff, they must be examined by nurses in the assessment of the client. When caretakers experience these feelings, it is a signal that client behaviors may be a triggering factor. Careful assessment is then necessary: the client's behaviors and manner of relating to staff must be examined to see whether there is evidence of resistance to treatment, sabotage of treatment, or demands for assistance in activities which could be managed unaided. Once behaviors have been identified and labeled, the next step in assessment is a determination of the client's need to act in this way. Understanding the client's need for this behavior leads to its acceptance and to assisting the client to explore other options.

Denial

Many defenses are naturally and appropriately used by clients to help them cope with their disease. De-Nour[6] lists denial, displacement, isolation of affect, projection, and reaction formation against aggression as the most common. He goes on to note that all these defenses are labile and brittle; therefore they can easily be shaken by any additional life stress. The clients are using almost all their psychic resources to deal with the illness and its treatment, and their ability to cope will decrease markedly with new stresses. It is important for the nurse to anticipate and assess the client for changes in coping and to determine how effectively these mechanisms are serving the client. Denial is a common and useful defense. However, of all the defenses used by the ill person, it seems to present the most difficulty to medical and nursing staff when it is used in such a way as to impair treatment. For example, there are many clients who consistently fail to stay on a reasonable diet because they cannot believe that what they eat and drink will affect their health. Anger[7] talks about this in terms of dialysis clients being *externally oriented,* that is, they perceive the illness and its resulting life changes as something that happened to them because of uncontrollable outside forces such as fate, or as *internally oriented,* perceiving the problem as coming from within and being affected by their own actions. The externally oriented client does not feel that his or her own action can affect this imposed disease. For such clients, it is very difficult to adhere to a treatment regimen which limits bodily comforts, life-style, and enjoyments as basic as eating when the disease is already so limiting.

It is also very difficult for some people to accept the fact that their bodies do not work like those of most other people around them and that they are in some way deficient. Therefore they engage in constant testing to try to prove to themselves that the deficiencies are not really there. The realization that one is chronically ill, possibly deteriorating, and experiencing many great losses is anxiety-provoking. If denial were not used to some extent, these people would be overwhelmed by their situation. Denial which enables the person to participate in life—maximizing opportunities for recreation and meaningful work—has positive value. However, denial of major requirements of the treatment regimen such as adhering to dietary restrictions and taking required medications faithfully is life-threatening. The degree to which clients can accept limitations and losses will be the degree to which they can limit denial. It is therefore important to assess the extent to which denial is being used as well as its compatibility with effective management of the health problem.

Anxiety and Depression

Anxiety and depression are two prevalent emotional states for the person with chronic disease. It must be stressed that these responses are usually based on the reality of having to adjust to many losses.[8] Anxiety and depression are normal and necessary feelings as a person works to adjust to the many changes presented by the illness and its treatment. It is also important to note that with chronic disease comes chronic deterioration, so that the person is continuously facing new losses. Nurses and family often expect a patient to "cheer up" after a while or to become less frightened about changes in procedure or bodily functioning. This expectation of the nursing staff comes from their own difficulty in facing anxiety and depression constantly and perhaps from a misguided notion that they should be able to dispel these feelings for the client. Family expectations are often derived from their need to have the sick member be more comfortable and to be themselves less pained and burdened by what they see their loved one experiencing.

For many people chronic anxiety and depression are part of the chronicity of their situation. This is not pathology requiring psychiatric intervention. It is a human response to devastating, continuous loss.

Assessment of anxiety and depression focuses on collecting data which will indicate the degree and extent of interference with the client's

- Ability to learn about how to manage the disease, such as the care of a shunt or pacemaker
- Ability to learn about which foods are to be avoided or limited and the quantities permitted
- Ability to follow directions concerning medications and their side effects
- Capacity to attend and relate to others or the environment versus total self-absorption, which limits the quality of life

- Capacity to interact with the environment and demonstrate motivation to engage in meaningful activity versus vegetative passive existence
- Capacity not only to cope daily but to see life as desirable rather than welcoming death

Chapter 18, Table 14-1 in Chap. 14, and the section on giving-up–given-up complex in Chap. 31 are useful guides in the assessment of anxiety depression.

Anger

Anger is a feeling commonly experienced by the chronically ill, but they have difficulty expressing it directly because of the degree to which they depend on family and professionals not only for basic needs but for survival itself. Their fantasy is that the expression of anger will lead to abandonment and rejection. These clients know that their lives depend on those around them, so that direct expression of anger is a risk they choose not to take, since the stakes are too high. However, unexpressed anger may be acted out in ways that sabotage treatment or create sufficient stress to cause other physical problems or psychopathology (see Chap. 26). If the client is able to express anger about the situation, the family, the caretakers, or the treatment program, the anger is less likely to be repressed or displaced. The assessment process focuses on determining whether the person is expressing anger, how the anger is being expressed, and whether the expression is being accepted by caretakers and significant others as a normal and necessary part of the process of dealing with the imposed losses. If the expression of anger is producing interpersonal problems for the client, steps can be taken to help all concerned to understand and accept the situation.

Interpersonal and Mechanical Relationship

The relationships of the chronically ill with those around them are easily interfered with by the amount of emotional energy that is expended in dealing with the stresses presented by the illness.

Family, friends, and business colleagues are viewing the client differently and feeling stress around increased responsibilities and perhaps role changes imposed by the illness. But there is also a rather unique relationship that must be considered in an attempt to fully understand the situation of the client with kidney failure: the relationship between the person and the machine.

Today, everyone is dependent to a large degree on technology. There would be no way to feed the population of the United States, for example, without a mechanized farming and transportation system. When they are ill, most people depend on technology for diagnosis and treatment, but they are not directly, intimately and regularly dependent on a machine for life itself. This, however, is the situation of clients on dialysis and those who have implanted pacemakers.

Abram[4] has studied clients who have been dialyzed and reports that they feel dehumanized by their dependence on a machine for what should be a normal function of their own bodies. These people do not feel entirely human. Some liken themselves to "zombies," people risen from the dead, or "androids," robots who appear human. On the other hand, Abram says clients project human feelings onto the machine, at times even having delusions that the machine is performing well or poorly with some direct intent to benefit or destroy them. Clients understandably feel a great deal of ambivalence about the machine and focus considerable frustration and anger upon the dialysis procedure. One client spoke of this relationship by saying, "I find it impossible to make friends with the monster."[4] Because clients to some extent incorporate the machine as a part of themselves, they also project their own feelings onto it. It should also be remembered that people on dialysis are often experiencing some organic brain syndrome from chemical imbalances in the body, and that the resulting confusion could increase the distortion in their minds concerning their relationship to the machine (see Chap. 30).

Given the reality that the person being dialyzed or using a pacemaker may have incorporated this technology into his or her body image, the assessment focuses on:

- The client's perception of the incorporation; whether the projected feelings interfere with active, cooperative participation in the treatment program or generate feelings which are frightening or have a negative effect on care
- Whether the client's perception is distorted to the point of delusional ideation and developing psychopathology, or organic brain syndrome, which may indicate a need for reevaluating the medical management or the client's adherence to the regimen requirements

The Family

Thus far we have discussed the impact of chronic disease and its treatment from the point of view of the person with the illness. No less involved, and certainly no less relevant, is the family and/or significant others of the person with the illness. People function not only as individuals but also as parts of a social system. The quality and substance of a person's life is largely determined by the quality and substance of relationships with other people. Each one of us has a number of people who are intimately involved with our self-concept and the purpose of our everyday activities.

The family of the person with chronic illness suffers fear and loss in much the same way as the client. There is constant fear about the permanent loss of the loved one through death. There are constant losses and changes in role and functioning in response to the changes in the client. The family is also going through a process of grief and mourning.

Family members use denial to cushion the feelings brought about by loss. They become depressed as reality overcomes denial and as they are burdened by extra responsibilities with the ill person. There is a very normal anger at the deprivation, fears, inconveniences, and burdens imposed by the illness and its treatment. And there is guilt over the anger because it is felt that one should not be angry at a person who is sick. There is also a sense of helplessness because one is not able to alleviate the ill person's suffering or bring back life as it used to be. There is a great frustration and mourning for all the dreams for the future that must be abandoned.

The family of the person with an identified illness must be included in the treatment of that person. The family system can be likened to a hand, with the fingers representing the members of the family. If something happens to one of the fingers to change its functioning and role, all the other fingers are affected and vice-versa. The changes are often subtle and complicated, but one cannot understand or deal with a person's response to illness without assessing, understanding, and dealing with the system of other people who are integrally involved with those responses.

An expectation for the continuation of rewarding family relationships, in spite of new stresses and many changes, is vital for the clients' motivation to deal with their illnesses and treatment. Therefore, the family is also the client as far as the nurse is concerned.

There are multiple situational changes for families over and above the changes in the client's status. Finances are usually a problem as work gets interrupted and the expense of treatment has to be met. Daily schedules and routines are altered for dialysis. The family's dietary habits may not be compatible with the client's needs, and there may be requirements necessitating the preparation of special meals in special ways. Relationships with friends change, sometimes gradually but usually in the direction of deterioration, resulting in a loss of this support system. Often social contacts are narrowed to the nuclear family. People find it difficult to deal with chronic illness, and the client may have limited energy, so that there is a mutual withdrawal.

The stresses on the family are very great, and hostile feelings toward the client are generated because of the burdens of the illness. These hostile feelings are sometimes acted out by the family toward the client in life-threatening ways: medical appointments are missed and dietary restrictions are not supported or perhaps even directly violated.

With home dialysis there is large, ominous equipment which serves as a constant reminder of the client's problem, its severity, and the responsibility it imposes on the family member or members who must assist the client.

Home hemodialysis poses increased problems for the relationship between the client and the person assisting with the dialysis, usually a spouse. The person doing the dialysis is constantly fearful that the loved one will die on the machine; and this is, of course, a real possibility. The client's dependency on this person is a burden for both and interferes with effective communication, especially of hostile or negative feelings. Anger is repressed but constantly fed by a situation in which the person doing the dialysing feels there is a great deal of "giving" and little "getting" in return.[9] Denial is the usual defense used to cope with the difficulties, and this, of course, interferes with the quality of the relationship. Home dialysis is known to be stressful, perhaps to the point of being contraindicated in some cases.

Children

Not enough is known about the reaction of children to a parent or sibling on in-hospital or home dialysis. Hoover[10] reports that children are exposed to vast changes and losses in family life; frightening scenes, such as hemorrhages; and frequent parental absence. The stress within the family is often characterized by inconsistency and instability in limit setting, giving of affection and demonstration of love, appropriate letting go, separation, and balancing of dependence and independence. Discipline is often a problem as children act out their angry and depressed feelings around the loss and deprivation in their lives. School performance may decline; aggression and withdrawal can increase if the child is unsupported.

The assessment of the family's response to the client's problems focus on:

1 Feelings generated and how they are being dealt with

2 Adequacy of support for all members

Table 28-1 Nursing Assessment Criteria for Positive Movement in the Process of Mourning

1	Effective expression of sad, anxious, and angry feelings
2	Periods of depression where the loss is faced and ramifications are felt
3	Resumption of some old and beginning of new relationships and activities, with recognition and integration of the loss as part of life

3 Ability to cope with changes in life-style, financial demands, and alterations in roles and relationships

The criteria used in the nursing assessment of clients and families to determine positive movement in the process of mourning the losses incurred by chronic disease are presented in Table 28-1.

Nursing Diagnosis

Analysis of the assessment data and examination of the broad goals provide the basis for conceptualizing the client's problems and formulating nursing diagnoses. The following are examples of nursing diagnoses representative of some of the major problems and needs confronted by these clients:

- Excessive and pervasive use of denial is interfering with adherence to dietary regimen, causing severe metabolic derangements.
- High levels of anxiety are blocking ability to comprehend content of teaching plan and to participate in the treatment regimen.
- "Nice guy" approach toward staff reflects inability to express anger and frustration when dialysis procedure causes problems.

- Withdraws from relationship with staff by feigning sleep and covering face with sheet during dialysis.

- Explosive, inappropriately directed hostility toward family members in increasing family disorganization and client's abandonment.

One young man with diabetes suddenly developed irreversible renal failure. His brow was always knit, his eyes were open wide, and his gaze darted from object to object in the room. He was sweating and sighing a great deal, but his only comments were that he was sure his kidneys would be fine, and any hour now the doctors would discover this too. This man is very appropriately in the initial phase of grieving for his lost kidneys. Part of him does not believe this loss has occurred, but somewhere there is a beginning realization of the loss as he exhibits anxiety and depression.

The nursing diagnosis in this case would be, "Client moving from phase of shock and disbelief into growing awareness that renal failure is irreversible."

Nursing Goals

When the data base regarding the client's and family's response to the chronicity of the disease and its ramifications has been assembled and analyzed, the nurse formulates goals which will provide direction in planning intervention and evaluating care. The following represent sample goals which would be established for clients with chronic illness who are dependent on technology for the maintenace of life:

1 Assist the client and family to cope effectively with the grieving process.
2 Prevent the development of psychopathology.
3 Assist the client and family to develop ways of coping effectively with the changes in body image, roles, relationships and life-style.
4 Help the client and family to participate actively and in a healthy way in the treatment regimen.
5 Help the client to integrate the loss.

Nursing Intervention

The Client

Clients coping with loss are dealing with feelings of disbelief, anxiety, anger, depression, and fear. They are using defenses such as denial, displacement, and identification to soften the impact of the loss so that feelings can be faced and worked through. The nurse's first responsibility is to understand the human feelings of grief and the process of mourning so that the client's emotional response can be understood.

Nurses must next examine their own feelings, defenses, and behaviors with regard to loss. This self-awareness is something that can only be achieved over time by examining responses to personal life events and client interactions to learn about oneself. It is of paramount importance, because without it the nurse is likely to allow personal feelings and responses to interfere with competent, objective nursing diagnosis and care of the client.

Acceptance of clients' feelings about the changes in their lives is the way in which the nurse can best support these people to endure the painful period of grief and continue on to some resolution of their loss. This can be a difficult task, because everyone prefers to avoid feelings like fear, despair, and anger. Genuine acceptance of whatever a person needs to feel supports that person's self-concept and prevents isolation. This support allows the person to work through the necessary painful feelings and resolve the losses.

In the case of the young man with diabetes and renal failure, the nurse need not confront his verbal denial. Instead, comments such as, "It must be very hard for you to believe this has happened to you" are most helpful, because they recognize, acknowledge and accept what is happening to this person. Such an approach should eventually encourage the client to talk about his anxieties.

When clients use denial to the degree that it interferes with treatment, the nursing intervention is aimed at helping them accept themselves as worthwhile. Illness does not diminish one's value as a person or one's dignity. The nursing task is to help the person confront, *a little at a time,* the losses imposed by the disease and to mourn these losses effectively (see Chap. 23).

Progression from initial denial to anxiety and depression does not go on at an even pace, and clients will at times fail to cooperate with the treatment program. These behaviors must be recognized as meeting a need for the client and not interpreted as a rejection of the nurse, the team, or the program. Reassessment of the client's physical, social, and psychological status may reveal precipitating causes for this pathological use of denial and indicate a need to revise the plan of care.

When the client displays anxiety and/or depression, the appropriate nursing intervention is acceptance of these feelings and constant reassurance about what is positive in the situation, so that these clients do not add isolation to their list of discomforts and have some help in keeping their feelings in line with reality.

The client should be encouraged to express all feelings, especially the difficult ones like anger and depression, because without expression the feelings become buried, only to reemerge at another time. Nurses need to let clients know that anger is a normal part of dealing with loss and that they can allow themselves to feel and express anger without fear of abandonment. If anger is repressed, expressed only indirectly through sabotage of treatment, or turned into sarcasm, the clients will become more depressed as they turn the anger inward and focus it on themselves. The sad reality is that staff often do withdraw from the angry client.

Nurses must expect some anger to be directed at treatment and at them as a part of that treatment. Becoming angry or defensive in return is not an objective response. Instead, the nurse should just acknowledge the anger and let the client express feelings. This kind of acceptance gives people permission to express themselves and work with their anger. Once again, it is helpful to remember that chronic illness and the effort to adjust to many traumatic life changes—in addition to being constantly fearful for one's very life— make any human being feel frustrated, anxious, and depressed. Anger will be expressed in some manner in such an uncomfortable situation, and it is most constructively expressed openly and directly.

The nurse, as the professional who spends the most time with the ill person, is responsible for understanding and treating the client's response to disease and treatment. This makes the nurse uniquely able to facilitate the expression of feelings, to explore alternative solutions to problems, and to clarify situations for the client. Ill persons will have continuous and often repetitive questions about their situations as they work to understand and accept the changes in their lives.

The nurse needs to support positive movement through the process of mourning and to support and advise constructive change as it occurs in the person's life. Through knowledge of human response and of the process of a chronic illness like kidney disease, the nurse facilitates adjustment (see Table 28-1 and Fig. 28-2).

The Family

The nurse should interview each family as a unit as soon as possible after admission of the ill person so that good communication and the flow of accurate information will be facilitated right from the start. The nurse needs to know how each member perceives and is affected by the illness, and what areas of strength and weakness need support and intervention as the family tries to cope. There should be periodic family meetings so that there can be accurate monitoring of the family's adjustment and, when necessary, intervention. In this way, crises can be prevented. Family group meetings[11] or group meetings of specific family members[9] have been found to be very useful ways of increasing communication; decreasing isolation, guilt, depression, and anxiety; and promoting constructive adjustment to the illness and its treatment. Psychotherapeutic nursing includes working with clients in groups.[12,13] Nonpsychiatric nurses should recognize that they can learn and use group process effectively with medical and surgical clients.

Regular home visits by the nurse can be an indispensable tool in the promotion of constructive family adjustment to dialysis, especially home dialysis. Difficulties for a family—both physical and emotional—are often much more easily recognized when the nurse can evaluate them in the home setting. Also, clients and their families live with their problems in their homes, so that it is often more effective to deal with the problem in that environment.

Families may need facilitation of their problem-solving and decision-making activities. Issues which need examination and areas for counseling often include allocation of resources (money, space, and time); rearrangements around division of labor; giving and receiving affection and esteem; limit setting and consistency in child rearing; understanding of feelings generated by the disruption in family life, that is, how various members express these feelings and how each may be supported in their resolution; and effective conflict resolution.

In particular, children need to be supported, helped to understand, and enabled to feel some control over the changes in their lives. They need to explore their fears and fantasies, expressing their concerns and needs verbally so that intellectual and emotional growth is not impaired.

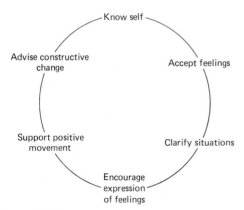

Figure 28-2 Cycle of nursing intervention during mourning.

Transplantation

Many dialysis clients eventually undergo renal transplantation. Like regular hemodialysis, this process of surgically replacing a damaged kidney with a healthy kidney from a living donor or a cadaver presents the client, living donor, and family with a unique psychological situation.

If a client is found medically suitable for transplantation, client and family are asked by physicians whether any family member is able and willing to give a kidney to the ill person, since the kidneys of relatives have a much lower rejection rate than the kidneys of cadavers. There are many personal pressures of responsibility and guilt that can be brought to bear on whichever person or persons are possible donors. This is a painful decision, usually made on an emotional basis *before* the donor has all the objective information from physicians.[14] If a family member does decide to donate a kidney, a great deal of attention and admiration is expressed toward this person by family, friends, and medical staff. This attention helps the donor get to the point of surgery. After surgery, the donor is initially quite ill and there is generally a moderate depression[14] as he or she deals with the physical and emotional loss of a body part. However family and staff attention generally shifts to the recipient, as everyone becomes concerned with the success of the "gift." Shortly after surgery, donors can be left feeling a lack of sensitivity to their needs.

The recipients of kidneys have a great deal of anxiety about the success of the surgery, since they have invested hopes of "cure" and freedom from the process of dialysis. If a family member was a donor, the recipient must deal with feelings about that person and having part of her or his body. If the kidney came from a cadaver, the recipient has another set of feelings, facts, and fantasies to deal with about the new organ. The process of incorporating this new body part is described by Muslin[15] as having three phases: at first the kidney is a *foreign body* and not yet a part of the client's body image. Then, as the kidney becomes invested with the client's emotions, it becomes *partially incorporated* and the client is

less preoccupied with it. Finally, with time and emotional investment, the kidney becomes *completely incorporated* and the client considers it a part of the self. This process is, of course, affected by the body's physical acceptance or rejection of the kidney. Emotional factors do affect this immunological response[14] and can affect the success of transplantation (see Chap. 26).

The nurse needs to understand the situation of donor, recipient, and family in order to deal with their responses effectively.

Life Satisfaction: Is It Worth It?

Today's medical technology is allowing many people to live with illness. The things that the person must do to survive, the treatment for the illness, and the day-to-day problems posed by the disease and treatment make people ask, *"Is it worth it?"* This is a very frightening, painful question because at its base lies the issue of the sacredness of life in relation to the quality of life. There is no simple answer. The individuals who have the illness make their decisions for themselves. Most dialysis patients speak of suicide at some point.[4] Suicide can be accomplished actively by cutting a shunt to exsanguinate or passively by ignoring dietary restrictions. It can even be accomplished unconsciously by insisting on a high-risk cadaver transplant for a "cure."[4] Levy[16] reports that suicide rates for dialysis clients, whether suicide is direct or indirect, are much higher than for the general population. He says they may not be different, however, from those for other groups of people with chronic diseases.

Suicide cannot be considered simply as an individual act. However, a person's view of the self is directly affected by the views of people closely related and by the environmental situation. Thus everyone has some input in the answer to the question of the worth of a person's life. Nurses have a professional responsibility to understand depression in their clients, to interact therapeutically with them, and to provide any possible supports in an attempt to alleviate the depression.

Nurses should determine when depression needs psychiatric assessment and intervention, that is, when the client is not sleeping and not eating; expressing hopeless, helpless feelings; and/or suggesting suicide. A life that may not seem worth living at one point may seem very much worth living with some interventions and changes in situation (such as relief from pain, correction of a misconception, or reconciliation with a spouse). There will be times, however, when in spite of all efforts, a person will decide that suicide is the only option.

References

1 John Bowlby: "Process of Mourning," *International Journal of Psychoanalysis,* vol. 42, pp. 317–340, 1961.

2 E. Kübler-Ross: *On Death and Dying,* Macmillan, New York, 1969.

3 George Engel: "Grief and Grieving," *American Journal of Nursing,* vol. 64, pp. 93–98, September 1964.

4 Harry S. Abram: "Survival by Machine: The Psychological Stress of Chronic Hemodialysis," *Psychiatry in Medicine,* vol. 1, pp. 37–51, January 1970.

5 Kaplan A. De-Nour and J. W. Czackes: "Emotional Problems and Reactions of the Medical Team in a Chronic Haemodialysis Unit," *Lancet,* vol. 2, pp. 987–991, November 1968.

6 Kaplan A. De-Nour et al.: "Emotional Reactions of Patients on Chronic Haemodialysis," *Psychosomatic Medicine,* vol. 30, pp. 521–533, September–October 1968.

7 Dianne Anger: "The Psychologic Stress of Chronic Renal Failure and Long-Term Hemodialysis," *Nursing Clinics of North America,* vol. 10, pp. 449–460, September 1975.

8 Jonathan W. Cummings: "Hemodialysis—Feelings, Facts, Fantasies," *American Journal of Nursing,* vol. 70, pp. 70–76, January 1970.

9 J. G. D'Afflitti and D. Swanson: "Group Sessions for the Wives of Home-Hemodialysis Patients," *American Journal of Nursing,* vol. 75, pp. 633–635, April 1975.

10 Phyllis M. Hoover et al.: "Adjustment of Children With Parents on Hemodialysis," *Nursing Times,* Aug. 28, 1975, pp. 1374–1376.

11 J. G. D'Afflitti and G. W. Weitz: "Rehabilitating the Stroke Patient through Patient-Family Groups," *International Journal of Group Psychotherapy,* vol. 24, pp. 323–332, July 1974.

12 Claire Fagin: "Psychotherapeutic Nursing," *American Journal of Nursing,* February 1967, p. 67.

*13 Penny Kossoris: "Family Therapy: An Adjunct to Hemodialysis and Transplantation," *American Journal of Nursing,* vol. 70, pp. 1730–1733, August 1970.

14 D. R. Freebury: "The Psychological Implications of Organ Transplant—A Selected Review," *Canadian Psychiatric Association Journal,* vol. 9, pp. 593–597, December 1974.

15 Hyman L. Muslin: "On Acquiring a Kidney," *American Journal of Psychiatry,* vol. 127, pp. 105–108, March 1971.

16 Norman B. Levy: "The Psychology and Care of the Maintenance Hemodialysis Patient," *Heart and Lung,* vol. 2, pp. 400–405, May–June 1973.

*Recommended reference by a nurse author.

29

Clients Dependent on Life-Support Systems

June N. Brodie

Learning Objectives

After studying this chapter, the student should be able to:

1 Identify the commonly used life-support systems that may generate feelings in clients and caretakers.

2 Discuss the ethical issues related to the maintenance of life.

3 Discuss the psychodynamics and behavioral response of clients dependent on life-support systems.

4 Discuss the nurse's response and personal reactions to such situations.

5 Apply the nursing process to the care of clients on life-support systems.

Health care in our society has become highly technological. The person who suddenly becomes critically ill is now placed in a special-care unit which may resemble the complex control room of a space project. Each year more and more highly technical, mechanized life-support systems are developed to monitor, treat, or restore life to clients who in the past would not have survived their deterioration or loss of physiological functions that are now assumed by technology.

In spite of the fact that special-care units are found in hospitals throughout our society, a review of the nursing literature reveals a paucity of data regarding the feelings of individuals dependent on life-support systems and an even greater dearth of information on the feelings and attitudes of those health professionals who provide care for these clients.

Life-Support Systems

The commonly used support systems which have potential for generating feelings in both clients and caretakers that will be discussed in this chapter include the Bird and Bennett respirators, hyperalimentation, and cardiac monitoring. Hemodialysis, which also falls into the category of life-support systems, is discussed separately in Chap. 28 because of the chronicity of these clients' problems. The focus of the present chapter will be the problems confronted by those acutely ill clients who face life-threatening situations and are dependent on technology for survival. We shall also consider the feelings that are generated in caretakers as well as the delivery of supportive care.

Nurses responsible for the care of acutely ill clients face unusual situations which challenge their personal value systems. They must have the ability to deal with the feelings generated by these clients and the capacity to confront a controversial social issue.

Respirators

The apneic client with increased hypoxia constitutes an acute emergency situation in which adequate ventilation must be instituted immediately. Mechanical ventilatory assistance is instituted using machines such as the Bird or Bennett respirator[1] attached to an endotracheal tube. These systems have the capacity to ventilate automatically (they may be machine-cycled), without client stimulation, or they may be patient-cycled. In the latter case, the client's own inspiratory effort turns on or trips the respirator to assist this phase of respiration.* Clients on this type of apparatus demand careful and close monitoring by the nurse. Any mechanical malfunction can mean loss of respiratory function and death.

Hyperalimentation—Total Parenteral Nutrition

Parenteral hyperalimentation is a method of providing a continuous infusion of required nutrients when clients cannot maintain themselves in a state of positive nitrogen balance or anabolism. This procedure is undertaken only by an experienced health team, since it is both complex and hazardous. However, it is a feasible method of providing the required hypertonic solution of glucose, amino acids, polypeptides, and other nutrients.[2,3]

Nursing responsibilities in connection with hyperalimentation are great and extraordinary vigilance is essential to the success of the procedure. These clients run a high risk of suffering life-threatening infections, hyperglycemia from too rapid a flow, inadequate nutrient supply from a flow that is not rapid enough, potentially fatal air embolism from the entry of air, and electrolyte derangement.

Cardiac Monitoring

Clients with cardiac disease who are vulnerable to potentially lethal arrhythmias require continuous electrocardiographic surveillance. This continuous monitoring alerts caretakers to early warning signs of these lethal arrhythmias so that immediate interventions can be instituted. The nurse supervising this monitoring must be able to recognize symptoms of cardiac problems and to interpret

*The student is referred to any standard medical/surgical nursing text for a more exhaustive discussion of these devices.

their implications so as either to institute immediate preventive measures, begin cardiopulmonary resuscitation, and/or summon assistance. In many instances these nurses must act quickly, efficiently and expertly to protect the client from anoxia, which would result in permanent brain damage or death,[2,4] and this is an awesome responsibility.

Context of Care

The numerous different types of intensive-care units (ICUs) which encompass an array of special disciplines, include the following: surgical, medical, coronary-care, stroke, pediatric, burn, neurological, critical-care, recovery and others. Many of these units resemble war bunkers and unfortunately—by design or otherwise—they are impersonal, windowless, highly mechanized centers that are overloaded with auditory and visual stimuli.[4,5] Providing care for clients in intensive-care settings demands split-second decision making and a variety of diagnostic, resuscitative, and therapeutic measures designed to ensure survival and, ultimately, optimal recovery.

Management of client care, out of necessity, assigns first priority to adequate cardiopulmonary ventilation; fluid, electrolyte, and nutrient balance; and the administration of pharmacological agents as necessary. Constant surveillance of clients is required. Second priority is assigned to the institution of rehabilitative/reparative care and the establishment of an interpersonal relationship with the client and family. Initially, the nurse-client relationship is unilateral because the client is either unconscious or the sensorium is seriously disturbed (see Chap. 30, under "Delirium").

Occasionally, nursing care in intensive-care units is limited to medical or surgical organ-oriented intervention. Fragmenting clients into their body systems and supplying care to each system is not only counterproductive for the client but also conflicts with the concept of the holistic nature of the person and the delivery of nursing care to the client as a unified individual interacting with the environment.

Maintenance of Life: An Ethical Issue

In recent years there has been a heightened awareness of the dying process and its impact on the client and family. People vary in the degree to which they fear death, but most are anxious about a prolonged and painful dying process. Some are further distressed by the increasing personal and financial burdens their illness places on their families and their concomitant loss of control over their destinies.[6] More and more, clients and families are expressing a desire to participate or have representation in the process by which decisions such as *not to resuscitate* are made.

People have fears about how death will occur, where, under what circumstances, and in the presence of whom. Some have a need to control these circumstances, particularly in relation to treatment during a terminal illness, when they may eventually be physically unable to make choices. Often wishes and preferred decisions concerning the use of technology to sustain life are discussed informally with family, clergy, and/or physicians. However, with this informal process the client's wishes may be overlooked or overridden by family or caretakers. Therefore an increasing number of persons are making *living wills,* or signed statements requesting that their lives not be unduly prolonged under certain circumstances. The legal status of these documents remains uncertain; they have not yet been universally recognized as binding. However, the state of California passed *The Right to Die Bill* in September 1976. This bill must be tested in court before its legality is assured. If upheld by the courts, it will permit a person to make an enforceable decision not to have extraordinary means used to preserve life under particular circumstances.

In 1977, leaders of the medical profession in New Jersey issued guidelines setting up a procedure whereby life-support systems could be withdrawn from clients who are in a vegetative, comatose state and for whom there is no hope of recovery. The guidelines provide for the establishment of a *prognosis committee* at each hospital composed of physicians in surgery, medicine, neurosurgery or neurology, anesthesiology; a pediatrician if the client is a child; and two physicians from outside the institution. A theologian and lawyer might also be appointed. This committee would either support or reject the attending physician's recommendation on the basis of their study of the client and records.[7]

While concerns regarding the inappropriateness of cardiopulmonary resuscitation of selected clients are now openly discussed, the method by which such decisions are made often remains covert.[8] Practices may vary among and within institutions and among physicians due to the ambiguous legal status of such a decision and to hospital policy. Generally, the position of the hospital is "pro-life"; that is, full resuscitation is to be initiated to preserve the lives of all clients. Limitations on this position must be clearly stated in the client's record. Hospitals tend to honor the competent client's informed acceptance or rejection of treatment, including cardiopulmonary resuscitation.[8]

Competence is based upon the client's understanding of the risks, benefits, and alternatives involved. However, even the client who is incompetent by this standard deserves representation in the planning conference.[9]

If the client is competent and makes the decision not to be resuscitated or to have life-sustaining systems used, this represents a deliberate choice. When the client is judged incompetent, then such a decision must be made with the agreement of appropriate family members and staff or the issue may be brought to court, where the decision will be rendered by a judge.[9]

Minors, who may be deemed incompetent, must be informed if a decision not to resuscitate or to use life-support systems is made; they have the right to reject such a decision. However, incompetent or not, the client should not be denied the benefits of the usual evaluation process.

In a situation where the competent client elects either the *order not to resuscitate (ONTR)* alternative—also known as a *no code* order—or the use of life-support systems, these decisions may not be overriden by the contrary views of the family; but family members should be informed of the client's decision if the client gives permission. When the family initiates a proposal for ONTR, it is the obligation of the previously established or newly formed committee to recognize that these wishes are not to be regarded as the client's choice.[8]

According to *A Report of the Clinical Care Committee of the Massachusetts General Hospital*,[10] the decision regarding whether or not to continue making maximum therapeutic efforts for clients who are judged to be hopelessly and irreversibly ill raises serious medical, emotional, legal, moral, and economic issues for the medical and nursing staff involved as well as for the clients and their families. Unless client-condition criteria are specified in advance for the initiation or withholding of life-saving measures during crises of failing organ systems, nurses, resident, staff, and physicians will feel particularly vulnerable if the responsibility of judging when not to intervene is left to them. The Clinical Care Committee has cautioned that any definitive act, such as turning off a mechanical device, is to be executed only by a designated physician after consultation with and agreement of the client's family and appropriate hospital committees where indicated. The responsibility for such a decision is the physician's.

However, more recently an interdisciplinary team approach has developed to manage the care of clients in intensive-care settings. This approach uses a team conference to facilitate collaboration and coordination of care. When such teams exist, the criteria used to guide decisions regarding the institution or discontinuation of life-saving measures and use of life-support systems are developed by the team and reflect the group's recommendation. This approach provides for the sharing of responsibility and would, on the surface, appear to be a rational and systematic decision-making process. However, a student of group process would recognize its limitations. In most instances, groups do make better decisions than individuals, based on the extent of potential input and expertise; but groups can also function irrationally and autocratically or too cohesively, and then the decision-making process is impaired. Whenever possible and appropriate, it is advisable to have the client and/or a member of the client's family participate in the decision-making process.[9]

Health professionals frequently object to having the clients or their families participate in meetings where crucial decisions are made concerning the clients' treatments or their very lives.[9] In support of their reluctance to have a client and/or family members participate in such conferences, health professionals cite such excuses as the lay person's inability to comprehend technical jargon, the probable inhibition of free discussion among the staff, the family's possible insistence on making unreasonable demands, and the ultimate obfuscation of client-centered goals.

Some of these objections are valid in the setting of a modern intensive-care unit; others are specious at best. Realistically, the fact remains that many of the clients who are placed in an ICU are not competent and cannot make responsible decisions, much less participate in a discussion determining the outcome of their very lives. Among those who cannot make an informed decision because they are deemed incompetent are the comatose, the very young, the confused, those suffering from organic brain syndrome, and the retarded.

Wright proposed that such incompetent clients might benefit from being provided with a representative member of the health-care profession who would be assigned to the client upon admission as an advocate and would function as an ombudsman between the client and the institution.[11] This client agent would perform the following tasks: maximizing communication, monitoring action, providing role support, and managing the client's exit from the institution. These tasks are outlined in Table 29-1.

In the event of a life-threatening situation—such as cardiac arrest, for example—the client agent should have discussed the alternatives with the client and family if this possibility had been known to exist. The client agent would then be responsible for communicating the decision of the client and/or family to the health team and/or

Table 29-1 Tasks of the Client Agent[11]

The communicative aspect emphasizes communicating hospital procedures and objectives to the client while conveying the client's goals and any complaints to the agency.

The action-monitoring component entails implementing decisions made by health professionals concerning the client and ensuring that the client's needs are met by the institution.

Role support includes providing for a consistent interpersonal relationship with the client to enhance the client's ability to cope with any alterations in health.

Exit management refers to the preparation of the client for discharge in the event that the client makes a sufficient recovery.

arranging for the team or committee to meet with the client and family to expedite the client's wishes.

It may happen that, after the ONTR[8] has been issued, the client's status is so altered that the order no longer seems applicable. Should this occur, the physician and health team must be informed without delay so that the initial decision can be rescinded if indicated. In such a situation, the client agent would be responsible for ensuring the explication of this process.

Psychodynamics and Client Behavior
Discontinuity
Many clients in intensive-care settings are in the acute phase of their illness and are suffering from some degree of delirium. The changes in sensorium that accompany delirium affect the way in which such clients perceive themselves and the environment (see Chap. 30).

The client's altered state of consciousness may have a physical or emotional basis, and the sense of continuity between past, present, and future may be disrupted. This sense of continuity, ordinarily taken for granted, only becomes conscious when it is interrupted. Then, it seems that the operations used in the past are no longer applicable and it becomes difficult to project oneself into a future which seems uncertain, bleak, or nonexistent.[9]

Clients who are transferred to an ICU postoperatively frequently have been prepared to some degree for the possibility of complications requiring special care. Nevertheless, their adaptation process resembles that of clients who were totally unprepared.[4] This apparent unpreparedness is often based upon the client's defensive dissociation to avoid or defend against an experience that may be emotionally painful. The client feels, at this stage, a need to retreat from full awareness of what may happen.

This defensive need to deny reality continues right up to the time when confrontation with the seriousness of the situation becomes unavoidable. At the point when awareness finally becomes possible, the shock phase of adaptation allows these clients to dissociate from their bodies. The subjective feeling is one of observing one's body being treated but not having any emotional response to the events or their meaning. This emotional retreat is a flight reaction which allows the person to conserve energy while under maximal physiological stress.

Following a period of unconsciousness, clients attempt to fill in the void in their experience retrospectively. Many will recall their situation without difficulty; others will use fantasies and distortions to structure and make sense of what has happened. According to Schnaper, a universal theme of these fantasies is that of being held a prisoner.[12-14]

Awareness of Alterations in Body Image

During the phase of emotional retreat, these clients become aware of changes that affect their body image. This mental picture and unconscious concept of their physical appearance also includes their perception of and investment in body organs and systems as well as their structure and function. Losses in organ or system functioning cause the client to feel incomplete or damaged, as if part of the self has been torn away (see Chap. 23).

With awareness of alterations in body image comes interest and concern about the technology that is sustaining life. Clients begin to acknowledge the situation and the losses incurred. Consequently, they begin to get in touch with their emotional responses, the feelings generated by their situation.

Helplessness

During a debilitating illness, especially one in which the control of life systems is surrendered to a machine, an individual—willingly or unwillingly—becomes dependent upon sources outside the self for assistance and support. Illness reactivates earlier conflicts and an awareness of unmet needs. Coupled with their present limited ability to control body functions and the environment, clients experience a sense of helplessness. They feel that they are incapable of doing anything about their situation but still anticipate that there will be some helpful response from others. As a result, clients in a dependent state see caretakers as protecting, nurturing figures even if their previous life experiences negate this expectation. Associated with the sense of helplessness is a fear of dependency on others in the environment or on nonhuman technology. For example, a client may express abject terror over the possibility that a staff member may accidentally trip over an electrical cord and dislodge it from the wall socket. This, of course, shows that the client has come to view the electrical cord as a lifeline.[15]

Hopelessness

In addition to feeling helpless and unable to control or change what is happening to them, these clients may also come to feel that no change in their situation is possible. Thus they will either remain for some indefinite time in the state they are in, deteriorate to an even more intolerable condition, or die.

An absence of hope impairs the person's motivation to participate in care and work toward health. Such clients exhibit listlessness, a lack of interest in others and the environment, and indifference to feedback on progress. They may say "It's no use" or "Why try." Fears of suffocation, cessation of the heartbeat, and starvation compound feelings of helplessness and hopeless-ness[15] (see Chap. 31).

Abasement

Clients who are dependent upon mechanical devices—such as hyperalimentation, cardiac monitoring, or respirators—may arrive at the ICU in shock, unconscious, near death, and unprepared for the ensuing experiences. Family members may also be unprepared for the sudden disaster that has befallen them. However, all these clients have one element in common: their surrender, temporar-ily or permanently, of a vital bodily function to a machine to sustain their very existence. When conscious, these clients—that is, all except the very young—are aware of the tenuousness of their position and of their utter dependence upon a machine and their caretakers to perform the nec-essary, often humiliating procedures which keep them alive. These clients see themselves as no longer competent, in control, or capable of func-tioning independently in their accustomed man-ner. The intrusion into body orifices of tubes to supply food and air and the imposition of incon-veniences such as bedpans and regulating elec-trodes, however sensitively accomplished, under-mines the client's self-confidence as a functioning, self-sufficient individual. The self-concept is dras-tically altered and coping abilities are severely stressed, no longer inappropriate, or unavailable.

Loss of Gratification

Commonly the client feels a loss of well-being when a vital organ is replaced by an artificial support system. At the same time the client experi-ences a diminution of important human relation-ships due to an inability to interact effectively with the environment for need satisfaction. These peo-ple are separated from family and role functions, which were once their sources of need satisfac-tion. Even simple gratifications such as eating, sleeping, breathing, and having the strength to care for oneself have been lost.

Reactivation of Memories

Clients may be reminded of other occasions in the past when they felt helpless, deprived, and unable to function independently. When such memories involve situations that were never adequately re-solved, symptoms of a neurotic conflict may be expressed. It is as if memories of earlier losses or failures,—crises that were never really mastered,—were reawakened by the client's pre-sent vulnerability and inability to cope. Enforced dependency in the past, particularly if needs were not met adequately, may have generated strong angry feelings or depression. These reactivated feelings may be as intense as they were when originally experienced. The clients' present help-lessness, dependency, and losses—particularly the loss of control—have the capacity in and of themselves to generate anger and frustration. If these painful feelings are further aggravated by reactivation of past feelings, the client may not be able to adopt the sick role and behave in ways that conserve energy (see Chap. 25).

Mobilization of Defenses

The crucial concern in terms of clients dependent upon life-support systems seems to be the ability to mobilize an adequate and appropriate system of defenses. The mobilization of defenses may occur more rapidly in situations where the client has had some chance to consider the possible outcomes. In situations where there has been no forewarning or preparation—such as accidents or fires—in which the client has been unconscious and awak-ens to total confusion, the client will attempt to structure an explanation for his or her plight. This attempt frequently includes a fantasy in which the client assumes the role of a bad child who is deservedly punished for a real or imagined "bad" act by imprisonment.[12]

The physiological demands on clients con-nected to life-support systems are great. Defenses which conserve energy and help clients to reduce their investment in emotional coping facilitate their assumption of the sick role and their commitment to the healing process. Some clients use the previously discussed dissociative reaction and experience a sense of unreality to avoid feelings, while others escape into sleep.

As their physical status improves, clients engage in the grieving process, mourning the losses they are experiencing. They also begin to hear and integrate reality-based information concerning their status and prognosis. The need for denial and dissociation lessens as the person becomes more stable physiologically and able to perceive progress toward health. Emotionally, clients often level off after an extended period of time in the unit. They have developed a sense of trust in their caretakers and a knowledgeable interest in the life-support technology. The environmental stimuli that were once anxiety-provoking and perhaps the causes of sleep deprivation are understood and accepted. The beeps and hisses may become comforting rhythms and less prominent in the clients' conscious perception of their environment. It would seem that once clients have settled into the unit and are feeling secure, they are confronted with the adaptational demand of transfer. Once the client's physical condition has been stabilized and the use of life-support systems is no longer required, these clients must deal with transfer to an intermediate or medical-surgical unit. The transfer and its anticipation generate anxiety in clients who have developed a sense of security in the intensiveness of care and the nurses' competent and rapid response to their distress. On the new unit, nurses are not as visible and the environment is quieter and more slowly paced. The client is visibly and geographically separated from the life-support system. All these environmental changes generate anxiety, hence trust in the caretakers and hospital system must be reestablished.

Problematic Client Behaviors

The stresses of illness, placement in an ICU, and attachment to a life-support system may be more than some clients can cope with adaptively. Maladaptive behavior and psychiatric symptoms may occur as a consequence of their physiological status, sensory disturbances, perception of the situation, and premorbid personality defects. Emotional sequelae may be exhibited by neurotic or psychotic behavior. Coping behaviors appropriate to the retreat phase may be extended beyond this stage and interfere with progressive acknowledgement and adaptation[5,12,16] (see Chaps. 24, 26, and 30).

Nurse's Response

In an intensive care unit, there are many emotional satisfactions for the entire staff in providing the necessary intensive and critical care. As a whole and in terms of the individual, this type of care encompasses great responsibility as well as the opportunity to gratify fantasies of omnipotence. On the other hand, the staff face enormous stress, often heightened by real performance pressures and fatigue. The transference and countertransference phenomena that occur affect the delivery of nursing care and whether it will be reflective of client needs.

When nurses have participated in saving a life, they project warmth, increased self-esteem, and a sense of omnipotence. However, when a client dies in spite of their efforts, they may experience a sense of failure, losing both self-esteem and a feeling of competence. In this instance they often become irritable, critical, and demanding. As a defense against further loss and threat to their self-image, they may tend to become less involved with clients interpersonally. The defenses used by nurses to combat these difficulties are denial, displacement, projection, repression, reaction formation, and passive aggression.[4]

In coping with the reactions of clients and their families, nurses are sometimes overwhelmed by their own feelings, anxieties, guilts, and fears; therefore they need to be cognizant of their own behavior patterns under stressful conditions.

Nurses, in intensive care units play an integral role both in planning care and giving it, on a day-to-day basis as well as in emergency situations. They must often act independently and quickly, depending on their knowledge and experience in making decisions which may mean life or death to the client. This awesome responsibility is both gratifying and potentially inundating. The ICU is a stressful work environment for nurses. The burden of responsibility, the machines, the stimuli, the turnover of clients, the critical status of the client population, and the concern for family place extraordinary demands on the nurses' coping capacity. There is a rapid turnover of nursing personnel in many special-care units as a consequence of excessive stress and—often—the lack of support from the system.

When assertive therapy is terminated, the nursing staff may complain about the decision because it conflicts with their philosophical base, motivation, and orientation to preserve life. At the same time, they may be critical of a decision not to terminate therapy on a client they feel has suffered extensively and for whom they see no hope of relief or recovery.

Bilodeau as well as Kellog and Curran[17,18] found that the sources of stress among nursing staff fell into the following categories: clients and client care, peer personnel, medical staff, the environment, families, personal difficulties, and conflicts with other areas of the hospital. Nursing staff frustration is manifested by fatigue, forgetfulness, hostility, depression, and guilt.

To defend against the feelings generated in a special-care unit, these nurses tend to perceive themselves as "special" professionals within the hospital system and to isolate themselves as a group from peers on other units. This is most clearly evidenced by their "groupy" behavior in. the cafeteria and at inservice education classes.

Many of the paradoxes, problematic situations, and maladaptive behaviors may be remedied by participation in interdisciplinary group conferences. Nursing staff in intensive-care settings need opportunities to ventilate feelings and receive support. A psychiatric nurse-consultant serving as a clinical liaison specialist can help the nurses plan care for problematic clients with maladaptive emotional responses and help the nurses themselves to explore and work through the feelings generated by this high-risk setting.

Planning Nursing Care

Planning the nursing care of clients dependent upon life-support systems begins with the prevention of complications and the preparation of clients, when at all possible, by providing explanations of expected procedures and outcomes. Presurgical clients who are at risk need to be told what kind of technology they may need, its purpose, and the possible need to be in an intensive-care setting. They should also understand how care there will be different from that of the unit on which they are presently located. As previously mentioned, clients who are given this preparation may initially indicate an apparent lack of understanding that they have been placed in an intensive-care setting; once the shock phase has been resolved, however, this prior knowledge helps them to cope more effectively.[9]

When clients are first admitted to intensive-care settings, the need for attachment to life-support systems requires immediate and assertive action; the client's physiological status and its assessment take first priority. The client's behavior and responses to procedures at this point are used as indicators of the client's physiological status. Data concerning the degree of anxiety are important in determining the need for interventions which will allay fear, assist adaptation, and facilitate cooperation. When the client's physiological status is stabilized, broader psychosocial needs and the implications of the disease process on the client's future life-style come into focus.

Assessment

The following assessment criteria can be used as a guide in identifying data which will be used to formulate nursing diagnoses and plan care:

1 Does the client's behavior suggest delirium? (see Chap. 30.)

2 Was the client prepared for admission to the ICU?

3 Is pain, fear of suffocation, or cardiac arrest the client's primary focus?

4 What is the client's behaviorial response to the life-support system?

5 What is the client's reaction to environmental stimuli such as alarms, beeps, or hisses?

6 What information does the client need to understand his or her health status, the life-support system, and the meaning of environmental noises?

7 What is the client's capacity to comprehend and deal with this information?

8 How can information be presented at the level of the client's need to know and ability to comprehend?

9 Is the client able to conserve energy by managing the emotional response effectively?

10 What is the client's perception of the cause of the illness?

11 Is the client's behaviorial response appropriate to his or her physiological ability to confront and acknowledge the situation?

12 Is there behaviorial evidence of a neurotic, psychotic, or otherwise maladaptive response?

Nursing Diagnosis

The nursing diagnosis is arrived at by a process of sifting, sorting, and analyzing data gathered from observations, physical assessment, laboratory reports, monitoring of the life-support system, and interaction with the client. The nursing diagnosis is a formulation of the problems and needs which emerge in response to the illness, the environment, and the life-support system to which the client is attached.

For example, several days after Mrs. Martin's admission to the ICU, she was physiologically stabilized. The nurse noted that whenever the client was observed, she had her eyes closed. When the nurse initiated interaction, she would open her eyes, look directly at the nurse, and then close her eyes again after the exchange was terminated. The nurse assessed this behavior as stemming from a need to avoid confronting the situation. The client verified this assumption by saying, "What I don't see don't bother me and I don't know about." Further exploration revealed that she was very frightened and had no idea why she was on this support system. The nursing diagnosis in this example is "Withdrawal behavior with continuing anxiety due to lack of understanding of health status and treatment program."

Examples of other nursing diagnoses which reflect the needs and problems of clients on life-support systems are given in Table 29-2.

Nursing Goals

Nursing goals for clients dependent on life-support systems include the following:

1 Establishing and maintaining communication with clients to maximize the exchange of information

2 Helping clients to deal with the feelings generated by their situation

3 Helping clients to understand what is happening to them, their life-support systems, and the environmental stimuli

4 Moderating sensory stimulation to maximize coping

5 Helping clients to conserve energy needed to cope with physiological problems

6 Helping the physiologically stable client to acknowledge losses, alterations in body image and self-concept; and the reality of the illness

7 Helping the client to cope with the anxiety generated by relinquishing the life-support system and transferring to another unit

Nursing Interventions

Nursing interventions for the care of clients on life-support systems are identified using the goals

Table 29-2 Client Problems and Nursing Interventions

Client problem	Nursing intervention
Disoriented	Initiate scheduled reality orientation program (to time and place) to be carried out during each shift. Identify client and self by name when approaching client. Place clock and calendar in view of client.
On admission, expresses fear and anxiety	Provide basis for development of trust. Reassure client, using continuous presence of nurses, frequent checks on support system. Emphasize client's ability to call nurse to bedside quickly.
Alert and anxious when support system checked	Explain purpose of system. Explain rationale for checks on system. Tell client the scheduled frequency of checks on equipment.
Exhibits alertness and anxiety in response to specific environmental noises.	Explain the cause of the specific noises and their purpose.
Shows effects of sensory deprivation	Initiate program of planned interaction on subject client chooses. Initiate program of comfort measures, including massage and efforts to relax client and maximize comforting touch.
Shows irritability and changes in the sensorium due to sleep deprivation	Schedule with client a period for undisturbed sleep. Explain that this period of sleep is needed to restore client's ability to cope. Reassure client regarding safety; explain that required monitoring will take place and only activities that can easily be put off will be postponed. Provide comfort measures to help client relax.
Expresses concern about altered body image	Explore at client's pace the extent and permanence of the changes and the feelings generated by them. Give reality feedback regarding extent of changes and prognosis for the future.
Expresses feelings of helplessness	Identify ways client can participate in care. Identify ways client can influence schedule of care. Identify ways client can control the environment.
Expresses feelings of hopelessness	Give client reality-based feedback on positive changes in health status. Identify ways that progress can be measured by the client.
Inability to communicate	Be certain client has call bell at fingertips at all times. Interact with client in such a way that client can agree or disagree nonverbally with perceptions, suggestions, or requests. Assess nonverbal behavior carefully and validate assumptions with client. Provide client with pad and pen for writing requests and responses.
Transfer anxiety	Gradually decrease frequency of technically oriented contact with client. Use time with client to explore feelings about transfer and to provide reassurance of safety and ability to cope. Give feedback that client can use as measure of progress and ability to cope outside the unit.

and diagnoses as a guide. Initially, interventions are directed toward conservation of energy, prevention of complications, and facilitation of effective coping. Table 29-2 provides examples of client problems and needs as well as nursing interventions which would either ameliorate or resolve the problems.

Nurses who are involved on a day-to-day basis with clients who are dependent upon life-support systems deal with individuals whose ability to communicate verbally is often impaired. The crux of nursing care is the ability to establish and maintain communication with the client. Knowing that the client often cannot communicate effectively,[17] the nurse must be attuned to the client's attempts to communicate. To communicate with a client who cannot talk or who may be delirious requires skill in anticipating, sensing, and observing nonverbal client behavior as well as inventiveness to establish a code of mutual, reciprocal understanding.

Once assertive emergency care has been initiated and the client is somewhat stabilized physiologically, the nurse needs to acknowledge the client as a person who feels threatened and is mobilizing defenses to cope with an overwhelming situation. Trust is an important component in developing a therapeutic relationship with a client dependent on a life-support system. The following are ways in which the nurse helps the client to develop trust and to feel more secure:

1 Ensure rapid accessibility to the nurse.
2 Be patient and gentle in providing care.
3 Prepare the client for all procedures.
4 Acknowledge the client's distress, pain, fear, anxiety, frustration, and other feelings.
5 Recognize early signs of prodromal pain and administer medications to alleviate or modify the pain.
6 Anticipate necessary comfort measures and provide them.
7 Answer questions openly, honestly, and directly and help the client deal with the content of these answers.
8 Provide reality-based reassurance.

When assertive therapy has been terminated because the client's status is hopeless, every effort must be made to help him or her live and die with dignity. Nursing interventions are focused on keeping the client pain-free, comfortable, and protected from feelings of abandonment and loneliness. Detachment from the environment and others is compensated by the "thereness" of the nurse

and continues with the client controlling the focus and extent of interactions.

Evaluation

Nurses in intensive care do not see the clients recover fully from their illnesses. Their contact with the client is brief, intense, and limited to the acute phase of the illness. Thus the goals used to evaluate the effectiveness of interventions are short-range in nature and, if the client's physiological status does not stabilize or improve, health-oriented goals are redefined toward helping the client to die with dignity.

Evaluation of the effectiveness of nursing interventions in intensive-care settings requires comparison of the client's status with the goals. Evidence immediately postadmission that there is conservation of energy and physiological stabilization indicates a satisfactory status. Data at a later point which indicate acknowledgement of the situation and effective management of feelings suggest that the client is adapting. Transfer anxiety is inherent in the situation; however, effective management of these feelings is reflected in the physiological status, the client's ability to verbalize feelings and work them through, and evidence of planning and problem solving regarding adaptation to the new environment. The clients' behaviorial responses to weaning or discontinuation of life-support systems may often indicate how they will deal with the transfer and how well they will master their fears.

References

1 A. Harvey et al.: *The Principles and Practice of Medicine,* Appleton-Century-Crofts, New York, 1972.
2 Eugenia Waechter and Florence Blake: *Nursing Care of Children,* Lippincott, New York, 1976.
3 Lillian Brunner et al.: *Textbook of Medical Surgical Nursing,* Lippincott, New York, 1970.

4   D. Hay and D. Oken: "The Psychological Stresses of Intensive Care Unit Nursing," *Psychosomatic Medicine,* vol. 34, pp. 109–118, 1972.

5   H. P. Rome: "The Irony of the ICU," *Psychiatry Digest,* 1969, pp. 10–14.

6   J. Brodie: "An Investigation of the Relationship Between General Fearfulness, Locus of Control, and Social Activity Among Retirees," in F. Downs and M. Newman (eds.), *Source Book of Nursing Research,* F. A. Davis, Philadelphia, 1977.

7   Alfonso Navarez: "Jersey Adopts Plan on Patients in Coma," *The New York Times,* January 26, 1977.

8   Mitchell Rabin, Gerald Gellerman, and Nancy Rice: "Orders Not to Resuscitate," *New England Journal of Medicine,* vol. 295, pp. 364–366, 1976.

9   Franklin C. Schontz: *The Psychological Aspects of Physical Illness and Disability,* Macmillan, New York, 1975.

10 "Clinical Care Committee Report of Massachusetts General Hospital, Optimum Care for Hopelessly Ill Patients," *New England Journal of Medicine,* vol. 295, pp. 362–364, 1976.

11 M. E. Wright: "Advocacy: A New Rehabilitation Role Function," *Rehabilitation Psychology,* vol. 18, pp. 89–90, 1971.

12 N. Schnaper: "Emotional Responses of the Surgical Patient," in *Tice's Practice of Medicine,* Harper & Row, New York, 1969, vol. 10.

13 N. Schnaper and R. Adams Cowley: "The Psychological Implications of Severe Trauma: Emotional Sequelae to Unconsciousness," *Journal of Trauma,* vol. 15, pp. 94–98, 1975.

14 N. Schnaper: "What Preanesthetic Visit?" *Anesthesiology,* vol. 22, pp. 486–488, 1961, editorial.

15 A. Schmale and G. Engel: "Object Loss, 'Giving Up,' and Disease Onset: An Overview of Research in Progress," *Symposium on Medical Aspects in the Military Climate,* U. S. Government Printing Office, Washington, D.C., 1965, pp. 433–443.

16 I. Janis: *Stress and Frustration,* Harcourt, Brace & World, New York, 1971.

17 C. B. Bilodeau: "The Nurse and Her Reactions to Critical-Care Nursing," *Heart and Lung,* vol. 2, pp. 358–363, 1973.

18 M. Kellogg and C. Curran: "Stress, Frustration and Crisis: Their Effects upon the Nurse," unpublished manuscript, 1975.

30

Response to Clients with Organic Brain Syndrome

Barbara Flynn Sideleau

Learning Objectives

After studying this chapter, the student should be able to:

1. Identify the causes and types of organic brain syndrome and the diagnostic process
2. Recognize the manifestations of organic brain syndrome
3. Assess the extent and impact of the client's deficits
4. Assess the client's adaptation to the deficits
5. Assess the nursing response to the client and family and its impact on the delivery of care
6. Formulate nursing goals for the care of the client and family
7. Formulate nursing diagnoses of the client's and family's responses to the illness and deficits
8. Intervene in ways that maximize the client's and family's coping and that preserve human dignity
9. Evaluate the effectiveness of nursing interventions

According to the American Psychiatric Association (APA), *organic brain syndrome* (OBS) is a mental condition characteristically resulting from diffuse impairment, from any cause, of brain-tissue function.[1] This diagnostic category is subdivided into eight types which further define the client's problem (see appendix).

The old, the infirm, residents of convalescent homes and the chronic alcoholics are the people one most often associates with OBS. It is true that these groups probably constitute the largest proportion of the OBS population; however, a surprising number of people in other age groups also fall into this diagnostic category. The incidence of OBS in children, as well as its management, is discussed in Chap. 38. In the adolescent and adult population, injuries due to accidents—on the highway and in industry, for example—as well as tumors of the brain take their toll. These young people or those in the prime of life face coping with deficits that require redefinition of goals and life-styles and sometimes drastic changes in socioeconomic status.

Organic Brain Syndrome

In addition to having deficits consequent to physical alterations in brain tissue, these clients may be diagnosed as psychotic or nonpsychotic. The psychotic client's functional impairment interferes with reality testing and the performance of independent daily living activities, while the nonpsychotic has a greater capacity to cope with the environment alone or with only minimal assistance. When an overlying psychosis is present, pharmacological and interpersonal therapeutic interventions are needed to alleviate the symptoms and enhance functioning.

OBS can also be categorized as either acute or chronic. When there is an acute brain syndrome, the onset is often sudden, with rapid impairment of orientation, memory, intellectual function, judgment, and affect. The client may be delirious or in a coma and, in some instances, an underlying psychotic and/or neurotic reaction will develop. The cause of acute OBS is usually a temporary, reversible, diffuse disturbance of brain function. With time and treatment, organic symptoms are resolved.

When a client is diagnosed as having chronic OBS, the onset is often but not always insidious. In some instances, acute OBS may deteriorate and become chronic. Consciousness is not usually impaired, at least in the early stages, but there is failing memory, intellectual impairment, and often disturbance in affect. The alterations in the brain tissue are irreversible; in some instances, the pathology progresses over time, intensifying and extending the symptoms.[1,2]

Causation

Brain-tissue dysfunction can stem from a variety of causes; these are listed in Table 30-1. Whatever the cause, symptoms of OBS include one or more of the following: excitement; vertigo; delirium; convulsions; stupor; coma; memory impairment; incoordination; visual impairment; ataxia; confusion; somnolence; hallucinations; anxiety; speech disorders; personality changes; irritability; alterations in sexual drive and activity; dementia; peripheral neuropathy; restlessness; sleep disorders; paranoid thinking; depression; suicidal ideation; loss of cognitive functioning; emotional lability; psychotic behavior; altered attention span; drowsiness; crawling sensations on limbs; delusions; confabulation; apraxia; agnosia; impaired judgment; euphoria; inability to think in the abstract; lack of initiative, foresight, inspiration, or fantasy; paucity of thoughts; lack of capacity for friendship, love, and social relations; rigid, stereotyped, and compulsive ways of dealing with the environment; combativeness; blunting of sensitivity to moral and social conventions; inappropriate behavior.[3-8]

Aging—complicated by pathophysiology, alcoholism, and trauma—probably accounts for the largest number of persons with OBS. A certain percentage of people with OBS are the survivors of a suicide, homicide, or accident. With increasing societal attention to environmental pollution and the efforts to enforce the Occupational Health and

Table 30-1 Causation of Organic Brain Syndrome

Categories	Examples
Volatile agents	Gasoline, aerosols, glues, paint removers, solvents, lacquers, varnishes, dry-cleaning agents, home cleaning products (alone or when mixed)
Heavy metals	Lead (paints, ceramic glazes, moonshine whiskey), mercury, arsenic, manganese
Insecticides	DDT, parathion, malathion, diazine
Circulatory disturbances	Atherosclerosis, infarction, hypoxia, hypoglycemia, hypertensive crisis, postcardiac surgery
Metabolic and endocrine disorders	Hepatic disease, uremic encephalopathy, porphyria, thyroid dysfunction, parathyroid dysfunction, adrenal dysfunction, nutritional disorders, Wernicke-Korsakoff syndrome
Senility	Alzheimer's disease, senile dementia
Progressive degenerative diseases	Parkinsonism, Huntington's chorea, multiple sclerosis
Brain trauma	Concussion, contusion, hemorrhage, thrombosis, penetrating wounds, blast effects, electrical trauma
Drugs	Sedatives, stimulants, psychotropics
Infections	Meningitis, encephalitis, neurosyphilis (tabes dorsalis)
Neoplasms, tumors	Astrocytoma, medulloblastoma, meningioma
Seizures	Petit mal, grand mal, focal seizures, psychic seizures

Safety Act, there is an increasing awareness of the damage to brain tissue caused by industrial chemicals. Occupational exposure to toxic substances may produce symptoms of OBS ranging from the mild and transient to those which cause severe destruction and dysfunction. People exposed to repeated courses of electroconvulsive therapy are also subject to permanent residual brain damage. Given so many possible causes and variations in symptoms, diagnosis requires an extensive assessment of the client.

The type of damage to brain tissue which results in OBS includes cellular damage; neuronal loss; neurofibrillary change; development of senile plaques; ischemia; microemboli; inhibition of cerebral enzymes; deranged cellular metabolism; proliferation of glial cells; depletion of dopamine; demyelinization; proliferation of cancer cells; and invasion by pathological microorganisms.[9]

In senile dementia (Alzheimer's disease), causation is still not clearly defined. Such changes of aging as brain atrophy, senile plaques, neurofibrillary changes, loss of glial cells, and loss of neurons are also found in senile dementia; however, in spite of these changes, many people remain alert and intellectually active into advanced old age.[9] When these losses do occur in the older person, environmental factors, underlying pathophysiological conditions, and other yet to be determined factors suggest multicausation. Dementia in the aging population appears to be on the increase. This presents a challenge to society as well as to researchers, who seek to identify contributing factors; and to nursing, which must identify the most effective ways of helping clients and their families cope effectively with the resulting deficits.[6]

Diagnosis

The diagnosis of OBS rests on data collected from a variety of sources. The behavioral assessment is based on direct observation of the client's behavior, descriptions and comparisons of behavior past and present provided by family or coworkers, the psychiatric interview, and the mental status exam. A physical examination and diagnostic laboratory tests provide information concerning underlying changes in physical structures and physiological functioning which may contribute to or cause symptomatology of OBS. Caretakers must take special pains to collect specific data about the client's place of employment, type of occupation, and potential for exposure to toxic substances. In the petrochemical industries, for example, the toxic effects of numerous products have only recently come to light; these toxic chemicals have affected both industrial workers and office support personnel. Psychological tests are also administered to assess the type and extent of the deficits. The types of tests and their purposes are listed in Table 30-2.[10,11]

Medical Management

Once the diagnosis of OBS has been confirmed, a variety of therapeutic modalities are employed to reverse, arrest, or ameliorate the tissue destruction. When OBS has been caused by toxic substances, the cellular damage cannot always be reversed. However, prevention of further exposure to the substance arrests cellular toxicity and destruction.[3] In the case of poisoning from heavy metals such as lead, the chelating agent EDTA may be prescribed. However, this is useful only in the treatment of acute poisoning and lead encephalopathy; it is not effective in chronic cases except in the presence of plumbemia. Unless treated immediately, mercury poisoning causes irreversible damage.

With metabolic and endocrine problems, treatment of the underlying disorders prevents irreversible neuronal damage. Hypoglycemic encephalopathies require interventions which focus on assisting the clients to better understand, accept, and manage their diabetes and life stress more effectively.

Circulatory disorders which contribute to the development of OBS require treatment of the underlying pathophysiology. Anticoagulants, vasodilators, and lipotrophic enzymes are used to alleviate the problems of atherosclerosis; however, no controlled studies have been conducted which clearly prove their value.[4,12] Other encephalopathies can usually be controlled or reversed by treatment of the underlying pathophysiology.[5] When OBS is related to inherited or acquired progressive degenerative disease processes, specificity of treatment is lacking and care is directed toward helping clients to cope effectively and comfortably within the limitations imposed by their deficits (see Chap. 38).

Brain traumas present a different picture. The reduction of increased intracranial pressure and removal of foreign objects or bone fragments may be all that is necessary to alleviate symptoms of acute OBS. However, where damage cannot be relieved or completely repaired, rehabilitation and retraining is employed to maximize functioning.[7]

Client Behaviors

The wide variety of behaviorial symptomalology associated with OBS reflects the complexity of the central nervous sytem. OBS is characterized by behavioral manifestations of the underlying tissue dysfunction or metabolic derangements. These clients may and often do exhibit psychopathological behavior along with the manifestations of their deficits. It is no simple matter to determine which abnormal behaviors are based solely on physiological deficits and which are maladaptive *responses* to the deficits—that is, due to previously impaired coping abilities. This difficult distinction requires extensive assessment by a team of specialists representing several different professions.

Client behaviors characteristic of OBS in which psychopathology may coexist may be classified as dementia, delirium, and paroxysmal disorders.[13]

Dementia

In this group of clients the OBS is characterized by amnesia, disorientation, impaired intellectual functioning, and affective dysfunction. These symptoms may also occur in delirium; in the latter, however, dysattention and a fluctuating level of awareness predominate.

Table 30-2 Psychological Testing[10]

Type of test	Purpose
General scales	To determine an index of general intelligence.
Reasoning and problem solving	To determine capacity for abstract reasoning and to identify reduction in behavioral flexibility.
Memory	To determine impairment of immediate memory (registration), recent memory (storage), and remote memory.
Orientation	To determine precision of temporal orientation.
Visioperceptive and visioconstructive	To determine ability to analyze complex stimuli and to translate perceptions into appropriate motor action.
Somatoperceptual	To determine right-left recognition, finger recognition, and responsiveness to double tactile stimulation.

Source: Adapted from A. Bentor, "Psychological Tests for Brain Damage," in A. Freedman, H. Kaplan, B. Sadock, (eds.), *Comprehensive Textbook of Psychiatry,* Williams and Wilkins, Baltimore, 1975.

Dysmenesia

Dysmenesia, which is an impairment in the ability to retain and recall information, is the most prominent symptom of dementia.[13] Initially the person may be forgetful and absent-minded. An example is the little old lady who puts the kettle on for a cup of tea and, while waiting for it to boil, forgets why she is waiting and decides to do a household chore. In the meantime the water boils away and the kettle handle or spout burns. If her sense of smell is poor, as is often the case in the older person, a fire may spread before she becomes aware of its existence. When dysmenesia progresses, the client remains, at least initially, able to recall events that occurred before the memory failure began. Such a client may reminisce in great detail about his life as a child or youth, the adventures of that time, his marriage, and the birth of sons and daughters. Dates are easily remembered, rooms described in detail, and social events recalled with attention to minor incidents. However, events of the recent past are either less easily recalled—with descriptions that are less precise—or no memory of them is available.

Memory loss may be very mild and almost undetectable, but with progression of the underlying destructive process the memory loss gradually extends to the remote past. Registration, storage, and remote memory may be lost, so that not only recent events but past ones as well are no longer recalled.[10,13]

Disorientation

Disorientation is closely related to dysmenesia. When disoriented clients do not know who they are, the time of day, the date, or to whom they are speaking, they must have dysmenesia or memory impairment as well. In its earliest stages, disorientation is characterized by an impaired sense of time.[13] For example, John was able to recall what work he had done the day before but not which tasks he did in the morning and which in the afternoon or evening. In Mrs. Quimby's case, the time confusion was manifested by her habit of arising in the middle of the night or very early morning and, thinking it was already daytime, preparing to leave her home to go shopping or to church.

As temporal disorientation increases, clients cannot recall the day, month, week, or year. They also have increasing difficulty orienting themselves to place and even to familiar surroundings, and they have trouble recognizing people they know.

This disorientation becomes more pronounced in twilight and as the night progresses. A strange environment, such as a hospital or convalescent home, can also aggravate this condition, as can abnormal levels of sensory input. Overstimulation can be confusing, and sensory deprivation may have an equally disturbing effect.[4]

One OBS client, a Mr. Simons, suffering from increasing disorientation and dysmenesia, walked away from his daughter's home. When he was picked up by the police at 3 A.M., wandering in the downtown district, he was unable to give either his name or his address and did not know the time, day, or year. When his daughter arrived at the police station to retrieve him, he refused to go with the "strange lady."

Impaired Intellectual Functioning
When abstract reasoning is impaired, the initial deficit may be mild and uneven. The affected person may be able to continue working for a considerable time if the job does not require decision making or the ability to deal with sensitive interpersonal situations. As the impairment progresses, it becomes more evident to coworkers and family because judgment becomes unreliable, decisions and behavior inappropriate. With progression of the disease process, speech becomes impoverished, social isolation increases, and self-care deteriorates.

For example, Mr. Adams, an investment broker, was noted for his conservative stance in managing his customers' portfolios. He first manifested his impaired judgment by selecting speculative stocks more frequently; but this went unnoticed initially. However, he began progressively to counsel investors away from blue-chip stocks until one day he advised a long-standing customer to close out his portfolio and invest all the cash in a risky company that produced avant-garde movies.

Many such people are highly defended against awareness and discovery of their growing impairment. Consequently they will provide long and involved rationales for their actions. In many instances, family, friends, and coworkers tend to deny the character changes until the behaviors become blatant or the social indiscretions embarrassing.

Affective Dysfunction
Emotional lability is sometimes a consequence of OBS. The person affected experiences strong emotion in the absence of either intrapsychic or environmental stimuli. The feeling tone may shift suddenly and excessively, without warning, from sadness and crying to euphoria and laughter, or the felt emotion may be inappropriate to the situation. When this occurs, it is disturbing to both the client and the family, particularly when they do not understand that it is a consequence of brain-tissue dysfunction.[2,14]

Other people with OBS manifest affective disturbance by exhibiting a blunting and shallowness of emotion or a lack of responsiveness.

Adaptive Response to Deficits
Many factors influence the way a person responds to memory failure, disorientation, and impaired intellectual functioning. One who is confronted with these losses has emotional reactions, undergoes personality changes, and makes efforts to adapt. The premorbid personality, the rate of deterioration, environmental demands, stresses, supports, and the state of health all affect the person's response to the deficit.[13]

According to Detre,[13] the most common manifestation of emotional disturbance seen in people with these deficits is an inability to modulate their emotional response.[13] Initial symptoms include anergia, declining interest, and alterations in affect. The person's difficulty in perceiving the outside world extends to the internal milieu as well. Because of this impaired sensitivity to the self, the range of emotional responsivity and the congruity between affective state and ideation may be disturbed. Since this disturbance is manifested by excessive and/or inappropriate emotional responses, lability, and blunting or shallowness of affect, it becomes difficult to discriminate between a maladaptive emotional response and alterations of affect caused by disturbance in brain tissue.[2]

Maladaptive responses are exaggerations of the ways in which the person coped in the past. Gregarious, outgoing people become more so, and their behavior often becomes socially obnoxious; while solitary and suspicious people become more withdrawn and paranoid. Often the personality that emerges because of the deficits and the emotional response to them is a caricature of the previous personality. Previous life events, stresses past and present, interpersonal factors, and the current environment influence the adaptive process.[14]

Initially such coping mechanisms as sublimation, denial, and repression serve to protect the person from confronting the deficits. However, with increasing impairment, these mechanisms become ineffective and inefficient and are replaced by more primitive defenses.[13] Rigid, negativistic behavior then predominates. Unable to defend against awareness of the deficits or to interact effectively with the environment for need fulfillment—a difficulty which is compounded by a constant misinterpretation and distortion of reality—the person is vulnerable to a *catastrophic anxiety reaction, profound depression,* or *assaultive aggressiveness.* Also, as anxiety increases, sleeping and eating problems develop, with consequent weight loss and susceptibility to other physical problems.

When these clients also suffer from visual impairment, hearing loss, or other complicating physical problems, social isolation may be greater. With increasing need deprivation there is physical deterioration as well as decreasing self-esteem and self-acceptance. Psychotic symptoms such as illusions, delusions, and visual hallucinations may emerge; or there may be neurotic symptoms such as depression, anxiety, obsessions, compulsions, or phobias[14] (see Chaps. 14, 16, and 18).

Compulsive ritualistic behavior is a common means whereby these people attempt to compensate for their disabilities (see Chap. 16). For others, alcohol abuse, promiscuity, and impulsivity develop as maladaptive responses to the impact of loss.[14]

The client's disturbed perception of the inner and outer environments creates a climate for the development of delusions. According to Detre,[13] the more cohesive delusions reflect the person's real-life situation and everyday irritations, particularly feelings of loss, helplessness, lonliness and abandonment.

An example of such a client is Mrs. Cremins who had been living with her son and daughter-in-law since her increasing forgetfulness began to worry her children. Preoccupied with the fear that burglars would break in and take her money, leaving her nothing, she squirreled her money away here and there around the house. She hid dollars in books, vases, pillows, and couch cushions and then promptly forgot where she had put them. After searching vainly one day for a particular envelope of money, she accused her daughter-in-law of taking her money and belongings.

The loss of her home and familiar surroundings and the resettlement in her son's home required adaptation beyond Mrs. Cremins's coping capacity. Her impaired thinking processes, the stress generated by the move, and the need to defend against recognition of her deficits created the need to link her daughter-in-law with her losses and to develop the delusion that her daughter-in-law was taking her possessions from her. What was particularly painful for the daughter-in-law was the element of truth that she had urged her husband to bring his mother into their home, fearing that her forgetfulness would result in an accidental injury or that she would set fire to her home while preparing meals.

The environment mediates the way in which people with OBS experience their deficits. If the environment makes demands on the individual which are beyond his or her ability to cope, disorganization will be accelerated and maladaptive behavior more apt to emerge. When support is inadequate—when the family or caretaking structure is rigid, demanding, confronting, or rejecting—it causes the person to feel isolated, abandoned, and anxious. If situational supports are adequate, flexible, accommodating, and focused on conservation of capacities and enhancement of strengths, they protect the person from unnecessary stress, anxiety-producing confrontations, and awareness of the deficits.

To protect themselves from full awareness of their disabilities, these people will deny their deficits. When a request is made such as "Clean your room" or "Make your bed," they may refuse to do so, not because they are truly negativistic but because they may not remember where their room is or how a bed is made. If pressured, they may not do what is requested but rather perform a *substitute task* with which they can cope, such as straightening the room in which they happen to be at the time.

These people may convey disorderliness in their dress or hygiene but be compulsively orderly in other areas of their lives. They may arrange holy statues on their dressers in a set pattern which, if disturbed for any reason, causes them considerable distress. Some carefully wrap or sew into bags odds and ends such as holy medals, buttons, broken jewelery, or other small items which they store carefully in specific places. Some tend to simplify their environment so that they will be able to negotiate it with a minimum of distress. Others hoard or save almost everything that comes into their possession, fearing that they will not be able to tell the difference between what is worth keeping and what is not.

Communication is an area these people can and often do control. By refusing to speak or to converse unless they themselves have chosen the subject, they attempt to manage the environment so as to avoid a confrontation of their deficits. A question may be met with stony silence, a rationalization about why they cannot answer, a fabrication of events rather than actual facts confabulation, or a tangential monologue that is not responsive but an attempt to bind anxiety.[12] One gentleman confronted the nurse, who was reminding him

that it was dinnertime, by replying "Stop hassling me! You don't want to help me, you only want to make me upset so I'll have to stay here."

Delirium

This term refers to a number of illnesses of organic origin that are usually reversible and characterized by dysmenesia, disorientation, and such disturbances of sleep-wakefulness regulation as insomnia, somnolence, fluctuating awareness, and dysattention.[13] It is a syndrome which is a *transient disturbance* of brain function characterized by a global impairment of cognitive processes. The level of consciousness is altered, but the person need not be out of touch with the environment. However, since thinking, memory, perception, and attention are disturbed, the ability to understand and interpret the internal and external environment in accordance with past experience is reduced.[2] This disturbed sensorium interferes with the person's ability to gratify needs. The disruption in the metabolic processes of the brain produces the behavioral symptoms; however, psychological factors strongly influence the content of the delirium.[2]

Manifestations of delirium vary widely. The person may be quiet and experience only brief periods of inattentiveness which are not easily detected. However, as the level of awareness decreases, responsivity to external stimuli slows and the impaired thinking becomes more evident. In the extreme, the person becomes delusional, enters a hallucinatory state, and statistically is apt to be moribund.[2]

The delusional thinking of these persons is poorly organized and the content of thought changes rapidly. The person tends to misidentify objects, people, or voices in the environment and then to generate hallucinatory experience. This misidentification also occurs in the form of *illusive pseudorecognition*. Clients suffering from a disturbed sensorium may, in a poorly illuminated room, mistake the nurse or other caretakers for people they have known in the past.[13]

Mr. Arthur, a client in serious metabolic disequilibrium, greeted the nurse one evening with the words, "Margie, how did you know I was here? I haven't seen you in years." Even as the nurse approached the bed and identified herself, he continued to relate to her as Margie, a friend from the past.

Four stages of delirium which delineate changes in the sensorium have been identified. In the *first stage* the person is restless and talkative, experiences distortions of time and space, has difficulty in remembering what is said or taught, is mildly suspicious, has increased sensitivity to stimuli, and exhibits moods which range from elation to irritability or bewilderment. In the *second stage* speech becomes incoherent and slurred; the ability to concentrate is even more impaired; and the disorientation to time, place, and person increases as misinterpretation of the environment becomes more marked. There may be overactivity which seems purposive, and emotional tone is labile.[13]

If the underlying problem is not resolved, the person enters the *third stage*. The hyperactivity continues but becomes purposeless, speech is disorganized, there is global disorientation, dysmenesia and easy distractibility predominate, hallucinations and delusions develop, and feelings of depression and fearfulness are pervasive. If the person enters *stage four,* the extreme of delirium may be manifested by either excitation or stupor or progress from the former to the latter. In either case, there is no meaningful relationship with the environment.[9,13] Delirium is a medical emergency. The underlying cause must be treated promptly if permanent damage to brain tissue is to be prevented.

Paroxysmal Disorders

Dysfunction in this group of persons originates in abnormal electrical discharges in brain tissue which interfere with the sensorium. Seizures are not a disease but a symptom of a problem in the central nervous system which is causing it to produce abnormal discharges. A seizure signals that neural, humoral, metabolic, and vascular regulatory systems of the brain are imbalanced[15] (see Chap. 38).

Client Behavior

In some seizure clients, particularly those who have been poorly controlled, there is an insidious dementia with narrowing interest, slowed mentation, and apathy.[14] These people may also be vulnerable to a variety of emotional disturbances which are complicated by family and societal attitudes toward seizures.[14]

Focal sensory, psychomotor, and autonomic seizures have psychiatric implications. These people are subject not only to alterations in consciousness but changes in cognitive and affective processes as well. They may become suddenly angry and paranoid and engage in bizarre behavior. Psychic seizures may also be accompanied by déja vu phenomena; dreamy states; changes in self-awareness; a sensation of growing larger or smaller; forced thought in which a phrase, melody, or scene occupies the mind; sexual arousal in the absence of stimuli; paranoid ideation; hallucinations; paroxysmal attacks of anxiety; or the impression that objects in the environment are growing larger or smaller. Such phenomena are similar to those experienced by the schizophrenic or the person labeled emotionally disturbed, and this fact has implications for adapation (see Chap. 16).

Adaptive Responses

Many people with seizure problems suffer from the psychotoxic effects of their anticonvulsant therapy; these include drowsiness, depersonalization, and dysmenesia. If these side effects are not remedied by alteration of dosage or drug, the person may develop disturbance of impulse control or judgment, depression, conversion symptoms, dissociative states, or delirium.[13]

Anticonvulsant toxicity and a history or repeated seizures have an impact on life-style and self-perception. They interfere with the attainment of personal goals and elicit fear and avoidance on the part of others in social situations. In addition, the symptoms contribute to the client's low self-esteem, low self-acceptance, fear of insanity, and difficulty in obtaining gainful employment.

The seizure-prone person, including the one who simulates seizures, is a member of a family system; consequently, when maladaptive behavior occurs, it is a symptom of the family's problems in coping with the disease process. Thus interventions are directed toward assisting the family to manage the interpersonal difficulties consequent to the paroxysmal disorder (see Chap. 11).

Nurses' Responses

Nurses respond to clients with OBS in a variety of ways depending on the client behaviors which emerge to cope with the deficits, the client's age, the nurses' perception of the client's ability to control the behavior and the nurses' view of the cause of the disturbances, particularly whether the client appears to be responsible for the underlying problem.

The seizure-prone client's social value is an important mediating factor in the development of a sympathetic response reflective of an identification process.

One such client, Carolyn, had just returned from a vacation and was sitting in the airport waiting room with college friends when a terrorist bomb exploded. When she had recovered from the blast injuries she was diagnosed as having residual OBS, as evidenced by impaired intellectual functioning, which ruled out further pursuit of her university studies and career aspirations. She also exhibited poor impulse control and affective lability. After medical discharge, she was transferred to a private inpatient psychiatric hospital. This attractive, gregarious girl was immediately well received by staff and clients. The senseless, traumatic destruction of her potential generated sadness and sympathy in the staff. In spite of her continual insensitivity in interpersonal relationships and disruptive impulsivity, the staff defended against frustration and diligently designed and implemented a wide variety of therapeutic plans to modify her behavior and help her function optimally.

Stash, age 48, was quite another case. A chronic alcoholic, he was diagnosed as having Korsakoff's syndrome. His history revealed early success and high achievement in the advertising world. As his affluence increased, so did his alcohol abuse. Initially he was well supported by his wife, who not only joined Al-Anon but became active in spite of the demands of three young children. Stash participated only sporadically in AA. Not only did his drinking increase but his abusiveness toward his wife and children became intolerable and his wife instituted divorce proceedings. A highly talented and creative person when sober, he had been offered job security by his boss if he would agree to participate in AA or another alcohol treatment program. Stash made an attempt but quickly sabotaged the plan and returned to heavy drinking. In time, he became a local derelict.

During Stash's psychiatric admission for detoxification, the staff avoided him when at all possible. Their efforts to explain unit rules and clarify his understanding were minimal. Meaningful communication was further thwarted by his invention of involved explanations because of impaired memory (confabulation). Staff felt that his frustrating behavior, deteriorated physical condition, and business and personal family failures were his own doing. They lacked interest and motivation for developing a plan of care. They tended to make few demands so that he remained relatively isolated and received little therapy and only impatient, insensitive care.

Many of the behaviors exhibited by OBS clients distance caretakers. Impulsivity, irritability, slowness to respond, and negativistic behavior generate feelings of impatience which, with time, grow into anger. Poor personal hygiene and inappropriate behavior may elicit feelings of disgust and the wish to avoid the client. These negative feelings may cause caretakers to succumb to pressured time schedules and sacrifice individual client needs; they may sometimes even coerce clients to conform when it is not necessary.

Responsibility, appropriateness, self-control, responsivity to others, social awareness, and rationality are attributes we assign to adulthood. These qualities are components of what we consider to be human dignity. When nurses must care for clients over time and watch irreversible, progressive deterioration of these human qualities, they experience feelings of impotence and helplessness. It can be depressing for nurses to work with perseverance and caring, only to find their clients becoming more vegetative, aggressive, or disorganized. The nurse's distress is, of course, compounded by the fact that there are no interventions available to arrest the progressive deterioration. As a defense against such feelings, nurses may appear to withdraw physically and emotionally from these clients. This response is often exhibited by the mechanical, technical, and impersonal way in which care is delivered.

Nurses respond to symptoms of delirium differently depending on the setting. In the hospital and when there has been a diagnosis, the symptoms are interpreted as a medical emergency and treated as such. If the symptoms begin when the client is not in a medical setting, they can be misinterpreted. If the dysattention, hallucinatory behavior, suspiciousness, talkativeness, elation, depression, or incidents of illusive pseudorecognition are not recognized as signs of acute and severe brain dysfunction, the nurse may respond with bewilderment and frustration or as if the problems were psychogenically rather than physiologically based.

Seizure disorders can also be misinterpreted. If the caretakers share the perception that there is an emotional component, the assessment process may be skewed toward interpreting data in a way that fails to attend to the client's needs. The nurse may become impatient and nonsupportive and the client may be baffled and anxious about the symptoms and lack of empathy from caretakers.

The responses OBS clients generate in the nurses who provide care are not preventable. They are real, unavoidable, and require ventilation.

However, these feelings need not interfere with the delivery of comprehensive, individualized, and sensitive care. Awareness that such feelings are developing is the initial step in their resolution. When nurses begin to get in touch with these feelings, client behavior can be examined in light of what is known about the effects of organic damage on functioning; this process will redefine the situation to some extent. Behavior which may have been perceived as purposively frustrating, inappropriate, and destructive may be redefined as the client's only available way of defending against deficits and the awareness of a changing self-concept.

Being able to "put oneself in *another's* shoes" is an important approach to understanding the client's dilemma and desperate need to protect and conserve the *self*. From this vantage point, the nurse's perception is altered. Empathy can emerge, and this expands and sensitizes the nurse's perceptions of client needs and environmental factors which influence coping.

Client impulsivity is yet another problem. Knowing that it is organically based is not always sufficient. The behavior may be provocative, disruptive, an obstacle to providing needed attention to other clients, and continuously frustrating. However, such situations need not be hopeless. Nurses can cope more cognitively than affectively if they are supported by a cohesive multidisciplined team which maximizes communication, plans knowledgeably and collaboratively, and evaluates plans nonjudgmentally, thus sharing the burden of helping the client learn some dimension of control.

Assessment

Clients exhibiting behaviorial symptoms of OBS are encountered by nurses in a wide variety of settings: emergency rooms, clinics, medical and surgical units in the general hospital; special-care units such as the intensive-care unit (ICU) or cardiac-care unit (CCU); convalescent and continuing care settings; psychiatric hospitals; mental health centers; or in their homes. These settings

Table 30-3 Case-Finding Assessment

1 Are there personality changes which can be observed over time or described in behaviorial terms by significant others?
2 Is the person oriented to time, place, and person?
3 Is there evidence of absent-mindedness which is creating problems or indicating potential problems of a serious nature?
4 Is remote memory more accessible than recent memory, and is there evidence of extensive use of confabulation to mask memory gaps?
5 Is the person's judgment becoming unreliable or dangerous to self or others?
6 Is speech more impoverished than it has been in the past?
7 Is self-care deteriorating?
8 Is there evidence of emotional lability or inappropriate affect, blunting, shallowness, or unresponsiveness in interpersonal relationships?
9 Is the sensorium disturbed?
10 Does the person exhibit behavior suggestive of a paroxysmal disorder?
11 Are there changes in the person's behavior which violate social conventions and have potential for causing embarrassment or being labeled deviant?

may alleviate or aggravate the display of symptoms. Nurses must be knowledgeable about symptoms characteristic of OBS and their causation so that they may be alert case finders and sensitive to the needs of their clients.

Nursing has a major advantage in the care of clients who are potential victims of OBS. In inpatient settings, nursing is provided with a 24-hour opportunity to observe and document the client's behavior in many situations and with various people. These data become a valuable base for the physician's and nurse's diagnoses as well as the planning, implementing, and evaluation of care.

Nursing is primarily concerned with client response to illness. Thus the assessment of clients suspected of or diagnosed as having OBS focuses on their behavior and their response to existing or progressing deficits. Table 30-3 is a general framework for assessing clients in a variety of settings to determine whether there is a possibility that OBS may be interfering with their ability to function optimally. Table 30-4 is a series of questions designed to elicit data which can be analyzed to determine how the person diagnosed as having OBS is coping with the organic dysfunction.

Table 30-4 Assessment of Client Response to Organic Brain Syndrome

1 What coping mechanisms is the client using to defend against awareness of the deficits?
2 Is the client becoming isolated and withdrawing from social contact with others?
3 Does the client exhibit affective dysfunction or increasing disorganization at certain times or in specific social situations?
4 Is inappropriate behavior elicited by specific situations or communications?
5 Does the client avoid situations which would expose the loss of intellectual functioning?
6 Do the client's deficits require protection from self-injury and the environment and interventions to preserve human dignity?
7 Are the client's family or caretakers flexible, supportive, and sensitive to the client's needs?
8 Are sleeping and eating problems developing or worsening?
9 Is the client's judgment and decision making becoming less reliable?
10 Is there behaviorial evidence that the delirium is worsening? (See stages listed under "Delirium.")
11 Is there evidence suggesting a toxic reaction to anticonvulsant therapy?
12 Is there evidence that the client with a seizure disorder is receiving secondary gains from the illness that interfere with effective functioning?
13 Is the client using substitute or negativistic behavior when requested to perform a designated task?

Planning

According to Yura and Walsh,[16] the planning phase begins with the formulation of the nursing diagnosis. During this phase of the nursing process, priorities are set regarding which problems require immediate intervention and which require long-range planning or attention at a later time. The problems that are identified—for example, *"Excessive drowsiness interfering with participation in unit activities"*—may not be under nursing's purview; if that is the case, a report or referral is made to those professional health-care providers with the requisite expertise.

Nursing Diagnosis

The data collected during the assessment process is analyzed, categorized, compared, and synthesized to determine the existence of problems and their extent. Once this work is completed, a decision is reached as to whether problems do in fact exist and whether there are areas where intervention would enhance existing strengths and assist the client to achieve the highest possible level of wellness given the existing organic damage. The nurse then formulates the nursing diagnoses which will guide planning and implementation[16] (see Table 30-5).

The following are sample nursing diagnoses of clients with OBS who are having problems adapting to or coping with their deficits:

1 Impoverished speech and shallow affect interfere with client's social and therapeutic relationships.
2 Irritability moves into aggressive assaultiveness when client is confronted with demands beyond his ability to perform.
3 Client is withdrawn and quiet. Her suspicion that her family is stealing her possessions while she is hospitalized is the focus of all interactions with others.
4 Impulsivity prevents client's participation in group activities off the unit.
5 Seizure client is controlling deferential family by managing her disease irresponsibly.
6 Abandonment by significant others is

contributing to the client's increasingly agitated depressive behavior.

Nursing Care of the OBS Client

There is a difference between reversible and irreversible OBS. In the former condition, nursing goals and interventions are directed toward (1) supporting medical treatment of underlying pathophysiology, (2) assisting the client to respond adaptively to the temporary deficits, and (3) reassuring the client that a return to wellness is a realistic expectation.

When OBS is irreversible, nursing goals and interventions focus on teaching the client new ways of coping. Thus retraining, when appropriate, takes top priority. Efforts are made to keep these clients mentally active, but always within the parameters of their limitations. Independent functioning is also fostered. These clients are never encouraged to explore feelings and must be protected against developing insight into their problems. It is very important to help them avoid awareness of their deficits and deterioration. This approach contradicts the nurse's usual way of helping clients adapt to alterations caused by illness. However, confrontation and recognition of deficits only heightens these clients' anxiety and encourages maladaptive behavior to emerge. Insight will only serve to damage the self-concept and interfere with a dignified decline.[18]

Clients with irreversible and progressively deteriorating OBS are a challenge to nursing regardless of the setting. Hospitalization often aggravates their symptoms, and increased disorientation often leads to noisy and disruptive behavior. The application of restraints to prevent the client from climbing over side rails will ensure safety but also usually increases the disruptive behavior unless a concerted effort is made to implement a program of reality orientation. Nurses working in convalescent homes may provide less direct care to these clients, but they are responsible for planning the care and helping the nonprofessional caretakers to understand the client's predicament and the importance of following nursing orders.

Table 30-5 Client Problems — Nursing Goals and Interventions

Client Problem: Disorientation, increasing demands on coping mechanisms.
Nursing Goal: Ameliorate disorientation and the concomitant increased demands; foster the development of less primitive coping mechanisms.

Nursing Interventions:
1 Frequently orient to time, place, and person, using clocks, calendars, and visual aids.
2 Establish a set, well-known routine for the client to follow.
3 Address the client by name and title (e.g., "Good morning, Mr. Tate") to reinforce a sense of identity.
4 Repeat basic information frequently during the day.
5 Orient the client when he or she wakes up during the night.
6 Do not agree with the confused client's incorrect statements, argue, or insist on your viewpoint.
7 Correct the client gently but not insistently.
8 Do not allow the client to ramble incoherently.
9 Respond to the client openly and honestly.
10 Create a calm, quiet, and unhurried atmosphere.
11 Speak slowly and distinctly.
12 Moderate or avoid stressful situations to decrease stimuli which would distort perceptions or cause sensory overload.
13 Convey warmth and concern.
14 Respond patiently and consistently.

Client Problem: Exhibits disturbed dysattention.
Nursing Goal: Ameliorate factors which contribute to dysattention.

Nursing Interventions:
1 Look directly at the client when communicating.
2 Position self in client's line of vision when communicating.
3 Give clear, distinct, simple directions in a step-by-step fashion.
4 Direct conversation toward concrete, familiar subjects.
5 Provide simple activities that will encourage purposeful motion.
6 Repeat messages slowly, calmly, and patiently until the client shows some signs of comprehension.
7 Vary media and/or words to fit the client's ability to comprehend the message.
8 Modify environmental stimuli which affect attention.

Client Problem: Social isolation with feelings of rejection and loss of identity.
Nursing Goal: Ameliorate factors which engender feelings of rejection and loss of identity and which would lead to greater behaviorial maladaptation.

Nursing Interventions:
1 Support statements in which the client describes the significant others as caring, concerned, and helpful.
2 Help the client to seek and accept reasons why the significant others' behavior is not meeting the client's expectation.
3 Encourage the display of mementos.
4 Actively listen to the client's viewpoints and perception of the past and present.
5 Modify environmental factors affecting feelings about significant others.
6 Help the client to maintain communication with significant others.

Client Problem: Dysmenesia, with increasing demands on coping mechanisms.
Nursing Goal: Alleviate factors affecting dysmenesia and the concomitant increased demand on coping mechanisms.

Nursing Interventions:
1 Give simple, clear, step-by-step directions even for routine, uncomplicated activities.
2 Interpret feigned deafness or refusal to perform certain tasks as a defense against memory loss.
3 Repeat policies, routines, and other information regarding daily living activities when the client's behavior suggests that he or she cannot remember this information.

Table 30-5 Client Problems — Nursing Goals and Interventions *(continued)*

4 Initiate assistance in the performance of a task if the client shows hesitancy or refuses to do it, giving verbal reminders for each step the client is expected to perform.
5 Avoid confrontation or exposure of fabricated stories or untruths and interpret these behaviors as defenses against memory impairment.
6 Interpret anger and irritability as possible defenses against the client's realization that he or she cannot cope with the demands of the situation.
7 Interpret difficulty with abstract reasoning and inability to conceptualize as a possible symptom of organic dysfunction and avoid making unnecessary and inappropriate demands.
8 Recognize negativistic behavior and substitute activities as a defense against dysmenesia; avoid confrontation.

Client Problem: Need to defend against catastrophic fear reaction, profound depression, or aggressive assaultiveness.
Nursing Goal: Avoids a catastrophic fear reaction, profound depression, or assaultive aggressiveness.

Nursing Intervention:
1 Support client's efforts to ignore or deny intellectual impairments.
2 Avoid confrontation of inappropriate behavior and probing for feelings.
3 Communicate in a way that does not increase the client's awareness of deficits or need for defensive coping mechanisms.
4 Accompany the client when he or she wanders, gently providing guidance back to the specified area.
5 Avoid use of restraints and/or incarceration, which will cause greater feelings of inadequacy and helplessness.
6 Interpret suspicious behavior as a possible regression to a lower level.

Client Problem: Loss of independent functioning.
Nursing Goal: Independent functioning maximized.

Nursing Intervention:
1 Support maintenance of personal hygiene through verbal step-by-step directions and avoid "doing for" the client.
2 Provide maximum personal freedom within the bounds of safety.
3 Accept compulsive orderliness as a way of structuring time and the environment.
4 Foster the maintenance of established daily living activities.
5 Actively listen to somatic complaints and help the client to remain physically active within medically defined limits.
6 Modify the environment to facilitate independent functioning.
7 Help the client perform a task only when there are data indicating sensorimotor impairment which would prevent the client from functioning without help.

Client Problem: Misinterpretation, distortion of reality, illusive pseudorecognition.
Nursing Goal: Maintains reality orientation.

Nursing Intervention:
1 Give reality-oriented feedback.
2 Avoid use of physical restraints, using "thereness" and calming verbal reassurance.
3 Support medical treatment for underlying medical problem.
4 Give reassurance that the client is safe.
5 Protect the client from excessive stimulation by reducing excessive noise level and restricting the number of people in the environment.
6 Provide a level of stimulation that prevents both excitement and sensory deprivation by modulating input.
7 Provide sufficient light in the client's room at night so that the client will be able to identify surroundings correctly and thus avoid developing illusions.
8 Have people who come in contact with the client identify themselves each time they enter the client's room.

When clients living alone show a degree of dysmenesia that threatens their safety, they need help in relocating to an environment which better meets their safety needs. In these cases, the nurse works with the client, the family, and in some instances social services in providing for safer living arrangements. If the person has been abandoned by his or her family and placement in a residential-care setting is necessary and desirable, then consistent caretakers sensitive to the client's needs may in some measure replace the lost family.

When these clients are living with their families, the first task the nurse may need to accomplish is to help the family stop denying the deficits. In the case of the older client, it saddens and distresses adult children to experience role reversal with their aging parents. Whether clients with OBS are young or old, their behavior may be frustrating and demanding, requiring continual supervision. Under such circumstances even a relatively healthy family will be stressed. As a result, symptoms of distress may appear in any one family member, they may be manifested in marital discord, or they may lead to family disorganization. The nurse may be able to help the family identify changes in their life-style, ventilate feelings, analyze responsibilities, clarify values, and examine both division of labor and allocation of resources. Once communication in these areas has been facilitated and issues have been examined, the family may be ready to effectively engage in problem-solving activities relevant to the difficulties engendered by living with a member having OBS. This helping process also includes helping the family understand that some of the client's behavior is a consequence of the organic pathology and of their need to defend against confronting these deficits. However, some abnormal behavior may stem from a maladaptive response to illness. Working with the family, the nurse helps them to understand the manifestations of the syndrome and to analyze the circumstances of daily living to identify situations which may tend to generate maladaptive behavior. Family members also need help in seeing how they are interfering or failing to

maximize the client's independence and participating in the development of maladaptive behavior. The family may also need assistance in looking at these data, developing awareness of their own and the client's needs, and planning ways to modify responses and relationships to extinguish maladaptive behavior and develop more effective functioning in all members. By engaging families in this problem-solving activity, present difficulties can be resolved and the family's ability to deal with problems in the future can be strengthened.

In some instances, the family is unable to care for the client at home and members must confront the decision to place the client in a residential-care setting. If the nurse has been working with the family for some time and deterioration was inevitable, then long-range planning regarding placement will have been initiated and feelings dealt with during the early phases of care. If the nurse enters the picture when the family is recognizing the fact that they can no longer manage the client in the home, then nursing interventions focus on helping the family with their decision-making process, the selection of a care setting, and the feelings generated by the placement. The placement and preceding period of decision making is always a crisis for the family (see Chap. 5). Guilt feelings usually predominate. In some families there is also blaming of a spouse, which is often based on denial of the client's status and an unwillingness to assume responsibility for the decision. The nurse intervenes by helping members ventilate feelings and develop an understanding of each other's burdens and position. Helping the family to recognize the client's deterioration and their increasing inability to cope can sometimes be accomplished by either identifying or helping them to identify significant incidents which illustrate the problem and need for placement.

Nursing care also focuses on supporting the pharmacological regimen often ordered for these clients. Psychotropics can be valuable in relieving symptoms of anxiety, impulsivity, hyperkinesis, depression, and paranoid ideation. Antidepressants are also useful in the management of psychomotor retardation and may improve intellectual functioning and social performance.[13] However, drugs with anticholinergic properties must be given with caution to avoid prostatic obstruction, constipation, glaucoma, and hypotension in older clients.[13] The nurse's documentation of changes in mood, behavior, and performance of daily living activities provides valuable data which will guide the physician's choice of drug and titration of dosage. If the client is living with family while on medication, the nurse teaches the family how to assess the client's response to the regimen, the side effects, and signs of toxicity (see Chap. 8).

Table 30-5 outlines examples of client problems, nursing goals, and suggested interventions.

Evaluation

Determination of the effectiveness of interventions is an important step in the nursing process. Validation of the effectiveness of the interventions includes not only objective data but subjective information as well if this is at all possible.

Carla, 18 years old, received severe head injuries in a car accident which left her with residual brain damage. Her impulsivity became intolerable for her family and a psychiatric admission resulted. Her first week on the unit was stormy. Temper tantrums—including the throwing of food and objects, the slamming of doors and the destruction of furniture—characterized her impulsivity. The nurses identified the need to institute measures to modify the most disturbing behaviors. The following plan and nursing orders were put into operation:

> Problem: Temper tantrums.
>
> Nursing Order: Immediate restriction to room for 1 hour following episodes of object or food throwing, screaming, or destruction of furnishings. Restraints to be applied if necessary to implement this measure.

During the initial assessment period, tantrums and their expression had been documented. Thus there was a baseline on the type and frequency of these outbursts. The nursing orders were followed consistently by all staff. The effectiveness of this intervention was evaluated by determining whether, after a specified period of time, the number of tantrums had decreased and their expressions were less destructive.

Initially Carla showed no sign of learning control. During this period the restrictions prevented her from attending a unit party, a van trip to the movies, and a volleyball game. During the succeeding days, the number of outbursts did not decrease, but the severity of their expressions was reduced considerably. In time and with support, she became able to verbalize that she felt anger but did not know why; at these times she would go voluntarily to her room until the feelings had subsided.

The effectiveness of the nursing care given to OBS clients is best reflected in the absence or decrease of pervasive anxiety, depression, and assaultive, aggressive behavior.

References

1 American Psychiatric Association: *Diagnostic and Statistical Manual of Mental Disorders* (DSM-11) 2d ed., American Psychiatric Association, Washington, D.C., 1968.

2 B. Sadock: "Organic Brain Syndromes," in A. Freedman, H. Kaplan, and B. Sadock (eds.), *Comprehensive Textbook of Psychiatry II,* Williams & Wilkins, Baltimore, 1975, vol. 1, pp. 1060–1064.

3 G. Peterson: "Organic Brain Syndrome Associated with Drug or Poison Intoxication," in A. Freedman, H. Kaplan, and B. Sadock (eds.), *Comprehensive Textbook of Psychiatry II,* Williams & Wilkins, Baltimore, 1975, vol. 1, pp. 1108–1121.

4 B. Sadock: "Organic Brain Syndromes Associated with Circulatory Disturbances," in A. Freedman, H. Kaplan, and B. Sadock (eds.), *Comprehensive Textbook of Psychiatry II,* Williams & Wilkins, Baltimore, 1975, vol. 2, pp. 1065–1077.

5 A. Dale: "Organic Brain Syndrome Associated with Disturbances in Metabolism, Growth, and Nutrition," in A. Freedman, H. Kaplan, and B. Sadock (eds.), *Comprehensive Textbook of Psychiatry II*, Williams & Wilkins, Baltimore, 1975, vol. 1, pp. 1078–1085.

6 D. Mulder: "Organic Brain Syndromes Associated with Disease of Unknown Cause," in A. Freedman, H. Kaplan, and B. Sadock (eds.), *Comprehensive Textbook of Psychiatry II,* Williams & Wilkins, Baltimore, 1975, vol. 1, pp. 1086–1093.

7 G. Peterson: "Organic Brain Syndrome Associated with Brain Trauma," in A. Freedman, H. Kaplan, and B. Sadock (eds.), *Comprehensive Textbook of Psychiatry II,* Williams & Wilkins, Baltimore, 1975, vol. 1, pp. 1093–1107.

8 A. Dale: "Organic Brain Syndrome Associated with Infections," in A. Freedman, H. Kaplan, and B. Sadock (eds.), *Comprehensive Textbook of Psychiatry II,* Williams & Wilkins, Baltimore, 1975, vol. 1, pp 1121–1131.

9 S. Solomon: "Clinical Neurology and Pathophysiology," in A. Freedman, H. Kaplan, and B. Sadock (eds.), *Comprehensive Textbook of Psychiatry II,* Williams & Wilkins, Baltimore, 1975, vol. 1, pp. 249–265.

10 A. Benton: "Psychological Tests for Brain Damage," in A. Freedman, H. Kaplan, and B. Sadock (eds.), *Comprehensive Textbook of Psychiatry II,* Williams & Wilkins, Baltimore, 1975, vol. 1, pp. 757–767.

11 G. Barnes and G. Lucas: "Cerebral Dysfunction vs. Psychogenesis in Halstead-Reitan Tests," *The Journal of Nervous and Mental Diseases,* vol. 158, no. 1, pp. 50–60, January 1974.

12 Thomas Ban: "Psychopathology, Psychopharmacology and the Organic Brain Syndromes," *Psychosomatics,* vol. 17, no. 3, pp. 131–135, July–August–September 1976.

13 T. Detre and H. Jarecki: *Modern Psychiatric Treatment,* Lippincott, Philadelphia, 1971.

14 M. Eaton, M. Peterson, and J. Davis: *Psychiatry Medical Outline Series,* 3d ed., Medical Examination Publishing Company, New York, 1976.

15 F. Ervin: "Organic Brain Syndromes Associated With Epilepsy," in A. Freedman, H. Kaplan, and B. Sadock (eds.), *Comprehensive Textbook of Psychiatry II,* Williams & Wilkins, Baltimore, 1975, vol. 1, pp. 1138–1157.

16 H. Yura and M. Walsh: *The Nursing Process,* 2d ed., Appleton-Century-Crofts, New York, 1973.

31

The Dying Process

Thomas Nolan

Maryann Bohner

Learning Objectives

After studying this chapter, the student should be able to:

1 Discuss the cultural milieu of death.

2 Assess client and family behavior.

3 Identify nurse's responses that facilitate client and family coping.

4 Assess environmental factors that affect client coping.

5 Intervene to help client and family cope effectively with the dying process.

6 Evaluate the effectiveness of interventions.

The Meaning of Death

The life process and dying are integrated into a universal rhythm.[1] One cannot speak about dying without also speaking about living. Indeed, a human being begins the process of dying from the very first moment of existence. Dying is as much a part of the life process as living. Dying and death are events that happen to each one of us. We can postpone death or gain reprieves, but ultimately we all must die. Many people react to this with the feeling that there is something morbid in paying attention to death. They comment that they are more interested in life than in death. La Rochefoucauld epitomized this viewpoint in his remark, "One can no more look steadily at death than at the sun."

In the course of our lives, we all relate in our own way to the knowledge that death is certain. Throughout human history, the idea of death has posed the eternal mystery which is at the core of our religious and philosophical systems of thought. And it is quite possible that this idea is the prototype of human anxiety. Insecurity may well be a symbol of death. Any loss may represent total loss of the self. One of mankind's distinguishing characteristics is the capacity to grasp the concept of a future, including the inevitability of death. And it is in this anticipation of death that each of us discovers the hunger for immortality.

In the presence of death, Western culture has tended to run, hide, and seek refuge in various forms of denial. Concern about death has been relegated to the tabooed territory heretofore occupied by sex and diseases like cancer or venereal disease. We have been compelled, in unhealthy measure, to internalize our thoughts and feelings, fears, and even hopes concerning death. In the twentiety-century, our thinking about the problem of death manifests profound contradictions. Our tradition assumes that a person is both terminated by death and capable of continuing in some other sense beyond death. Death is viewed by some as a wall, the ultimate personal disaster, and suicide as the act of a sick mind; by others death is seen as a doorway, a point in time on the way to eternity.

Cultural Milieu of Death

The prospect or fact of death has been interpreted in many ways in our culture. Most of these interpretations come to us as part of our heritage from previous generations, earlier cultures. Yet they are also part of our own contemporary culture. We are more likely to accept some alternatives than others, and our own cultural milieu may be generating significant new variations on ancient themes while also developing new approaches.

This society tends to foster the idea that it is futile to contemplate death; at the same time, it communicates that the only proper way to conduct one's life is through the daily contemplation of that inevitable moment toward which one is moving.

It is believed by some that fear of death is instinctive, deeply rooted in human nature; others contend that no one can truly accept or even understand the proposition of mortality.

Healthy people who contemplate death do so with nervous laughter, composure, denial, resignation, intensity, indifference, doubt, or certainty. Critically ill people and others who face imminent death maintain silence, sometimes an agitated silence and sometimes a stoical, tranquil, or enigmatic one. Or they face death with desperate maneuvers, eager anticipation, dread, apathy, or mixed feelings.

Death as a Background of Life

Four conditions from the past have contributed significantly to the general background of life against which interpretations of death have emerged. The *first* and most obvious condition was the rather limited life expectancy that has confronted people throughout most of history. Relatively few people survived beyond the years of early maturity. A *second* and related condition was exposure to death, to the sight of dying and dead persons and animals. The average person had relatively little insulation from witnessing death. A *third* condition was the sense of possessing relatively little control over the forces of nature. The world was an untrustworthy abode, comfortable and dependable at some time but at others crushing and devastating to its inhabitants. For many centuries, people had rather limited resources for altering the unfavorable circumstances in which they frequently found themselves. The *fourth* factor is that psychosocially, the concept of individualism was poorly developed in the ancient world. The person was primarily a social component, a unit that fulfilled an expected role within the dictates of custom. One's lineage and station in life were of primary importance. The extended family and the clan, tribe, or city provided the needed strength and continuity. Most persons in most societies were not expected to make individual decisions about basic issues or ultimate matters, nor was the emotional satisfaction or fate of the individual as an individual considered to be of primary significance. The well-being of the individual was important chiefly as it related to the carrying out of obligations for the group.

Thus, in earlier cultures, the individual's hold on life was quite precarious, with death occurring within what we now regard as the first half of the life-span. Dying and death were visible, and one generally did not expect to exercise control over the environment. All these factors seem to have provided an important part of the context for earlier interpretations of death. Whatever myths and other conceptualizations of death have developed must be considered against these background conditions of life.

The Death System

Words and actions concerning death may be considered as jointly constituting a system. All societies have developed one or more death systems through which they have tried to come to terms with death in both its personal and social aspects.[2]

The Egyptians of antiquity developed a death system that was quite explicit and detailed. Their *Book of the Dead* and the Tibetan counterpart with the same title provided outlines of a comprehensive death system cast largely in the form of prescriptions for funerary practice.[3,4] This system was intended to transmit a relatively integrated approach that would enable individuals to think,

feel, and behave with respect to death in ways that they might consider to be effective and appropriate. The Egyptian system offered an explicit world view which was sponsored by the governing authorities, shared by the community, and linked to individual behavior in specific terms. Within this system, the individual's belief was the community's belief. The individual was not alone. People had important actions to perform in the total death situation, ranging from the dying process through the care of the dead.

These actions were important from the standpoints of both the individual and the community. The individual's actions were important because, according to the prevailing belief, one's sacrifices and rituals actually affected the sequence of events connecting life in this world with the life after death. From the standpoint of a psychologically oriented observer, such actions were important not because they had any actual effect upon the fate of the deceased or on future relations between the deceased and survivors but because they performed functions vital to individuals and their society. The most important function seemed to be that of giving people something to do in situations that otherwise might have exposed them to feelings of utter helplessness. Belief in magical control over the powerful forces of death and the afterlife further encouraged the Egyptians to think of death as an event that was well within their province of action.[3]

The American System of Death

American society today differs from most earlier cultures in that we no longer have to contend with limited life expectancy, constant exposure to death, a feeling of helplessness against the powers of nature, and a lack of individualism. Life expectancy in the United States today is more than twice as great as it was for most of our ancestors on this planet. We are less likely to regard death as a knife at our throat or a scourge at our child's bedside. Death stands at a more reassuring or *proper* distance from the young and middle-aged adult. It is old people, not we, who die! This line of reasoning is, of course, highly biased in the direction of youth. We are a youth-oriented society. The power and glory belong to the young. Increasingly, then, death is becoming detached and transposed from the valued core of society: the young. We could say, in a sense, that natural death is becoming obsolete. It is an event that happens only to those people who have already become obsolete.

Illness and death, just like illness and recovery, is a sequence that is becoming removed from household management. Americans pull through or die on the crisp white sheets of an institutional bed. There is now a choice regarding how children will or will not be informed of death. Not so many years ago there was no choice: children saw what was happening because death occurred in the home and was part of the family experience.

As a society, we are insulated from the perception of death. The insulation is not perfect, yet we are protected from the sights of dying and death to an extent that could not have been imagined in most previous cultures. The dying-death sequence in our own culture is increasingly handled by teams of specialists. The hospital people and the burying people are licensed experts. They perform their functions in special settings, inviting us to participate only at certain approved stages of the process. Our participation is peripheral, and we can, in fact, opt out of the dying-death sequence completely if we so wish.

Even within hospital walls there are implicit rules and choices. Hospitalized clients are not supposed to die just any place at any time. It is deemed important that they not expose other clients, staff, or visitors to the phenomenon of death except under carefully specified circumstances. The obliging terminal clients will first provide clear evidence, either through clinical symptoms or laboratory findings, that their condition is worsening. This enables the hospital administrative process to add their names to the "danger list." Then clear signs of further deterioration or jeopardy require either that special treatments begin in a private room on the present ward or, preferably, the transfer of the client to an intensive treatment unit.

Death is expected. The approved sequence is winding to its finale. The chaplain and other non-hospital personnel can enact their roles in the customary manner. This reflects a *technological ritual of death.*

Those involved feel a sense of discomfort and sometimes even express rage when a client dies in the wrong place at the wrong time. We have become very fond of the insulation our culture offers us from the perceptual impact of death. Even the death specialists, to whom we have delegated the responsibilities that formerly were our own, demand a certain insulation.

This general situation is also related to our attitude toward the physical environment. The growth in scientific knowledge and its visible technological applications has greatly increased our ability to reshape the world. This has led us to expect control and mastery of events. We implicitly assume that, with the help of science and money, we ought to be able to solve any problem in which we care to invest sufficient time and resources.

The point is not how far we can go in sweeping death back from our daily lives; we have already gone a long way in that direction. Our present difficulties stem mainly from the expectation that technological answers can be found for all problems, from the idea that people can remove or remake whatever stands in the path of their desires, including death.

Finally, we no longer participate in a society that is dominated by tradition, lineage, or accepted dogma. The older systems of social control without our culture have lost much of their ability to shape our behavior and to support us in times of crisis. These systems have never been adequately replaced.

We experience this situation of freedom and responsibility with anxiety. The individual is the primary unit now, and people are free to pursue their own self-actualization. But they also face more doubt and anxiety than did their ancestors, who grew up in a milieu which had firmly entrenched ideas and practices regarding life-and-death matters. Increasingly, individuals are held responsible for their own ideas and actions. Decisions that once were almost automatic must now be made without guidance from tradition.

These decisions are particularly evident in the realm of death. The orientation of healthy people toward their own death, the orientation of the dying person, and people's attitudes toward funerary practices are no longer predictable or constant; therefore they call for decisions by the individual. Death, in this sense, has become decontextualized. There is not the reliable, heavily reinforced social fabric that enabled the ancient Egyptian to know that the right thing was being done in the right way. The need to make individual decisions arises more often for those who encounter death repeatedly in their professional lives. It also weighs upon people in various walks of life who occasionally find themselves in life-and-death situations. Decisions and responsibilities, then, are salient characteristics of our relationship with death in the present cultural milieu, and not everybody accepts the responsibility for making and abiding by their decisions.

Client Behavior

When someone is faced with the prospect of terminal illness, that person and, later on, the family members experience the process of anticipatory grief. Anticipatory grief is a reaction to loss before the actual loss takes place and may take the same form as a reactive grief (see Chap. 23). The person faced with declining health grieves for the self and the inevitable separation from significant others (see Chap. 28).

Individual differences in response to the threat of illness—such as helplessness, disability, pain, or separation—are based on differences in personality patterns which are derived from past experiences. Kübler-Ross has identified five stages through which most terminal patients pass.[5]

Denial

Denial, used by almost all clients, functions as a buffer after unexpected, shocking news. It allows clients to collect themselves and, with time, to mobilize other, less radical defenses. This kind of denial is characterized by remarks like: "No, it can't happen to me . . . there must be some mistake . . . it just isn't true . . . we'll call in a better physician. . . . " The same mechanism is at work when someone passes the scene of an accident on the highway and subconsciously feels that "It can happen to anyone else, but never to me." An athlete who suffered a severe heart attack denied the reality of the disability and the possibility of personal death by doing chin-ups in the hospital room even after the physicians repeatedly limited his physical activity. Denial is usually temporary, to be replaced by partial acceptance.

Avoidance is a more subtle form of denial that is used by people confronted with death. The dying client may appear to be externally well adjusted to the fact that death is near, but when physicians visit, such clients choose to talk about anything else except their condition; they even avoid answering direct questions about their situation. A woman with radical breast mastectomy could describe in detail the muscles that were removed but adroitly avoided talking about her missing breast.

Staff who are uncomfortable with the dying process may participate in this avoidance. They may relegate such clients to the room farthest from the nurse's station, rationalizing the decision by saying, "It's quieter and the client will be more comfortable." They may also avoid the client's predicament by failing to initiate communication about the client's perception of the prognosis or its impact on his or her life-style and future. This game of avoidance occurs when staff, family, and client know the seriousness of the illness but there is a mutual unwillingness to talk about it. This *conspiracy of silence* is further reinforced by visitors who also deny the facts. When the client, in spite of obvious deterioration, asks, "Don't I look better today?" such a visitor will hastily reply, "Yes, you *do* look much better."

Denial can be seen in a variety of client behaviors. There may be an unwillingness to look at or examine the operative site or to look in the mirror. One such client, who had had a colostomy, refused to watch or participate in his colostomy care; he would pull the over-bed television set up to his face to block his view of the procedure.

In another example, a woman had a large fulminating mass on her left breast which replaced all normal tissue and was twice the size of her right breast. When asked by the nurse why she had postponed medical evaluation, she replied, "It's really nothing. It's only slightly uncomfortable when I sleep."

Anger

When the first stage of denial and avoidance cannot be maintained any longer, it is replaced by feelings of anger, rage, envy, and resentment. In the dependent client, anger often stimulates feelings of guilt and fear of retaliation. It is frightening for clients to express anger to the caretakers or family members upon whom they feel dependent for survival. To control or hide anger, clients may withdraw from all self-assertive behavior and become emotionally inaccessible. Or such a client may become the classically "difficult patient," the one who is uncooperative with staff, who complains about everything and never seems satisfied. Some clients may show overt anger, if they feel safe enough, toward family or staff.

Usually, however, the anger is more subtly expressed. One superficially sweet little old lady, during her terminal illness, frustrated the nursing staff to "wit's end" because she would neither swallow her pills nor spit them out. She would just let the pills sit in the back of her throat. This was her way of controlling the last manipulable piece of her life.

The client may feel guilt over hostile thoughts and feelings and overtly angry behavior. Clients may view their illnesses as punishments visited upon them for past sins, though they usually cannot tell what they have done that is so bad.

Clients are often distressed over their anger and do not always understand its derivation or how to resolve it. One young man prayed out loud on the day before he died that God would forgive him

for trying to bite the nurse who routinely gave him his injection. This prayer was his way of expressing guilt for his angry feelings and an attempt to resolve the hurt he felt he had caused.

Angry clients are often exasperating and generate hostility in their caretakers. Staff are tempted to retaliate in kind, but if they did so they would, of course, further isolate and alienate clients who are already overwhelmed by the dying process (see Chap. 17).

Bargaining

The third stage, that of bargaining, is helpful to the client for brief periods of time. Bargaining is an attempt to postpone pain or death by offering good behavior. It sets a self-imposed deadline and includes an implicit promise that the client will not ask for more if this postponement is granted.

Most of these bargains are made with God and are usually kept a secret or mentioned only implicitly. It is not uncommon to hear, "I prayed to God that if He would let me live, I'd go to church every day for the rest of my life." The husband of a dying wife said, "If she gets better, we'll go on the vacation she has always wanted." One mother whose deterioration was becoming more evident said, "I only want to see my children graduate from college and starting their own lives." Psychologically, promises like these may be associated with guilt for not attending church more regularly; for feeling as though one has not done enough for one's family, treated them badly; or, in the case of the family, feelings that one has not done enough for the dying family member.

Sense of Loss and Depression

When the terminally ill client can no longer deny the illness and begins to have more symptoms, the numbness, stoicism, anger, and rage are replaced with a sense of great loss and a feeling of deep depression, which may be reactive and/or preparatory (see Chap. 18).

Reactive depression may be the response to change of body image, financial burdens, inability to function, and/or loss of job. Preparatory depression occurs in anticipation of impending loss and is necessary to facilitate acceptance. The client is in the process of losing everything and everybody; the spouse or other survivors, on the other hand, are losing only one person, the client. This preparatory depression is more silent than reactive depression, in which the client has much to share and requires many verbal interactions. This silence is difficult for the client's family and other visitors to accept because they instinctively want to cheer up the client. But nothing could be more hollow than the sometimes banal efforts that well-wishers make to humor those who are on the verge of losing their entire world. Such efforts are thin disguises for the anxiety that stalks beneath.

Acceptance

If clients have had enough time and have been given some help in working through the above stages, they may enter a phase in which they are neither depressed nor angry about their fate. This acceptance is not a happy stage. It is almost void of feelings. When dying clients have found some peace and acceptance, their range of interests diminishes. They wish to be left alone, or at least to have shorter visits, and are no longer in a talkative mood. Communication becomes more nonverbal than verbal. Occasionally the dying person can actually articulate what is happening and can do so casually, and this startles those present.

One young man, the day before his death, greeted the nurse who came to give morning care with "You know, I'm dying!"

Even though these clients are realistic, accepting, and at peace, they usually still leave the possibility of cure open. It is this glimmer of hope, a form of temporary, partial denial, which maintains them through long periods of suffering.

The Giving-Up–Given-Up Complex

Engel has identified a complex of behaviors that seem to contribute to the emergence of life-threatening disease and persist throughout the downhill course of illness. This set of behaviors is referred to as the *giving-up–given-up complex.*[6]

In clinical and phenomenological terms, Engel delineates the characteristics of the complex as follows:

1 It has an unpleasant affective quality, expressed in such terms as "Too much," "It's no use," "I can't take it anymore," "I give up." It encompasses two different affective qualities: helplessness, where these feelings are ascribed more to failures on the part of the environment; and hopelessness, where feelings are ascribed more to one's own failures and include a sense of being beyond help from others.

2 The self is perceived as less intact, less competent, less in control, less gratified, and less capable of functioning in a relatively autonomous fashion.

3 Relationships with significant others are felt to be less secure and gratifying; the client may feel given up by these or may give up the self.

4 The external environment may be perceived as differing significantly from expectations based on past experience, which no longer seems as useful a guide for current or future behavior.

5 There is felt to be a loss of continuity between past and future and an inability to project oneself into the future with hope or confidence. Hence the future may appear relatively bleak or unrewarding.

6 There is a tendency to revive feelings, memories, and behavior connected with occasions in the past which had a similar quality.

This description represents a composite of overlapping phenomena, not all of which are represented to an equal degree in every client. Hence it is called a complex, having configurational, temporal, and quantitative aspects. It may exist very briefly or for an extended period of time, may begin or end abruptly or gradually, may wax and wane over a period of time, and may be of greater or lesser intensity.

Helplessness and hopelessness have been identified as characteristics of two distinct types of the giving-up–given-up complex. These affects reflect ego awareness of an inability to defend against a loss of two different types of autonomy. *Helplessness* reflects a loss of ego autonomy combined with a feeling of deprivation; it results from the loss of gratification from an other-than-self object. *Hopelessness,* on the other hand, reflects a loss of autonomy accompanied by a feeling of despair; it comes from an awareness of the self's inability to provide the desired gratification. Not all life situations which engender true hopelessness or helplessness evoke giving-up–given-up responses. Central to the giving-up–given-up complex is the psychic perception of failure or unavailability of resources; hence real, threatened, or symbolic psychic object losses constitute the most common provocative situations. The giving-up–given-up complex is only one of innumerable possible responses to loss and is not employed by everyone in the same situation. Hence, the giving-up–given-up response is not present in all terminal cases; when it is, however, it seems to hasten death. It seems that there is a direct connection between the giving-up–given-up complex and the various biological processes that occur at the same time.[6]

Family Behavior

The client's family, by their reactions, significantly influence the client's response to the illness and the dying process. Families experience parallel stages of resolution. However, the dying client's problems have an end in view, while the family sees its problem as continuing. The tendency is to hide feelings from the patient in an attempt to keep a smiling face and a front of make-believe cheerfulness.

Most terminally ill people *know* they have a disease with a poor prognosis, and they know when death is imminent. However, both the family, unable to confront the reality, and the client often attempt to deny the client's knowledge of the facts and to prevent the caretakers from discussing the predicted death with the client. The conspiracy of silence, born of the wish to be protective, condemns both the client and family to an inauthentic relationship. This loss of openness deprives both of the support and the interactions which would facilitate dealing with feelings.

One young woman, dying of cancer, said to the nurse, "Please don't tell Mom and Dad how sick I am; I don't want them to be upset." Later that day, the parents instructed the same nurse, "We don't ever want our daughter to know what she has, or that she is dying."

An absence of communication denies the client the right to separate from loved ones and life in an orderly manner and to share a part of the living experience.

Some families may proceed through the grieving process more quickly than the client. Consequently their feelings and behaviors are incongruent with those of the client, who may feel abandoned. On the other hand, clients may reach the stage of acceptance and be at peace with themselves and the world when families have not yet have reached this point; consequently the families will feel closed out of the clients' world.

When death occurs suddenly, with little or no forewarning, members of the deceased's family are generally told about the death in a historical perspective. In such instances the family is the client. They need help in working through the shock, anger, and guilt. Their feelings of helplessness are heightened by the fact that they have not been able to "do anything" for the deceased. They may be overwhelmed by guilt feelings rooted in prior conflicts with the deceased or aroused by their failure to recognize the seriousness of the deceased's illness. Family members need to know why and how the person died and what was done to help. This information helps family members not only to actualize the loss but also to feel that everything possible was done to save the deceased's life. Nurses who have not directly cared for and have had no interpersonal contact with the deceased are more insulated emotionally; they do not have to deal with feelings of personal failure. Therefore they may be better able to develop a supportive relationship with the family.

Nurses' Responses

Research Findings

LeShan's study of nurses' responses to terminal cases revealed that nurses took longer to answer calls from clients with terminal prognoses than from those who were less seriously ill. They lacked awareness of this "undemocratic" behavior.[7]

Kastenbaum found that verbal behavior also reflects the professional's discomfort with the topics of dying and death. Nurse's responses to clients who brought up the subject of their death ("I think I'm going to die soon"; "I wish I could just end it all") were classified according to five categories:[8]

1 *Reassurance* "You're doing so well now. You don't have to feel this way." "You're going to be feeling better soon, then you won't be thinking this way. You'll be feeling more like your old self again."

2 *Denial* "You don't really mean that." "You are not going to die. You're going to live to be a hundred."

3 *Changing the Subject* "Let's talk about something more cheerful." "You shouldn't say things like that; there are better things to talk about."

4 *Fatalism* "We are all going to die sometime, and it's a good thing we don't know when." "When God wants you, He will take you. It's a sin to say that you want to die."

5 *Discussion* "What makes you feel that way today? Is it something that happened, something somebody said?" "Could you tell me why? I'd like to know."[10]

Fatalism, denial, and change of subject were the most frequent responses. Only 18 percent of the total group studied indicated that they would enter a discussion with the client and explore thoughts and feelings. It would seem that unless nurses are sensitized to the needs of the dying client, helped to develop communication skills and clarify their own feelings about death, then these clients are unlikely to find a nurse who is able and willing to help them verbalize and deal with the dying process.

Those who were inclined to "turn off" the client often explained that they did not like to see their clients looking so glum. Mention of death was equated with a state of fear or surrender that was unacceptable to the nursing personnel. The nurses felt that clients should want to live and should expect to live. Therefore, they considered it appropriate to try to get the client's mind off death. Some of the respondents were direct enough to say "Death talk bugs me." In general, silencing a client who speaks about death seemed to derive from both a humanistic ("I like to see them happy") and self-protective ("It shakes me up to talk about death") viewpoint. When the facts of the situation were too obvious to permit an easy denial, then the fatalistic response was deemed appropriate. This response came naturally to those attending personnel who held it as a personal belief.

Those who tended to follow up the client's remarks about death with an open discussion had a problem-solving orientation. They viewed the client as expressing emotion and asking for psychological assistance, hoping that maybe an answer or help of some kind could be found.

Further inquiry revealed that nurses experienced many feelings about their terminal clients but tried not to let them show, even when, as a client deteriorated, their feelings became stronger.[8] However, nurses are not always able to insulate themselves from the emotional implications of their work. It is typical for nurses to care about what their clients are experiencing and common for them to believe that they should not "give in" to their feelings, even to the extent of letting them show to others.

In such instances nurses may be trapped by their role image. If the prevailing professional ethic disapproves of the expression of feelings or the nurses believe this to be true, then fear of censure serves to suppress and repress emotional responses to clients.

In Kastenbaum's study, the typical nurses considered themselves to be devout people with a strong belief in some form of life after death. This included the conviction that they would be personally accountable to God after death. Very few nurses agreed that we are each entitled to do as we like with our lives as long as no one else is hurt, or that suicide is nobody else's business.[10] Few reported that they had ever wished someone else to die, and few were in favor of "mercy killing" under any circumstances. Most of the nurses agreed that "the length of people's lives is pretty much decided when they are born, and that no matter what you do, when it's your time to go, you go."[8]

This cluster of attitudes and beliefs was discernibly different from that of staff members at the same hospital who had different educational and occupational backgrounds. It seems fair to suggest that the ethnic, religious, and socioeconomic background that people bring with them to a situation affects the way they think and behave when they become caretakers. The degree of influence that background and the professionalization process have on practice has yet to be studied adequately. However, it is probable that personal background and professionalization come together at certain points to emphasize a particular behavior. For example, the nurse may, because of a particular ethnic heritage, have a fatalistic outlook on death. If this is reinforced by an agency ethic not to show emotion on the job, then for that person it may be easier to control the outward expression of feeling than it is to live with the feelings that continue to percolate inside.[10]

Attitudes and Values

When nurses have difficulty coping with the emotional needs of terminal patients, it may reflect an inadequate preparation. In such instances they fall back upon whatever guidelines are available from other sources: the life-and-death orientations that have been learned within a particular ethnic and socioeconomic background; the pressure of colleagues to conform to their definition of what constitutes a "good" nurse; personal experiences and quirks. The influence of these orientations will be lessened if the nurse has had guidance, supervision, and sensitization to client needs; if communication skills have been developed, and if the nurse has a broad knowledge base as well as a theoretical framework to guide practice.

When nurses sense inadequacy in themselves in caring for the dying—if they have not developed an awareness of how they perceive death or worked through the concomitant feelings—they tend to become invested in routines and rituals of a technical nature that help them to defend against anxiety. This approach denies the client's emotional and social needs and may serve to alienate and isolate the client. Moral, ethical, and legal considerations, including the client's *right to know*, may be overlooked.

Enormous attention may be given to techniques of life-prolongation and to the most tenuous hopes of recovery while little effort is made to provide comforts to the dying. It is difficult to strive to keep clients alive at all costs and simultaneously to help them die in a dignified and comforted manner. These conflicting goals become more difficult to resolve if the nurse fails to attend to the nurse-client relationship, exploration of the thoughts and feelings of both the nurse and client, and the primacy of the client needs and rights.

Authority and Control

While it is important not to get involved in power struggles with clients, this is especially true in the case of dying clients. Sometimes nurses become very withholding when it comes to the delivery of pain medication. Or, conversely, they become pushy in an effort to see that a client takes medication. The issue quickly becomes one of who is in charge rather than of doing what is best for the client, even though the nurse may say, "I'm doing this for your own good."

Perhaps the reason why nurses are so controlling around a dying patient is that, since the client is losing control over everything, their own anxiety is high. The loss of the client's control reminds nurses of their own potential loss of control; because of this reaction, the nurse works overtime at being "in charge" on the unit.

Identification

Some nurses develop a strong identification with their terminal clients. The projective identification and the transference and countertransference phenomena are potentially disruptive to the quality of a relationship which would otherwise be facilitative, therapeutic, and supportive (see Chap. 22).

Transference is a distortion of the client's perception of the nurse. The dependency and regression that occur in illness, along with personal physical care and comfort given by the nurse distort the relationship. Feelings generated in the client have their roots in past childhood relationships of a similar nature. These feelings and the resulting behavior are normal; they are not directed at the nurse personally but are distortions of the present based on remembrances of the past.

By the same token, it is natural for the nurse to have distorted feelings about the client. This distorted perception of the client is the countertransference phenomenon. These countertransference feelings are heightened when the dying client reminds the nurse of a relative or friend who has died.

Countertransference and transference can be both positive and negative. The feelings generated may be warm, supportive, and nurturing or hostile and rejecting. These feelings and their consequent expression may interfere with sensitive and accurate need assessment and delivery of care.

When the nursing staff has invested considerable time, energy, effort, and feeling in the care of a terminal client, the death of the client causes acute feelings of loss. Consequently, they may react with anger which is not recognized. Since they are unaware of the roots of this feeling, the anger gets projected onto others. This is often evidenced by the staff's irritability toward ancillary help, housekeeping, or another department with whom they interface.

Nurses who care for dying clients may fall victim to rescue fantasies. Clients of *high social value* have a greater potential for generating these fantasies in their caretakers. Such fantasies prompt nurses to try to help the client whether or not the "help" they wish to give is appropriate or desired. When this happens, the nurse's needs are not congruent with the client's needs. Mr. Adams, a client with terminal cancer, worked persistently and with great effort at self-care and maximum independence. Mr. Cook, his nurse, motivated by a rescue fantasy that his care made the client comfortable and the dying process peaceful, intervened to foster dependence and regression. These interventions met Mr. Cook's need to be helpful and needed, but they generated anxiety and helplessness in Mr. Adams.

Chronic helpers do things for others constantly and without being asked. They operate under the assumption that what they do is helpful, never checking to see whether their interventions *do* actually help the client to cope more effectively. Their behavior is indicative of their underlying dependency needs. Their helpfulness engenders inappropriate dependency in the client, which blocks the client from assuming responsibility and maintaining mastery. This dependency generates feelings of helplessness and anger in the client. Caretakers are puzzled and hurt when their "help" is rejected or sabotaged by the client. The helper's dependency need is not being met and the client's compensatory independence is not being effected. Thus feelings of rejection, failure, and anxiety surface. Such helpers may say, "What a fool I am for letting myself be used," or "Look what it gets you, when you're kind and helpful." The theme becomes "I'm not approved of, therefore I must be bad." The development of self-awareness is the most effective way of preventing and/or managing rescue fantasies and chronic helpfulness.[9]

Certain areas of the hospital setting have been designated as posing high emotional risks. The emergency room, intensive care, cancer units, and coronary care units are the most prominent. Nurses working in these areas are often exposed to the death of clients of high social value. This bombardment of the nurse's emotional system elicits and requires a strong defense system to secure ego integrity. Consequently nurses working in these areas employ a variety of maneuvers which serve to distance them emotionally. They may interact minimally and/or superficially, avoid gathering data about the client's premorbid life-style, or avoid developing a relationship with the family. Preoccupied with the very necessary physical ministrations and technical procedures, they defend against experiencing the client's predicament and humanness. Supervision, consultation, and team conferences can be useful and supportive to nurses, helping them to deal with their feelings constructively and to manage them effectively while caring for the dying client.

The Nursing Process
Context of Care

"Terminal care" generally refers to the care of clients who are dying and in the final stages of their lives. Yet the fact is that the presence of death, near-death, or fear of death characterizes many situations in which nursing personnel interact with clients and families but where the definition of the dying client may not be explicit.

There are at least four types of situations in which nurses come into contact with persons facing death. *First,* there are situations involving terminally ill people who require direct physical ministrations or assistance in matters of daily living. Some care is available to people in their homes, but there has been a definite trend toward the institutionalization of persons who need these services. More recently, efforts have been made to establish a hospice in the United States modeled after St. Christopher's in England. The purpose of the hospice is to help people live through the dying process, experiencing it with strength, confidence, and alertness; to provide these people with dignity and respect; and to help them find meaning in their lives through the experience of dying.[10]

The *second* type of contact occurs in situations where nursing personnel provide life-prolonging and sometimes intensive care to individuals who are facing the possibility of death, or

sometimes, imminent death. Hospitals are organized primarily to promote the saving of lives, and this activity assumes critical importance on units like the coronary care unit, where rapid action can make the difference between life and death. Here top priority is given to recovery-oriented, medically delegated nursing tasks, and "comfort care" is essentially relegated to a secondary position. There are other wards where death is a frequent visitor, but there the work is less dramatic in character because the period of dying tends to be slow. This pattern is common with cancer, cystic fibrosis, and progressive neurological disease. Often these clients are in and out of hospitals several times before they enter for the final admission, that is, before the hospital becomes the permanent abode because care at home is no longer possible. On some of these units, there are increasing numbers of clients who are socially dead because they have suffered partial or complete loss of brain activity yet who are biologically alive and sometimes kept among "the living dead" with the assistance of life-prolonging machinery (see Chap. 29).

A *third* context for interaction occurs when those injured in accidents or natural disasters are brought into a centralized emergency-care setting for immediate help. The demand for this type of service has grown tremendously in metropolitan areas, where the accident rate is increasing. In the case of mass disaster—as may occur with fires, floods, hurricanes, and earthquakes—the demand for care can sometimes be overwhelming and beyond the capabilities of the services normally available to a given community. Nursing personnel in emergency wards work with the reality of unexpected and sudden death almost on a daily basis, and they are often in contact with families in psychological shock or the early stages of grief.

Finally, there are numerous contacts with people who have chronic and life-threatening diseases. These clients may be at various stages of incapacitation and thus have different requirements for assistance in coping with the psychosocial and physical problems imposed by long-term illness (see Chap. 27). Different approaches to client care are needed when the disease is newly diagnosed and still viewed as curable, when signs of disease progression appear, and when the terminal stage becomes apparent.

Assessment

Assessment of the dying process requires nurses to focus on themselves, the client, the family, and the environment. The data base which includes significant information from these four areas assists the nurse to formulate and set goals and priorities as well as to plan and implement sensitive and effective nursing care.

The Nurse

1 What is my perception of death and the dying process?
2 What was my first encounter with death and what effect did it have on me?
3 What are my thoughts and feelings about the client?
4 How does this client's behavior affect me? Am I spending as little time as possible with the client or am I devoting more time than I would with another client with the same problem?
5 Have I been able to reach out to the family? How does this aspect make me think and feel?
6 In my relations with other caretakers involved with this client, do I collaborate, act defensively, or see the client as only mine?

The Client

1 How is the client behaving?
2 Has the client been told the diagnosis and prognosis? What was the response?
3 What is the client's affect? Is it appropriate?
4 What needs is the client presenting?
5 Does the client have realistic expectations and are the resources for meeting these available?
6 How is the client's physical status contributing to the client's psychosocial status?
7 In what stage of the dying process is the client? Is there evidence of maladaptive responses which will interfere with need-fulfillment and resolution of the grieving process?
8 Does the client feel supported by significant others?
9 Is the client where he or she wishes to be? If not, why not?

The Family

1 What is the family's perception of the diagnosis and prognosis?
2 What feelings are being experienced by family members?
3 What influence do these feelings have on the dying person?
4 How do family members communicate? What influence does this style of communication have on the dying person?
5 What are the family's needs? What resources do they have for gratification of these needs?
6 How does the family respond to the dying person? What is the impact of this response on the dying person?
7 How does the family relate to the caretakers? How do caretakers respond? Is this response helpful?

The Environment

1 What is the context of the dying process?
2 Is the environment designed to assist the client to cope effectively with dying?
3 Is the client's room set off from others?
4 Is relief from pain and discomfort readily available?
5 Does the client participate in planning the care?
6 Is there a staffing pattern which facilitates communication with the client? Do staff have adequate time to spend with clients? Do the staff have ample opportunity to develop an ongoing relationship with the client and family?

The problems of clients vary a good deal and are dependent upon a combination of circumstances, including (1) the stage of illness (early, middle, late); (2) the type of assistance that is needed (lifesaving care, direct physical care, teaching-socialization, emotional support); (3) the amount of time that is involved (short-term, long-term, or permanent contact); and (4) the social context in which care is provided (ambulatory care, home care, institutional care).

Nursing Diagnosis

Nursing diagnoses are formulations of what the nurse sees as the client's problematic response that requires nursing intervention. They are so stated as to identify the problem and define it conceptually and thus provide a basis for the development of the nursing-care plan.

The following are examples of nursing diagnoses:

1 Prognosis is poor, client is reactively depressed and withdrawing from staff, family, and friends.
2 Dependence on staff and family is generating anger in the client, which is expressed in verbal attacks that cause withdrawal behavior in recipients and result in isolation of the client.
3 Continuous, intense pain is generating heightened anxiety and demanding behavior.
4 Infrequency of family visits is increasing client's depression and isolating behavior.
5 Impaired family communication is blocking client from resolving unfinished business matters and causing the client to be anxious.
6 Client approaching death is communicating only minimally with family, causing them to feel confused and helpless.

Goals

The goal of terminal nursing care, as with any other kind of nursing care, is to help the client live as fully as possible. This may mean that nurses assist the client to carry out the prescribed regime; beyond that, it means that the goal of nursing is to help the client reach out for a fullness of being that is always possible despite biological limitations against which medicine may be helpless.

While there are differing circumstances and conditions within the broad context of terminal care, the following goals encompass the broader aspect of the dying process:

1 *Assist the client and family to cope effectively with the fear of the unknown that accompanies confrontation with death*   Aside from pain, loneliness, and abandonment, one of the things clients fear most about dying is the unknown. Death itself is *the* great unknown. Even though some clients have a strong religious belief in a life hereafter, the experience of making the transition from this life to the next is still unknown and frightening. Such fear of the unknown can extend and be generalized to the hospital and nursing procedures.

2 *Assist the client to cope with the pain and discomfort of the 'physical disease with dignity and a sense of mastery*   In the latter stages of many terminal illnesses, pain is a constant companion. Pain itself is the strongest antagonist to analgesia.[8] Pain can exclude all other living, requiring only endurance until relief comes. Relief from pain need not mean loss of conscious awareness and alertness.

3 *Assist the client and family to maintain hope*   Hope is frequently confused with magical solutions. People sometimes say that they do not want to tell clients they are dying for fear of taking away their hope. Hope involves more reality than magic. Hope can be maintained right up to the moment of death; it does not mean taking death away but rather supporting the dying person to the end. Most dying people know the truth, whether they are told or not. Thus, their hope is taken away when they try to talk about reality and find family members engaging in avoidance. With hope, clients can *live* until they die.

Humankind cannot bear very much reality and often need a "day off[10]"; thus intermittent periods of denial occur.

4 *Assist the client and family with the grieving process* Mourning is not forgetting. It is untying each knot that holds the person or thing and the memories to the self. Grief is a personal experience and a part of the matrix of humanity. Grieving has psychological, sociological, and somatic components. People need relatedness to one another to survive, to experience life, and to die.

5 *Assist the client to live until death occurs* There is a time to live and a time to die. Death asks for our identity, and meaningfulness is crucial. Being a part of life is often difficult, but to experience it is to truly live.

Planning Care-Intervention

The delivery of nursing care to the dying requires an attitude of attention and an atmosphere of security and caring.

Clients experiencing the dying process have explained that they fear being abandoned while at the same time feeling distressed over being burdens to their families. As they confront the inevitability of death and physical deterioration, much of the effectiveness of nursing care is contingent upon the quality of the nurse-client relationship (see Chap. 6).

The Right to Know

As previously mentioned, terminal clients know they are dying. Nevertheless, when the diagnosis is made initially and when complications arise during the illness, the client has the right and the need to be told. This does not mean that the client will necessarily show evidence of *hearing.* Even if there has been direct and truthful communication, the client may act and speak in ways that deny the reality. However, the facts have been given and the brain has recorded the message. When the client is able to cope with the message and its implications, it will be recalled in part; then the client will seek confirmation of what is feared but yet known to be a possibility.

When the diagnosis is made initially, the goal of medical treatment generates optimism. The client is usually eager to talk and there is a minimal need for defenses.[15] Clients at this point are able to articulate their need to know; they readily ask questions about what they are able to deal with. Open and honest answers in response to these questions lay the foundation for quality communication throughout the dying process. However, the client may not be able to handle all the implications of the condition; therefore it is important to respond to what is asked but to find out how the client perceives and experiences this information before offering further elaboration.[11]

If there have been open channels of communication and support, the client will continue to ask questions when the disease process has advanced. However, the questions are now different. The client may complain to friends or ancillary staff but never ask the nurse or physician, who could give the correct information. Areas of communication that still exist focus on symptoms and remedies. Clients who were formerly open and direct exhibit a "loss of memory" for previously discussed facts and implications. Such clients are often compliant and seem to project a "nice guy" image, which is a defense against fears of rejection and abandonment (see Chap. 22).[11]

During this phase the nurse supports the denial and provides the desired information regarding the client's complaints. Patience, acceptance, and reassurance which enhance the nurse-client relationship will help the client to be less fearful of abandonment. Because the client is suppressing and repressing anger toward the caretakers, it is important to determine when, where, and how this tension is being released. If the family are receiving the major portion of this anger, they may need support to understand and deal with it effectively.

In the terminal stage, when the disease process is irreversible and deterioration is evident, fear and loneliness predominate; they are then replaced by positive withdrawal and acceptance.

These clients tend to be uncommunicative verbally but retain a need for continual support. They do not want to talk about death or dying but will explore the possibility that their death may have a meaningful purpose. Even though these clients do not express their anxieties or fears easily and tend to withdraw, it is essential that the nurse continue to communicate, sometimes with words and at other times by touch and presence.[11]

Pain

Pain—the anxiety it produces and the fear of it—is a major concern of the terminally ill. Chronic pain is very different from acute pain, not only in duration but also in quality. Saunders defines chronic pain as a reaction between the stimulus and the whole individual. To many, the pain has no meaning; in this instance it must be seen as an illness in its own right. The pain is often intolerable and unrelenting. As previously indicated, pain is a powerful antagonist to analgesia. When pain is experienced, anxiety is heightened; this, in turn, intensifies the pain. Thus pain control is essential if the client is to cope with it and feel some degree of comfort. Saunders recommends anticipating pain *for* the client and stresses the importance of this. These clients must be monitored very closely for the early prodromal signs of pain; their patterns of relief and distress must be defined. If the nurse administers pain-relieving medications and institutes comfort measures before the pain has reached the client's conscious awareness, the client is provided with maximum relief continuously. In this way, the clients are not reminded of their dependence on the caretaker, since they do not have to watch the clock or ask for pain relief. Addiction is not an important issue or concern in the care of the terminally ill. When pain relief is consistent and accompanied by sensitive caring, tolerance and ever-increasing dosages do not seem to be a problem. Dosages are usually maintained at levels which permit the client periods of drowsiness and periods of alertness until the disease itself clouds the consciousness. If periods of alertness without pain can be provided for the client, the client will have a greater opportunity to participate in life and its remaining pleasures.[12]

Feelings

The dying person experiences the broad spectrum of human emotion; this can be both rewarding and painful. The feelings which present the greatest problem to the client and caretaker are fear, anger, anxiety, and depression. Each of these feelings and caretakers' responses are discussed in Chaps. 14, 17, and 18. However, when the client who is experiencing these feelings and generating others that present obstacles to care is a terminally ill person, there are other ramifications. There is usually no underlying neurotic component when anxiety and depression accompany a real and catastrophic situation. Therefore the usual approach to working through these feelings—which is helpful when there is a neurotic basis—is not applicable in relieving the client's distress. The reality of the client's death and the absence of remedies generate feelings of inadequacy, helplessness, and insecurity in the nurse. However, the emotions the client experiences need not be overwhelming and can be resolved. Identification of the factors which are contributing to an intensification of the feelings associated with the normal stages of resolution and grieving is the first step toward intervention. Once these factors have been identified and labeled in the nurse-client relationship, joint problem solving offers the client an opportunity to master what has previously caused helplessness and hopelessness. The more the client is able to control and modify the environment, even indirectly, the more feelings of anxiety, depression, and anger are ameliorated.

One hospitalized woman, dying of cancer, had difficulty falling asleep at night. She watched television until the early morning hours and had slept only a few hours when the hospital routine required her to be awake for early-morning care and breakfast. Fatigued and anxious about her condition, she felt depressed and helpless. Had she been able to control her environment—to eat, sleep, and participate in her care in a way that met her individual needs—her anxiety and feelings of helplessness could have been greatly reduced.

Another woman in the same predicament lashed out at staff angrily and was quickly labeled the "difficult patient." Staff began to avoid and isolate her. In response, she too began to withdraw, intensifying her feelings of anxiety, guilt, and abandonment. This cycle of mutual withdrawal is preventable if client behavior is assessed within the environmental context and as an expression of need.

Dependency on others generates conflict and anger. The anger felt and expressed by the dying person activates fear of abandonment and guilt, which in turn fosters depression. Minimizing the client's perception of dependency and need to be dependent while also maximizing the client's power to control what is happening lessens the client's need for defenses and feelings of distress.

Sexuality

The dying client is a human being, with all the feelings that go with being human. Sexuality is a part of one's total identity, and the fact that clients may be dying does not reduce them to asexual beings. Consequently, it should be expected that dying clients may sometimes want to express themselves sexually. This expression may take the form of genital behavior, speech, or touch; it may be overt or covert. Its occurrence should not disturb nurses unless they are already uncomfortable with their own sexuality or sexual feelings.

When clients experience a critical diagnosis and prognosis, they may well wonder about their sexuality. Their sexual identity may be challenged: they may wonder if they are still attractive, if they will ever have sexual desires again, if they will be potent, or if they can tolerate sexual activity.

Clients who exhibit flirtatious or seductive behavior may really be calling for attention or an expression of warmth or tenderness. It may be a bid for approval, since some clients may see

flirting as a way of paying the nurse a compliment. Clients may be testing themselves in a male-female relationship by flirting. Or they may be asking the nurse "How important am I to you?" "Do you care about me?" "Do you think about me when you're off duty?" Flirting may also be a way for clients to gain control over a nurse when they are fast losing control in other areas of their life. This may be all the more true if they have discovered that the nurse is anxious about flirtatious behavior. It may be the client's way of picking on the nurse's "weak spot."

Clients who have undergone mutilative surgery, chemotherapy, or increasing deterioration need factual information on the potential and/or extent of change in their sexual functioning. Feelings about the change and its impact on life-style and relationships must be explored; the client needs support in adjusting to the imposed changes. Alternatives to the expression of sexuality must also be identified and explored. Inappropriate sexual behavior is minimized or eliminated if sex education and counseling are initiated early in the disease process and continued until satisfactory and comfortable adjustments and adaptations have been made.

When clients are seductive and flirtatious, it is important for the nurse to set firm limits on this behavior without communicating rejection. Nurses who are aware of their own feelings, are secure in their own sexual identity, and are sensitive to clients' needs will be better able to help clients deal with their sexual feelings appropriately.

Clients who are hospitalized for any period of time and have been sexually active should be provided with opportunities to express their sexuality and to have the requisite privacy. Their rights as sexual beings should be respected.

Family-Client Relationship

When the family wishes to deny the client information about the disease process and prognosis, they must be helped to understand why it is important for them and the dying person to have an open and honest relationship. They must be reassured that the person who is dying has a tendency to hear *only* what he or she is able to cope with at that time.

Initially, the family needs support when talking to the dying person about issues that provoke their fears and generate anxiety. A nurse who listens empathically and explores fears, fantasies, and feelings will help the family: to understand what the dying person is experiencing, to deal with its own problems, and to support the client through the dying process.

Families who mourn prematurely or who are overwhelmed by their feelings of inadequacy, helplessness, and hopelessness may withdraw from the dying person, leaving him or her isolated and abandoned. Some of these families will visit less frequently, offering transparent excuses, while others will continue to visit faithfully but will tend to talk among themselves, excluding and even discussing the dying client as though he or she were not present. In such instances, the nurse—who may initially feel anger toward the family—must work at understanding why they are behaving in such a manner and must reach out to them to help them deal with the feelings generated by the situation. The family may need to learn how they can still communicate with and support the dying person by their presence. If the client's acceptance and consequent withdrawal is contributing to the dynamic, the family needs help in understanding this phenomenon and in finding ways to continue communicating their care and support to the dying person.

The client's physical deterioration and helplessness may generate helplessness, anxiety, and a need to be useful in family members. In such instances the nurse may enlist the help of family members rather than excluding them when giving physical care to the dying person. Family members can help the nurse to provide such care and comfort measures as bathing, turning, massaging, and feeding. This participation in the nursing care may help the family deal more effectively with their feelings. It gives them a sense of having done something for the person, which will help them later, after the client's death, in their own grieving.

Altered Body Image

Clients who have suffered an alteration of their body image due to radical surgery or the ravages of disease experience a crisis and must engage in the grieving process (see Chap. 23). Initially, when confronted with the reality of the alteration, they will experience a period of denial, including a retreat from reality, and/or they may have fantasies about their body and its functions in its earlier, healthy state. Some people may experience a temporary euphoria and/or may rationalize what has happened to them. With a healthy course of events, the client will eventually acknowledge the reality of the new image and redefine the self. This means cooperating with the goals that are set, the treatment plan, and the care given. The client's personal goals will be realistic. The crisis is successfully resolved if the client tries new coping mechanisms and sets out with a renewed sense of worth. It is unsuccessfully resolved if the client permanently tries to avoid reality, regresses in behavior, and withdraws from social contacts.

During the actual crisis of physical alteration, the client should be encouraged to mourn. The process includes facilitating acknowledgement and expressions of anger, rage, depression, and phantom pain.

The client should be encouraged to peek at the dressing if surgery has been involved and to feel the stump if there was an amputation. This will help the client actualize the loss. The client will watch others' reactions closely; the nature of these reactions will influence the client's own perception and acceptance of the loss.

If the client exhibits denial, reinforcement or argumentation are neither useful nor therapeutic. When denial is present, it is a defense against more anxiety than the client feels able to cope with; it must not be shattered by another. Interventions which reassure the client, increasing self-esteem and self-acceptance, will in time diminish the need for such a defense. The client will then slowly and carefully begin to confront well-defined bits and pieces of reality. The client who copes successfully with these bits and pieces will be encouraged and motivated to venture further in acknowledging his or her loss.

Hope

Hope is a very personal experience and a mediating process which influences perception. Failure and success tend to be cumulative. These outcomes contribute to a schema which is a perceptual set, telling the person that he or she will succeed or fail in an endeavor (see Chap. 18). The nurse who cares for the client expressing hopelessness must direct activities toward building and evoking a hopeful, high-order schema. This includes emphasizing the client's strengths and intervening to desensitize the client to that which is feared and provokes anxiety. To accomplish this, the nurse must build a relationship in which the client has confidence that the nurse will consistently facilitate the satisfaction of needs. When the client has confidence in the nurse, the resulting feeling of security encourages risk-taking behavior. If goals are simple, attainable, and graduated, the client will build and strengthen the schema of hope as success is experienced. Success begets success. Clients' participation in defining and reaching goals in itself increases their sense of mastery, thus reducing anxiety and supporting movement toward goals. This reduction of anxiety, the activity, and the mastery all serve to diminish feelings of hopelessness.

Evaluation

The effectiveness of nursing interventions is assessed using the predetermined client and family behaviors identified in the goals as criteria. Evidence that the goals have not been attained requires reassessment of needs and reexamination of the interventions and rationales. If goals have been satisfactorily attained and related needs met, then higher-order needs will emerge. These will call for assessment and subsequent reinitiation of the nursing process.

References

1 M. Rogers: *An Introduction to the Theoretical Basis of Nursing,* Davis, Philadelphia, 1970.

2 R. Kastenbaum and R. Aisenberg: *The Psychology of Death,* Springer, New York, 1972, p. 9.

3 H. M. Tirard: *Book of the Dead,* Oxford University Press, London, 1910.

4 W. Y. Evans-Wentz: *The Tibetan Book of the Dead,* Oxford University Press, New York, 1960.

5 E. Kübler-Ross: *On Death and Dying,* Macmillan, New York, 1969.

6 G. Engel and A. Schmale: "Psychoanalytic Theory of Somatic Disorder," *Journal of the American Psychoanalytic Association,* vol. 15, pp. 344–365, 1967.

7 M. Bowers, E. Jackson, J. Knight, and L. LeShan: *Counseling to the Dying,* Nelson, New York, 1964.

8 R. Kastenbaum: "Multiple Perspectives on a Geriatric 'Death Valley,'" *Community Mental Health Journal,* vol. 3, pp. 21–29, 1967.

*9 S. Rouslin: "Chronic Helpfulness: Maintenance or Intervention," *Perspectives in Psychiatric Care,* pp. 25–28, 1963.

*10 C. Saunders: "The Last Stages of Life," *American Journal of Nursing,* vol. 65, no. 3, pp. 70–75, March 1965.

*11 R. Abrams: "The Patient With Cancer—His Changing Pattern of Communication," *New England Journal of Medicine,* vol. 274, no. 6, pp. 317–322.

*12 C. Saunders: "The Moment of Truth," paper presented at Yale University School of Nursing, April 28, 1966.

*Recommended reference by a nurse author.

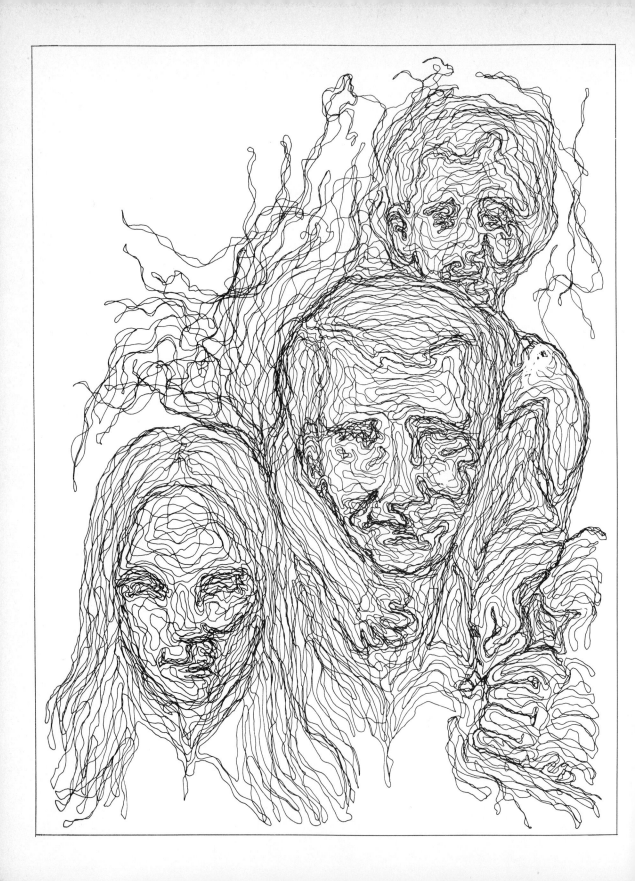

Five

Nursing Management of the Family System

Chapter

32

Promotion of Mental Health in Families

Ann Bello

Alice Marie Obrig

Learning Objectives

After studying this chapter, the student should be able to:

1   Identify the structure and function of families
2   Describe the options available to an individual or couple in the childbearing years
3   Describe the common assessment factors for individuals in the childbearing years
4   Discuss the basis for evaluating nursing intervention with the couple who have decided not to become parents
5   List the emotional tasks undergone by the childbearing couple during pregnancy, labor, delivery, and the postpartum period
6   Describe the nursing process in pregnancy and the postpartum period
7   List the assessment factors which are less important for the traditional couple than they are for the working mother, the single parent, or foster care
8   Formulate a plan of nursing intervention for families in the childbearing cycle

Structure and Function of Families

Family Structure

For many middle-class Americans, the term "family" brings forth a mental picture of a married couple and their children. This grouping is termed a *nuclear family*. The nucleus in which one has been a child is termed the *family of orientation*; while the family in which one is the parent is termed the *family of procreation*. An *extended family* consists of the nuclear family and others related by descent, marriage, or adoption.

The traditional middle-class pattern for the nuclear family calls for the husband to work and the wife to stay home and care for the house and children. In this arrangement, the husband has the single career in the family. The wife, regardless of her education, does not pursue a career, although she may work before children are born. One of the most common variations is for the wife to pursue a career, either continuously or intermittently, throughout the childbearing cycle.

Variations in the traditional middle-class pattern include the following:

1 The nuclear dyad—couple with no children in the home—with either a single career or dual careers
2 The single, previously married parent—one adult with one or more children—with or without a career
3 Single adult living with parent or alone
4 Three-generation family
5 Kin network—groups of nuclear families living close enough to exchange goods and services

Groups in the American society are experimenting with other family structures such as these:

1 Communes—households of one or more monogamous couples with children, all sharing common facilities
2 Communes—households of adults and offspring, usually with a charismatic leader
3 Unmarried parent and child
4 Unmarried couple and child
5 Unmarried couple
6 Homosexual couple

Family Functioning

Regardless of the seeming similarity of the visible structures, each family develops a unique personality and methods of performing the tasks that society expects. The behavior, beliefs, values, and goals shared by the family are distinguishing characteristics. Once the family's method of functioning has been identified, their behavior is to some degree predictable and characteristic.

The family develops a division of labor among the family members so that relationships are orderly. They make provision for caring activities such as cooking, child care, etc. The family develops a system of leadership; this may be vested in one member, or responsibilities for different functions may be divided. To perform the functions society expects of them, families need long-term stability. These social functions of the family include the following:

1 Meeting the basic needs of the family members
2 Helping the members to understand their roles
3 Enabling the members to learn control and to solve the conflicts of dominance versus submission and of autonomy versus dependence
4 Gaining acceptance within and outside the family
5 Developing a support system in the kin network and extended family
6 Resolving the conflict of flexibility versus rigidity
7 Allocating the family's resources
8 Dividing the work of the family
9 Socializing among family members
10 Placing family members in the larger society
11 Producing new members (children) in the family

12 Adding members to the family by marriage or by choice

13 Releasing family members to start new families

Formation of New Families

Young adults, having passed through the first five stages of development as defined by Erikson,[1] are faced with the sixth: intimacy versus isolation. They must decide whether or not to align themselves to another individual in a significant relationship. If a commitment is made, its depth must be explored. The couple must select the family structure which will best fit their needs. Pressure for a decision comes from all sides, especially from the parents, who look forward to being grandparents. To reach a rational decision, the young adults must look at themselves as individuals who are exploring their life goals.

Napier suggests that in choosing a partner, an individual takes unconscious yet careful account of the complex trends in the partner's and his or her own family of origin.[2] The marriage choice represents an attempt at growth. The choice may add new information to the model of each individual's family of origin, which will disrupt the patterns each learned in their family. Thus the first 6 to 12 months of marriage are often spoken of as being difficult. This is the period during which the couple work at synthesizing the new information into a schema that is congruent with their mutual needs. The initial conflict can contribute to the growth pattern, or it may produce lasting sources of tension between the couple. Complementary patterns in each family of origin can combine to make the emerging family more satisfying to the couple than was the family of origin. The potential for conflict in the relationships increases in proportion to the divergence in the backgrounds of the partners.

Once they have made a commitment to each other, the couple enter the stage of the *emerging family*. The members of the emerging family need to develop ways of collaborating that minimize their individual differences and those of their families of origin.

The new family begins to develop rules for living based on individual differences and similarities. As the partners perform the family tasks, rules begin to emerge to regulate behavior and communication. Jackson defines this process as *quid pro quo* (something for something).[3] There is a give and take in negotiations to define the rights and duties of the partners. The bargaining occurs on an unconscious level and is not necessarily overt. According to Haley, each new situation encountered by the partners is dealt with by establishing explicit or implicit rules.[4] Some of these rules govern the marital dyad, while others are established for the children and enforced by the parents. Marital conflict often centers around disagreement about these rules.

Having passed through the developmental stages of courtship and marriage, the emerging family next faces the major decision of whether to become parents and, if so, when. Figure 32-1 indicates the choices available regarding parenting options. Before making a decision, the couple must assess both the resources available and the goals and life-style they hope to have in the future. Resources include financial status, support systems available, current health status, technology available to help them achieve their goal, and their reasons for wanting a child.

Common Factors in the Assessment of Childbearing Families

Recurring patterns of assessment factors can be identified in various situational and developmental crises. Factors to be evaluated regarding the decision about having children are outlined in Table 32-1; they include:

1 Client's reasons for taking the new step or considering the change. The reasons should be rational and well thought out.

2 Knowledge about the situation. This needs to be factual and complete enough for problem solving.

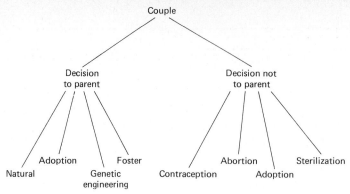

Figure 32-1

3 Support systems available to the individual and family to cope with the decision. The support system includes the extended family, kin network, peers, and community resources.

4 Potential effect on the individuals and the unit. This involves consideration of the effect on balance of power, family roles, family and individual goals, identity, and feelings of self-worth.

5 Intracouple agreement on the action to be taken.

6 Current status of communication between the couple, the extended family, and significant others.

7 The role religious beliefs have in the life of the couple. Exploration needs to be done on how strongly the beliefs are held and how important they are to the couple.

8 Current life-styles of the couple and their planned life-style in the immediate future. This includes regularity of hours, size and condition of living quarters, income, etc.

9 Couple's degree of motivation or commitment to the decision.

10 Couple's physical health.

11 Couple's personal characteristics and attitudes.

Assessment of these factors will enable the nurse to identify the strengths and weaknesses of the individual and the marital unit. From this identification will come the nursing diagnosis and nursing intervention.

Much of the nursing intervention in the childbearing family is aimed at primary prevention, that is, by anticipating the kinds of problems that are likely to arise and by providing the sort of guidance and support that will help the family to avoid problems.

Decision Not to Parent
Postponement of Parenthood

Among the reasons for deferring childbearing are the following: fears of pregnancy and/or labor and delivery; fears of parental responsibility; pressure from society, in which childbearing is less popular every year; and disagreement when one partner wants a child and the other does not. Any one or more of the resources needed for responsible parenthood may simply not be available at the current time. For example, a couple may lack money or housing, be in school, or may be pursuing their own challenging careers; they may therefore choose to defer childbearing until they have achieved their current objectives. When couples

Table 32-1 To Parent or Not to Parent

Assessment factor	Nursing diagnosis	Intervention
Clients' reasons to parent or not to parent.	Reasons are rational (e.g. finances, maturity of relationship, etc.).	Support reasons (see Chap. 6).
	Reasons are irrational (e.g. fear of pain).	Explore basis for reason (see Chap. 6).
Health.	Couple in good health.	Support health habits.
	Health problems (e.g. diabetes).	Guidance on significance of health problem and treatment.
Intraunit agreement		
Couple.	Agree on decision to parent.	Support decision.
	Disagree on decision to parent.	Explore basis of disagreement.
Extended family.	Agree with couple's decision.	Support their agreement.
	Disagree with couple's decision.	Explore basis and methods of coping with long-term disagreement.
Supporting people.	Supporting people are present.	Identify and affirm support systems.
	Supporting people are absent except for a few friends; no kin network.	Explore community resources.
Knowledge needed to make a decision.	Clients have sufficient knowledge about parenting.	Answer any questions clients may have.
	Clients have insufficient knowledge about parenting.	Supply information and make sure clients understand it.
Potential effect of parenting		
On woman.	Maturing effect.	Provide psychological support.
	Regressive effect.	Assess maturity levels on Erikson scale; explore problem areas.
On unit.	Will strengthen the unit.	Support strengths.
	Will weaken unit.	Explore causes, look for options.
On lifestyle.	Decision will fit lifestyle.	Support decision.
	Decision will not fit lifestyle.	Explore lack of fit.
In relation to religious beliefs.	Decision fits couple's operating beliefs.	Support decision.
	Decision does not fit couple's religious beliefs.	Explore lack of fit.
Current communications		
	Current communications are open.	Support communication patterns.
	Family is not communicating freely.	Explore dysfunction and facilitate open communication.
Motivation, commitment, and other considerations		
	Present in both partners.	Support commitment.
	Absent in one or both partners.	Explore other options.

decide to postpone parenthood, several options are available to them.

Contraception

When a couple desire contraception (defined as reversible prevention of conception), the next question is where to obtain it. The facility they need may be as close as their physician's office or hospital clinic. Or they may prefer a freestanding clinic such as the network of family planning clinics. The Planned Parenthood League has pioneered in services which provide adequate education for each and every client as well as methods of contraception.

The role of the nurse in these facilities involves assessing the knowledge and attitudes of the couple, assisting them to decide on the best method, helping them to get the knowledge and practice they need to use their chosen method effectively, providing regular checkups, and—lastly—serving as a resource for the answers to questions.

To do this, nurses must be clear about their own feelings. For example, if one believed that contraception was wrong or unhealthy, it would be difficult to assist others in a positive way. The nurse may need to refer the couple to other helpers in such cases.

Having resolved their own feelings, nurses are then in a position to assess, diagnose, and intervene in the couple's behalf. Assessment factors for decision making in contraception are outlined in Table 32-2.

While nurses will need to look at each assessment factor individually, they also need to look at the total picture to arrive at the final diagnosis. The more agreement among each of the diagnoses, the surer the nurse will be when reaching the final diagnoses.

Sterlization

For the couple who have completed their family, who have decided against children, or who face a high risk of having a genetically damaged child,

sterilization (permanent contraception) may be the solution. For those families who elect sterilization, the current options are vasectomy, tubal ligation, or an elective hysterectomy. Recent developments in laparoscopy have made tubal ligation easier and the hospital stay shorter; in some cases it may be 12 hours or less. Sterlization is still considered a permanent procedure although research on its possible reversibility is continuing.

Any elective alteration of a person's own body is certain to have a psychological impact. Therefore, sterilization should be discussed by the couple over a period of time in order to be sure that its effects on their relationship will be positive. Possible changes which sterilization and the absence of more children may bring to the family should be assessed. Table 32-3 summarizes the areas which should be considered.

Before beginning to assess the family, nurses need to clarify their own beliefs and be sure their personal knowledge is up to date. Nurses themselves need to go through the same list of assessment factors as the family in order to clarify their feelings.

Problem Pregnancy

The couple faced with an unwanted pregnancy comes face to face with the problem of deciding whether to have the child. Modern science and societal changes have given them the options to avoid parenthood at later stages than was possible in past generations. The options for abortion, adoption, or keeping a baby are often confusing because of the strong feelings and values associated with childbearing and child-rearing. Nurses may find themselves experiencing the same confused feelings as do clients. These feelings arise from societal values and support, religious values and beliefs, and the woman's emotional needs or basic maternal instincts.

Thus there are several main areas of difference in assessment between the decision to postpone parenthood when it is made after conception instead of before conception. These are the areas

Table 32-2   Decision Not to Parent

Assessment factor	Nursing diagnosis	Intervention
Reasons for contraception.	Rational reasons.	Support rational reasons.
	Irrational attitudes.	Explore attitudes.
Partner's attitudes toward contraception		
Need for contraception.	Agreement present.	Support agreement.
	Agreement absent.	Explore disagreement.
Who is responsible (he, she, both).	Agreement present.	Support agreement.
	Agreement absent about assumption of responsibility.	Explore options.
Knowledge about reproduction, sex, and contraception		
Reproduction	Adequate.	Reinforce knowledge and provide further information.
	Inadequate or distorted by myths.	Supply information where inadequate; clarify misconceptions.
Physiology of sexual response.	Adequate.	Reinforce knowledge and provide further information.
	Inadequate.	Supply information where inadequate.
Contraception.	Adequate.	Reinforce knowledge and provide further information.
	Inadequate.	Evaluate learning; supply information.
Couple's lifestyle		
Regular hours, living conditions (privacy, storage), bathroom facilities, income.	Lifestyle limits choice.	Discuss limitations.
	Lifestyle does not limit choice.	None.
Motivation to space or limit the number of children.	Strong motivation to postpone.	Explore sources of motivation.
	Weak motivation to postpone.	Explore sources of motivation.
Preferred method.	Preferred method indicated or not by couple.	Supply indicated method.
Religious belief.	Limits choice or does not limit choice.	Support and explore choices and limitations.
Personal attitudes and characteristics		
Feelings about various methods (e.g. remembering pill, touching genitalia, parents' and peers' experiences, safety of various methods).	Attitudes about and characteristics of method limit choice.	Explain limitations imposed by attitudes.
	Attitudes about and characteristics of method do not limit choice.	
Communication between couple.	Couple is currently communicating feelings.	Support good communications.
	Couple is currently not communicating feelings.	Facilitate improved communications.

Table 32-3 The Nursing Process and Sterilization

Assessment factor	Nursing diagnosis	Intervention
Reasons for wanting sterilization (e.g., factors of health, age, genetics, income, family size, housing, career goals.	Reasons are rational and realistic.	Support reasons.
	Reasons are irrational and unrealistic.	Explore reasons, help couple clarify their reasons.
Feelings (his and hers) about sexuality.	Feelings are compatible with sterilization.	Support feelings.
	Feelings are not compatible with sterilization.	Explore degree and significance of conflict.
Effect of sterilization on balance of power in family.	Sterilization will change balance in family.	Explore effect on family.
	Sterilization will not change balance of power in family.	Support balance.
Effect of sterilization on family roles.	Sterilization will change roles in family.	Explore effect of role change on each partner and on family.
	Sterilization will not change roles in family.	Support balance.
Effect of sterilization on feelings of self-worth.	Sterilization will decrease feelings of self-worth.	Explore feelings, delay sterilization.
	Sterilization will increase or create no change in feelings of self-worth.	Support feelings of self-worth.

Knowledge of effect of procedure

On sexual functioning.	Knowledge sufficient to make decision.	Support decision.
On sexual drive.	Knowledge not sufficient to make a decision.	Supply information and evaluate understanding.
Knowledge about anatomy and physiology of reproduction.	Knowledge adequate to understand explanations.	Support.
	Knowledge inadequate to understand explanations.	Supply information and evaluate understanding.
Assess postdecision feelings and family functioning.	Couple has positive feelings.	Support feelings.
	Couple has negative feelings.	Explore and assist couple in making necessary changes; referral as needed.
Communication between couple.	Currently communicating feelings.	Support communication patterns.
	Currently not communicating feelings.	Act as facilitator, being careful not to be triangled into the situation (see Chap. 11).

of religious belief, societal and family support, and the potential effect of the woman and the family.

Table 32-4 summarizes these and other areas which are involved in the decision to parent or not to parent after conception has occurred.

Therapeutic Abortion

When the nurse and the couple have completed the assessment in Table 32-4 and the couple has decided that abortion is the chosen option; the nurse can begin to collaborate with the client as to

Table 32-4 Pregnant: To Parent or Not to Parent

Assessment factor	Nursing diagnosis	Intervention
Religion.	Religion limits options.	Explore open options.
	Religion does not limit options.	Explore all options.
Potential effects on woman.	Decision will have a maturing effect.	Support decision.
	Decision will have a negative effect.	Define problem areas, provide counseling and referral.
Potential effects on family.	Decision will facilitate a closer relationship between family members.	Encourage close relationships.
	Decision will cause increased separation and distancing between family members.	Explore cause, suggest possible family therapy.
Support systems		
Expectant father.	Father supports decision.	Include father in planning.
	Father opposes decision.	Counsel with father alone and as a couple to promote consensus.
Extended family.	Supports decision.	Include some members in planning.
	Opposes decision.	Explore reasons for opposition.
Peer group.	Supports decision.	Consider including in planning.
	Opposes decision.	Explore reasons for opposition.
Kin network	Supports decision.	Encourage help.
	Opposes decision	Explore reasons for opposition.

the time, place, and method of abortion.

Community resources for counseling and abortions are increasing. Freestanding women's clinics are available to counsel women and perform first-trimester abortions. Such clinics often have arrangements with local hospitals for the performance of second-trimester abortions. Many hospitals have abortion clinics. In some states, legislation permits doctors to perform first-trimester abortions in their offices, using accepted protocols.

Financial help for the procedure is usually available from Medicaid or from some medical insurance companies. Freestanding clinics may be the least expensive source of abortion for the woman with limited resources.

The nurse can serve as a resource person in helping the couple or the woman alone before, during, and after the procedure. The nurse should encourage the couple to talk about their percep-

tions of the procedure and should answer their questions. This is important in clearing up misconceptions about the procedure, its effects on future childbearing and future sexual relations. The nurse should clarify who will help the client, who will come with her and pick her up after the procedure, and who will help her at home. The nurse should also serve as a good listener and provide emotional support, for the couple may need help in expressing their feelings at each stage of the process. These emotions may range from guilt through confusion, anger, and depression. Follow-up studies on women who have undergone elective abortions have shown that if they have had sufficient support for their decisions, there are no measurable emotional sequelae.[5]

The nurse can help the couple prevent further unwanted pregnancies. Repeated unwanted pregnancies may be a sign of pathology and hence may require referral for psychiatric care.

Placement for Adoption

Adoption is an alternative not only for the young unwed mother but also for the married couple who have experienced contraceptive failure after completing their family or the young couple who are not ready to begin one.

When a decision is made that adoption is in the best interests of the child and the couple, help will be needed by the couple or woman in implementing the decision. Referral to a licensed adoption agency, in order to provide the best placement for the infant, is in order. Homes for unwed mothers are still available, but their numbers are decreasing. For support during pregnancy, groups such as Birth Right supply counseling and financial aid.

In counseling the couple, the nurse must realize that the giving up of a baby is experienced as a loss and that the couple, especially the woman who will carry the child for 9 months, will need to resolve these feelings. (See Chap. 23.) This is true not only before the baby is born but also after placement of the baby, before the child is legally given up.

Additional pressures come from a society which expects any couple to want and keep their children. However, the couple can be helped to ask themselves whether this philosophy is congruent with their needs (see Chap. 33).

Decision to Parent
Natural Pregnancy

Having made the decision to parent after realistically assessing the changes this will bring about in their lives, the couple then have the opportunity to choose a style of care, the type of institution, and a provider who practices their chosen style of care. The modality that is selected depends on intangibles such as power, ethnic considerations, and knowledge. If the couple feel that all decisions regarding reproduction are the woman's, she will make the decision. In some ethnic groups the grandparents are responsible for the decision. The isolation of the nuclear family may lead the couple to make a decision based on the advice of friends.

When the distant extended family learns of the decision, they may or may not support it. The degree of support received has an effect on the family's coping patterns.

Several alternatives exist which have in common a philosopy of family-centered care. This allows the couple to define their roles in the childbearing process, such as allowing the father's presence in labor and delivery and allowing both parents unlimited access to the infant. It also provides siblings access to the mother, father, and new baby during the childbearing process.

This philosophy of care is available in different types of settings or institutions. The one which has most recently returned to the urban health-care scene is the maternity home or childbearing center. Couples attend classes and finally have a wide-awake delivery by a nurse-midwife. The mother breast-feeds her baby, and they share the same room. Mother and baby leave the center within 12 hours of delivery. The center "operates with rigid rules on the mother's physical condition and with enormous latitude in procedures."[6] Mothers with complications make a short trip to the nearest hospital.

Another mode of care which is being popularized purely because of consumer satisfaction, and by word of mouth, is home delivery. However, home deliveries will probably always be fewer in number than those performed in hospitals and maternity centers.

The most widely used mode of care is hospital delivery. For many couples, the reason for choosing a particular hospital is not the scientific excellence of care but rather the warmth and interest centered on the family.

Couples who have defined the style of care they want must make a careful search of their area to find the providers who will meet their needs. They may choose an obstetrician or a nurse-midwife. The provider may be located in an individual or group practice or in a public clinic.

In order to find a provider who will meet their expectations, the couple need to decide (1) on a particular style of care, (2) whether there is a preference for a caretaker of a particular sex or training, (3) on the degree of the participation they want in decision making, (4) on the amount of time they hope the provider will spend with them, (5) on the amount of money they have to spend, and (6) how far they can travel.

After an initial interview, the couple can change their minds. It is important for the husband to feel that he can trust the provider. It is not uncommon for the husband to find that he is jealous of the depth of his wife's attachment to her male obstetrician.

In addition to understanding what is involved in a couple's choice of style of care, institution, and provider, the nurse must know the dynamics of the psychological tasks of pregnancy and their normal sequence.[7]

The first trimester is occupied with the psychological process of *incorporation* of the fetus into a woman's concept of her own body. As she begins to care about the fetus as an extension of her body, a woman turns inward and begins to consider her own needs. The increase in narcissism or concern with self manifests itself in the woman's need to detach herself from previous commitments. This may be upsetting to family, friends, and associates who have come to depend on her. She may also experience increased sensitivity and changes in her personality. Changes in sexuality and emotions require that the couple communicate their respective interpretations of the shifting pattern of emotional states.

Also, in this phase a woman often becomes concerned with the past and with her relationship with her mother. Now that she is to become a mother herself, she must begin to sort out the input on mothering from her past and decide what is necessary and what is not. She begins to see herself as an individual rather than as a daughter. This change in viewpoint may enable her to develop a new adult-to-adult relationship with her mother, but the change may be a problem for the prospective grandmother if she sees her only role as a human being in being a mother who is needed by her children.

The emotional changes in the woman may be due to hormonal and metabolic alterations as well as to psychogenic factors. She may experience changes such as nausea and mood swings even before she knows she is pregnant. Her increased fatigue in the first trimester decreases her ability to handle stress. The petty annoyances which she might once have overlooked now take on major proportions. If this is a second or subsequent child, the other children may become confused by changes in the mother's behavior. The nurse may need to interpret the expectant mother's fatigue to the couple and help them plan rest time for her.

The next recognizable psychological task generally occurs during the second trimester. It is described as *differentiation,* or the task of recognizing and acknowledging that the fetus—whom she has accepted as present in her body—is not part of her. This begins with the momentous experience of the baby's first movement.

It is with this unseen but distinct being that the couple now develops a relationship called *attachment.* This involvement is very real, so that the loss of the baby from this point on brings not only physical trauma but also psychological grief and mourning (see Chap. 23).

The woman often develops an increased concern about and interest in her husband. She wants and needs to know that she can depend on him. His sharing in the experience clearly is important. "Feel the baby move," is a familiar demand directed at him.

The baby's movement is the first proof the husband may have that the baby is real. This may awaken in him fears about his adequacy as a provider and fears for the safety of his wife and the infant. He is beginning to view his wife as a mother, and this may awaken feelings he may have had about his own mother. At the same time, the expectant wife is continuing to resolve her feelings about her relationship with her mother. Both are striving to shake off the last adolescent dependence on their parents and to stand on their own. The extent to which they accomplish this task of achieving independence will influence their new roles as parents (see Chap. 11).

During this second trimester, the couple may have to make sexual adjustments. Frequently, the wife feels an increase in sexual desire; but as the trimester progresses, the expanding abdomen may interfere. This requires adjustment by both partners. They need to discuss their feelings about sexual relations and to adjust positions so that the sex act is satisfying to both. The adjustment in position again can bring up the issue of dominance and social and ethnic role orientations when dealing with reproductive functions. For example, how does a wife who is oriented to a passive role in sexual relationships use the superior position?

As the third trimester approaches, the couple's view of the fetus or fear of hurting it may cause difficulty in their sex life. The changing sexual desires of the woman may confuse the husband. She may desire relations more or less often than before.

The third trimester usually coincides with third task: *separation*. Here the mother prepares for delivery, and her main interest is the baby. Dreams, fantasies, and everyday conversations are likely to include the baby. The couple's ability and willingness to name the baby says much about their anticipation of the birth of a separate and distinct individual to whom they are becoming attached. Thus the first stage of becoming a parent is well under way.

Couples tend to have very definite views of their infant. These ideas may relate to looks, age, future skills, and the couple's unfulfilled wishes. They visualize the baby as being at a specific age and having a distinctive personality. They become attached to this view, and if the infant does not fulfill their expectations, they may go through a period of mourning for the fantasized infant before they are willing to accept the real one.

The couple's perception of the fetus may be an indication of how the parent-child relationship will develop. If the couple view the fetus as a problem which interferes with their life, they may continue to view the child as a problem. If the feeling toward the fetus is positive, then their initial reaction to the infant is usually positive.

Couples may also see in the infant a chance to fulfill their unrealized dreams. They may invest the fetus with the talents and abilities needed to fulfill these dreams. As long as these expectations are adjusted to reality, this can be a healthy process. When the fetus is considered to be in physical danger, however, the mother does not form a mental image of the baby. This lack of attachment in pregnancy may pose problems if the child is born and lives.

Last but not least, the third trimester is accompanied by an inescapable anxiety about the coming labor and delivery. No matter how slight the impulse to worry, the coming event looms large as the completion of the process of pregnancy nears. Couples use many coping mechanisms in an attempt to channel the anxiety concerning approaching labor.

Constructive coping mechanisms will enable the couple to develop the skills necessary to manage labor, delivery, and parenting. Among them coping activities are the following: (1) caring for other infants, (2) attending parent-education classes, (3) attending classes preparing for labor and delivery, (4) gathering infant-care items, (5) preparing and freezing meals for after delivery, (6) housecleaning, (7) maintaining open communications, and (8) other activities the couple can share. Couples who are having difficulty in dealing with anxiety may become aimless in their activities and may arrive at labor and delivery without preparation.

As the due date approaches, constructive coping activities fade into insignificance; at this point the desire to have the pregnancy over becomes dominant. The woman begins to tire of carrying the extra weight and of having people say, "Are you still around?"

The extra body weight is the most striking of the developmental changes in body image which are especially prominent at this time. The changes bring highs and lows. Buying (or letting out the seams of) maternity clothes can bring deep emotional satisfaction if the baby is a planned and wanted one. But it can also be the cause of feelings of ugliness and clumsiness, especially if the woman is ambivalent about this pregnancy or is receiving little or no emotional support from her husband, friends, or relatives. Other cues to the mother's reaction are her comments about negotiating her enlarged body through familiar spaces which magically seem to have shrunk. One example is pushing a shopping cart through the supermarket checkout counter, where most women are surprised that they do not fit as easily as before. If the woman is really unhappy about her pregnancy, this discovery can be an upsetting event. Whether happy or sad, the woman wonders whether she will ever be the same size again. Will she ever get her figure back?

Other physical changes which occur during pregnancy may be either delightful or burdensome, depending on the couple's stability and desire for this child. Chloasma, or the mask of pregnancy, can be seen as imparting either a healthy suntanned appearance or a disfiguring brown skin rash. Striae or stretch marks appear on the abdomen and breasts. If the couple highly prizes physical appearance and "youth," striae, which are very visible in a bikini, are highly undesirable. This is especially true since they, unlike chloasma, do not disappear completely.

Another concern for the couple is preparation of the siblings for the coming of the new baby and the mother's absence from home for a few days. The extent of the preparation will vary with the age of the children, but all questions about the childbearing process should be answered honestly and simply. Correct terminology should be used to avoid future confusion. The emotional and physical changes which the mother undergoes have a marked effect on her husband and children. In other words, her responses set up responses in the family, and the *resonance phenomenon* set up in the family leads to the term "the pregnant family."

The pregnant family's progress through pregnancy and the postpartum period can be assessed and dealt with through the nursing process, as shown in Table 32-5.

Labor and Delivery

After 9 months of anticipation, the couple arrive at the childbearing center full of apprehension. During a first pregnancy, there is a particular fear of the unknown, which is deeper than any knowledge. The couple have probably heard many stories about labor and delivery and do not know which ones to believe. Here at last is the culminating event for which they have been exercising, studying, and preparing. For a couple approaching labor and delivery, the experience can be overwhelming as they feel a loss of control over what is occurring. The deep emotional significance of the appearance of new life in itself makes labor and delivery momentous. This is especially true for the couple who have had past disappointment; the event then becomes a confirmation of their ability to have children.

The onset of labor also makes the couple more fully aware of their changing role. There is no turning back; they are about to become parents. This thought may increase the feeling of apprehension.

It is only natural that such a momentous event will be more meaningful if it is shared with someone who cares deeply, who is able to recreate the scene because he or she was there. This is far different from trying to describe the delivery later. The classes and exercises have set the scene for this sharing; continuing it through labor and delivery seems to be a logical sequel. When the woman wakes up in the middle of the night wondering whether she is experiencing false labor or the real thing, she will find it helpful to receive reassurance from someone who remembers what the instructor said in class. Later, after being admitted to the center, she may be comforted by having a familiar person at hand to coach her in breathing.

As labor advances, a woman is very dependent on others for her physical needs as well as for emotional support. She is apprehensive and uncomfortable, unable to do anything for herself. She becomes aware that "this is it." The contractions continue unabated despite her momentary, frightened wish to withdraw. She may well feel "caught," somewhat as a soldier does when under fire, he feels an urge to run away.

Having mastered the most painful phase of labor—the transition phase during which the cervix dilates to 8 to 10 centimeters—the couple may

Table 32-5 Nursing Management During and After Pregnancy — "Normal" Physical and Psychological Progress

Assessment factor	Nursing diagnosis	Intervention
Health of mother, fetus, infant.	Mother and fetus have no problems.	Support: primary prevention.
	Mother and fetus have problems.	Appropriate treatment of problems; evaluation of effect.

Effect of pregnancy and postpartum

On woman (e.g., new feelings, body rhythms, etc.).	Woman is adjusting and adapting.	Support adjustment patterns.
	Woman is not adjusting to changes during or after pregnancy.	Explore feelings and disturbances.
On couple (e.g., feelings about each other).	Feelings have changed.	Explore direction of change.
	No change in feelings.	None.
Daily physical activity, sharing time.	Realistic changes being made.	Explore direction of changes.
	Changes are not realistic; i.e., mother healthy but resting all day.	Counsel regarding exploration of unrealistic changes.
On other family members (siblings, grandparents).	Changes in feelings or behavior are extensive.	Explore changes in feelings or behavior.
	No changes in feelings or behavior.	None.
Family functioning.	Changes in functioning.	Explore direction and impact on family.
	No changes in functioning.	Support current patterns.

Family's knowledge about practical preparations for childbirth and baby care

	Sufficient knowledge to allow action.	Answer any questions that arise.
	Insufficient knowledge.	Teach family and evaluate their understanding.

Current status of communications and expression of feelings

	Open communication, sufficient expression of feelings.	Support communication patterns and expression of feelings.
	Insufficient expression of feelings; closed communication.	Explore problem, help establish more effective communication.

Presence and use of support systems in family

Present.	Sufficient (i.e., family nearby and willing to help).	None.
	Insufficient (i.e., family unable to help).	Explore, counsel, interview supporting people.
Effectiveness of use.	Effective (i.e., help when needed).	None.
	Not effective.	Interview supporting people.

Developmental tasks of the pregnant and postpartum periods

	Accomplishing developmental tasks.	Support; anticipatory guidance.
	Not accomplishing developmental tasks.	Explore; counsel; teach developmental tasks.
Parenting expectations and planning for child-rearing.	Realistic plans.	Support plans.
	Unrealistic plans.	Explore; counsel; teach realistic plans.

derive real satisfaction from delivery. The satisfaction of having delivered without anesthesia (except perhaps for a local) is a universal one. Thus, the prepared couple who have shared this experience are likely to come to the joyful moment of holding their newborn, well prepared for events to follow. However, those who have not lived up to their mental image of what the well-prepared couple should do may experience feelings of failure and dismay after delivery. Their self-images as competent individuals may be shaken. There are several ways in which their expectations may be disappointed. For example, they may be disturbed by the doctor's need to use forceps or a vacuum extractor or by having to have the baby delivered by caesarian section.

A second problem emerges when a woman's behavior does not accord with her self-image. If the labor is a long one or if it is just too much of a burden for her nervous system, her loud cries and restless behavior may be much more upsetting to her than to any of the providers present. The couple may feel they are total failures, and these negative feelings may overflow onto their images of themselves as parents. If they could not deliver the infant without assistance, how can they raise it?

The woman without any knowledge may come to labor and delivery having heard many stories about the pain and dangers of childbirth. She has no facts with which to counter her fears. Since she is unprepared, she is not likely to have anyone with her to share her labor and delivery experience. The woman may prefer to have her sister present rather than her partner, but she may be unaware that this is possible. Her anxiety level may be so high that she is unable to comprehend what is being said to her. One method of coping is to regard this as a crisis which is the initiation into womanhood. Survival is the requirement, and culturally accepted modes of behavior in childbirth, such as screaming or moaning, provide reassurance that she is one with the women who have gone before her.

Nursing intervention during labor and delivery depends on continually assessing the couple's reactions during the stages of labor. Each stage is characterized by expected physical changes which are accompanied by more or less predictable emotional reactions.

The Postpartum Period
Following the delivery of the infant, the family undergoes profound physical and emotional changes. The infant adjusts to extrauterine life and performs its own vital life functions. The mother's body begins to adjust to not being pregnant and completes the physical changes necessary for breast-feeding.

The process of attachment begun during pregnancy continues. Signs of the healthy progress of mother-infant attachment include these:

1 Mother inspects baby (a) to make sure it is whole, "all there"; (b) to identify this baby as it really is, and to adjust her fantasies to the reality; (c) to identify common characteristics with the families or origin.
2 Mother seeks eye-to-eye contact with the baby. This is facilitated by the baby's fixed gaze during the first hour.
3 Looking is accompanied by progressive touching and stroking, first with fingertips, then with the whole hand. Mother then embraces the baby and holds it close to her body.
4 The baby is held so that mother and baby are in the *en face* position (eyes of mother and baby in the same vertical plane).[8]
5 Mother takes care of baby, as by feeding and changing diapers. Women who are going through the process of attachment after delivery may develop anxiety if they do not feel immediate mother love. They wonder if they are normal. If offered the infant to hold, they may refuse and prefer just to look. Caplan believes that many mothers experience this delay in feeling mother love and regards it as normal.[9]

Movement through the tasks of attachment is

facilitated by initial and continued contact between mother and infant. One advocate of initial close contact between mother and baby is Dr. LeBoyer. He claims gains in adaptation for the newborn whose entrance into this world is "eased" by a warm bath and soothing massage.[10]

In addition to the task of attachment, mothers have other psychological tasks to perform; these are described best by Rubin.[11] The first stage in the postpartum period is *taking in.* This period lasts 2 to 3 days; during it, the mother's primary concern is with her own needs. She reacts passively and initiates little activity. Adequate sleep and rest are major needs in this period.

So that the mother may have sufficient energy to meet the needs of the infant, the nursing staff must mobilize the environment to meet the mother's hierarchy of needs as outlined by Maslow (see Chap. 1). She needs periods during which she does not have to care for anyone else. She has been through a period of biological stress, and within a few days she will be putting out large amounts of energy in caring for her newborn at home.

In addition to needing rest, the mother needs to have opportunities to talk about and relive her labor and delivery experience. This includes clarifying the events which took place and should lead to the feeling that she has met the challenge successfully.

If the dependency needs of the taking-in phase are well met, the mother will be ready to progress to the next stage, that of *taking hold.*

The taking-hold period lasts about 10 days. During this time, the mother is concerned with her need to resume control of her life in all its phases. She wants to be viewed as competent. It is important to her that everything function well, her own body as well as that of the infant. She seems ready to organize herself and her life. As a mother, she now wants to be in command of her situation. But when problems occur, they are likely to reduce the mother to tears. This sudden emotional frailty may bewilder her husband. He is at a loss to explain what has happened to his confident wife, who seems to have lost her common sense. The wife, in turn, may see the nurse as the perfect mother. The nurse is the one who can get the infant to burp in a few seconds after the mother has spent 10 minutes trying. When the nurse diapers the baby, they stay on; when the mother does so, they fall off. She feels that she is being judged and must measure up in everyone's sight, especially in that of her mother and mother-in-law. To maintain her self-esteem, she must be as good a mother as they are.

At this time she may want to have the infant with her as much as possible. If the concept of rooming-in and its advantages to the development of the parent-infant attachment have been explained before delivery, mothers will often be eager to have the infant with them. On the other hand, if the infant is suddenly brought to the room to spend the day and mothers are unprepared, they may view the infant's arrival as an indication that the nursing staff do not want to care for the infant.

Rooming-in

Advantages	Disadvantages
1 Facilitates attachment	1 Decreases mother's rest
2 Increases caretaking skills of mother and father, such as bathing, diapering, handling	2 May be culturally unacceptable to patient or her husband
3 Increases knowledge of infant's rhymthic patterns of sleeping, eating, etc.	

To meet the needs of the family, rooming-in needs to be flexible. The mother needs sufficient exposure to the infant to develop caretaking skills and attachment but not so much as to interfere with the meeting of her own basic needs.

During this phase, the mother needs praise and encouragement for her efforts. The "helping others" should provide support for *her* efforts rather than doing the tasks themselves. They must understand the need for adequate rest in this phase as well. Exhaustion in the pursuit of perfection can be damaging to mental as well as to physical health. This is a danger with first babies as well as when the mother has no help in coping with her new family.

The final phase, that of *letting go,* is initiated in the postpartum period and follows through the life of the child. The mother will begin to see the infant as an individual rather than as an extension of herself. Mothers who are making satisfactory progress in the task of letting go will recognize the need for increased independence at various stages of growth and development.

The woman experiences many conflicts within herself during the third phase. She must balance her dependency needs against those of the infant. This may prove a problem if the mother has not previously mastered her own developmental task of dependence versus independence. If a mother has not developed independence in some spheres of her own life, it will be difficult for her to allow independence to develop in the child.

Such a woman may think of the perfect mother as one who always loves her infant, whose infant wakes, eats, and sleeps but never cries. This is probably in direct contrast to the reality of the situation, in which an infant may cry from time to time for no apparent reason. The mother may be amazed at how much she resents the infant when it interferes with her needs. The baby cries when the mother wants to sleep or fusses when the couple are about to eat dinner. This feeling of resentment may be particularly strong if the mother has had no contact with infants and does not realize that such behavior is normal and will subside.

A third internal conflict which may materialize is that between the roles of mother and wife. The woman who has formerly been able to serve quiet, candle-lit dinners may, in the initial weeks, find it difficult to have her hair combed and her lipstick on when her husband arrives. If she accumulates guilt over not meeting her own expectations, this will increase her communication problems with her husband.

A potential source of conflict exists when the postpartum mother has a tubal ligation for which she was not totally ready, either intellectually or emotionally, or for which she does not receive substantial support and acceptance from husband and relatives. If the mother has not made a positive, internally integrated decision for sterlization, she may handle her conflict by spoiling her last child and retarding its movement into independence.

Because of her inner conflicts, the reality of caring for a new infant, and the hormonal changes in her body, the woman may experience a period of depression following the birth of the infant. The mother may frequently feel very tired or find herself crying for no apparent reason. The rest of the family may be puzzled; they expect her to be happy with the infant. This period of postpartum blues usually lasts only a few days. The others in the environment can be most helpful if they try to meet the woman's dependency needs so that she will have the energy to meet those of the infant. Extra rest is frequently helpful. Depression which is not relieved by simple measures may require psychiatric referral.

While the adjustment of mother and infant are occurring, the couple must also adjust to new relationships. The family has now formed a triad (see Chap. 11). The husband and wife have to adjust their relationship with each other to include this new member. The readjustment occurs both after the first child and after each subsequent child.

The period of readjustment may be difficult for the couple. The husband may feel jealous of the new infant and all the attention it is receiving. If the relationship throughout pregnancy, labor, and delivery has not been a shared one, he may feel abandoned by his wife. If she has had an episiotomy, she will be too uncomfortable for the first 3 or 4 weeks to have sexual relations, and the unprepared husband may find this, too, difficult to accept. If the couple are isolated from the extended family and have not developed a strong kin network, the husband may have to help his wife with the household chores after he has worked all day at his job. The increased responsibility without any immediate, tangible rewards may strain the relationship.

The children may also be experiencing the

strain of a new relationship. If this is not a first child, the sibling(s) will have to adjust to sharing the limelight. Visitors frequently sweep by the older children in their hurry to see the infant. The mother is often tired from caring for the infant; she may have less time and less physical and psychic energy to devote to the older children. The older ones resent the loss of the mother's time and may feel displaced in her affections. They may show their feelings by acting out or by adopting regressive, infantile behavior.

In addition to dealing with internal conflicts and feelings, the couple begin to take on or expand the parental role. The parents' response to the infant after the initial contact is governed by many factors. Most people gain their knowledge about parenting from their own parents. They are also influenced by sociological factors such as social class, ethnicity, religion, and community.

One influence on parenting has been the exposure of fathers to childbirth education. This increased exposure to their newborns has increased their attachment to and engrossment[12] in the infant. Thus, men who are more involved in the care of their children develop an interest in increasing their parenting skills.

The process of parenting goes through many stages in its development. Parents must first learn the cues the infant gives to its needs. Then they must accept the stages of growth and development and the child's increasing need to be a separate individual. As the child begins to develop independence, the parents must accept the child's need to reject them without deserting the child. And, finally, the parents and child must build their own separate lives.

The primary role of the nurse in the postpartum period is to mobilize the environment to meet the needs of the developing family. To do this, the nurse needs to assess the family's strengths and weaknesses. The nurse should look at the physical health of the mother and infant. After these data have been collected, a nursing diagnosis can be made and the nurse can plan with the family for their care. This is explained in Table 32-5.

Problems in Becoming a Parent
Death or Impairment
The parents who experience a fetal or perinatal death or who have a defective child go through the five stages of mourning (see Chaps. 37, 38, and 39). They need the nursing staff to support them and listen to them. They mourn not only the child they have actually lost but also the perfect child they had visualized.

High-Risk Infants
If the infant is high risk instead of being a healthy, full-term baby, then the couple and the nurse encounter other problems. Perhaps the most common high-risk infant is the premature baby (born less than 38 weeks after conception or weighing less than 2500 g.

Normally women have time to become psychologically as well as physically prepared for labor during the last few weeks of pregnancy. However, premature labor is different in many respects: (1) it occurs earlier, (2) there is an air of an emergency, (3) the husband may be excluded, (4) increased use of fetal monitors and tests creates a feeling of danger, (5) there are an increased number of people watching the monitor and not the client.

The rapid removal of the high-risk infant to a special nursery can retard the normal attachment process by (1) making the mother feel that she may lose her infant, so that the mother begins to withdraw from the relationship she has established with the fetus; (2) making it more difficult to see, touch, and care for the infant—a difficulty that is increased by the special equipment. And in addition to having disturbances in attachment, the mother is left to deal with her feelings alone.

If the baby is small, the mother may experience feelings of failure and depression. This may be manifested by teary sadness or by anger. If the baby has medical problems, the mother may blame them on the care she has received. Often she searches her own actions to find a cause.

Another common feeling is loneliness. This

may be partly due to the fact that the mother cannot take care of her baby when others care for theirs and that she may have to go home without the infant. Perhaps the staff tend to avoid her because they are unsure of what to say. They are accustomed to focusing on the relationships in a happy family (see Chap. 39).

During this period, the father is also experiencing deep feelings. He is concerned for his wife and infant. If he has been excluded from the delivery room, his concern is first for his wife and then for the infant. As the first of the two to see the infant, he may be startled by its size and by the complexity of the equipment used. He needs support and explanation of each procedure. It is to him that many of the initial decisions concerning medical care will fall. Asking him to make the decisions without consulting his wife may disrupt communication between them. While in most cultures the mother is allowed to express her feelings, the father is expected to be stoical and to support her. In order to accomplish this, he needs the support of the nurse. The husband is also faced with the task of explaining what has happened to the other siblings, the family, and friends.

The emotions both parents feel may take several forms. They may express general anger with the situation, blaming each other or the caretakers. They may make insistent bids for reassurance and attention. They may be unable to communicate with each other and may withdraw from each other.

The parents' method of coping with the emotions evoked by the infant's problems generate feelings in the nursing staff caring for the family. Outbursts of blaming and anger may cause the staff to withdraw at a time when the parents most need support. The staff needs to look at its actions in light of the parents' needs.

Some avenues of intervention which may help to answer the family's needs are as follows: (1) change high-risk nursery rules to allow parents into nursery; (2) change rules to allow parents to touch, handle, and possibly feed or diaper baby; (3) make referral for nursing support at home.

Infertility

The couple who have decided to have a child and are unable to conceive will feel frustrated. Their self-concept will be altered and, doubting their sexual potency and fertility, they may begin to search for an answer to their difficulty. An extensive work-up of both partners may or may not uncover the reason for their inability to conceive. Most obstetricians will not do any infertility work-up without the active participation of both partners, but sometimes the husband is reluctant to participate. He may find the possibility of being the cause of the problem more of a threat to his masculine pride than he can face.

During the period of the work-up, the couple need support, and they need to be able to express their feelings and frustrations. If, after the work-up is done no cause is found or the cause is not amenable to treatment, the couple need help in exploring the alternatives open to them: remaining childless, acquiring a child by other means such as *genetic engineering,* or adoption.

Genetic Engineering

Still in the experimental stages are test-tube conceptions with subsequent implantation of the embryo into the uterus of a woman desiring pregnancy. Depending on the problem causing infertility, the ovum and the sperm may or may not be those of the couple desiring parenthood. AIH is artificial insemination with homologous sperm (the husband's). Unfortunately, AIH is usable by fewer couples than is AID (artificial insemination by donor). AID is legal in only about six states; the other states require that the couple adopt the child. The legal restrictions are indicative of the deep feelings and religious-cultural issues generated by the idea of fathering one's own child. The important sense of continuity involved in inheritance from one's own father is also disrupted by AID.

Assessment of a couple considering AID should particularly emphasize (1) physical examination for infertility; (2) the couple's reasons for wanting AID; (3) their feelings about it; (4) their knowledge of the legal implications of adoption, divorce, inheritance, etc; and (5) other common assessment factors as indicated (see "Common Assessment Factors" and Table 32-1).

After diagnosis and goals have been established, the intervention needed will become clear. Counseling sessions may be numerous, and perhaps each partner may need to be seen alone. After conception, counseling is continued to enable the couple to work through their feelings. This helps them to sort out the normal feelings of pregnancy from any remaining misgivings about AID.

Resources to obtain AIH and AID are infertility clinics and private doctors' offices.

Adoption

Since 1960, adoption has been more widely discussed. Couples who can have their own children are looking to adoption in order to keep population growth down. During the same period, the number of young, healthy infants available for adoption has decreased. This decrease is a result of the pill, abortion, and the fact that unwed mothers are increasingly choosing to keep their babies. Available children tend to be older, of mixed racial backgrounds, or handicapped. In addition to couples looking for children to adopt, there has been an increase in single persons who want to adopt. The changing values and expectations of society have opened this possibility. Society has become more willing to allow individuals to choose unique life patterns.

The adoptive process may be a long one with a sudden climax. If the couple apply for adoption through an agency, there is usually an exploratory interview in which the process is explained and the motivation for adoption is probed. Then the couple or individual may have a series of in-depth interviews in which motivation for adoption, family health, income, life-style, relationship with others, and life goals are probed. Home visits are part of this procedure. If the prospective parents are approved, there is still a waiting period before a child is placed with them. If an infant is desired, the wait may extend to several years. When a child is suddenly available, the parents may have only 1 or 2 days to gather necessary equipment. The agency will supervise the placement before the adoption is final.

After the adoption proceedings, the parents are usually left to cope with the new family member on their own. They face the same difficulties as biological parents do, plus some that are unique to adoption. They will go through the same process of attachment as natural parents, but it may be prolonged by some feelings of ambivalence about the adoption.

One task of the family is telling the child that he or she is adopted. There is general agreement that the child should be told and that the telling should be done by the parents. The question of what is the best age to tell the child is open to discussion. The young child has active fantasies and little vocabulary with which to discuss his or her feelings. On the other hand, the longer one waits, the greater the likelihood that the child will get the facts from another source. The parents need to hear all the pros and cons of each age and to be supported in their decision about the best time at which to tell their child. The revelation should be as matter-of-fact as possible, and the explanation will need to be repeated as the child grows older. The young child may be confused by the concept of two mothers; another term, such as "lady," may be used for the biological mother.

Another task of the adoptive family is to help the adoptee to develop his or her identity. This may include the adoptee's need to know more about the biological family and possibly to meet the biological parents. The adoptive parents may feel threatened by this search for identity and may fear they will lose the child. They need to be helped to see that this search is normal and nonthreatening and that, if it is handled well, it may tighten the adoptive parent-child relationship.

The nursing practitioner usually does not become involved with the family until after the adoption. The family may then request advice on routine health maintenance or want to discuss a seeming difficulty. These families are at greater risk for mental health problems because of the adoption; the parents may need help in distinguishing problems which are unique to adoption from those which are developmental in origin.

Some adoptive parents may be insecure. This is almost the only group of parents who need someone else to approve their parenthood. A larger number of adopted children than one would normally expect appear on mental health clinic rolls. This may be a result of the insecurity of adoptive parents or of the need to sort out developmental problems. Some parents may fear that the behavior is a result of the "bad" genes of the biological parents. These parents need counseling to sort out the behaviors and to recognize normal growth and development (see Chap. 5). Sometimes the behavior of the child is a result of the parents' anxiety.

The nurse working with these families should assess their strengths and weaknesses. The strengths can then be enhanced by counseling. The nursing diagnoses and goals can be agreed upon with the family. Home visiting may be an excellent way to assess the family's natural functioning and to give direct assistance in parent education. Many of these parents would benefit from attending either classes in infant and child care or parent-effectiveness training groups with older children (see Chap. 33).

Potential Problems in Parenting
Single Parents

The term "parents without partners" has become a familiar one for divorced or widowed people who are trying to be parents without the support of husband or wife. With the rising divorce and marriage dissolution rate, there has also come a continued drop in the marriage rate and an increase in the number of people 25 to 34 years of age who have never married. So, in addition to the formerly married, the ranks of single parents also include the never marrieds, both young and mature, who are bringing up children alone. Together

they account for a drop of almost 5 percent in 5 years in the number of children under 18 living with both parents. In New York City alone there are 212,000 recorded single-parent families.[15]

To begin assessing the needs of these families, nurses need to be aware of their own feelings about divorce, illegitimate children, homosexual parents, or single adoptive parents. Nurses may find that their feelings are different for each group. These feelings need to be sorted out and acknowledged.

While the assessment of the single-parent family should include all the common assessment factors previously cited, special emphasis needs to be placed on (1) the support systems available to the single parent; (2) the use of the support in the extended family or kin network as well as financial support; and (3) the potential effect of single parenthood on the individual involved. This includes assessment of such factors as the child's feelings, growth, and development. The diagnosis, to be useful, should pinpoint the areas where the parent and/or the child is presently coping or not coping well or can be predicted to have difficulties in the future. For example, the parent may need job training, child-care facilities, or a consistent base of support.

Direct support may be most helpful when it comes from a group of adults in similar positions. Resources such as Parents Without Partners or the Single Parent Family Project (SPFP, sponsored by the Community Service Society of New York City) are available.[15] The SPFP not only refers parents to needed services and to single-parent discussion groups but also helps clients organize to meet their own needs in the areas of health insurance, day care, and housing. There are also newly created centers for the widowed. The unwed teenage mother can sometimes find assistance from the continuing services of her high school's division for unwed mothers.

Working Mothers

Mothers are increasingly working outside the home for reasons ranging from economic necessity to self-fulfillment. The child-development litera-ture of the 1950s and 1960s suggested that a large quantity of continuous mothering by the mother was necessary for the normal development of the child. More recently, however, evidence has been pointing to the fact that it is the quality rather than the quantity of parenting that is important.

Quality parenting can generally be described as that behavior of the parents which promotes the healthy growth and development of the child, leading him or her to grow into a responsible and happy adult. Among the factors which contribute to quality parenting are the mother's emotional state, agreement between parents, stable care arrange-ments, a stable family, and a basically flexible personality in the child.

Hoffman and Nye feel that the mother's emo-tional state is the key factor. If she works willingly or stays home willingly, there is little or no negative effect on the child. The one who suffers is the child whose mother is doing what she does not want to do.[16] Chess and Thomas suggest that the only child who may have difficulty in adjusting to a working mother is the child who has difficulty in adjusting to any change.[17] Another important fac-tor is consensus among marital partners as to whether the wife will work and, if she does, how the household chores will be handled. If, tired from work, she is too busy with household chores to have time for the children, they may then suffer. This is of special concern to the working mother who is also a single parent.

The main nursing role with the working mother may be to provide anticipatory guidance and to help her sort out her feelings about working. Why is she working? How does she feel about it? The nurse also needs to help the mother assess the adequacy of the care arrangement. The nurse may have to interpret the latest findings to the mother and serve as a parent advocate to the community at large. The nurse also works for the establish-ment of adequate child-care facilities in the com-munity, whether in private homes or in day-care centers. She may be involved in the assessment of children at the centers. If a difficulty is found,

possible causes beyond the fact of the mother's working should be explored.

Foster Care

"Foster care" refers to the placement of a child in a home for "board and care," usually by a state welfare commission or by a recognized social agency. Placement is usually made because of a problem such as death, illness, incompetence, or lack of sufficient support in the natural family. The placement is usually regarded as temporary, with the placing agency retaining the right to remove the child when it sees fit. The temporary nature of this arrangement frequently leads the child to have problems in developing intimate child-adult rela-tionships. The adults in the situation are often reluctant to develop any deep emotional commit-ment to the child. The foster child feels the imper-manence and insecurity of this arrangement, which clashes with the need for emotional consis-tency. The child may also have feelings of aban-donment and guilt, feeling that placement is a form of punishment for something bad that he or she has done.[18]

The assessment of the situation requires a careful evaluation of the effects of foster care on the child (see Table 32-6).

Currently, there is increasing pressure for strengthening the child's right to be permanently adopted if the biological parent displays only minimal interest. In some states, one postcard a year from parent to child is sufficient to prevent permanent adoption. The parent need not ever visit the child. Such a relationship over a long period of time is hardly beneficial to the mental health of the foster child.

Stepparents

Stepparents have neither a biological nor a legal relationship to the children of their spouse. Howev-er, there develops an emotional relationship which may be positive or negative.

The difficulty of the stepparent role may be

Table 32-6 Foster Care: Its Effects on the Child

Assessment factor	Nursing diagnosis	Intervention
Reason for placement.	Placement should be continued.	Support, communicate strengths of placement.
	Placement should be terminated.	Explore change, pinpoint obstacles to continuation of placement.
Child's current communications with biological parent, foster parent, extended family peers.	Open, effective communication.	Support open communication.
	Poor, absent communication.	Assess, diagnose, intervene to improve communication.
Task of period stage of growth and development.	Child is at or ahead of appropriate stage.	Support, identify strengths of child, provide anticipatory guidance.
	Developmental lag observed in child.	Identify developmental lag, plan intervention (see Chap. 33).
Child's and parent's knowledge of placement.	Child and parents have accurate information about placement.	Support knowledge.
	Child and parents do not have accurate information about placement.	Explore information sources.
Support systems present.	Systems are sufficient (i.e., family is nearby and willing to help).	None.
	Systems are insufficient (i.e., family is unable to help).	Explore and counsel.
How support systems are used.	Systems used effectively (i.e. help when needed).	None.
	Systems are not used effectively.	Interview supporting people.
Future prognosis of child placement.	Parent has improved quality or maintained high parenting.	Support positive parenting change.
	Parenting patterns not improved by placement.	Consider changes in permanent parenting arrangements.

due to the fact that the stepparent is usually living with one of the biological parents.[19] Thus, unlike the biological or adoptive parent, the stepparent does not necessarily share the other parent's influence over the child. The opinions of the stepparent are often seen as opposed to those of the biological parent. However, in most cases a balance is worked out.

Families in which a balance has developed between stepparent and child usually do not come to the attention of the nurse. Those families with a diagnosis of family dysfunction will usually come to the attention of health and welfare services.

Factors which are particularly relevant to assessing stepparent relationships are (1) the reasons the stepparent relationship was formed, (2) the adequacy of knowledge about parenting and growth and development, (3) impact of change on family relationships, (4) the way the stepparent is defining the relationship, (5) roles the absent biological parent plays in relationship to the child, (6) decision for the arrangement and how it was made,

(7) whether there are siblings separated between two households, (8) presence of stepsiblings and their ages, and (9) relationships among parents and children.

References

1 Erik Erikson: *Childhood and Society,* Norton, New York, 1963.

2 Augustus Napier: "The Marriage of Families: Cross Generational Complementarity," *Family Process,* vol. 10, pp. 373 and 394, 1971.

3 Don Jackson: "Family Rules," *Archives of General Psychiatry,* vol. 12, p. 589, June 1965.

4 Jay Haley: *Strategies of Psychotherapy,* Grune & Stratton, New York, 1963.

5 "Psychiatric Sequelae to Term Birth and Induced Early and Late Abortion," *Family Planning Perspectives,* Fall 1973, p. 13.

6 Nadine Brozan: "New Childbirth Centers: Baby Born in Morning Was Home by Evening," *The New York Times,* March 27, 1976, p. 30.

7 Arthur Colman and Libby Colman: *Pregnancy: the Psychological Experience,* Herder & Herder, New York, 1971.

8 Mary Lou Moore: *The Newborn and the Nurse,* Monographs in Clinical Nursing, no. 3, Saunders, Philadelphia, 1972.

9 Gerald Caplan: *Concepts of Mental Health and Consultation,* Children's Bureau, U.S. Department of Health, Education, and Welfare, 1959.

10 Frederick LeBoyer: *Birth without Violence,* Knopf, New York, 1975.

*11 Reva Rubin: "Puerperal Change," *Nursing Outlook,* vol. 9, no. 12, December 1961.

12 Martin Greenberg and Norman Morris: "Engrossment: The Newborn's Impact Upon the Father," *American Journal of Orthopsychiatry,* vol, 44, pp. 520–531, 1974.

*13 Chloe Hammons: "The Adoptive Family," The American Journal of Nursing, vol. 76, no. 2, pp. 251–257, February 1976.

14 Betty Jean Lifton: *Twice Born: Memoirs of An Adopted Daughter,* McGraw-Hill, New York, 1975.

15 Jean Forest, Coordinator of Single Parent Center, Community Service Society, 105 East 22 St., New York, N.Y. 10010. Personal correspondence.

16 Louis Hoffman and Ivan F. Nye: *Working Mothers: An Evaluative Review of the Consequences for Wife, Husband, and Child,* Jossey-Bass, San Francisco, 1974.

17 Stella Chess, Thomas Alexander, and Herbert Birch: *Your Child Is a Person,* Viking, New York, 1965.

18 Freud, Anna, Joseph Goldstein, Albert Solnit: *Beyond the Best Interests of the Child,* Free Press, New York, 1973.

19 Maddox, Brenda: *The Half-Parent: Living with Other People's Children,* M. Evans, New York, 1975.

*Recommended reference by a nurse author.

33

Secondary Prevention in Families with Infants and Children

Jane N. Gorman

Learning Objectives

After studying this chapter, the student should be able to:

1   Recall two major limitations in the delivery of mental health services to children
2   Explain (or give examples of) the two etiologic categories that relate to secondary prevention
3   List at least seven early warning signs of stress for the infant or young child and for the school-age child
4   Describe four components of the family assessment and three components of the child assessment
5   Given case material and the use of Table 33-1, identify problems related to parenting, the family situation, and/or the child's behavior or characteristics and organize the appropriate interventions into a unified treatment plan
6   Outline three steps in the mental health referral process

The Joint Commission on the Mental Health of Children has estimated that 10 to 12 percent (approximately 10 million) of those under 25 years of age are in need of mental health services. However, only about 5 to 7 percent (approximately $\frac{1}{2}$ million) of the children who need mental health care are being served.[1]

The kinds of services that are needed depend on the causes or characteristics of the emotional and mental disorders found in the population. The Joint Commission reported five categories of problems that are considered to play a role in the genesis of emotional and mental disorders:

1 Faulty training and faulty life experiences
2 Surface conflicts between children and parents which arise from such adjustment tasks as relations among siblings, school, social and sexual development
3 Deeper conflicts which become internalized within the self and create emotional conflicts within the child (the neuroses)
4 Difficulties associated with physical handicaps and disorders
5 Difficulties associated with severe mental disorders such as the psychoses, severe mental retardation, etc.[1]

Of the children who need treatment, 80 percent suffer from emotional disorders related to the first two categories. These children, whose problems are less severe, can generally receive sufficient help from a variety of people who work with them, including public health and school nurses.[1] It is this group that is the focus for secondary prevention.

Of those whose disorders are related to the remaining categories, 10 percent show deeper conflicts (category 3) and need help ranging from outpatient services to residential care; 5 percent show physical handicaps (category 4) and require specialized facilities and intensive care; and 5 percent suffer severe mental disorders (category 5) and require more intensive care, often institutionalization.[1] The tertiary level of prevention is applicable to these categories.

Limitations in the Delivery of Services

There are two major limitations in the delivery of mental health services to children. As already mentioned, the existing mental health services are reaching only 7 percent of the identified population in need.

The other major limitation in services is the neglect of the group aged 3 years old and under. Many children disappear from professional surveillance during the period from birth to entry into school or preschool programs. The various mental health disciplines have not focused training on the assessment and treatment of children who suffer from emotional disorder in the first years of life, and families do not take advantage of existing services. Yet the first 3 years of life are the most crucial in the life of a child. The foundations of development in all areas—physical, intellectual, language, emotional, social—are laid down at this time; likewise, barriers to normal development can be erected during this period. The effects of such early emotional and experiential deprivation can be seen in much later periods.[2,3]

Children under 3 are rarely exposed to responsible adult observation outside the family. Since all children do not attend preschool programs, society has no clear responsibility for the child until he or she reaches school age. Consequently many problems of development go unnoticed until the child enters school. By this time the maladjustment patterns may be deeply entrenched and difficult to treat.[1,2]

Assessment

The goal of secondary prevention is to provide remediation of mild, early behavioral manifestations of maladaptation. Early case finding is essential to meet this goal. As members of the health team, nurses are in contact with infants, children, and parents throughout the developmental cycle. Although specific forms of treatment may be provided by professionals·with specialized psychiatric training, the opportunity for early case finding and intervention is associated primarily with nonpsychiatric roles, such as public health, school, and pediatric nursing.

Settings for Case Finding

The main settings for early case finding are prenatal and postpartum services, well-child and pediatric outpatient services, pediatric inpatient services, homes, nursery and elementary schools, and adult mental health services.

In the prenatal period, assessment of expectant parents' resources, needs, and limitations in assuming the parental role should begin. Observations of parental responses and handling of the newborn at the time of delivery and during the early postpartum period provide valuable data for planning immediate intervention or referral for follow-up. Continuity of care from delivery through the initial parent-infant adjustment phase, particularly in the first 3 weeks, is important to establish professional availability during a time when help is most frequently needed.[4] The well-being of the mother has profound significance for the well-being of the infant and for the formation of a strong mother-infant bond. If adequate support is not being provided for the new mother by family members or friends, the mother's needs should be assessed and appropriate interventions carried out (see Chap. 32). Nursing visits to homes provide a unique opportunity for early case finding and intervention, and this setting has potential for reaching the neglected group below age 3.

Health professionals in outpatient and inpatient pediatric settings should be alert to the early warning signs of stress (see the section entitled "Selected Client Behaviors" in this chapter) and to difficulties or distress experienced by parents.

As mentioned earlier, nursery and elementary schools are usually the first settings in which children are exposed to responsible adult observation outside the family. Health professionals can observe children directly, or they may function as consultants to teachers for early case finding among the school population.

Adults who receive mental health services may also be parents and, if so, assessment of parenting adequacy should be made on behalf of their children. Children are considered at risk if their parents are mentally ill, alcohol or drug abusers, or mentally retarded.[5,6] In addition, a family crisis, financial problems, poor living conditions, a pending divorce or separation, or other disruptions of family functioning may lead to a handicapping home environment for children.

Family Assessment

Family assessment based on the current functioning of the family includes information about current stressors, needs, and problems as well as current resources and strengths (see Chap. 5). Inquiry into the following areas will provide a picture of the current functioning of the family: the current situation, the family constellation and roles, the history of problem solving and coping with stress in the family, and parenting knowledge and skill.

Assessment of the current situation of the family includes obtaining information related to the economic and living conditions of the family, the health status of each family member, recent or impending stressful events or major life changes, and the family's perception of the current family problem.

Data on the family constellation include the name, age, and sex of all persons in the living unit, persons temporarily out of the living unit, and persons who exert influence on or provide support to the family. Identification of the person or persons who fill the following roles should be made: economic provider, primary parenting figure, support person for the primary parenting figure, marital-type relationship for each adult, adult emotional support relationship for each child, and peer support relationships among the children. Among the support relationships, the absence of a support person for the primary parenting figure is the most detrimental for effective parenting;[7] and the absence of an emotionally supportive adult for a given child is the most damaging for the well-being of that child.

The history of previous problem-solving experiences and ways of coping with stress in the family provides information about family strengths, weaknesses, and stability. Important areas to cover concern the early marital history and the parental adaptation to the first child.[8] The health history of each pregnancy, the parents' response to each baby, and the sibling adjustment to each new baby are factors in the resolution of common maturational crises faced by most families. Other life crises that may have occurred are family illness, parental disharmony, unemployment, home disasters, and death in the family (see Chap. 5).

The assessment of parenting knowledge and skill is useful in planning intervention, since treatment frequently consists of imparting and demonstrating healthy and effective child-rearing patterns.[9] (See Chap. 32.) Ideally, parents should have basic knowledge of the needs of children as they progress through the developmental cycle. For example, the curiosity drive of an infant or small child leads to exploratory behavior that can be bothersome to parents; yet an absence or curtailing of opportunities for exploration and manipulation of the environment is detrimental to the intellectual development of the child. In addition to understanding the needs of children, parents should be able to tolerate—and, one hopes, enjoy—the child's unfolding behavior in order to perceive needs accurately and to respond positively.

Other important elements of successful parenting are the use of age-appropriate child-rearing techniques, for example, setting limits appropriate to the child's developmental gains; general parental agreement and consistency in child-rearing attitudes and practices; and the sharing of responsibility and provision of mutual support between parents.[10]

Parents' expectations for their child may not be appropriate for the child's actual behavior, temperament, or potential. Unrealistic or inappropriate expectations interfere with the parents' selection of age-appropriate child-rearing techniques and can contribute to disagreement and inconsistency in the handling of conflict or areas of difficulty (see Chap. 36).

In summary, the identification of difficulties in parenting includes: (1) identification of gaps in the parents' understanding of child development and needs; (2) identification of limitations in the parents' understanding of age-appropriate child-rearing techniques; (3) identification of limitations in the parents' ability to recognize or discriminate among needs, to meet needs or tolerate behavior, or to use specific child-rearing skills effectively; (4) identification of incongruities between parents' expectations and the child's actual characteristics; (5) identification of areas of inconsistent discipline or handling of behavior by parents; and (6) identification of areas of conflicting child-rearing attitudes and practices between parents.

Parenting may also be interfered with by situational factors such as unfilled role functions in the family, family crisis, marital disharmony, neurotic needs of parents (see the section entitled "Psychodynamics/Family Dynamics" in this chapter), or severely dysfunctional family patterns (see Chaps. 11 and 34).

Child Assessment

Assessment of the child for early intervention differs from both screening and a comprehensive psychiatric examination. Deeper in scope than screening, this assessment seeks to determine the developmental level attained by the child and to identify problems that may interfere with the development of sensorimotor, language, or psychosocial skills. Unlike a comprehensive psychiatric examination, assessment does not explore or evaluate the intrapsychic levels of functioning. The elements of the assessment include developmental testing, interviewing of parents, and observations of the child in a variety of settings.

Developmental Testing

The current developmental level of an infant or young child is assessed through standardized testing procedures. Several developmental tests exist, each measuring development in four main areas: gross motor abilities (integration of the CNS and the musculoskeletal system), communication skills (comprehension, expression, hearing, and speech), fine motor skills (eye-hand coordination), and personal-social behavior (self-care and interaction with others).[11] The Denver Developmental Screening Test[12,13] is the most widely known by nurses; it is also familiar to pediatricians, social workers, and psychologists.

The Denver Developmental Screening Test is used for detecting developmental delays during infancy and the preschool years. As with any testing, one must bear in mind that the results can be influenced by the rapport established by the examiner and by factors related to the child's psychosocial environment.[14,15] A brief description of the administration and scoring of the test is found in DeAngelis.[15]

Testing of the school-age child frequently consists of evaluating problems in learning. Emotional problems are usually associated with impaired school achievement; but in the cases in which specific learning disabilities (e.g., impaired visual or auditory memory) are found, the emotional problems are secondary. To gain a comprehensive picture of the child's learning difficulties, a battery of tests is selected that is sensitive to the child's overt problem areas.[16] This testing is usually done by a clinical psychologist or an educational specialist.

Parent Interview

Parent interviews cover three main areas: the parents' perception of the child's current functioning, the child's developmental history, and the child's history of previous episodes of behavioral difficulty or difficult life experiences.

In the interview the parents are encouraged to describe their perceptions of the child's current behavior and adjustment. From this discussion, one can learn whether or not the parents feel there is a problem; if so, how severe they feel it is; and whether they have considered or sought help.

To gain a picture of the child's previous progression of development, a brief history is useful. The developmental landmarks that parents can usually report are holding head up, sitting without support, crawling, saying "Dada" or "Mama," walking alone, using short sentences, and achieving bowel and bladder control. Although the parents' memory of the actual months of occurrence of these developmental landmarks may not be accurate, one can get an estimate of their occurrence and of the parents' ideas about the appropriateness of the time of occurrence.

In addition to information about sensorimotor and language development, inquiry about interpersonal behavior provides information about the child's psychosocial development. Some of the psychosocial adjustment tasks the parents should be asked about involve separation from mother, sibling rivalry, socialization with peers, and adjustment to school.

Possible relationships of current behavioral and adjustment problems to the child's past development and experiences can be discovered by inquiring about previous areas or episodes of difficulty with troublesome or inadequate behavior or the occurrence of difficult life experiences (e.g., hospitalization or major illness, separation from mother during infancy or early childhood). Sometimes a current problem behavior first occurred during a difficult life experience, and through secondary gain the behavior persisted as a habit. (See the section entitled "Psychodynamics/Family Dynamics" in this chapter.)

Observations of the Child

Observations of the child at home, at school, in a play situation, and interacting with peers can provide data about the child's relationships with parents, other family members, peers, and teachers; the child's play and exploratory behavior; the child's presentation of self (e.g., hostile, aggressive, withdrawn, shy); and the child's characteristic mood. Observations over a period of time are helpful to distinguish between enduring behavioral characteristics and transitory reactions.

From the testing, interview, and observations one can identify problems related to (1) specific developmental lags or learning disabilities, (2) difficulties in the mastery of psychosocial adjustment tasks, (3) problem behavior which has become established as a habit, or (4) difficulties in relationships.

Vulnerability/Trauma Risk Factors

Children are considered at risk because of certain vulnerabilities that they possess or because they have been exposed to traumatic situations. Factors potentially contributing to risk are genetic (e.g., familial schizophrenia), reproductive (e.g., prematurity), constitutional (e.g., temperamental type), developmental (e.g., medical problems at a given stage), physical health (e.g., acute or chronic illness), environmental (e.g., psychotic parent), or traumatic (e.g., physical abuse, separation from mother).[5]

"Difficult" Child Syndrome

Thomas, Chess, and Birch have identified a type of vulnerable child they labeled the *difficult temperamental type*. Such a child is characterized from early infancy onward by irregularity in bodily functions (e.g., unpredictable sleeping and feeding schedules), high intensity of reactions or responses, a tendency to withdraw in the face of new stimuli, slow adaptability to changes in the environment, and negative mood. "Difficult" children comprised 10 percent of the study sample. Approximately 70 percent of the children with the "difficult" temperamental cluster developed behavior problems, in contrast to 18 percent of the "easy" children.[17]

However, when parents can maintain consistent approaches based on an objective view of the child's reaction patterns, the child is able to adapt slowly to step-by-step demands for normal socialization.[17] Thus, these children require a high degree of consistency and tolerance in their upbringing; their parents may need help in defining and understanding the child's special needs as well as support in handling the day-to-day behavior.

Cumulative Stress from Major Life Events

The death of a parent is a major life event that is clearly traumatic for a child. What is less frequently considered is the cumulative stress from a number of life events or changes. Coddington developed a life-events questionnaire and scoring system for children.[18,19] Examples of high-ranking life events for preschool or elementary-school-age children are death, divorce, or marital separation of parents; jail sentence of parent for a year or more; marriage of parent to stepparent; death of a brother or sister; serious illness requiring hospitalization of the child; acquiring a visible deformity; serious illness requiring hospitalization of a parent; birth of a brother or sister; and mother accepting full-time employment outside the home.[18]

The frequency or severity of stress from major life events determines the amount of readjustment required by the child. With increased levels of stress from recent life events, more time is required to accomplish readjustment. A few high-stress events or several lower-stress events occurring within a single year may overload the child's capacity to adjust to the changes. In a study of the significance of life events as etiologic factors in the diseases of children, the research team found that, compared to normal children, 2 to 3 times as many children in each patient group (rheumatoid arthritis, general pediatric hospitalization, surgical patients, and psychiatric patients) had an overload of stress from life events prior to the onset of the disease.[20]

Children's responses to change and their ability to readjust are influenced by their strengths, weaknesses, and resources. For example, a child characterized by a "difficult" temperament would be likely to respond with great intensity and to adjust quite slowly to life events or changes. A child who has emotional support during the period of readjustment to major life events is more likely to have a favorable outcome.

Selected Client Behaviors: Early Warning Signs of Stress

The client behaviors of concern in the secondary level of prevention are those that indicate mild, early manifestations of maladaptation. Because crystallized and circumscribed symptom pictures are unusual in very young children, the Joint Commission on Mental Health of Children has identified early warning signs of stress. From infancy through age 5, these are:

1 Disturbances in eating, elimination, and sleeping: too much or too little food intake and sleep, disturbances in cycles of tension and relaxation, appetitive disturbances (food avoidances, ingestion of nonedibles, pica), conflicts with parents around these areas
2 Delayed or disordered growth: poor weight gain, retarded skeletal growth, and failure to thrive, which may occur even when food intake is adequate
3 Specific organ-system symptoms: vomiting, rumination, poor absorption of food, diarrhea, constipation, skin rashes, wheezing and rhinoarrhea, etc.
4 Delayed acquisition or deviant nature of specific developmental steps: motor skill and activity, control over sphincters, communication (verbal and nonverbal), and intellectual growth
5 Delayed or disturbed relationships with others
6 Loss of previously acquired skills or regression in levels of psychosocial organization
7 Disturbances in the capacity to play
8 Accident proneness
9 Fears of familiar and new situations, doubts about one's own capacity for mastery
10 Mood disturbances: overreaction to minor stress, sadness, prolonged anger, lack of tolerance for frustration, etc.[2]

Berlin outlined the following early warning signs for the young school-age child:

1 Difficulty in separating from mother to go to school
2 So-called school phobia (refusal to attend school)
3 Temper tantrums

4 Marked isolation
5 Asocial, hostile, and impulsive behavior
6 Inability to relate to teachers or classmates
7 Problems in learning[21]

Three additional signs of stress for school-age children identified by Bower are:

1 Inappropriate types of behavior or feelings under normal conditions
2 A general, pervasive mood of unhappiness or depression
3 A tendency to develop physical symptoms, pains, or fears associated with personal or school problems[22]

The early warning signs of stress indicate that the infant or child's adaptive equilibrium is altered; however, the nature of the stress must be determined by further assessment of the child and the family. One must also determine whether the difficulty is transitory, within the range of individual differences, or an early manifestation of maladaptation.

Three factors to be considered in weighing the significance of early warning signs are the *extent* or severity of the behavior, the *duration* of the behavior, and the *number* of early warning signs present. If any one sign is manifested to a great extent or has persisted over a long period of time, further assessment of the child and family is indicated. Likewise, if more than one early warning sign is present, further assessment is needed.

Psychodynamics/Family Dynamics

At the beginning of this chapter, five etiologic categories of emotional and mental disorders were presented. The two categories that pertain to the secondary level of prevention are faulty training or life experiences and surface conflicts between children and parents around adjustment tasks. Faulty training can result from unclear or contradictory expectations, inconsistent discipline, reinforcement of undesirable or developmentally unproductive behavior, or the lack of reinforcement for positive or developmentally appropriate behavior. Faulty or inadequate life experiences can block the child's achievement of developmental tasks because of unmet developmental needs; for example, the lack of a continuous relationship during infancy can interfere with the development of trust and the ability to form normal attachments.

Externalized situational conflicts—such as difficulties with siblings, school, or parent-child relations—may not be easily distinguished from deeper, internalized conflicts (neuroses) initially. The persistence of symptoms, despite the efforts of the child and others to change them, is a cardinal clue to intrapsychic conflicts.[23] Thus, if the first line of intervention (i.e., problem-focused intervention) fails to bring about a change in the problem behavior, the possibility is that deeper conflicts are involved. Likewise, with problems in parenting, if problem-focused interventions are not successful, the possibility exists that the parents' practices are sustained by their own neurotic needs.[9] It is also possible that problem behavior manifested by an infant or child can be detected early enough for secondary prevention but that the problems interfering with parenting are longstanding and require more intensive or prolonged treatment.

In assessing problem behavior in a child, another distinction to be made is between the original factors related to the *development* of the maladaptive behavior and ongoing factors related to the *maintenance* of the behavior. For example, a child might have begun to show clinging, dependent behavior at age 3, when displaced by a sibling, but—long after the original situation has been mastered—the behavior continued because it was rewarded, either positively or negatively. Parents are often unaware that negative reinforcement, such as excessive criticism, can maintain the very behavior it seeks to suppress.

Nurses's Response to Child and Family

The nurse who is relating to children with behavioral manifestations of maladaptation should be sensitive to the children's feelings or concerns about their adequacy, differentness, problems, or special situations. Although infants and very young children may not be aware of their standing in relation to other children, older children are often acutely aware of being singled out. Professionals should avoid talking about children in front of them or their peers. On the other hand, it is appropriate for nurses to point out that they are interested in the child, aware of his or her special needs, and available for support or help.

In working with the family, the nurse should avoid taking a critical stance but instead attempt to establish a relationship of collaboration in problem solving and intervention. Even in the case of referral, a positive rapport with the family is important to ensure cooperation in following the referral and acceptance of the referral agency by the family.[24]

Nurses may have to deal with their own feelings of anger or frustration when they identify limitations in the care and handling of children. In extreme cases, in which the home environment is severely handicapping for the child, prompt intervention on behalf of the child's basic needs or safety is required (see Chap. 36); however, in most cases the nurse should be aware that parenthood is an enormous task. The Joint Commission report stated: "In our complex, demanding, and fragmented society, it has become more and more difficult to be an effective parent, whatever the family's socioeconomic status."[2] Most parents are trying to do the best job with their children that they can, and they are often aware of their shortcomings. Thus, support and understanding are essential in establishing a trusting and receptive relationship with the family.

Assessment of Environmental Factors

The delivery of mental health services to children and families occurs in the context of a larger environment. Both families and providers are affected by economic, social, and cultural factors.

For example, in a study of the treatment of psychological disorders among urban children, less than 50 percent of the seriously impaired children were referred; however, referral rates were sharply higher among more educated mothers.[25]

In terms of availability of services, economic factors greatly affect the lower-income working families who are not eligible for medical assistance. Many health-insurance plans do not provide adequate coverage for psychiatric services, and there are not enough low-cost programs to meet the needs.

Maternal employment is another major economic factor affecting the mental health of children. One-fourth of the mothers of infants and toddlers, one-third of the mothers of 3- to 5-year-olds, and one-half of the mothers of 6- to 17-year-olds are employed.[26] Many of these children are inadequately cared for while their mothers work, and many child-care arrangements lack the stability that children, particularly those under 3 years of age, need. The younger the children, the more they are dependent upon a consistent and continuous relationship with one person.[2] Thus an important area to assess in families with a working mother is the adequacy of the child care that is provided. For an infant it is, of course, important to establish continuity, but the caretaker must also be willing to enter into a responsive, nonrejecting, and stimulating relationship with the infant.[27]

Social factors that affect the behavior of clients and providers are changing family patterns, sex roles, and life-styles. Many recent changes in family-life patterns call for the reinterpretation of assumptions about the nuclear family. Only approximately 40 percent of the United States population lives in the traditional nuclear family.[26] The divorce rate in this country increased 135 percent between 1962 and 1974. In 1974 more than a million children below the age of 18 were affected by divorce.[28]

Just as the providers of mental health care cannot assume that the intact family is necessarily normal or healthy, one cannot assume that the single-parent family is dysfunctional. In either case, an objective assessment of family resources

and functioning is needed. Likewise, changing patterns of child care within the family must be evaluated as they relate to children's needs rather than to traditional roles.

Cultural factors influence communication and interaction between clients and providers in several ways. Cultural differences exist in values concerning behavior, attitudes and practices of child rearing, and patterns of using outside help for problems. Although families and subcultural groups have the right to hold differing child-rearing attitudes and philosophies, some basic principles of effective child rearing transcend these values. For example, whether the family values conformity or creativity, a child still needs clear, unambiguous messages about what kind of behavior is expected. The developmental stage of a child should be considered in determining expected standards or levels of behavior at specific ages.

Nurses and other health-care providers should be aware of their own values and their feelings about various child-rearing attitudes and practices. When these practices are harmful (e.g., excessively punitive or rejecting), professionals must be prepared to intervene; however, where attitudes and practices are merely different from one's own, one should attempt to convey acceptance and understanding so as to facilitate a collaborative relationship with the family. Consultation with a professional from the client's subculture can be used to gain information about cultural patterns and viewpoints as well as insight into the family's needs and behavior.

Application of the Nursing Process in Secondary Prevention

Assessment of the family and the child provides information about the significance, and possibly the origins, of the early warning signs of stress or problem behavior exhibited by the child. This information is useful in determining the most effective level in the system for intervention, i.e., focus on the parenting, on the family situation, or on the

Table 33-1 Guide to Treatment Planning for Early Signs of Stress or Problem Behavior in Infants and Children (Secondary Prevention Level)

Nursing diagnosis	Interventions
Parenting	
Insufficient knowledge or understanding of child development and needs.	Parent education classes; individual counseling.
Insufficient knowledge or understanding of age-appropriate child-rearing techniques.	Parent education classes; individual counseling.
Inability to assume an appropriate parenting role in relation to the child's needs.	
Inability to recognize or discriminate among needs.	Assist with problem solving; provide an effective parenting role model; provide supervision and validation.
Inability to meet needs or tolerate behavior.	Provide support to parents, assist parents to express feelings about parenthood and about the child; make use of community resources for support (e.g., day care).
Inability to use specific child-rearing skills effectively (e.g., limit setting).	Provide general rationale and principles, demonstrate appropriate use of skill, discuss outcome of parents' attempts.
Inappropriate expectations for child.	Assist parents to become aware of expectations and feelings about child, correct misconceptions about child development and needs, assist parents to accept child.
Inconsistency in handling behavior.	Assist parents to identify unclear or contradictory cues for behavior, to establish clear expectations and rules, and to set and enforce appropriate limits.
Conflicts between parents in child-rearing attitudes and practices.	Assist parents to identify areas of conflict, to explore feelings, and to resolve conflicts; assist parents to share responsibility for child rearing and to provide mutual support.
Family situation	
Lack of support for the primary parenting figure.	Reinvolve withdrawn family member to fill the support role; establish alternate source of support.
Lack of adequate or stable adult emotional support relationship for child.	Assist parent or family member to support; provide a corrective relationship (e.g., foster grandparent).
Family in crisis.	Crisis intervention.
Marital disharmony interfering with parenting.	Referral for marital therapy.
Neurotic needs interfering with parenting.	Referral for family or individual therapy.
Severely dysfunctional family (e.g., drug addiction, psychotic parent, child abuse or neglect).	Advocacy for the child; referral to appropriate agency for management of family problems.
Child behavior or characteristics	
Significant developmental lag; learning disabilities.	Referral for evaluation by specialist; facilitate entry into specific remedial program if indicated (e.g., infant stimulation, special classes); provide support for child and family.

Table 33-1 Guide to Treatment Planning for Early Signs of Stress or Problem Behavior in Infants and Children (Secondary Prevention Level) (continued)

Nursing diagnosis	Interventions
Difficulty mastering a psychosocial adjustment task (e.g., separation from mother, sibling rivalry).	Assist parents to establish and implement a program for gradual mastery; utilize goal-directed play sessions.
Problem behavior which has become established as a habit.	Assist parents and/or teachers to establish and implement a behavior-modification program.
Inadequate or unsatisfactory peer relationships.	Arrange for group therapy or activity group to foster the development of effective peer-relating skills.
Difficult temperamental type.	Assist parents to cope with infant's irregularity in eating and sleeping patterns, to understand the child's reactions and needs, and to follow appropriate principles of handling; use community resources for support.
Incomplete adaptation to recent major life events.	Provide for a support relationship until adaptation has occurred; use play sessions to allow expression of feelings (e.g., grief, anger, or helplessness over a loss by death or divorce).

child's behavior or characteristics. Problems and interventions related to these levels are outlined in Table 33-1.

Each of the problems can be exhibited to a mild or extreme extent. The clinical example which is described below illustrates several interrelated problems, each present only to a mild extent; nonetheless, the resulting behavioral problems were highly distressing to the family.

Clinical Illustration of Early Case Finding and Intervention

A woman who was receiving public health nursing visits for major health problems had also reported problem behavior with her 4-year-old son, Randy. He had recently become disobedient, inconsiderate, mean to his younger brother, and frequently angry.

The assessment of the child revealed a normal but active boy who could not comfortably comply with the quiet, sedate standards of behavior expected by the mother and successfully met by the older sister. The family assessment indicated that the family was poor and somewhat isolated, but the parents were stable and intelligent. They lived in a third-floor apartment located on a busy urban street, and the three children spent most of their time indoors.

The parents had not had difficulty with Randy during his infancy or toddler period, but as he moved into the heightened activity level characteristic of 4-year-olds, his boisterous behavior became intolerable to his mother. Although this mother had demonstrated effective parenting in many areas, she lacked knowledge of an aspect of the normal developmental needs of a 4-year-old child. She had inappropriate expectations for her son's behavior and could not meet his needs for a broader range of activity and experience.

Because the identified problems affecting parenting were present to a mild degree, the intervention was direct and effective. After allowing the mother to ventilate her feelings of exasperation and failure, the nurse presented relevant developmental information and discussed the concept of individual differences among children in relation to the mother's inappropriate expectations for Randy. The mother readily understood the implications; however, her health problems prevented her from taking Randy to a playground or other setting to meet his needs for increased activity. A nearby, low-cost preschool program was recommended to provide an outlet for Randy's need for more activity through play with other children his own age and to provide some respite for his mother.

Initially Randy was reluctant to separate from his mother, and he held back from interacting with the other children. His mother needed support to continue taking him to the play group at this time, but within a week he had mastered entry into the program. Follow-up evaluation a month later revealed that Randy had come to value the preschool program highly, and his mother reported that his behavior at home was no longer a problem.

Nursing Diagnosis

The problems listed in Table 33-1 are a guide to making the nursing diagnosis or problem list. More than one problem may exist in a given case. Additional family problems may be identified which relate to the health status of family members, economic and living conditions, stressful events or major life changes, or problems with other family members. For example, the major health problems of the mother in the clinical illustration would be included in the family problem list along with the specific problems related to parenting.

A complete problem list, therefore, includes (1) a description of the behavioral indications of stress or disturbance seen in the child; (2) identified problems associated with parenting, the family situation, or the child's behavior or characteristics; and (3) other problems impinging on the family.

Planning Nursing Care

Planning nursing care involves defining behavioral problems, identifying nursing interventions, and specifying goals.

Defining behavioral problems

Depending on the perspective of the person who identifies a child in need of assessment and early intervention, behavioral problems may be stated as signs of stress (see the section entitled "Selected Client Behaviors" in this chapter), troublesome behavior (e.g., bullying, lying), or inadequate behavior (e.g., withdrawal, learning difficulties).

Secondary Prevention and Remediation

Anticipatory guidance is the major intervention used to accomplish goals related to prevention. Parents can be prepared for emerging developmental stages in their children, and children can be prepared for impending life events or changes in the family.

The interventions suggested in Table 33-1 are remedial in nature, but their purpose is also to prevent more complex or additional handicapping problems from developing. Each intervention is specific for an identified problem; however, as problems may be identified in several areas, an integration of the interventions must be made.

Many of the interventions involve several steps in order to deal with both affective and cognitive components. Generally the affective level must be dealt with, at least in part, before clients can use information or engage in problem solving. In dealing with the affective level with parents, the nurse might provide emotional support, help the parents ventilate their feelings, reflect back feelings, clarify conflicting feelings, verbalize certain feelings or thoughts for the parents, or offer gentle confrontation of inconsistencies in attitudes.[23]

The process of establishing rapport and working through the affective and cognitive components of an intervention will usually take several sessions. Four sessions were used in the clinical example: two for ventilation of feelings and problem solving and two for support around beginning the preschool program. Two additional transitory problems arose during the intervention: difficulty separating from mother and difficulty relating to peers.

In addition to interventions for the problems related to parenting, the family situation, or the child's behavior or characteristics, appropriate interventions for the other problems impinging on the family must be planned.

Goals

The major goals of early intervention for the child are to improve the actual condition or behavior; to provide for continued normal development; and to prevent the recurrence or worsening of stressful or problem behavior.[2] Similarly, the goals for the family are to correct the limitations in family functioning, particularly those that affect parenting; to provide for continued normal functioning; and to prevent the recurrence or worsening of problems (see Chap. 11).

Specific treatment goals should be expressed as the remission of problems, and these goals should be described with behavioral criteria. The specific goals in prevention should be expressed in terms of normal development or functioning in light of the child's characteristics and the family situation.

Evaluation Process

In the initial evaluation of the effectiveness of the intervention, data are obtained that relate to the behavioral criteria which were established to indicate a remission of the child's problem behavior or signs of stress. The extent of improvement, lack of improvement, or worsening of the child's adaptation should be described in all areas of the child's functioning, both at home and at school.

Families should be followed up at least once a few months later to determine the effectiveness of the intervention over time and its generalization to other potential problem areas which might have arisen.[29]

Tertiary Prevention

In working toward early case finding, members of the health team may also encounter infants and children who show marked impairment in functioning or whose symptoms do not improve with secondary-level intervention. In these cases, the nurse's role is to facilitate a referral for specialized treatment and to act as a liaison between the family and the referral agency. Before discussing the referral process, criteria for tertiary prevention will be presented (see Chap. 34).

Criteria for Prolonged Treatment or Hospitalization

Tertiary prevention is indicated for an infant who shows numerous signs of disturbance, who has severe physical defects, or whose mother cannot assume an appropriate mothering role.[30] The preschool child who is severely disabled developmentally—with emotional, intellectual, or social defects—should be referred for specialized treatment.[30] Other indicators of the need for referral in the child over 3 are behavior that is dangerous to the child or to others, bizarre behavior, night terrors at age 5, bowel incontinence (daytime regression after control), loss or lack of speech, no personal interaction, or severe separation anxiety (terror)[31] (see Chap. 34).

Additional referral criteria for children are a severely handicapping home environment (e.g., severe marital discord, family disintegration) or seriously disturbed parents; extreme intensity, frequency, or chronicity of the child's symptoms (e.g., marked regression); severe school or learning problems; withdrawal and isolation from social relationships; severe loss or absence of impulse control leading to frequent acting out in the community; and the persistence of problem behavior or signs of stress despite secondary-level intervention[23,30-33] (see Chap. 36).

The Referral Process

Referring a family for mental health services is a complex process involving several elements. The agency selected must be appropriate so that the needs of the family match the services of the agency. The family, however, may not be aware of their need for mental health services, or they may have concerns or misconceptions about mental health care that prevent them from seeking help.[34] Thus a referral involves a preliminary process in which the family is assisted to understand and accept their need for help and given support and encouragement to seek appropriate services.

Three steps have been identified in the preliminary process of bringing about parental cooperation in providing mental health services for children. These steps are (1) acknowledging the reality of their child's emotional disturbance, (2) overcoming their concerns about using mental health services, and (3) dealing with reality issues in seeking and starting these services.[24] Often a series of interviews is necessary to establish rapport and to work through these steps.

In helping the parents to acknowledge the reality of their child's emotional disturbance, the nurse can clarify and support the parents' concerns about their child's behavior and provide information about the seriousness of the problem and the need for prompt intervention. If the parents are unaware of their child's symptoms or if they distort or minimize the significance of the distress signals, they may be using denial to avoid accepting the reality of their child's problem. These parents need help to work through their feelings before they can act on a referral.

Families often have concerns about using mental health services, and they may have distorted ideas about what these services are like. The nurse can encourage family members to express their perceptions and concerns and then correct misconceptions by providing accurate information about the helping agency and the helping process. To help bridge the gap between the known and the unknown, the nurse can compare the preliminary interviews to the kind of help that the agency might provide.

Once the need for help is admitted and conflicts about using mental health services are reduced, the nurse can assist the family with reality issues in seeking and starting these services. When an appropriate agency has been found, the nurse can facilitate the family's actually going to the agency by acting as a liaison between the family and the agency. A personal phone call to the referral agency on behalf of the client, to establish contact with the agency and to arrange for the initial appointment, is an effective referral method. Assistance with other practical problems, such as providing for a bilingual interpreter, will also increase the likelihood of a successful referral.[24]

After the initial appointment has been made and the family has had contact with the referral agency, a follow-up visit is useful to convey continued interest and concern for the family and to deal with any remaining issues or problems that may have arisen around seeking or using help.

References

1   Joint Commission on Mental Health of Children: *Crisis in Child Mental Health: Challenge for the 1970's,* Harper & Row, New York, 1970, p. 251.

2   Joint Commission on Mental Health of Children: *Mental Health: From Infancy Through Adolescence,* Harper & Row, New York, 1973, pp. 11, 78–79.

3   Reginald S. Lourie: "The First Three Years of Life: An Overview of a New Frontier in Psychiatry," *American Journal of Psychiatry,* vol. 127, pp. 1457–1463, May 1971.

4   T. Berry Brazelton: "Anticipatory Guidance," *Pediatric Clinics of North America,* vol. 22, pp. 533–544, August 1975.

5   E. James Anthony: "A Risk-Vulnerability Intervention Model for Children of Psychotic Parents," in E. James Anthony and Cyrille Koupernik (eds.): *The Child in His Family: Children at Psychiatric Risk,* Wiley, New York, 1974, vol. 3, pp. 99–121.

6   Sharon B. Sloboda: "The Children of Alcoholics: A Neglected Problem," *Hospital and Community Psychiatry,* vol. 25, pp. 605–606, September 1974.

7   Nathan W. Ackerman: "The Principle of Shared Responsibility of Child Rearing," *International Journal of Social Psychiatry,* vol. 2, pp. 280–291, Spring 1957.

8   Gail J. Donner: "Parenthood as a Crisis: A Role for the Psychiatric Nurse," *Perspectives in Psychiatric Care,* vol. 10, pp. 84–87, April–May–June 1972.

9 Harvey H. Barten and Sybil S. Barten: "New Perspectives in Child Mental Health," in Harvey H. Barten and Sybil S. Barten (eds.): *Children and Their Parents in Brief Therapy,* Behavioral Publications, New York, 1973, pp. 1–20.

10 Ira D. Glick and David R. Kessler: *Marital and Family Therapy,* Grune & Stratton, New York, 1974, pp. 18–21.

11 Helene Thorpe and Emmy E. Werner: "Developmental Screening of Preschool Children," *Pediatrics,* vol. 53, pp. 362–370, March 1974.

12 William K. Frankenburg and Josiah B. Dodds: "The Denver Developmental Screening Test," *Journal of Pediatrics,* vol. 71, pp. 181–191, August 1967.

13 William K. Frankenburg, Arnold D. Goldstein, and Bonnie W. Camp: "The Revised Denver Developmental Screening Test: Its Accuracy as a Screening Instrument," *Journal of Pediatrics,* vol. 79, pp. 988–995, December 1971.

14 Anne Anastasi: "Psychological Testing of Children," in Alfred M. Freedman, Harold I. Kaplan, and Benjamin J. Sadock (eds.): *Comprehensive Textbook of Psychiatry,* 2d ed., Williams & Wilkins, Baltimore, 1975, vol. 2, pp. 2070–2087.

15 Catherine DeAngelis: *Basic Pediatrics for the Primary Health Care Provider,* Little, Brown, Boston, 1973, pp. 86–98.

16 Reginald S. Lourie and Rebecca E. Rieger: "Psychiatric and Psychological Examination of Children," in Silvano Arieti (ed.): *American Handbook of Psychiatry,* 2d ed., Basic Books, New York, 1974, vol. 2, pp. 3–36.

17 Alexander Thomas, Stella Chess, and Herbert G. Birch: "The Origin of Personality," *Scientific American,* vol. 223, pp. 102–109, August 1970.

18 R. Dean Coddington: "The Significance of Life Events as Etiologic Factors in the Diseases of Children: I. A Survey of Professional Workers," *Journal of Psychosomatic Research,* vol. 16, pp. 7–18, March 1972.

19 R. Dean Coddington: "The Significance of Life Events as Etiologic Factors in the Diseases of Children: II. A Survey of a Normal Population," *Journal of Psychosomatic Research,* vol. 16, pp. 205–213, June 1972.

20 J. Stephen Heisel, Scott Ream, Raymond Raitz, Michael Rappaport, and R. Dean Coddington: "The Significance of Life Events as Contributing Factors in the Diseases of Children: III. A Study of Pediatric Patients," *Journal of Pediatrics,* vol. 83, pp. 119–123, July 1973.

21 Irving N. Berlin: "Children in the Seventies: Developmental Findings and Recommendations from the Joint Commission on Mental Health of Children," in Irving N. Berlin (ed.): *Advocacy for Child Mental Health,* Brunner/Mazel, New York, 1975, pp. 11–26.

22 Eli M. Bower: *Early Identification of Emotionally Handicapped Children in School,* Charles C Thomas, Springfield, Ill., 1960, pp. 8–10.

23 Dane G. Prugh and Anthony J. Kisley: "Psychosocial Aspects of Pediatrics and Psychiatric Disorders," in C. Henry Kempe, Henry K. Silver, and Donough O'Brien (eds.): *Current Pediatric Diagnosis and Treatment,* Lange Medical Publications, Los Altos, Calif., 1970, pp. 465–492.

*24 Jane N. Gorman: "Delivery of Mental Health Services to Children of 'Resistive' Parents," *Journal of Psychiatric Nursing and Mental Health Services,* vol. 11, pp. 3–8, May–June 1973.

25 Thomas S. Langner, Joanne C. Gersten, Edward L. Greene, Jeanne G. Eisenberg, Joseph H. Herson, and Elizabeth D. McCarthy: "Treatment of Psychological Disorders Among Urban Children," *Journal of Consulting and Clinical Psychology,* vol. 42, pp. 170–179, April 1974.

26 Angela Barron McBride: "Can Family Life Survive?" *American Journal of Nursing,* vol. 75, pp. 1648–1653, October 1975.

27 Ann D. Murray: "Maternal Employment Reconsidered: Effects on Infants," *American Journal of Orthopsychiatry,* vol. 45, pp. 773–790, October 1975.

28 Joan B. Kelly and Judith S. Wallerstein: "The Effects of Parental Divorce: Experiences of the Child in Early Latency," *American Journal of Orthopsychiatry,* vol. 46, pp. 20–32, January 1976.

29 Peter D. McLean and James E. Miles: "Evaluation and the Problem-Oriented Record in Psychiatry," *Archives of General Psychiatry,* vol. 31, pp. 622–625, November 1974.

*30 Patricia C. Pothier: "Developmental Reactions in Infancy and Childhood," in Marion E. Kalkman and Anne J. Davis (eds.): *New Dimensions in Mental Health-Psychiatric Nursing,* McGraw-Hill, New York, 1974, pp. 58–95.

31 H. Paul Gabriel: "Identification of Potential Emotional and Cognitive Disturbances in the 3- to 5-Year-Old Child," *Pediatric Clinics of North America,* vol. 18, pp. 179–189, February 1971.

*Recommended reference by a nurse author.

*32 Claire M. Fagin (ed.): *Nursing in Child Psychiatry,* Mosby, St. Louis, 1972, p. 148.

33 Alan J. Rosenthal and Saul V. Levine: "Brief Therapy with Children: A Preliminary Report," *American Journal of Psychiatry,* vol. 127, pp. 646–651, November 1970.

34 Olga R. Lurie: "Parents' Attitudes Toward Children's Problems and Toward Use of Mental Health Services: Socioeconomic Differences," *American Journal of Orthopsychiatry,* vol. 44, pp. 109–120, January 1974.

Chapter

34
The Family with a Psychotic Child

Nada Light

Learning Objectives

After studying this chapter, the student should be able to:

1 Discuss the etiologic theories of childhood psychosis
2 Assess the behavior of the child and the family as well as their mutual interaction
3 Identify their response and its effect on the delivery of care
4 Discuss the types of psychotherapeutic interventions
5 Formulate nursing diagnoses for the responses of the child and family to the illness and treatment
6 Formulate goals for the management of behavioral problems and family dysfunction
7 Intervene in ways that will maximize the child's and family's coping
8 Evaluate the effectiveness of the interventions

A great deal has been written about the profound disturbances of childhood, perhaps because of their dramatic bizarreness and the pain they generate in those who must live with and treat these children. This concerned response appears to be disproportionate to the actual numbers afflicted. For example, The Joint Commission on the Mental Health of Children in 1970 identified the various groups of children needing mental health services, and barely 10 percent of those identified were considered psychotic.[1]

Definition

Several basic issues remain unresolved in the theoretical understanding of childhood psychosis. Whether it is a disease entity with specific symptoms or a descriptive term for a group of profound disturbances in a child's relationship with others and maladjustment to reality has yet to be determined. The term "psychosis" has a legal definition, a factor that must be weighed carefully when identifying and labeling a child's behavior. When a child reaches school age, placement in a school becomes an issue. Lingering prejudices and fears about psychosis exist in most communities and may influence those who come in contact with a child so labeled. However, more positively, the identification of a child's disturbance may also open opportunities for special treatment, education, and understanding.

The origins of psychosis remain obscure, and the prevailing hypotheses about them are not congruent. Systematic research is sparse, hampered by the small numbers of subjects, the diversity of the subjects' backgrounds, and the variety of the treatments received.

In psychotic disorders of childhood, basic personality development is extremely distorted. Disturbances are seen in thinking, affect, perception, motility, and speech. Reality testing and object or human relationships are disturbed. A child can become psychotic at various levels of development. Basic personality functions such as individuation and relatedness to people are dis-

Table 34-1 Categories of Psychosis in Childhood

Stage	Psychosis
Early childhood (birth to 3 yr)	Infantile autism Symbiosis
Middle childhood (3 to 7 yr)	Atypical childhood psychosis
Late childhood (8 to 12 yr)	Childhood schizophrenia

turbed in the very young child, while the older psychotic child may lack an integrated personality, show arrested development, or fail to achieve adequate reality testing. The psychotic preadolescent may demonstrate severely distorted social relationships, lack a sense of identity, or show disturbances in thought processes and other aspects of ego functioning.[2]

Table 34-1 presents the categories of childhood psychosis in chronological order of appearance in the developmental scheme.

Etiological Concepts

The issues of etiology as well as exact classification plague the categories of childhood psychoses. The various existing hypotheses postulate organic causes, disturbances of the parent-child relationship, and multicausation.

The Organic Hypothesis

The work of Rimland[3] and Bender[4] suggests that the symptoms seen in childhood psychoses are the result of an impairment in the reticular formation of the brainstem. Those who oppose the organic hypothesis do not account for the widespread neurophysiological changes that are seen even in the absence of severely faulty parenting. Bender defines childhood schizophrenia as a biological disorder in central integration and in behavioral maturation processes, with a lag characterized by embryonic features, especially plasticity.[4] She views the parenting difficulties as a result of living with a severely disturbed child.

The Parent–Child Relationship Hypothesis

The concept of *the schizophrenogenic mother* flows from work at the James Jackson Putnam Center in Boston. Rank[5] and her colleagues developed a research project which used as its client population families composed of disturbed parents and a psychotic child. Three broad conclusions can be drawn from their work:

1 The mother-child relationship was disturbed in the first years of life and was characterized by unusually high ambivalence in the mother.

2 The father-child relationship was disturbed.

3 The infants had suffered severe gastrointestinal and respiratory embarrassments in infancy. A current traumatic event centering around separation from the parent precipitated the acute psychotic symptoms.[5]

Kanner's[6] work at Johns Hopkins supports the theory that childhood psychosis is parent-induced. In his work on infantile autism, Kanner developed the concept of the *icebox mother.*[6] The mothers of Kanner's autistic clients were cold, detached, and interested in their children only intellectually. These same mothers were often quite different with other children in the same family. The empathic bonding that takes place in the first years of life was absent in these disturbed mother-child relationships, which consequently produced psychosis.

Multiple-Causation Hypothesis

Mahler[7] and Escalona[8] in their respective work include an emphasis on constitutional predisposition. They each understood that an infant who was "different" could elicit irrational responses from the parents, especially as the mother and father grew more perplexed, discouraged, and tired of trying to understand the child's needs. Even Kanner in his later work acknowledges multiple causation.

Eisenberg[9] suggests that the intellectual inadequacy seen in disturbed children may be the outcome of an organic limitation or cultural deprivation. Affective inadequacy may reflect an organic dysfunction, affective deprivation, or some combination of these factors.[9]

Goldfarb's[10] position is the clearest endorsement of both the organic and nonorganic hypotheses. He views the whole area of childhood psychosis on a continuum where, at one end, the preponderance of data suggests that the etiology of a particular child's disturbance is organic; at the other end of this continuum is a group of children who by history and assessment have a more environmentally induced psychosis.[10] Thus, the children found at midpoint on the continuum contribute more evidence *against* either single-causation theory. Examination of clinical data points to multicausation based on inadequate nurturing, environmental deprivation, and an organic predisposition.

Incidence

Autism has a higher incidence in first-born male children and in children whose histories include perinatal complications. These children appear to be born to families with well-educated and bright parents. Rimland characterizes the autistic child as the equivalent genetically of a homozygote for high intelligence associated with a special vulnerability to various types of anoxia during pregnancy and delivery.[11]

Few autistic children are seen. Kanner has seen 150 cases in 19 years; these represented only 1 percent of all the children he evaluated.[12] Bender, in her 20-year study at Bellevue, diagnosed 8 percent of all children seen as schizophrenic; this includes autism as a subgroup of schizophrenia.[13] These figures are significant, since these centers attract larger numbers because of their specialized interests in treating these children.

Client Behavior
Infantile Autism

Infantile autism is a neurological, perceptual, physiological dysfunction and psychotic behavior state in the very young child.[11]

While the diagnosis of autism almost never occurs in the first year of life, developmental histories have indicated that disturbed behavior patterns of feeding, elimination, and sleeping have existed from birth. The average period of several months needed by the normal infant to establish physiologically stable patterns appears absent in these babies. Their parents may describe irritable sleeping in a very young infant which evolves into long periods of night screaming. Night feedings may be maintained for an inordinate amount of time. Independence in toileting and a growing awareness of the process of elimination may be absent.

Auditory peculiarities are also present. For example, some of these babies avoid responding to normal cues such as loud noises and people's voices. Yet these same babies may be fascinated by and attentive to music. Often these children are mistaken for being deaf, a possibility that must not be overlooked.[11]

Motor developmental milestones are usually normal in autistic children, but peculiarities do exist. For example, a love of motion in many forms dominates the mobile infant. These children have an *excessive* interest in riding, swinging, turning, and spinning. Further self-stimulation is seen in rocking and head banging. Special gaits, arm flapping, jumping, and walking on tiptoe may also be present. Often the clumsiness in fine motor development gives way to unusual grace as the child develops.

Language development in the autistic child is altered, but this is not the simple developmental lag that is seen in Down's syndrome. Autistic speech is characterized by echolalia, where the last phrase or word is repeated, and developmental aphasis. The latter disorder can take a variety of forms and confuse the diagnosis. For example, fragments of speech, confused word meaning, lack of abstract word meanings, and difficulty in understanding sound productions are all problems of developmental aphasia. However, when the whole child is examined, altered language development coupled with disturbed perceptual-motor and interpersonal development confirm autistic behavior.

Of greatest concern is the abnormally developing relationships with people. The social smile first appears as a reflex in the normal child, but in the autistic child the smiling response *remains* a reflex. Other social cues are absent in the growing baby. For example, there are no anticipatory behaviors from the child when the parent approaches—arms are not extended toward the parent—and there is an absence of molding to the parent's body when the child is held. The infant seems more content to play alone and does not seek the parents during the crawling and early toddler stages. Further, if the child is hurt and therefore cries, comforting offered by the parents does not console the child (see Chap. 32).

An autistic child's play is also peculiar. Toys and objects are handled in a restricted way. Form is everything. Toys that are smooth, spin, reflect light, and sparkle, as well as puzzles with odd shapes, are all sources of inordinate fascination. The giver of the toy holds little meaning for the child.

In the second and third years, visual-perceptual alterations are demonstrated clearly. The ability to separate figure from background develops slowly. Peripheral vision is preferred over central; thus, the characteristic eye avoidance involves looking past people and objects. However, moving objects are recognized more easily than stationary ones, such as a dog on television or live dog as opposed to a picture of a dog in a book. This is further demonstrated by older autistic children who, when studying the characteristics of a stationary object, do so by moving it up and down or moving their heads from side to side. Very complex visual stimuli—including people—are avoided; this may account for some of the interpersonal avoidance. This response suggests a defense against a flooding of perceptual stimuli.

Abnormalities of mood are most apparent by the third and fourth years. A remote and aloof distance is now obvious. Interestingly, by 5 or 6 years an increase in affection toward familiar people has been observed, but any new person or situation evokes a withdrawal reaction. Emotional outbursts of tears, rage, stamping, or kicking occur as a reaction to frustration, fears, changes in the environment, or for no apparent reason. Bursts of giggling and laughter may also occur without provocation.[11] Autistic children often lack the fear of real dangers such as height and moving cars. Yet, they fear the harmless, such as the wearing of shoes, a particular piece of furniture, bathing, or brushing the teeth.

The establishment of some meaningful speech by 5 years is a good prognostic sign. After this age, few autistic children develop the ability to use language as a communication tool, and neurological maturation in other deficit areas is minimal. Eventual institutionalization is usually necessary.

Few studies have looked at the autistic adolescent or young adult, and no systematic research data are available. However, the lack of interpersonal development means that autistic adults are unlikely to marry or have children. Most remain in the custodial care of their families or institutions.[14]

Symbiosis

Symbiosis is a relatively new category of childhood psychosis. Mahler used the term to refer to an intrapsychic rather than a behavioral condition; she was referring not to physical clinging but to a primitive cognitive-affective feature of the infant, where differentiation between self and mother has not taken place.[15] Mahler was concerned that the young psychotic child never felt a wholeness of self and a sense of human identity. She viewed autism and symbiosis as two extremes of disturbances in identity: primary infantile autism as a frozen wall between the child and the human object and symbiotic psychosis as a fusion, meeting, or lack of differentiation between the mothering one and the child[16] (see Chaps. 11 and 32).

Because of the developmental nature of the first year, the clinical symptoms of symbiosis may not be readily apparent until the period of normal symbiosis, although grossly distorted, ends. The child begins to sense this impending separation. Retrospectively, the parent describes the child's unusual dependence on the mother. When this real or fantasized threat occurs to the mother-child relationship, the child shows intense separation anxiety, for example, panic tantrums, clinging, and regressive behaviors often accompanied by the giving up of speech. The latter may be the symptoms of most concern that bring the child to a clinical setting. By then, other psychotic behaviors may have developed, such as emotional aloofness, autistic behaviors, reality distortions, and autoaggressive behaviors.

Atypical Development Psychosis

There remains a group of children who cannot be called autistic and who do not have a symbiotic tie with a parent. Their symptoms develop in the later preschool years or early latency, before the age of 8 years, which is generally accepted as the demarcation point for childhood schizophrenia. Features of autism and symbiosis may be present, but adaptive behavioral strength is also present. Rank and her associates studied a group of preschoolers and their parents. A summary of their observations of these children revealed that all (1) lacked contact with reality, (2) had little or no communication contact with others, and (3) lacked integration and uniformity in personality development; for example, the children demonstrated single well-developed functions along with many that were crippled or arrested.[5]

Symptoms included withdrawal from people, mutism or use of language for autistic purposes, alternating impassivity and violent outbursts of rage or anxiety, identification with inanimate objects or animals, and excessively inhibited or uninhibited expression of impulses.

In families with an atypical child, a disturbed relationship with the parent in the first years of the child's life appeared to exist, but there was also a current traumatic event that triggered the psychotic symptoms. Events like a physical illness, separation from a parent, birth of a sibling, a family move, sexual molestation, and observations of violence initiated the intense anxiety and resulting ego fragmentation (see Chap. 6).

Further symptoms include stereotypic rituals, grimaces, and tics, all appearing without external stimulation. If some expressive language remains, the quality of the voice is peculiar, high pitched, and raspy, suggesting a faulty feedback process within the child. Eye focusing is disturbed; the child may explore objects intently, give fleeting glances to people, or not focus at all. Motor development may be above average for the age or the opposite, that is, it may be awkward, stiff, and rigid. Ritualistic movement may be seen, such as rocking, compulsive touching of self or others, mechanical handling of objects, and excessive mouthing and spinning of objects. Eating habits are usually disturbed in the extreme, as shown by limited food choices, gluttonous stuffing, or pica.

These children may relate first to inanimate objects, then pets, and finally people. Rank's working hypothesis is that the child experienced a highly ambivalent parent during the years antedating the burst of atypical psychotic behaviors. This process may have been one of rapidly alternating overgratification and needless frustration coupled with a lack of nurturance and appropriate sensory stimulation. Historically, the infant may be described as fretful, sleepless, tense, and excessively demanding. While the infants continued to demand that basic needs be met, they eventually gave up, feeling helpless and hopeless. A gradual withdrawal into their own isolated world may be misinterpreted by the parents as calming down, finally being able to play alone and not needing as much attention.[5] Some of these observations may seem at first to describe the developing autonomous behaviors of a normal preschooler; however, this isolation is premature and may be misunderstood by the parents. Parents burdened by their own psychiatric disturbances may not have the coping mechanisms to understand the problems developing within their child (see Chap. 36).

Childhood Schizophrenia

The Group for the Advancement of Psychiatry (GAP) has designated the psychoses of later childhood "schizophreniform psychotic disorders" to differentiate them from the schizophrenias of adulthood.[2] Not all children who have what can be called a schizophreniform episode become adult schizophrenics. Childhood schizophrenia differs from the adult disorder in the following ways: (1) regression is not as marked because the child does not have fully matured behaviors; (2) hallucinations are rare; (3) bizarre motor behaviors are seen more frequently in children (e.g., whirling, hand flapping, sudden bursts of aggressive and sometimes self-mutilating behaviors). The type differentiations of adult schizophrenia cannot be applied and are not recognizable in childhood because personality trends are then not well developed (see appendix).

Bender[17] points to the marked disturbances in the vegetative rhythms and neurological system as another way of differentiating this disorder from the adult type. She cannot support the faulty parenting hypothesis as a primary cause of pathology because of the pervasive malfunction in the autonomic nervous system and motor areas as well as language deficits, faulty affectional responses, and perceptual problems. Further, Bender[17] feels that the extreme anxiety seen in these children is the *result* of their organic problems.

However, one piece of research indicates that some of the visual-motor disturbances that appear to be organic may be environmentally induced or reinforced. Fish and Hagin[18] studied several infants born to schizophrenic mothers in institutions. Thus they were able to follow the development of these infants closely. At age 3 to 4 months, normal infants begin to touch their hands together and to notice (see) this act themselves. This tactile-motor pattern results in linking vision and touch by a double feedback system: (1) eyes see what hands feel (that is, each other), (2) each hand is being touched and is touching.

The children born to these mothers did not begin this visual-motor pattern until 6½ months.

Therefore, they had continued to explore objects without visual-motor linking. The critical lesson here is that the infant learns the difference between touching self and touching objects that are not self.[18] The researchers were unable to demonstrate clearly whether constitutional predisposition or faulty environmental stimulation was the prime causative factor. However, they went on to wonder whether the severity of the disintegration seen in schizophrenia was due partly to this type of faulty experience. Even without any clear etiology, this piece of research has strong implications for assessment of the visual-motor development of infants at risk and for the designing of appropriate interventions if needed.

Childhood schizophrenia is not a unitary disease entity but a label indicating a dramatic deviation from normal ego functioning. These children lack the normal guides necessary for self-regulation, for achieving an identity, and for differentiating inner from outer experiences (see Chap. 23). The onset of a schizophreniform psychotic experience can be gradual or sudden. In dysfunctional families, symptoms may not be recognized until the child's behavior reaches crisis proportions.

Nurse's Response

Nurses have expectations of how the child at different age levels should respond to verbal and nonverbal messages related to teaching and learning, nurturing, and social interactions. But the bizarre behavior of the psychotic child disappoints these expectations and challenges the nurse's repertoire of skills in caring for sick children.

Touch and relatedness are important components of nursing intervention. There is a natural inclination to hold, stroke, and cuddle young children and an expectation that the child will accept and respond to such contacts. Autistic children have difficulty relating to others and tolerating gentle touching. They may respond to nurturing behavior by becoming agitated or running away.

Responses of this kind make nurses feel frustrated and incompetent as well as anxious to avoid interactions with disturbed children.

Bizarre behavior and the absence of affective and social responsiveness are learned distancing maneuvers employed by the child. If nurses are not aware of how the disturbed child uses these maneuvers as a defense or of the feelings these behaviors generate in themselves as they attempt to deliver care, they participate in the distancing process and block the development of a therapeutic relationship.

Disturbed children who engage in self-mutilating behavior also generate strong feelings in their caretakers. It is abhorrent to watch other human beings, particularly children, mutilate their bodies or rip their hair out by the roots in a purposeful but irrational manner. Nurses who must care for such children experience mental pain, frustration, and at time even anger at the child as well as the parents, whom they may perceive as the root cause of these extreme disturbances. The prevention of self-mutilating behavior may initially require the application of physical restraints. The feelings of the caretakers mediate the manner in which such restraints are applied and the approaches taken to help the child control behavior and express feelings in more appropriate ways. If anger and frustration predominate, the nurse's response is apt to be punitive. Behavior which reflects loss of control and aggressive assaultiveness causes nurses to fear for their own safety as well as the possibility that they might overreact and harm the child while applying restraints.

Having to sit with a restrained psychotic child who cannot communicate in a rational manner creates feelings of helplessness in the caretaker. This feeling, as well as a sense of hopelessness, also pervades the nurse's feeling tone when rapid recovery does not occur or if the child does not display observable progress over time.

The disturbed child often exhibits exceptional precocity or ability in a particular area, such as mathematics. These special talents may mask the underlying cognitive and affective disturbances.

When nurses begin to recognize the discrepancy between the exceptional ability in a very circumscribed area and the massive underlying psychotic disturbances, they may become puzzled and confused. They must then confront the challenge of sorting out the healthy dimensions of the personality—the child's strengths—from the weaknesses which require therapeutic intervention.

Awareness that the autistic child's behavior may stem in part from perceptual disturbances helps the nurse to become more accepting and to work within the limitations of the child's deficits.

The etiological hypothesis which influences the nurse's perception of the child's problem also influences the nurse's view of the family in relation to the problem. If the nurse believes that inadequate parenting or deprivation has contributed to the child's difficulties, then anger toward the parents is experienced. This feeling increases the nurse's tendency to exclude the parents from participating in the child's care and thus deprive them of valuable opportunities to receive teaching and counseling (see Chap. 36). Such situations also lead the nurse to entertain *rescue fantasies* which are unrealistic and interfere with the development of a more effective family unit.

Assessment

The setting, the presenting problem, and the nurse's role may modify the assessment process. Regardless of whether the child is in a hospital unit, a residential setting, or the community, an ongoing assessment which includes the child, the family, and/or the caretakers is required. A child in crisis with distraught parents may require a modified and condensed assessment until a more thorough evaluation is feasible later on. The nurse may function as a primary care-giver, a liaison to others directly responsible for care, or a member of the treatment team.

The nursing interview is the major tool in the nurse's assessment of a disturbed child. Ideally, a brief meeting with the parents and the child begins the contact and sets a clear goal of gathering information about the family unit in order to solve or alleviate part or all of the presenting difficulties. The nurse can observe the interaction between parents and child and hear their respective views. A separate interview with each is needed for several reasons. For the parents, this is an opportunity to express their special concerns about their child without the inhibiting and shaping influence of their child's presence. Marital and family problems and needs may emerge more spontaneously. And last, the parents can provide an understanding of their child's past development.

The child too needs a chance to be seen without direct parental influence. The nurse can observe the differences in the child with and without the parents' presence. Some children may not separate easily from a parent; with them, information gathering must be done cautiously and tactfully over a period of several joint interviews until a physical separation is possible. Young children will be unable to clearly tell what is troubling them or their family. However, the nurse can listen with a third ear as the child answers nonloaded questions about a child's world; the nurse can also observe the way play materials are manipulated. Even a very disturbed child without speech or interactional language may be observed in order to gather primary data.

Bringing the family unit back together at the end of the interview, provides the nurse with an opportunity to articulate observations and interventions that may be useful. While a nursing diagnosis or complete understanding of the issue is rarely possible at the end of an initial interview, the family will have observed and experienced a systematic process and the beginning of a therapeutic relationship will have been established.

In addition to the nursing interview, the data base may include information from other disciplines. For example, a psychiatric exam may identify psychopathology that requires the use of psychotropic drugs. Psychological assessment through intelligence testing and projective techniques can identify strengths and weaknesses in cognitive and personality functioning that may be useful in designing a treatment plan (see Table

30-2 in Chap. 30). A general health exam is necessary, especially in the very young child where concurrent problems involving hearing, vision, and kinesthesia may exist. This physical assessment is also mandatory when placing a child on medication. Self-mutilization, toileting problems, seizures, and other abnormalities with a mixed etiology must be clearly identified and organic bases either ruled out or treated appropriately. Finally, any past records from other treatment facilities or agents may be helpful in gaining the scope needed for effective planning.

The nursing assessment focuses on the child's response to the problems posed by the physical deficits and affective disturbances as well as on the child's ability to interact effectively with the environment and with other people. The data bases needed for planning care include the following:

Infantile Autism

1 Is there evidence of developmental lag?
2 Is there a lack of responsiveness to people, with avoidance of eye contact?
3 Does the child engage in self-stimulating rather than interactive behavior?
4 Does the child exhibit a strong problematic response to new people or situations?
5 Does the child respond with inordinate fear toward neutral, harmless objects but lack fear of real danger?
6 Is there an absence of relief when the child is given comfort and nurturing after a painful or distressing experience?
7 What activities diminish distress when the child is upset?

Symbiosis

1 Do incidents of separation elicit excessive anxiety and problematic behavior?
2 Does the child exhibit temper tantrums inappropriate to the developmental age?

3 Do the parents exhibit problems or express fears about normal separation from the child?
4 Is the child's speech appropriate to the developmental age?

Atypical Developmental Psychosis

1 Is there covert evidence of symbiosis or autism?
2 Do the child's verbal messages or behavior seem out of touch with reality?
3 Is there a paucity of communication with others: caretakers, parents, peers?
4 Is the child becoming socially isolated—withdrawing from family and peers?
5 Does the child exhibit ritualistic behaviors or report obsessional thoughts?
6 Does the child make inappropriate facial expressions or lack appropriate affect?
7 Are there language disturbances?

Childhood Schizophrenia

1 To what extent are the child's body boundaries intact?
2 Does the child exhibit impulsivity?
3 What is the degree of regression?
4 Does the child engage in self-mutilating behavior?
5 Is there evidence of bizarre behavior?
6 Does the child exhibit outbursts of aggressive or assaultive behavior?
7 Can the child distinguish between reality and fantasy?

Management Approaches
Biological Interventions

Electroconvulsive therapy with children has been supported by Bender. She feels that children can tolerate this treatment better than adults and that it can help the child to utilize and accept the adjustive psychotherapies.[19]

Drug therapy is used in conjunction with educational and psychotherapy modalities. The more potent but less sedative of the major tranquilizers are better tolerated by young psychotic children. Barbiturates tend to disorganize the severely disturbed child and may have a paradoxical effect. Several principles guide the use of these drugs with children:[20]

1 As the child grows, not just the dosage changes but also the response to the medication.
2 Side effects can be severe.
3 Regular laboratory evaluations and physical exams must be a part of the larger treatment plan.

Milieu Therapy

Milieu therapy can include both educational and psychotherapeutic modes. Emphasis is on the whole experience and environment, and therapy can take the form of half-day, whole-day, or residential care (see Chap. 9). If the program is educationally oriented, the thrust may be to habilitate and educate the child using the teacher-pupil model. Classroom experiences focus on visual-motor training, language skills, socialization through group projects, and other ways of remediating learning disabilities. Daily activities become learning situations. Behavior modification techniques have been useful in shaping more functional behaviors.[21]

Psychotherapy

Individual, group, and family therapies have all been used to treat the psychotic child (see Chaps. 6, 8, 10, and 11). These can be used within community and residential settings, and occasionally one or more is employed in association with drug therapy on a private basis.

Cause usually dictates treatment. However, the lack of agreement in this area has meant the development of many treatment approaches. No one modality appears to be better than another; in fact, client histories seem to indicate that some children have reconstituted without treatment. An eclectic treatment plan can be formulated to manage problems.

Treatment Planning

A comprehensive list of problems is drawn from the data base and used in formulating a treatment plan. Areas to be considered concerning the child and the family are listed below:

The Child

1 Chronological age and developmental functioning
2 Current severity of psychopathology
3 Secondary physical handicaps (e.g., low intelligence; chronic illness, like asthma)
4 Treatment setting being considered (i.e., home, school, residential)

The Family

1 General health of members
2 Economic and living condition
3 Concurrent capacities to handle child's pathology
4 Concurrent problems with other members
5 Family's need for a disturbed child to remain psychotic (e.g., dysfunctional marriage)

Goals

Long- and short-term treatment goals must be arrived at with the family. Short-term goals usually center around the amelioration of current symptoms and dysfunctional behavior patterns. Long-term or major goals include the family's acceptance of their psychotic child and the need for a structured therapeutic treatment program. Currently, the major treatment goal is to help the child remain in the community with a combination of the available therapies or—if hospitalization is necessary—to employ this approach judiciously. Community mental health centers can provide the various psychotherapies; school systems can support partial hospitalization programs and "mainstream" emotionally disturbed children in selected academic areas.

Regardless of the setting selected, dynamic treatment planning is necessary because of the unexpected events in a family and the development of the child. For example, some families may be able to care for a disturbed preschool child but not an autistic adolescent.

Throughout the treatment process, nursing is involved in helping with the implementation of the treatment program, assessing progress and appropriateness of the program as changes occur, and collaborating with other professionals to develop or revise the program.

Nursing goals should be congruent with the overall treatment plan and reflect the interdisciplinary, collaborative efforts and coordination of services. Each classification of childhood psychosis defines the child's dysfunction behaviorally and physiologically. Thus the nursing goals for children and their families in each classification will differ.

A broad treatment approach with an autistic child would work toward the following:

1 Helping the child to establish meaningful interpersonal relationships
2 Encouraging the child to develop an effective mode of communication
3 Helping the child to achieve reasonable conformity to the social structure of the environment
4 Encouraging the child to develop autonomous self-care according to developmental potential
5 Helping the family to deal effectively with their feelings and the child's behavior

Since the underlying problem in symbiosis is fusion with the mothering figure, nursing-care goals focus primarily on assisting the child to differentiate. These goals would include:

1 Helping the mother to manage the anxiety of the separation process
2 Helping the mother to gradually invest energy and interest in areas outside her nurturing role
3 Gradually increasing the child's tolerance of separation from the mother
4 Helping the child to develop satisfying relationships with others
5 Helping the parents to examine and work through their impaired communication patterns and improve their ability to resolve their conflicts effectively
6 Helping the child to maximize the independence appropriate to developmental stage

The goals for the child with atypical developmental psychosis focus on maximizing available strengths and resolving conflicts which are precipitating or perpetuating the deviant behavior. The following goals would be appropriate for this group of children:

1 Maximize the child's reality orientation and minimize the need to use pathological coping mechanisms.
2 Help the child learn to communicate with others in a comfortable and satisfying way.
3 Foster the development of identity.
4 Help the child work through the conflict which precipitated the psychotic behavior.
5 Help the child relinquish antisocial and bizarre behaviors which are isolating.
6 Strengthen the family unit so that family members will be able to satisfy one another's needs effectively.

The underlying basis of childhood schizophrenia is still being disputed. Despite the lack of agreement on theoretical formulations regarding this childhood disturbance, nursing goals can be established to help the child function more effectively. The following goals would be appropriate to the care of such children:

1 Help the child to behave as maturely and responsibly as possible in defined areas.

2 Help the child to gain control of bizarre behavior, using various interventions to limit or extinguish these behaviors.

3 Help the child to: maximize potential in motor performance, use of language to communicate needs and receive feedback, and affectional interaction appropriate to chronological age.

4 Help the child to cope effectively with perceptual deficits.

5 Help the family unit to understand the child's problem, support the treatment program, and engage in effective decision making and problem solving.

Nursing Intervention

The nurse may function in both psychiatric and nonpsychiatric settings. The latter may include schools, public health nursing agencies, well-child clinics, emergency rooms, and inpatient pediatric units. In these settings, the nurse can apply the knowledge of childhood psychoses as a case finder and/or supportive professional to the treatment process. Community mental health centers and outpatient child psychiatric clinics are now recognizing the prepared nurse as a primary therapist who can render direct therapy to the psychotic child or disturbed parent of a psychotic child. Partial hospitalization programs have utilized the nurse as a therapeutic role model, supporter of health, and parent liaison. The nurse in a residential center can also provide a holistic approach to the child, enabling child-care workers to function more effectively.

Whatever the setting, the first step is to identify problems and establish goals. Then nursing diagnoses must be arrived at which will guide the selection of interventions. Table 34-2 lists selected nursing diagnoses and interventions for the autistic child.

Parental support is an imperative part of the nursing care of an autistic child. Autistic children

Table 34-2 Nursing Diagnoses and Interventions for the Autistic Child

Nursing diagnosis	Interventions
Lacks interpersonal relationship	Positive reinforcement of eye contact (e.g., with candy, favorite toy), no matter how brief. Replace this reinforcer as quickly as possible with a social reward that is comfortable for the child.
Is disinterested in human contact.	Planned gradual deliberate intrusion into the child's solitude to force the beginnings of social interaction.
Lacks a communication mode.	Mouth any sounds or word fragments uttered by child. Consider the use of deaf-signing as a language tool with children who have little or no language.
Is restless, distractible.	Seek pharmacotherapy evaluation. Excessive movement can be reduced with improved neuromuscular efficiency and better concentration on tasks.
Has phobias.	Plan with parents gradual exposure to change needed in the environment.
Has obsessional attachments to particular objects.	Plan with parents gradual withdrawal of these transitional objects.
Shows anxiety associated with intense muscular stiffness; is nonverbal.	Use body massage to relax stiffened muscles if the child can tolerate this tactile approach. The message is an active process intended to provoke a nurturing interaction similar to early infancy stimulation.[14]
Shows autoerotic behavior.	Repatterning process: Determine when behavior occurs, using observations and parental assistance. Intervene *prior* to these times with alternative motor patterns.

are handicapped children, and their parents suffer the guilt and ambivalence experienced by all parents who are faced with a special child (see Chap. 38). Autistic children do improve with growth, again pointing toward the *maturational-lag hypothesis* of Bender. Parents have usually experienced an excessively long period prior to a diagnosis of autism in which they have spent sleepless nights and been in a state of chronic anxiety. They have felt depressed, angry, resentful, and at a loss to understand the nature of their own child. Although Kanner's *ice-box mother* does appear in a few cases, the question of whether the problem originated in the mother or the child is in this instance academic. Did the mother become turned off by the strain of relating to an infant who had unbalanced rhythms, felt uncomfortable in her arms, was not soothed by her *mother measures,* avoided eye contact, and did not smile responsively? Or was the mother unable to respond to her special infant because of her own needs and problems? The guilt generated by blaming a parent or having the parents accept a *blaming process* may be counterproductive to treatment. Where disturbed parenting methods exist, these should be identified and replaced by more healthy approaches through parent education, role modeling, and supportive counseling.

Since the very young child may not be eligible for a day treatment program, home treatment techniques are an area in which the nurse can be helpful. Suggestions may be needed by the family regarding expanded and protected play space, safer and more practical furniture until destructiveness is controlled, methods of feeding, and satisfying other family members' needs. The advantages of home treatment even for an older child include the following:[22]

1 Parents are more relaxed in their own homes.
2 Problems at home require different management than clinic/office problems.
3 Home treatment is cheaper than institutionalization.
4 If a child does experience prolonged hospitalization, there is marked regression

when the child is discharged home, thus diminishing valuable time and treatment gains.
5 Greater progress over time has been observed in homes where there has been increased parental involvement.[15]

Schizophreniform and atypical children exhibit psychotic behaviors which reflect their anxiety. Since their behavior may be unmanageable in the home situation, hospitalization may be required until they are better able to cope within the family system. Table 34-3 lists selected nursing diagnoses and interventions which can be utilized either in the home, in day care, or in a residential setting.

The boundaries of the psychotic child may be fluid—unfixed and undefined. Even though the nurse may have a comfortable way of using touch to achieve closeness with clients, physical contact must be used judiciously with the disturbed child who may be overwhelmed by closeness but may nevertheless desire some safe contact or connectedness.

The nurse may be directly responsible for administering medications. This task potentially contains elements of both positive and negative effects on the child. For example, the more disorganized child may feel relieved to have control facilitated by the medication and to feel less anxious; the occasional child who has hallucinations may experience relief at feeling stronger than, for example, an auditory command. However, other children may be highly anxious about ingesting oral medication, viewing this as an invasion or intrusion of their bodies. Injections become a difficult procedure for a child who has a limited capacity to comprehend that the nurse wants to be helpful. Nurses can also be particularly useful in transmitting and reinforcing essential knowledge about the medications that are used to parents and child-care workers.[21]

If the nurse is caring for a psychotic child in a nonpsychiatric setting—for example, a general pediatric surgical or medical unit—the procedures used in treating the child will require specialized approaches and explanations. Routine hospital care can disorganize a normal youngster and can

Table 34-3 Nursing Diagnoses and Interventions in the Schizophreniform and Atypical Child

Nursing diagnosis	Interventions
Lacks self-awareness.	Reinforce any behavior which differentiates the child from the environment, e.g., eye contact, self-feeding (putting something that is outside inside), exploring an object or person.
	Reinforce by providing repetitive chance to reexperience desired behavior.
	Reinforce with food and/or secondary object valued by child, but moving to social reinforcers.
Repetitive behavior patterns as a response to high anxiety (self-destruction, self-mutilation, head banging, biting excessively, scratching self, autoerotic manipulation).	Identify possible stimuli and eliminate them.
	Program of repatterning through physical exercise can interrupt and refocus this autoerotic and/or destructive behavior.
	Develop outer stimuli more interesting and satisfying to child than own body and bodily sensations.
	Protect child from injury by proper restraint (e.g., place child's back against front of caretaker and hold securely and/or make selective use of restraints to protect body and maintain integrity). Carefully determine whether restraints increase or decrease anxiety response.
Fecal soiling and urine incontinence in the absence of an organic basis.	Rule out any organic basis (e.g., poor anal sphincter muscle tone or renal anomaly).
	Toileting is a means of promoting social responsiveness and body-function awareness. Assess developmental potential to accomplish this self-awareness task. Steps in training follow sequence for a normal toddler except that each step may take a longer period of time and special explanations may be necessary.
Inability to manage changes or separations.	Anticipatory planning where possible to provide for gradual introduction of change and sensitization to separation experience.

certainly do the same more readily to a child who depends on routine to manage anxiety. Therefore special efforts must be made to help the child comprehend the situation and cope with the anxiety it generates. It is helpful to limit the number of persons providing care so that the demands on the child to adjust to strangers are minimized. The presence of familiar objects and favorite toys also helps to reduce the strangeness of the environment. With these children and those diagnosed as autistic, it is very important that all who are providing care be taught about the management of behavior problems and special personal rituals. These nursing orders will provide greater consistency in caretaking and lessen the possibility of provoking anxiety-producing situations which will further stress the child.

Many families cannot move beyond placing blame and feeling guilty about the presence of a disturbed child in their midst. These feelings often take the covert form of overprotection or unwillingness to relinquish part of the child's care to outside resources when available. The nurse can provide supportive counseling during this period of adjustment. The provision of daytime relief through schooling, weekend care, overnight camps, and occasional babysitting reduces the family's oppressive feeling that they have "no options." While a few children may have a schizophreniform psychotic episode and reconstitute with minimal residual problems, the child who is severely disorganized early in life generally remains chronically disturbed. This burden becomes intolerable for some families as the child grows and hope of major change and improvement disappears. Eventually placement in an institutional setting becomes the only choice when family growth is compromised. Support during this decision and process is essential if the family is to be left feeling that it can continue to function without being

Table 34-4 Nursing Diagnoses and Interventions: The Disturbed Child's Family

Nursing diagnosis	Intervention
Inability to handle feelings and attitudes about having a severely disturbed child in the family.	Parental counseling to establish an understanding of the child.
	Family meetings with those members having the most contact with the child.
	Serve as a therapeutic ally and advocate to the family.
	Act as an information resource.
	Provide support by listening empathetically and clarifying feelings and conflicting values.
Dysfunctional parent or parent relationship that precipitates disturbed behaviors in child.	Assess dysfunctional dynamics and determine counseling or therapy needs.
	Explore problem areas that can be ameliorated by parent education, financial assistance, better decision making, and activities which will better meet needs of family members.
	Provide a role model for more effective behavior with child client.
	Serve as a role model for more effective communication patterns within family.
	Make appropriate referral for treatment unless nurse functions as a primary therapist and is available as a treatment agent for the family.
	If parenting process causes severe disorganization in the child, consider recommending removal of child to a foster or residential setting.
Inability to cope with or accept the idea of separation from a child who needs residential placement.	Provide a forum for family to discover and explore their feelings about placement.
	Arrange for family to have contact with their child in placement.
	Provide supportive counseling after placement to help with working through feelings of loss, guilt, and mourning.
	Provide any special assistance needed to help siblings and other family members deal with their particular grief reactions.
Excessive guilt, anger, and blaming within the family, centering around or precipitated by the presence of a disturbed child.	Help family to explore these attitudes by identifying the presumed source and providing an alternative point of view about the process.

burdened by excessive guilt and a sense of failure.

Table 34-4 presents the nursing diagnoses and suggested interventions for treating the family of a disturbed child.

Evaluation

Evaluation is an important dimension in the delivery of effective services. The nurse uses the goals and nursing diagnoses as guides to measure whether or not the selected interventions have been effective in ameliorating or eliminating symptoms of distress in the child and family. They are also used to determine whether the child and family are functioning in a more effective, healthy fashion. Of course, in such evaluation allowances must be made for deficits that cannot be corrected or that can only be ameliorated by normal maturation over time.

The following case studies of three children illustrate the behavioral dysfunction, the family dynamics, the management of the problems, and the evaluation of change.

Case Study 1

Maria Arno was a beautiful, curly-haired 3-year-old with dark Italian features. On the first encounter with the nurse, Maria walked past her and made comments directed at the nurse's knees. Her poor eye contact continued until persistent interventions were made to help her focus on human faces. These measures included bending lower to facilitate eye contact and allowing Maria to explore the nurse's face with her hands. These interventions helped Maria begin to relate to the caretaker.

 . Maria's developmental history revealed several distressing experiences. She was her parents' only and first child, and Mrs. Arno had been overwhelmed by her newborn daughter's care. She was afraid to change the baby's diapers; thus Maria lay unchanged in her crib until her father returned, late at night. Mrs. Arno was also anxious about feeding Maria, "because she cried when I tried." At last Mrs. Arno's anxiety became so great that she feared destroying and abusing Maria and sought help from a mental health clinic nearby (see Chaps. 33 and 36). Maria's father was reluctant to get involved in the recommended parent-child program; therefore disturbed parenting continued. When Mr. Arno became frustrated with his daughter's finicky eating habits, he force-fed her. When she cried, he pulled her hair. Maria banged her head and rocked excessively from early infancy. Mrs. Arno could not cope with Maria's toddler activity and had kept her in a crib for most of the day. Thus Maria's large-muscle and fine-motor coordination were below age level. She made peculiar high-pitched sounds, ran on tiptoe, flapped her arms, and had violent temper tantrums that required much protection from banging her head on the floor. When she examined toys, she usually held them close to her face, rotating them and her head sideways.

A seizurelike behavior pattern resembling petit mal could be elicited only by a certain storybook, yet no EEG abnormality was found. When the book was read, Maria would begin flapping her hands, fall backward, and make orgastic mouth movements. Despite all these behaviors, Maria attracted interested people like a magnet and became a special client (see Chap. 22). This was fortunate, as her mother felt helpless at the time treatment was first begun and could offer Maria little nurturance (see Chap. 33).

Mrs. Arno attended a mothers' group and also received individual therapy. Family therapy was tried, but Mr. Arno and his parents, who resided in the same apartment, resisted involvement by labeling Mrs. Arno "the sick one" and terminating contact. A staff member became a strong transference person for Mrs. Arno, who had lacked consistent early mothering herself (see Chap. 36).

A classroom experience was the primary treatment modality with Maria; however, an unusually sensitive teacher, a small clinic, and a healthier maternal relationship were important adjuncts. Maria was eventually toilet trained at $4\frac{1}{2}$ years by her teacher, since Mrs. Arno's preoccupation with her own bathroom habits prevented her from helping to train Maria. (Mrs. Arno was still being spoon-fed milk of magnesia at night by her husband, and stronger cathartics were administered when necessary.) The use of laxatives had been a lifelong pattern for Mrs. Arno, and her problem was aggravated somewhat by phenothiazine therapy. After she was trained, Maria burst forth with expressive language overnight. Sadistic biting and mouthing of all objects declined as Maria relaxed in the classroom, and her language developed into a powerful tool to help her get basic nurturance from those around her.

Treating children as inanimate objects remained a problem until Maria's third year of treatment, when a girl her age became her first friend. This child presented Maria with a healthier and more flexible ego to incorporate. No medication was required for Maria, but Mrs. Arno has remained on phenothiazines to reduce her anxiety. While Mrs. Arno had no history of psychotic decompensations, she had experienced borderline periods of disorganizing and paralyzing anxiety (see Chap. 14). Both mother and child were very dependent on the clinic and staff. The final treatment goal was to help them move on to more independent functioning. After 3 years of treatment, when Maria was about to enter school, a comprehensive evaluation was done. While psychotic features remained, her intelligence was average and she demonstrated a capacity for relating to peers and adults. Impulse control was improved, and Maria could go on trips with her classmates without requiring two adults to restrain her from darting across the street. Termination from the clinic took the form of a gradual weaning. Contact days were reduced, the pair were helped to plan neighborhood trips together, and Mrs. Arno was allowed to use the classroom as a day-care center so that she could venture out alone. This separation process took 6 months. When the day finally came, Mrs. Arno and her family left the intensive therapeutic milieu feeling shaky but able to function more independently. Mrs. Arno continued to attend an aftercare evening group at a related clinic and planned eventually to return to work.

Case Study 2

Terry was brought to the clinic by her maternal grandmother because her behavior had become increasingly bizarre. She had no friends, and when she was together with other children she provoked fights. Terry had no idea why the children did not like her and felt very sad about their rejection. In addition, Terry was sometimes found standing by open windows with one leg out, looking very confused. She was failing school and felt worried about being left back.

Both 10-year-old Terry and her 8-year-old brother Albert had been subjected to multiple and rapidly shifting caretakers from infancy. Their mother would leave them with friends and then disappear for days. Finally their grandmother, Mrs. Canner, obtained legal custody of both, but by then Albert had burned their apartment and had been sent to a residential center where he lived for over 9 months. Their mother would call up and drop by unexpectedly from time to time, but this would only disorganize Terry still further.

On interview, Terry had difficulty knowing what was real and not real in her life; she became lost in retelling her dreams and suddenly panicked into a frozen immobility. She would begin a sen-

tence and get caught up in the rhythm or a certain word. Loose associations to television characters interrupted any train of thought. When asked to draw a person on subsequent interviews, she would confuse parts of the figure with herself and her therapist.

Albert's return to the home appeared to further disrupt Terry's tentative functioning. Residential placement was suggested to Mrs. Canner, whose own ambivalence about keeping these two very disturbed children further upset Terry. Therefore phenothiazines were prescribed for both children, individual therapy with separate therapists began for each, and supportive counseling for Mrs. Canner was provided to help her reach a more satisfactory decision about the children. Mrs. Canner continued to encourage her unreliable daughter's visits because this was her only respite. However, the assignment of a homemaker helped Mrs. Canner to give up her fantasy of seeing her own disturbed daughter return to mother these children. Placement finally became more palatable to Mrs. Canner and current treatment was focused on separation feelings.

Case Study 3

Mrs. Ruiz brought her son John to the clinic because "he wouldn't let her do anything without him." He was 2½ years old, and she had begun to notice that his clinging and irritability were getting worse, his speech was still babyish, and he now refused to stay with anyone, even his father. He remained aloof from other children and became violently tearful when his mother encouraged him to play with others. During the first interview, Mrs. Ruiz tried to leave to use the bathroom, but John lay on the floor gasping, sobbing, and flailing uncontrollably. When she offered him comfort, he remained inconsolable.

Mrs. Ruiz could add nothing remarkable about John's development except that his speech had never progressed beyond mama-dada. However, she felt that she knew what he wanted and depended on other cues. Further, Mrs. Ruiz, born into a Polish-Jewish family, had been isolated from her extended family and now lived in a hostile, poor neighborhood of different ethnic and religious background. She had married a Hispanic man who feared her socializing and had no friends or family of his own. A friend had once tried to baby-sit to give Mrs. Ruiz an opportunity to go out while John slept; however, he had cried endlessly when he found his mother gone. Thus Mrs. Ruiz gradually gave up this one respite.

A pediatric neurology examination revealed that John had no organic abnormality. While phenothiazines were recommended, it was decided to try a drug-free trial of psychotherapy, since this had not been attempted before. Mrs. Ruiz and John were enrolled in a mother-child program which met three times each week. Observations of the pair revealed an intense mutual sensitivity. For example, if Mrs. Ruiz's face registered disturbance, John would burst into tears and literally cry for her. A separate group therapy experience was offered to Mrs. Ruiz. In the beginning, John sat under his mother's chair in an open doorway leading to his classroom. Gradually, he was tempted away by his teacher and the other children for brief moments. His speech advanced to naming objects and forming simple sentences in the presence of others but not with his mother. While his social skills were primitive at best, John began to relate to the other children. Mr. Ruiz and Mrs. Ruiz's one friend were also included in treatment because their help was needed to pull Mrs. Ruiz into adult group activity. After 10 months of treatment, Mrs. Ruiz could sit in another room and have her lunch. John still needed to check on her whereabouts, but Mrs. Ruiz could at last manage to get "out of sight," although only briefly.

References

1 U.S. Congress, Joint Commission on The Mental Health of Children: *Crisis in Child Mental Health: Challenge for 1970's,* Harper & Row, New York, 1970.

2 Committee on Child Psychiatry: *Psychopathological Disorders in Childhood: Theoretical Considerations and a Proposed Classification,* Group for the Advancement of Psychiatry, New York, vol. 6, report no. 62, June 1966.

3 Bernard Remland: *Infantile Autism,* Appleton-Century-Crofts, New York, 1964.

4 Lauretta Bender: "The Brain and Child Behavior," *Archives of General Psychiatry,* vol. 4, pp. 531–548, 1961.

5 Beata Rank: "Intensive Study and Treatment of Preschool Children Who Show Marked Personality Deviations, or 'Atypical Development,' and Their Parents," in Gerald Caplàn (ed.), *Emotional Problems of Early Childhood,* Basic Books, New York, 1955.

6 Leo Kanner: "To What Extent Is Early Infantile Autism Determined by Constitutional Inadequacies?" *Proceedings of the Association for Research on Nervous and Mental Diseases,* vol. 33, pp. 378–385, 1954.

7 M. S. Mahler and B. J. Gosliner: "On Symbiotic Child Psychosis," *Psychoanalytic Study of the Child,* International Universities Press, New York, 1955, vol. 10.

8 S. Escalona and P. Bergman: "Unusual Sensitivities in Very Young Children," *Psychoanalytic Study of the Child,* International Universities Press, New York, 1948, vols. 3 and 4.

9 L. Eisenberg: "The Autistic Child in Adolescence," in Charles Reed, Irving Alexander, and Silvan Tomkins (eds.), *Psychopathology: A Source Book,* Harvard University Press, Cambridge, Mass., 1958.

10 William Goldfarb: *Childhood Schizophrenia,* Harvard University Press, Cambridge, Mass., 1961.

11 J. K. Wing (ed.): *Early Childhood Autism,* Pergamon, London, 1966.

12 Leo Kanner: "The Specificity of Early Infantile Autism," *Zeitschrift für Kinderpsychiatrie,* vol. 25, pp. 108–113, 1958.

13 Nic Waal: "A Special Technique of Psychotherapy with an Autistic Child," in Gerald Caplan (ed.), *Emotional Problems of Early Childhood,* Basic Books, New York, 1955.

14 Marian K. De Myer et al.: "Prognosis in Autism: A Follow-up Study," *Journal of Autism and Childhood Schizophrenia,* vol. 3, no. 3, pp. 199–246, 1973.

15 Margaret S. Mahler, Fred Pine, and Anne Bergman: *The Psychological Birth of the Human Infant,* Basic Books, New York, 1975.

16 Margaret S. Mahler: "Thoughts about Development and Individuation," *Psychoanalytic Study of The Child,* vol. 18, pp. 307–324, 1963.

17 Lauretta Bender: "Twenty Years of Clinical Research on Schizophrenic Children with Special Reference to Those under Six Years of Age," in Gerald Caplan

(ed.), *Emotional Problems of Early Childhood,* Basic Books, New York, 1955.

18 Barbara Fish and Rosa Hagin: "Visual-Motor Disorders in Infants at Risk for Schizophrenia," *Archives of General Psychiatry,* vol. 28, pp. 900–904, June 1973.

19 Lauretta Bender: "The Development of a Schizophrenic Child Treated with Electric Convulsions at Three Years of Age," in Gerald Caplan (ed.), *Emotional Problems of Early Childhood,* Basic Books, New York, 1955.

20 Magda Campbell: "Biological Interventions in Psychoses of Childhood," *Journal of Autism and Childhood Schizophrenia,* vol. 3, pp. 347–373, 1973.

21 Dean Critchley: "Nursing Interventions with the Disturbed Latency Aged Child," in Claire M. Fagin (ed.), *Nursing in Child Psychiatry,* Mosby, St. Louis, 1972.

22 Patricia Howlin et al.: "At-Home-Based Approach to the Treatment of Autistic Children," *Journal of Autism and Childhood Schizophrenia,* vol. 3, no. 4, pp. 308–336, 1973.

35

The Family with Adolescent Adjustment Problems

Katharine J. Burns

Learning Objectives

After studying this chapter, the student should be able to:

1 Assess the adolescent's growth and development
2 Assess family dynamics
3 Intervene to prevent the development of an adolescent adjustment reaction
4 Apply the nursing process to the management of problematic adolescent adjustment behavior

Adolescence is a social phenomenon as well as the stage of physical, psychological, and emotional development and integration which forms the basis for maturity. It is a developmental stage characterized by accelerated growth and emotional turmoil.

There is a delicate and intricate balance in the relationship between parents and adolescents. The two separate but interacting aspects of the parent-adolescent dyad are the physical and the relational aspects. The child possesses certain characteristics of its forebears and has a unique relationship with the parents; this relationship, in turn, is influenced by the family's cultural and environmental background and its ongoing dynamics.

In childhood there is a strong and necessary dependence on the parents for protection, nurturing, and need fulfillment. As the child approaches and proceeds through adolescence, this dependence is relinquished and there is movement away from the family and into society. The evolution of the child into and through the adolescent stage of development is a dynamic process within both the individual members and the family system. Thus the adolescent and family are in continuous reciprocal interaction and flux and must be viewed as a psychosocial unit.

The plurality of factors which must be considered to understand and analyze the adolescent-family dynamic and the growth and development process include the physical and emotional characteristics of the individual members; the mores, attitudes, values, and life-style of the family; the social milieu; and the relational dynamics. Each of these factors influences family functioning and the adaptation of individual members.

Adolescence

In our society today, there is continual reference—in professional journals, conferences, television, and magazines—to the newly emerged "youth culture." This culture is most dramatically evidenced in the changes in clothes, hairstyles, and language. Sex and age differences are no longer as clearly distinguishable by hair and dress styles as they were in the past. The various movements of the 1960s—civil rights, human rights, the antiwar movement and women's liberation—escalated these changes. These social convulsions of the sixties occurred at a period of time when the investigation of adolescence as a stage of development was in its infancy.[1]

Adolescence has always existed as a process, but it was not until the 1950s that we began to see it as a unique yet vital developmental stage in the life cycle and a bridge between childhood and adulthood.

Information and theories about adolescence are still somewhat incomplete when compared with our knowledge of earlier developmental stages. According to Erikson, what is known is intertwined with the influence of greater societal issues. The normal maturational crisis of adolescent development cannot be completely separated from contemporary social crises, for these two issues define each other and are interdependent on one another.[2]

Adolescence is an important phase in the life cycle in that it incorporates—psychosexually, interpersonally, and cognitively—the past years of development into a new and different gestalt in preparation for an adult identity. With the onset of rapid physical and hormonal changes, children may feel that they are turning into completely different people.[3]

The latency child is industrious in work, play, and peer relations. At this stage the child lives in a psychobiological moratorium. The child's involvement in the physical environment and in learning about it is the most important aspect of this stage of life, during which the child is still being protected and nurtured by parents or significant others. This stage of development forms a self-contained world characterized by a preoccupation with hoarding, superstitions, collecting, and counting.[3]

Drastic changes psychologically, biologically, and socially occur with the onset of adolescence. However, these changes do not always manifest in a uniform, integrated way. There are delays in some areas, while overlapping and acceleration occur in others. Physical maturation may be rapid and complete much earlier than emotional or social maturation. The artificial division into early, middle, and late adolescence provides a framework for examining the growth process, but there are no clear-cut boundaries between these substages. The divisions can be seen more clearly in some social classes and cultures than in others. These stages are more evident in young people who continue their education but less clearly defined in those who leave school at an early age and are exposed to the pressures of a complex society. Post-high school training usually means extended socioeconomic dependence on the family, thus prolonging the late adolescent stage; whereas the adolescent in our society who either leaves high school or graduates and goes to work achieves financial independence more quickly.

The division of adolescence into three stages is also indirectly supported by the educational system in our society. School progress is to a great extent determined by chronological rather than maturational age. However, this division presents problems for some, because considerable discrepancies can occur between chronological and maturational age. For example, in any group of 15-year-old adolescent males, physical maturation can vary widely. Some will appear immature, small, and more childlike, while others may clearly resemble adults. The males in this latter group may shave and have deepened voices.[4]

Early Adolescence
Physical Changes
Early adolescence begins with the onset of secondary sex characteristics and the experience of having a close, special friend. It is initiated by biological and endocrinological changes which prepare for and promote the concomitant changes within the intrapsychic, cognitive, and interpersonal subsystems of the personality.

Although the exact chain of events is extremely complex and some information is as yet unclear, it is known that in prepuberty there is an increase of estrogen in girls and androgen in boys. These biological changes occur in boys sometime around the age of 13. The penis, testes, and scrotum increase in size and the first downlike pubic hair appears. For girls, the biological changes occur sometime around age 11 and are seen in a rounding of the hips, budding of the breasts, and the appearance of pre-pubic downlike hair.[5]

Between 11 and 13 years of age, girls are taller than boys of the same age. They also tend to have temporary puppy fat.[4] The menses are often irregular at first and do not necessarily indicate the capacity for pregnancy. The shape of the boy's larynx changes, deepening the voice; but initially the deeper voice tends to be uneven and sudden breaks in pitch occur frequently. The boy's hips become slimmer and his body more muscular. Downlike hair appears on the upper lip and at the hairline at the side of the face. In both sexes the endocrine changes also include the activation of sweat glands and the facial oil glands. The increased activity of the sebaceous glands predisposes the early adolescent to suffer from acne and blackheads, which constitute a very disturbing alteration in their body image.

Behavior and Dynamics
These important physical changes cannot be separated from psychological development. The chemical changes cause increased sensitivity and awareness of the genital areas, while the changes in the body shape, size, and contour increase general body awareness. These body changes dramatically alter the body image and self-concept.

Early adolescents are uncomfortable about their bodily changes. The need to gain control over their bodies and impulses at the same time they are separating from the family system is problematic. The rapid physical growth and change in body image alters the perceptual system; therefore these youngsters are often clumsy and self-conscious. Girls often dress in loose-fitting, unfeminine garb to hide their developing bodies, and they often engage in giggling fits in the presence of boys. The males withdraw into their own same-sex groups.

The child's identity no longer fits its self-perception. The young person is in effect "half child and half adult." Thus early adolescents exhibit behavior which is quite contrary to that seen in latency in that they are less rational, less mature, less predictable, and more egocentric.[5–7] They are extremely active physically because of their increased libidinal energy, which is not always directed into socially acceptable behavior.[8] For example, Katy came home from school obviously upset. Her mother empathetically commented, "You look upset, did something happen?" Katy responded with a flow of anger: "You don't understand . . . its my business! Stop nosing in!" Then she stomped upstairs and slammed her bedroom door.

Early adolescents become concerned with freeing themselves from dependence on their parents. The peer group is used as a support in their struggle for freedom. Besieged by sexual and aggressive impulses, they enter a period of psychic turmoil. Struggling with their own sexuality, they deny their parents' sexuality but are preoccupied with it. It is emotionally painful to them if their parents have another child. This blatant evidence of their parents' sexual activity often makes them feel shame.[4]

For example, when Carla's mother became pregnant, Carla did not mention the fact to her friends. When the pregnancy became obvious and Carla was questioned by her girl friends, she became angry and refused to talk to them.

During this intrapsychic upheaval, these young people are involved in thoughts and feelings reminiscent of the oedipal phase. Although these reactivated feelings may be quantitatively the same, they are now very different in character due to the adolescent's increased awareness of being physically more like an adult.

The parent-adolescent relationship becomes strained by the adolescent's striving for independence and the way in which they undertake this process. Conflict is a common occurrence as the young person fluctuates between dependent, childlike behavior and independent, mature functioning, and it is certainly made worse by the adolescent's sadistic attacks and masochistic sufferings when rules are enforced or discipline is applied. As the parents attempt to relate to the ever-changing moods of their early adolescent, they are apt to say, "I don't know you anymore . . . I don't know what to do with you." Such messages reinforce adolescents' perceptions of their changing self-concept. Parental limit setting and concern are met with intense argumentativeness or dramatics characterized by a flood of confused and incoherent complaints and grievances.[8] Confusion in communication, feeling, and relationship is evidenced by both sides on the new battleground.

Ian's parents, for example, refused him permission to go with his friends to a local shopping center on a school night. Ian accused his family of treating him "like a baby." Both Ian and his parents got into a shouting match. The wrangling deteriorated as the parents attacked Ian for his irresponsibility toward household chores and his poor grades in English. Ian countered with accusations that his parents were alcoholics, although they had only a single cocktail before dinner every night. Both Ian and his parents lost track of the initial issue as they tried to find vulnerable targets in one another.

Adolescents begin to become intolerant of parents. They disparage the parents' dress, lifestyle, friends, and way of doing things. The parents cannot drive the right way, cook well, or dress appropriately. In the young adolescent's view, the parents are ignorant and insensitive. At times, the adolescent's "put down" of the parents seems cruel, unfounded, and insensitive. Adolescent diatribes often threaten the parents' self-concept as "good" parents and generate anger. The parents often ask themselves, "What have I done wrong? Do I deserve this treatment?" If adolescents are forced to suppress this rejection and to maintain a primary identification with the parents, the process of separation and differentiation is hampered and they experience increasing anxiety.

Adolescents verbally resist and reject parental beliefs, values, and standards. They may become reluctant to bathe and vehemently refuse to wear clothes selected by the parents. Instead, they prefer the careless dress code of their peers, often looking somewhat disheveled or mismatched by parental standards. The clothes they select must conform to what is "in" with the peer group. The adolescent becomes recalcitrant about participating in the household chores or maintaining his or her room, which is often kept in chaotic disorder. These reactions and behaviors are, in effect, the early adolescents' way of defending against the sexual impulses they are experiencing. These behaviors are a direct means of expressing the concomitant aggressive drives; they also reflect the disorganization of the superego in preparation for adult restructuring. Finally, the conflict between adolescents and their parents is part of their struggle for autonomy and separateness.

During early adolescence, boys assess their masculinity in relation to others of the same sex and age.[4] They are preoccupied with their bodies, and masturbation is an important activity in the development of self-awareness and sexual feelings (see Chap. 12).

In early adolescence, boys are particularly intolerant of control exercised by female authority figures and see such control as a threat to their emerging masculine identity.[4] When illness strikes, male adolescents can be very difficult clients. Enforced inactivity robs them of a major avenue for discharging tensions. The treatment regimen is often seen as a form of parental control and represents loss of independence. Their ambivalence and fear regarding dependence and independence are often manifested in irritable noncompliance.

Impulse control is a major problem, particularly for the male. Frustration escalates to anger or tears easily. When adolescents are threatened or perceive themselves as being treated unjustly, they exhibit their anger loudly and vehemently.

They consider justice and fairness very important; when they encounter what they see as injustice, they will shout and slam doors.[1,4]

Girls confront the dependence-independence issue somewhat differently. They want independence but still need to maintain a degree of dependence, particularly on their mothers. While the male's fight for independence is waged primarily outside of the home, the female's struggle takes place mainly within the family system. Girls attempt to form alliances with their fathers against their mothers. Their preoccupation with their bodies leads them to focus on physical attractiveness, and their puppy fat is very distressing to them. In early adolescence, girls are often moody and tense, and daydreaming is an important part of their mental lives. They differ from boys in that they can use the parents for support and do not always need the peer group to the same degree. They develop their sense of femininity by appraising their body configurations and comparing them to those of other females; femininity is also cultivated through their relationships with their fathers or other older men in the family who care about them but are not interested in using them sexually.[4]

The early adolescent begins to move away from intimate contact and relationship with the parents and to some degree replaces them with peers and other adults. The new adult figures become idealized; in choosing them, adolescents are attempting to identify with their parents but in a less sexualized manner. They project some of their previous adoration and respect onto the idealized person, who may be a teacher, coach, youth-group leader, a television star, or a music celebrity. The intensity of the adolescent's feelings toward the idolized adult allows for a release of sexual energy which is displaced onto an object that is less remindful of the oedipal relationship with the parents. This displacement of feeling also allows early adolescents to desexualize the parents while at the same time permitting them to gratify their curiosity about the sex lives of adults as well as to pursue their own sexuality.

For example, Peter developed an interest in photography and joined the school camera club. Mr. Corey, the faculty adviser, became a "Pied Piper" for several boys including Peter. They admired his dress, opinions, and life-style. The group gathered in his home room after school each day to talk about photography, school, and world issues. Sometimes, they would kiddingly question Mr. Corey about his ski trips and dates with another teacher.

Peer relationships are important in the development of the early adolescent. These relationships are more intense and exclusive than friendships in latency, but each may last for only a short time before being replaced by another close relationship. Initially these friendships are most often with peers of the same sex; thus this period is also identified as the normal homosexual period. At this stage there is intense rivalry, teasing, and aggressive behavior toward peers of the opposite sex.

Girls dramatize these relationships by acting like tomboys or being openly seductive or sadistic toward boys. This behavior may appear to be heterosexual in some respects, but it is not acted on and serves as a defense against identifying with the preoedipal mother.

Boys turn to peers of the same sex for friendship also partly in defense against reactivating feelings toward the mother. They interact very little with girls their own age.[8,9]

The early adolescent also chooses friends of the same sex as a narcissistic identification in order to avoid uncomfortable feelings about the changing self-concept and to gain feelings of self-worth. Same-sex friendships and activities also help the early adolescent avoid the exciting and anxiety-producing presence of the other sex, avoid loneliness, increase self-esteem, and gain support during the separation and differentiation from the family. Within the context of the peer group, adolescents are able to explore their own sexuality and developing identity.[8,9]

Moralistic and conservative values and beliefs continue to influence the adolescent perception of sexuality. These societal constraints concerning sexual experimentation, premarital sex, and masturbation may not inhibit behavior but often generate guilt and anxiety if they are violated.[10]

The chum relationship, as it becomes consolidated, is in essence a prototype of all future love relationships. The intense drive for intimacy is both strong and frightening. Chum relationships facilitate mutual validation of personal self-esteem and are absolutely essential if the individual is to gradually deal with the issue of intimacy, to modify the impact of earlier parenting, to expand interpersonal relationships, and to grow socially.

Cognitive Development

During this stage of development, the cognitive structures undergo change.[11] The capacity for different types of formal thinking and abstract thought develops.[4] The early adolescent begins to explore ideas and thoughts about what is experienced and can now rationalize about the causation of events.

Adolescents' preoccupation with their changing bodies, their relationships, and their fantasy world often interferes with academic work. They have particular difficulty with rote learning at this time, but their potential for imaginative thinking is great. For these reasons they may go through a period in which they become less able to concentrate on work efficiently.[4] They may become frustrated and frustrating. Academic achievement may slip, causing parental concern and usually generating conflict.

Needs of the Early Adolescent

In spite of their wild and dramatic protestations, these adolescents expect and need some limit setting and enforcement of parental standards. They are not yet able to cope with total freedom and independence and if it were given would feel overwhelmingly anxious. The conflict and struggle are a part of the growth process for both the parents and the adolescents. The way the conflict is managed has greater importance than its existence. Adolescents need gradual, supported movement toward independence and a climate that tolerates the "noise" made in striving for autonomy. They need, *first,* interest and emotional involvement and, *second,* external control of their behavior by the adult world that is founded on mutual respect rather than fear.[4]

Adolescents need a school as well as a home environment that is safe and secure. They will test the limits of each system and need to find firm and rational boundaries. The educational setting must be one that is conducive to the exploration of intellectual and emotional issues and which provides opportunity for physical activity.

Midadolescence
Physical Changes

The physique of the midadolescent is different from the earlier stage in that it is more developed in height and weight; also, the incidence of acne is greater. Males develop facial and body hair, genitals increase in size, and there is a more developed musculature.[4] There is also a concomitant increase in awareness of sexual feelings.

The rounding of the female's body contours increases. Estrogen production is increased and pregnancy is possible. The girl's voice changes in timbre as the ovulatory cycle stabilizes and growth stops.[4] Girls also experience a strong upsurge of sexual feeling, which is related to the hormonal and bodily changes.

These body changes, which are noticeable to others, heighten the adolescent's awareness of being more like an adult and become an intense preoccupation.

Behavior and Dynamics

Adolescents at this stage of development react with anxiety, fear, and apprehension when confronted with biological maturation and the capacity to engage in sexual activity. At the beginning of midadolescence, girls may develop "crushes" on older girls or women to defend against a lack of

readiness for emotional involvement with boys. They may also exhibit an interest in mothering small animals or children. Boys may have a special same-sex friend, but their needs are adequately met in a same-sex group which also continues to serve as a defense against involvement with girls.

In time, both sexes experience the wish to experiment and to test out their sexual capacities. The boy's drive is directed toward conquest and confirmation of his physical capacity. Love, tenderness, and intimacy are not primary. In girls, these needs are reversed. Their primary concern is a tender, loving, intimate relationship; sexual exploration and excitement are secondary.

Sexual permissiveness is a dilemma for this age group. Family pressures are great, but subtle societal messages and peer pressure are in conflict with the family position. The double standard concerning the sexual behavior of males and females still exists in our society. Families tend to be less protective and more tolerant of the sexual behavior of their sons than they are with regard to that of their daughters. The risk of teen-age pregnancy and an out-of-wedlock child often worries the parents and results in restrictive and overprotective behavior toward daughters, which generates intense conflict. The daughter envies the loving relationship between her parents and is acutely aware of her own needs for love and affection. She becomes angered and confused by her mother's perception of males as predatory and dangerous.

Girls mature more rapidly than boys, so they are more likely to be interested in boys 2 or 3 years older than themselves.[4,12] It is at this time that girls experience their first love, which usually terminates in considerable emotional upheaval.

The teen-ager falls in and out of love often or may have two love objects at the same time, investing both with intensely romantic feelings. These multiple short-term romantic friendships allow teen-agers to express their new genital lust as long as there is no anxiety imposed by the attitudes of family, significant others, or society. In time, genital lust is integrated into the self-system, which is the composite "me" developed out of the involvement in maintaining a sense of security within the self, through interpersonal interraction with others.[13]

The parent-adolescent relationship continues to be strained and conflicted. The parents and adolescents have conflicting needs and struggle with the separation and differentiation process. Both must work out the adolescents' questioning of family attitudes as well as religious and cultural mores and beliefs. The adolescents' sexuality may threaten the parents, who may see their own sexual potency declining. Responsibility is often a hot issue. Parents and adolescents struggle over what, how much, and how it is handled.

Academic achievement becomes somewhat more manageable. Some adolescents busy themselves in schoolwork and books as a way of avoiding confrontation of their emerging sexuality and relationships with the opposite sex. Bill, for example, did poorly in junior high school, but his academic performance showed a marked improvement in high school. He spent long hours studying and preparing projects. However, in spite of parental encouragement, he refused to attend school dances or parties.

Identity formation is a major task that must be confronted. These adolescents begin to examine their relationships to peers, parents, and society and to think about the roles they hope to assume. They begin to think seriously about career choice and often seek employment for the first time. Adults outside the family continue to be important and meaningful. Sometimes another set of "parents" is found, who will provide a home away from home. Young people are often better able to talk with and—more importantly—listen to these adults, whose viewpoints they not only tolerate but often respect.

Cognitive Development
Cognitive processes are consolidated into a more unified and consistent self-concept. The adolescents' thinking processes are now incredibly more logical. They are capable of demonstrating wisdom, understanding, and empathy. However, this fine intellectual ability has little effect on their behavior. The preoccupation with lofty ideals and love is continually being redefined but does not yet help the adolescent to find a place in society.[8]

Needs of Midadolescents
Midadolescents need adult models with whom to identify, and this identification process may be either conscious or unconscious.[14] They may adopt mannerisms, communication styles, and personality traits of significant adults without becoming aware that they are doing so. They may also consciously imitate mannerisms, interactional styles, and personality traits because they admire the way particular adults present themselves or deal with people.

Adults have a responsibility in this identification process. Adolescents tend to tune in to and adopt the behavior they observe, and this may be a negative identification. Rather than incorporating the ideals recommended by the parents, they tend to pick up the discrepancies between what the parents say and what they do. It is the "what they do" that is incorporated; and the "what they say" ideal is ignored or rejected. For example, a parent may warn a youngster about alcohol abuse and issue prohibitions against drinking; but if that parent then "ties one on" after a hard day at work or at a party, conflicting messages are being sent and the adolescent is more apt to notice and identify with the drinking behavior than the content of the lecture against alcohol.

Midadolescents also need a secure and stable environment that makes demands appropriate to their capacities. A midadolescent can be a competent baby sitter for a defined period of time but is not able to assume total child-rearing responsibility for younger siblings. Such responsibility is too great. It distracts these young people from their own need fulfillment.

These youngsters also need stable relationships—"Stability" meaning more than continuity of relationship with the people in the environment. Divorce and the death of a parent can be extremely upsetting, but emotionally absent parenting can be equally destructive. The adolescent needs the parental figures to argue, struggle, and clarify so as to further the development of personal identity. A parent who is physically present but overpermissive and/or uninterested does not provide a climate conducive to identity formation.

School and career choice are often problematic for these youngsters. They need support, acknowledgement of the difficulties in these areas, and help in applying a problem-solving approach to these and other dilemmas. They also need opportunities to learn how to relate to the opposite sex, and to develop a positive view of themselves as attractive and competent as people.

Late Adolescence
Physical Changes
Late adolescence is essentially a stage of psychosocial development; however, the male, more often than the female, continues to grow physically.[4]

Behavior and Dynamics
The time a person takes to proceed through this stage of development depends on social class, economic status, and the family influences. For those who enter universities or post-high school vocational schools, this stage of adolescence will be extended since they will continue to be economically dependent on their families. Those who enter the working world directly will assume socioeconomic responsibility for themselves and enter adulthood sooner.

At this stage, the clumsiness of earlier adolescence has disappeared. Older adolescents have gained control of their adult bodies and have integrated the adult body image. Males maintain their interest in competitive sports, either by active participation or as passive spectators.[15]

The heightened emotionality which characterized earlier periods has tended to subside. Anger is the most easily aroused emotion and is most often generated when self-assertion is blocked or when the individual's usual pattern of activities is interrupted. The angry responses are now under control and are expressed verbally, particularly through sarcasm.[15]

The person at this stage of development has fewer intimate friends but a broader social circle. Interests are no longer centered on same-sex friends and groups; rather, they are shifted toward developing opposite-sex relationships. The number of friends is of lesser importance, but the "right" friends are of greater concern. Late adolescents have well-defined expectations for friends of both sexes. The major concerns of the late adolescent are appearance, independence, career, and relationships with the opposite sex.[15]

The conflicts between parents and late adolescents diminish in number and intensity. The young people still need support and caring from their parents and other significant adults, but these relationships no longer hinge on dependency and control.[4]

Late adolescence involves a series of transitional experiences which contribute to the final consolidation of identity. People at this stage employ a variety of techniques such as vacations, study abroad, or extended visits to friends' homes to facilitate their separation from the family of origin. When they first leave home to live at college or in an apartment with friends, they may return home to visit frequently. During these visits, they often provoke arguments with their parents, particularly just before they leave, as if to reassert their own need to separate and their ability to do so.[4] For example, toward the end of a semester break and shortly before returning to college, Paul would often provoke an argument with his parents, which left them feeling confused and angry.

The maturity of the late adolescent is evident and can be measured by the capacity to be loving, to wait for emotional satisfaction, to consider the future, and to control aggressive and hostile impulses.[4] The degree of maturity in the physical, emotional, and intellectual spheres still varies due to the individual differences in the rate of progression through adolescence, but the disparity between maturational and chronological age is not as great as before.

Late adolescents seek loving relationships

with members of the opposite sex. They are, at this stage, better able to understand the depths and variations of another's mood and are capable of emotional trust. However, they still maintain a degree of concern about performance expectations in social life and sexual relations and also about their attractiveness.

The major theme at this developmental stage is the tension between self and society. Late adolescents have developed a relatively defined sense of who they are, but they must now find places for themselves in society. They feel ambivalent about this process and its possible effects on their personal identities.

Assessing their strengths and weaknesses, they test, challenge, and confront the attitudes of the older generation. They experience both estrangement and omnipotence. They are alienated from others and experience loneliness; at the same time, they have the opportunity to live in a world designed by themselves, which suggests a powerful sense of being able to create a "new society" without the old values and inhibitions. As they struggle to integrate themselves in society, they are constrained by the facts of history; but they may become part of that very history when their struggle is recognized and accepted as intrinsic to the period.

The sense of identity takes on a different definition as late adolescents emancipate themselves from the family of origin and begin to participate in the world. This synthesis, whereby both self and society can be affirmed—wherein both remain autonomous yet related to reality—is now established. A process of individuation occurs in which neither the self nor society are lost.

The success and ease with which the adolescent moves into adulthood depends on prior successes in negotiating earlier developmental tasks, the family's capacity to facilitate separation and differentiation, and society's capacity to absorb each new member. Social organizations are significant in the reinforcement of late adolescents' mental health, since they reinforce both personal and cultural identity and provide a feeling of personal and social continuity.

Cognitive Development

Late adolescents have consolidated abstract thinking and deductive reasoning. Their intellectual processes operate on a mature, adult level. For some, this is a period of increased interest in pursuing knowledge and examining ideas critically and logically.[4]

Needs of Late Adolescents

Adolescents at this stage are still separating and differentiating from the family. They exhibit stability in their life-styles and relations with others and need to have a supportive environment to facilitate the maturation process. Friction with parents tends to center on the acceptance of responsibility, use of money, dating, and choice of friends. Late adolescents still need the counsel and the support of family, but in the form of advice rather than imposition.

To prepare themselves for a place in the larger society, these young people need sound information, support, and encouragement so that they may pursue their interests and develop the skills needed for socioeconomic independence.

Selection of friends, dating, and sexual activity are areas of concern; however, people at this stage are most resistant to interference or comment from parental figures. Social insight and sensitivity are greater at this stage. When opportunities to use and develop these qualities are found, the young person's growth in social competence is enhanced.

Adjustment Reactions to Adolescence

"Adjustment reaction to adolescence" is a diagnostic classification (see appendix) which includes the emotional and behavioral difficulties encountered by the young person who is negotiating the adolescent stage of development. The symptoms tend to be acute, transient, and mild if the young person is supported through this developmental period.

Symptoms fall into *four* areas of functioning: (1) affective (anxiety, depression, psychosomatic complaints, phobia, acting out); (2) characterologic (schizoid trends, immaturity, aggressivity, passivity, obsessive compulsivity); (3) cognitive (under- or overachievement); and (4) psychosocial (conflict with family, school, or society).[16] The emergence of these symptoms is related to the successes and failures the adolescent has experienced in negotiating earlier developmental periods, the quality and quantity of immediate stresses, and the quantity and quality of available environmental support from family, school, and community.

Dynamics of Adjustment Reactions

The emotional turmoil of adolescence can be escalated by any one or several of the previously identified causes. The anxiety may be manifest, easily identified, and labeled by the adolescent, or it may be expressed in the form of depression, school failure, or acting-out behavior. When the adolescent's behavior is grossly out of line, socially unacceptable, or destructive to the self or others, the emotional disturbance is the basis.

Depression is usually described as a state of sadness, retarded psychomotor activity, and social withdrawal, reflecting a low energy output. Adolescents may exhibit the classical symptomatology of depression, or they may express their depression through violent, aggressive, and acting-out behavior. Hostility and aggression are considered by many to be the underlying factors in the psychogenesis and psychodynamics of depression. The adolescent's energy level is greater because of the increased libidinal energy characteristic of this developmental stage; thus the depression could conceivably reflect this higher energy level and be masked by hyperactivity, attacks on the environment, and impulsive acting out.[17]

Depressed adolescents often suffer from a chronic feeling that they are unable to live up to the idealized image they have pictured for themselves. As a result, the self-esteem, self-confidence, and self-acceptance of depressed adolescents are poor. These attitudes, of course, undermine ambition and the aggressive seeking-out behavior that might help them to find the gratifications and happiness they feel themselves to be missing.

By acting out in the immediate and larger environment, adolescents are escaping from their feelings of despair and hopelessness. Although this may not make them feel satisfied or happy, it does provide a defense against feeling unhappy. However, in some youngsters, this dynamic may be combined with the insatiable need for security or attention, whatever the price. It does not matter if the price is punishment as long as the behavior brings the needed attention. This behavior may be very similar to that described by Sullivan[18] in his concept of *malevolent transformation.* In his view, some youngsters are *conditioned* to behave negatively, and such conditioning begins in early childhood. It is then that they learn that they can satisfy their need for tenderness and attention by being "bad." Later, they may find that their needs are not met, and then the "bully syndrome" emerges in all social relationships. This has a profound effect during adolescence, when peer relationships are extremely important. Lacking the necessary skills and means to replace parents with peers and to gain satisfaction from friendship, the adolescent is left without a viable support group.

The disturbed adolescent carries along the primitive identification models of childhood, in which there are both ego and superego deficits. With impoverishment in both these psychic structures, the youth is unable to achieve self-satisfying human relationships within the broad societal constructs. This failure provokes feelings of rage, helplessness, and hopelessness; hence "negative self-identity" is acted out in the environment through dissocial behavior.

Family Dynamics

When adolescents have difficulty negotiating this developmental stage, the parent-child relationship is to some degree dysfunctional. A stable, nurturing, and need-fulfilling relationship was impaired in prior developmental stages. Given the maturational crisis of adolescence, the family system is further disorganized and less able to help the youngster through the normal upheavals and emotional turmoil of this stage. Parents are in conflict concerning their own aging, the separation and differentiation of their adolescent, the rejection of their values and beliefs, and the adolescent's sexuality. These parental uncertainties and ambivalences affect the way adolescents perceive their positions and self-concepts as emerging adults.

Restrictions which may have been easily enforced in the past generate fury and family chaos. Parents may overreact to these resistances and battles either by becoming overrestrictive or by throwing up their hands in surrender and pursuing a line of permissiveness and nonresistance. The greater the family's rigidity and lack of knowledge about the growth process and the less their respect for the autonomy and individuality of the child, the greater the conflict and the greater the potential for an adjustment reaction. Blurred gender and generation boundaries increase the adolescent's anxiety and the need to defend.

Adolescents who are anxious, depressed, and/or participating in an unhealthy family dynamic manifest their distress in a variety of self-destructive ways. These young people are not born basically "bad" or "mad" but are the by-products of their environment. Their intrapsychic problems are related, at least in part, to a family, school, and/or community system which interferes with their effective progression through the development stages. Their self-concept and the consequent behavior is formed by taking on the negative attitudes of significant others toward the self that others display toward them.

Sullivan[18] postulates that the child can develop *malevolence* when love is not the predominant experience in the child-parent-other relationships. This occurs when the child who needs tenderness and performs activities that should evoke it is not only denied tenderness but also treated in ways that generate anxiety, emotional distress, and/or physical pain. Adults may take advantage of their authority positions and make the child feel even more wretched by laughing at, ignoring, or ridiculing the child or by actually abusing the child physically. This provokes feelings of helplessness.

When adults fail to meet the child's need for affection and approval, the child develops a malevolent attitude toward others and sees itself as living among enemies.

As these youngsters proceed through adolescence, they are unable to trust others, particularly adults. They are conditioned to perceive any evidence of benevolence as a threat, a sign of impending trouble, and a cue that tells them to assume a malevolent defensive posture.[19] This attitude about self and others becomes a vicious cycle as these youngsters attempt to protect themselves and their feelings. They relate to the world in a hostile, destructive, and self-destructive manner.

Some of these youngsters are generally isolated and immature. They—as individuals or in groups—maintain no clear alliances or friendships with others.[20] They are hedonistic in that they are most concerned about themselves and material desires and pleasures, and they are generally able to rationalize their behavior and actions on the basis of their own individual pleasure principle. However, youngsters of another type are primarily "dissocial." They develop close loyalties with others within a group or gang, all of whom demonstrate disregard for the conventional social order or moral codes, usually as a result of having lived most of their lives under abnormal moral conditions.

In the psychoanalytic framework, Szurek[21] and Johnson[19] postulate that the personality organization of these youngsters is warped in that the superego or conscience is not effectively helping them to assess the demands and moral codes of their society. The psychic structure of superego evolves out of the primary relationships the child had with parents. That is, children develop a conscience through the parent-child relationship. Throughout this process, limits or prohibitions should be consistent and not enmeshed with overwhelming guilt or anxiety. The child should be allowed to express needs in an assertive manner, and the parents' response must be one of educating and assisting the child to gain reward and satisfaction for more appropriate behavior.

However, Szurek[21] states that on occasion the

parents, because of their own neurotic needs, in essence actually encourage the delinquent acting out of a particular child or of all their children. The parent or parents unconsciously encourage the antisocial or amoral behavior of the child. This encouragement is initiated and maintained by parental behavior toward the child which is either excessively domineering, dependent, or erotic, thereby satisfying the parents' own neurotic needs to the neglect of the child's needs.

Steirlin[22] has categorized family dynamics which interfere with the adolescent's progress through this stage of development as either centripetal or centrifugal. His framework speaks to the issue of separation and the way transactional modes in the family system interfere with the process. Age-appropriate transactional modes are out of phase in these families. They are either too intense, inappropriately mixed with other modes, or too distancing.[22]

Centrifugal Dynamics

When the centrifugal dynamic is operating, the family employs a binding mode of transaction. Members operate under an unspoken assumption that needs can be satisfied *only* within the family system. The outside world is viewed as dangerous and unsatisfying. This dynamic sets up insurmountable barriers between the family and society and, in a collusive way, forces members to remain within the family. It fulfills some needs for security, support, and nurturing, but it does so at the expense of individual ideas, feelings, experiences, and behavior. Members are prevented from separating and differentiating, which is destructive to the development of individual potential and freedom.[22]

The binding process corrals the members through the affective, cognitive, and superego levels. The affective binding is accomplished by offering the adolescent too much regressive gratification and thus infantilizing the youngster.[22]

The awakening libidinal drives and the oedipal conflict are blocked from resolution in peer and societal relationships. The parents, particularly the opposite sex-parent, become the focus of

reactivated symbiotic and incestuous feelings. Anxiety increases in youngsters who are blocked from moving away, and it must be defended against, yet it is not possible to run away or rebel without feeling guilt and increasing anxiety. Even if these youngsters do manage to reach out to others, their ingrained, well-learned, excessive demands for regressive gratification are intolerable and unacceptable to peers or adults outside the family. These young people often turn to drugs or alcohol to quiet aggressive and sexual drives and to enable them to tolerate the smothering family life. Since the substance abuse does not, at least initially, interfere with the mutual parent-child dependence, it is often covertly and unconsciously supported by the parents.[22]

Binding on the cognitive level occurs when the parents interfere with the adolescent's self-differentiated awareness and self-determination. The parents attribute to the adolescent feelings, needs, motives, and goals that disconfirm the child's position in these areas. Such an attribution process interferes with the ability of adolescents to perceive and differentiate what they are experiencing, want, and need by injecting meaning or by withholding meaning. For example, when the daughter is angry because she cannot select her own clothes, the parent tells her she is just nervous, thus substituting anxiety for anger and disconfirming the daughter's own perception of the events and her feelings about them. The withholding of meaning is usually accomplished by the parents who are silent or cryptic. Without reality-based feedback and shared perceptions, the adolescent is cognitively isolated and immobilized. The developing cognitive skills are blocked and distorted, leaving only fantasy, supposition, and untested hypotheses rather than logic and rationality.[22]

Parents also bind by interfering with the process of loyalty transfer. These parents paint a picture of self-sacrifice, concern, and love. Any investment of feeling or interest in others is seen and interpreted as a rejection of them. The parental message to the adolescent is clearly, "How can you treat us like this and leave us? We live only for you." Consequently, if these adolescents attempt to initiate the normal separation process of this developmental stage, they feel guilty about abandoning their "loving" parents, who cannot exist without them. The conflict between parental requirements and developmental need fulfillment is intolerable and they see self-destruction or incorporation back into the family system as the only alternatives.[22]

Centripetal Dynamics

In this dynamic the parents are also coping with their own crises. The problems inherent in their adolescent's growth process are not the focus of their interest and are burdensome. Concerned primarily with their own needs, goals, and desires, they lack both the energy and the motivation to help the adolescent.

These parents do not want their children; instead, they want to pursue desired changes in their own lives.[22] They may not be ready or able to confront their own aging process. They may exhibit this expelling mode by becoming totally absorbed in their own recreation or work and simply ignoring their adolescents. They set no limits and provide no stability or support, and they may be unavailable physically and emotionally. If the youngster runs into problems at school or with the law, the parental posture is, "What do you want me to do? I can't follow him [or her] around."

These youngsters may or may not be neglected or deprived materially. Some live in the most luxurious of homes and are provided generously with food, clothes, money, and transportation. Others lack even the bare necessities of life: warmth, food, warm clothing, and a safe home. In either circumstances, they are seen by the parents as nuisances and also see themselves in that light.

In some instances adolescents are thrown out of the house; in others they run away because they are aware they are unwanted. Sometimes the parent or parents leave—if not permanently, then for extended periods of time—leaving their children without financial support.

Youngsters caught in this dynamic are left to spend their time as they wish. They collude in the lack of communication. They say little or nothing about their feelings, expectations, or activities and the parents ask no questions. The family may simply coexist under the same roof. All the relational aspects of family life are minimal or absent.

Some of these young people, left to their own devices, exhibit delinquent behavior, become drug abusers, or create violent turmoil in the home. The school authorities or police confront the parents, who choose not to take active steps toward helping their children. Enraged that their lives are being disrupted, they expel the adolescent from the family system through a psychiatric commitment, surrender of guardianship, placement in a boarding school, or refusal to allow the youngster back into the home.

Delegating Dynamics

Parental developmental crises contribute to the emergence of the delegating dynamic. These ambivalent and conflicted parents select neither the centripetal nor centrifugal solution to the problematic adolescent growth phase.[28] They are caught between their wish to consolidate existing relationships and positions and their desire to be rid of the adolescent. Consequently, they send conflicting messages to their adolescents: "Leave, but don't leave." They send the adolescent out on a mission as a proxy, while at the same time they hold on. The adolescent incorporates this ambivalence.

Stierlin[22] has identified four types of missions that adolescents may carry out to serve the ego needs of the parents: (1) helping (work around the house, financial support of the household); (2) fighting (support of embattled parent); (3) scouting (serving as parents' experimenter); and (4) preserving (protecting fragile parents from conflict, activating emotions, and ambivalence).

The parent may vicariously enjoy and covertly support the acting out of dissocial impulses. The adolescent's dissocial behavior *or* successes in school vicariously fulfill parental fantasies or are experiences they were deprived of in their own youth. The adolescent's behavior is not directed toward self-fulfillment but toward the affective and ego needs of the parents. The parents may push the adolescent into the world to experiment with the single life to test out what this life-style is like before they decide to pursue a divorce and a similar life-style.[22]

When the parents have punitive and restrictive superegos, they may ascribe any one of three superego functions to the adolescent: (1) to serve as ego ideal, (2) to provide self-observation, or (3) to serve as a conscience.[22] If the first alternative is selected, the youngster's career choice will fit parental expectations and their own unfulfilled dreams regardless of the adolescent's personal preference. When given the self-observation mission, the adolescent must behave in ways that are contrary to the family's values and be "mad" or "bad." If the third alternative applies, these adolescents will be covertly encouraged to exhibit behavior that justifies punishment. The adolescent tends to exhibit dissocial behavior similar or comparable to that of the parent in the past. The premarital pregnancy of a daughter and consequent maternal punishment resolves the mother's own guilty feelings about her out-of-wedlock pregnancy.[22]

Client Behavior
Overt Depressive Behavior
Adolescents may initially manifest underlying depression through indifference toward themselves, others, school, and social activities.

This apathy or indifference may be followed by overactive garrulousness and activity. The adolescents search frantically for someone or something that will not only keep them busy but will be entertaining, satisfying, or fun. There is an ability to work diligently in trivia and be happy without interruption for a time, possibly a long time, but then there follows a period in which they cannot be alone, nor can they be productive in any activity, even their most favored ones. A sense of restlessness and boredom sets in which cannot be shaken, regardless of the environmental stimulation. They avoid being alone in order to defend against conscious awareness of their depression. They may complain of fatigue and sleep a great deal but still exhibit periods of inexhaustible energy. These physical complaints are more extensive and pervasive than an occasional period of low energy. Extremes in energy level are related to the internalized conflicts with which they are trying to cope.[20]

Since depression in adolescents is often masked, its depth is often not recognized. Suicide is a significant problem among teen-agers. As startling as the statistics are, they do not reveal the full extent of the problem because of the failures in reporting. Overdoses and accidents with firearms and cars are often the result of a conscious or unconscious wish to die. The suicidal behavior usually follows a number of stresses and crises which tax an already weakened ego structure. The loss of a meaninful relationship, suspension or expulsion from school, an unwanted pregnancy, or an injury may aggravate the depression. Rather than rebel, these youngsters withdraw emotionally into themselves and see no solution to their problems except their own extinction.

Eddie, age 17, dropped out of school after repeated suspensions for the possession and selling of pot and for disruptive behavior. He drifted around with a loosely organized group and had a minimal relationship with his family. The night his girlfriend broke off their relationship, he killed himself by driving his motorcycle into a stone wall at full speed.

Low Academic Achievement
These youngsters may find it difficult to concentrate, particularly on their academic studies. This easy distractibility, may first be noticed by school authorities, teachers, and guidance counselors when assignments are not completed, daydreaming in class becomes noticeable, and tests are handed in without answers. On the other hand, it may become evident only after an extended period of time in which failing grades become the norm, whereas average or above may have been more common previously. As the adults, parents, and school authorities place more pressure on them to "succeed," these teen-agers begin to internalize the belief that they are not able to learn

and begin to think about dropping out of school, or they cut classes even though they may be in the school building on a daily basis.

They have no purpose or goal in life and are unable to seek out an adult for support or identification. They may want to succeed but are unable to mobilize themselves purposefully or persistently. There may be spurts of interest and achievement, but apart from these isolated incidents the overall picture is one of withdrawal, apathy, and isolation. These youngsters may join loosely organized groups of peers or remain loners. If they associate with a group, there is no real involvement or friendship. There is no loyalty to the group or another individual, only a tangential association which reinforces feelings of loneliness, alienation, and low self-esteem.

They may choose to drop out or continue through high school, meeting only the minimum requirements for graduation. They may continue through life ill-prepared and with a perception of themselves as failures.

Acting-Out, Impulsive Behavior

The adolescent who acts out often does so impulsively. One minute these youngsters can be charming, agreeable, outgoing people, and the next minute they are raging furies if limits are imposed, expectations not met, or underlying conflicts and the concomitant anxiety triggered. When overcome by rage, they may provoke physical altercations with parents, peers, or adult authority figures such as teachers, policemen, or—if they are hospitalized—caretakers.

If confined to an inpatient setting, adolescents may suddenly decide to "elope" (run away) rather than be confronted by members of their therapy group, participate in a family meeting, or follow through on discharge plans. If they remain in the community, they may feel overwhelmed by anxiety or anger and impulsively steal a car for a joyride or vandalize a home or public building. They seem unable to control their affect sufficiently to think through the consequences of their actions.

The unpredictability of their behavior and the risks they take challenge caretakers. In group sessions, if they are angered by feedback from another member, they may stomp out or smash furnishings.

Karen was scheduled to be discharged on Friday. Unable to verbalize her fears about returning home, she panicked and impulsively eloped from the hospital, thus further aggravating the discharge crisis. She returned to the hospital voluntarily, feeling depressed and confused about her impulsivity.

Acting out also includes sexual behavior which violates the social norms for adolescence. During midadolescence, homosexual episodes may occur as youngsters attempt to deal with overwhelming feelings of object hunger.[16,23] These adolescents may experiment with homosexuality or heterosexuality. Some are covert and their activities are discovered by accident; while others blatantly flaunt their behavior, to the discomfort of everyone. Some adolescents frantically seek closeness and affirmation of their sexuality in a series of sexual encounters which only leave them feeling lonelier and less accepting of themselves. The negative opinions of others concerning their promiscuous behavior reinforce their own poor self-concept. Even though they may find that their behavior fails to satisfy their needs for love and belonging and only aggravates their depression and anxiety, they seem unable to break the pattern.

When these youngsters come into treatment, they do not readily surrender this behavior. They use sex to dampen the feelings of loneliness and anxiety—feelings which may be intensified by the therapeutic process.

Laurie's seductiveness and overt sexual behavior toward the male staff and clients disrupted the unit. She required close supervision, which angered the other clients, who felt that her monopoly of staff attention decreased their opportunities for therapy and help.

Substance Abuse

When adolescents suffer from chronic emotional pain, they seek ways to diminish the intensity of their feelings. The substance they choose may vary, but the use of a drug to numb feelings is most often learned in the home. These youngsters watch their parents or other significant adults cope with work frustrations and use alcohol or drugs for recreation. The drug-taking behavior is also reinforced by television, radio, and magazines. Commercials and advertisements "push" a variety of remedies to ease the tensions of daily living and to induce sleep. The adolescent watches the adult world use drugs to escape from rather than cope with problems.

Initially these adolescents may tap their parents' liquor supply or steal their tranquilizers or sleeping pills. Once they experience tension release from experimenting with what is available in the home, they seek out peers who either sell or who can make contact with suppliers of drugs and marijuana or an older youth who can purchase alcohol.

Young adolescent abusers may use pot exclusively but are more likely to eventually experiment with whatever capsules or pills they can acquire. They often mix these drugs with alcohol, even though they know it is dangerous. Glue sniffing, LSD tripping, skin popping, and cocaine sniffing may all be tried for varying periods.

These young people will acknowledge the risk involved in taking "street" drugs, but they tend to shrug it off with a comment such as, "I've never gotten burned." Their risk taking and apparent lack of concern reflects their underlying depression and self-destructive tendencies.

Most often such youngsters are hospitalized only to avoid imprisonment after arrest for possession or selling; because parents have had them committed; because an LSD trip led to a psychotic episode; or because they had frightening blackouts or anxiety attacks after heavy use of alcohol. Thus they are unwilling clients and initially invest much time and energy in devising ways to escape or to have drugs brought in to them. They resist the imposition of hospital rules and policies, examining their feelings, exploring their behavior, and planning realistic changes in coping patterns and life-style.

These adolescents tend to be manipulative; if there is any divisiveness in staff, they find it and use it to cause disruption. Hospitalization does not mean the end of drug use for these clients. They will plot and plan to either smuggle in drugs or alcohol themselves or have it brought in. Hence they require careful surveillance of their activities and visitors.

Runaway Behavior

According to the DSM classification runaways characteristically escape from threatening situations by fleeing from them. They are typically immature and timid. They feel rejected, inadequate, lonely, weak, abandoned, worthless, helpless, and hopeless[24] (see appendix).

Adolescents leave home for a variety of reasons: sometimes to fulfill the vicarious wishes of their parents and sometimes to escape intolerable feelings and fears generated by the home situation. There are those who leave home in a fit of temper, go only a short distance, and return in a day or two. These youngsters are more apt to run away after a family argument during the warm weather, when the hardships are not as great. Many in this group attend school regularly. They may not attend classes, but they will be in the building during the school day. They sleep in friends' homes or vans or in empty houses in the community. Some have part-time jobs and, with the help of friends, they manage to eat regularly. In time they return home only to repeat the runaway behavior sporadically. They hunger for affection and are seething with suppressed and repressed anger. They have had little opportunity in their families to express their anger directly. If they steal, it is usually only from the family to finance their running away.

Some youngsters leave because they have been overtly rejected or subjected to incestuous advances by an alcoholic parent or stepparent. They feel unsafe and/or unwanted. These homes have often provided few opportunities for socializing experiences and, as a consequence, these youngsters have a history of problems with school or police authorities. Their parents are not likely to protect them from the authorities. When their youngsters run away, these parents—unlike the parents in the other group—make little or no effort to locate them or bring them into treatment. If the children are hospitalized, this is done after the parents have been pressured by the authorities or the youngsters have been remanded by the courts.

Once the runaway pattern becomes routinized and unrelated to external events, the freedom to run becomes essential and confinement or restriction of any kind is seen as punitive, even if applied in a supportive way.[24]

During hospitalization, elopement is always a risk. The treatment structure exerts a continual force, and the urge to run away is strong. However, the adolescents themselves see the problems they experience as centered in the family. If family therapy is initiated, they may feel more hopeful, but they are sensitive to their parents' willingness to participate and work in therapy. If the adolescents sense reluctance or resistance to an open and honest confrontation of the family problems, they feel the situation is hopeless. In this instance they are apt to act impulsively and attempt to elope.

Unsocialized Aggressivity

According to the DSM classification, these youngsters' behavior is characterized by overt or covert hostile disobedience, quarrelsomeness, physical and verbal aggressiveness, vengefulness, and destructiveness. They exhibit temper tantrums and will steal and lie if given the opportunity (see appendix).

These young people have often grown up without stability, discipline, or opportunities to become socialized. They are not only aggressive but lack sexual inhibitions as well. Persistent enuresis even into early adolescence is not uncommon, reflecting the overall lack of control.

They are hostile, uncooperative, and provocative. Their belligerence, defensiveness, and tendency to withdraw—compounded by a history of deprivation and disorganization—distances caretakers. The impulsive and unpredictable verbal and physical hostility has been learned in the family system and seems ingrained. They have deep-seated inner feelings of self-hatred, depression, and helplessness.

These youngsters will strike out at anyone who interferes with what they want to do or say. Eddie, a well-developed 15-year-old, was playing cards with three other adolescent clients on the unit. He insisted on being dealer, and when the others resisted, he grabbed the smallest boy and began punching him in the face and head. When the nurse and aide intervened, Eddie shifted his physical attack to them and had to be placed in restraints.

These youngsters often have long histories of delinquent behavior; their patterns of violence and stealing may continue during hospitalization. Bart was caught "red-handed" stealing money from another client's wallet. In spite of confrontation and anger from staff and clients, he seemed unconcerned. Several days later, he was caught again trying to jimmy open a cabinet where the nurses locked their belongings.

Nurses' Response

No other group of clients can elicit a wider variety of feelings in the caretakers than the mercurial adolescents. Their unpredictability is both a challenge and a burden. The competitive struggle and testing of limits taxes the nurses' patience. Repeated violation of limits frustrates and angers staff. Progress toward self-control for these clients is a slow process, and the staff may become impatient and angered by the lack of improvement or the sabotaging of the treatment plan.

These clients may feign meekness and, given their family histories of deprivation or abuse, they elicit sympathy in the caretakers, who may entertain rescue fantasies. However, their compliant, meek behavior may be short-lived. As the therapy proceeds and the need for conformity to hospital structure is made clear, these adolescents may become sullen, negativistic, hostile, and/or violent. Caretakers become frustrated and angry when they must deal with impulsive acting out and monosyllabic responses to their interventions.

The adolescent's constant testing of people and limits seems endless. Attempts at exploring underlying conflicts may be met with intellectualizations or social criticisms which only serve to increase frustration and a feeling of fruitlessness in the nurse.

These youngsters attempt to put the nurse in various authority roles and try to provoke exasperation and hostility, and they are often successful. Regardless of whether they display open opposition or negativistic silence, they manage to provoke anger in the nurse (see Chap. 17).

The violent, aggressive, assaultive, and impulsive behavior of adolescents often frightens the staff. The enforcing of limits is dreaded in anticipation of the turmoil that will follow. If there have been physically violent episodes during the hospitalization or in the past history of a given client, nursing staff are wary and may tend to ignore disruptive behavior and the enforcement of established limits. The nurses fear for their own safety as well as that of the other clients.

If restraints are prescribed, they may be used inappropriately when the nursing staff are fearful. Psychotropics may also be used to excess to avoid confrontation of aggressive behavior.

Nursing staff may also be reluctant to extend the adolescent's privileges, thereby increasing dependency and impeding progress toward self-control and assumption of responsibility. Unwittingly, nurses may assume a punitive parental role, which replicates the family dynamic and escalates the adolescent's anger.

The family may be equally frustrating and anger-provoking. Their resistance to participating in the treatment program or their sabotaging of it infuriates staff. If they abandon and reject the adolescent, the staff may side with the adolescent, thus further distancing the family and isolating the adolescent.

If the adolescent's behavior is obnoxious toward parents who appear to be supportive in spite of their child's rejection, staff may be sympathetic toward the parents and side with them. If staff align with either side, they alienate the other and only divide the family into warring factions, thus impairing the differentiation process.

Identification with either the adolescent or the parent is problematic (see Chap. 22). The young nurse with unresolved adolescent issues may identify with the client. Consequently this nurse may support the adolescent's rebellious behavior toward authority figures, and this can be destructive to the unit's stability and therapeutic effectiveness. The older nurse may identify as a parent figure. If this nurse fosters dependency or takes a punitive, disciplining posture, the adolescent will be prevented from taking advantage of the opportunity for growth offered by the therapeutic process.

Assessment

The adolescent with an adjustment reaction is problematic, and so is the family. To understand the full extent of their problems and to intervene effectively, the nurses' data base must include information about the adolescent and the family system. The following is a guide for the assessment process:

The Adolescents

1 Do they see a problem?
2 To what do they ascribe the problem?
3 What is their perception of the problem?
4 Is there evidence of developmental disturbances?
5 What do they think will remedy the problem?
6 How do they relate to peers and authority figures?
7 What is their motivation for change?
8 What are their fears and fantasies about changing?
9 How do they define and describe their relationship with their parents?

10 What feelings are they aware of?

11 Can they identify what situations trigger activating emotions?

12 What problematic behavior do they exhibit?

13 How do they relate to caretakers?

14 Was there a precipitating event for this hospitalization? If so, what was it?

15 How do they distance people and reinforce their poor self-concept?

16 What needs are met by the maladaptive behavior?

The Family

1 Do they see a problem?

2 What is their perception of the problem?

3 What do they feel will remedy the problem?

4 What are their perceptions of the adolescent's development?

5 How do they describe past separation events in the adolescent's life?

6 Are they willing to participate in the treatment process?

7 What is the quality of the marital relationship?

8 How do they define and describe their relationship with their adolescent?

9 How do they relate to the staff?

10 What needs are met for the parents by having a dysfunctional adolescent?

Planning Nursing Care
Primary Prevention

The problems which precipitate an adolescent adjustment reaction have their roots in early childhood. Healthy family functioning and member growth and development may be facilitated by nursing interventions which assist families to cope effectively with the decision to parent, integrate the child into the family, understand growth and development, adapt to change, engage in authentic conflict resolution, and recognize and meet member needs. Chapters 11, 26, and 32 discuss the application of the nursing process to helping families function effectively, particularly in relation to child rearing and nurturing.

Secondary Prevention

When symptoms of adolescent adjustment reaction occur, the turmoil and pain is distressing to all participants. When symptoms first appear and if they are mild, counseling on an outpatient basis may help family members enhance strengths and ameliorate weaknesses. In some instances, parents need to understand adolescence as a developmental stage and a growth process. The nurse assesses the parents' knowledge of adolescence and provides the necessary information. The normal behavioral and emotional responses of their child may have been misinterpreted or mismanaged. With knowledge about the norm, the parents are better equipped to cope more appropriately. However, feelings are not always resolved by the provision of information alone. The nurse must also help the parents and adolescent articulate their feelings and needs in a way that can be "heard." The nurse gives family members feedback on how their communications are received and encourages members to do the same. For example:

John: (Yelling) Stop treating me like a baby. Keep your damn hands off of me and quit the nagging.

Nurse: John, when you shout like that I don't really "hear" what you say. I get angry when I'm yelled at and I think that's how your parents react too. Is that true Mr. and Mrs. Bok?

Mr. Bok: Sure I get angry. And if he keeps it up he'll be sorry.

Nurse: So you get angry too, and when this happens, it sounds like you threaten John, which probably escalates his anger. Is that true John?

John: Sure I get madder . . . he can't boss me around anymore.

Nurse: I'm wondering how each of you could

tell the other how you feel, but in a way that the other could hear and understand and maybe work out the problem by finding another solution.

John: I don't like being told so many times to take out the garbage or do my homework.

Nurse: Why do they tell you so many times?

John: Because I forget.

Mrs. Bok: He needs to be reminded, but when we tell him, he blows up and there's a fight.

Nurse: Sounds like John doesn't object to the chores but does have a problem remembering and being reminded.

John: Yeah, that's right.

Mr. Bok: That's about it.

Nurse: Well then, if you could find a way of remembering or reminding other than by telling, the problem might be solved. Has anyone ideas on how this could be done?

By helping family members see how they participate in the conflict, the nurse refocuses the problem from being one person's burden and presents it as a shared difficulty. In this instance, the nurse focuses on the central issue and then attempts to help members look at the conflict as a problem for which a solution can be sought.

Parents may be helped to empathize with their children's difficulties if they are helped to get in touch with the struggles and distress that accompanied their own adolescence. It can be useful to facilitate reminiscence and recall of how the parents felt and responded. The parents also need to explore their feelings about their relationship and the changes they are experiencing. Interventions which help parents share needs, feelings, and concerns facilitate parental communication. Often the focus of their interactions has been their problematic adolescent. Refocusing onto their relationship defuses the parent-child conflict and provides an opportunity for them to explore their relationship as well as confront and resolve their conflicts. Both the parents and the adolescent may resist this type of intervention because the adoles-

cent has been protecting the parents from this very activity.

The adolescents often need help in modifying and controlling their responses to irritating situations. By providing feedback and enforcing limits, the nurse initiates a socialization process directed toward helping the youngsters learn ways of interacting which are less abrasive, so that expressed needs can be heard by significant others.

Limit setting is a problematic issue for both the adolescent and the parents. Parents may adopt an inconsistent and unstable permissive stance in order to protect themselves from the conflict which occurs when they attempt to enforce limits. Other parents may be at the other end of the continuum, enforcing restrictive and inappropriate limits. The nurse models and facilitates the negotiation process as a way of defining and implementing limits. Both parents and adolescents must be helped to listen to and analyze the other's position. Sometimes each can be helped by role playing the other's position or by alternating roles.

The adolescent needs to assume responsibility and to separate from the family gradually. The nurse helps each client explore how changes in these areas are experienced as well as the fears and fantasies that go with such changes.

Tertiary Prevention

The adolescent may be hospitalized if symptoms become so pronounced that the family can no longer tolerate the chaos, the school system pressures the family, or the law becomes involved because of delinquent behavior. When this happens, the dysfunctional family patterns may be well-established and the resistance to change strong. Both the parents and the adolescent may express a desire to change the situation, but underlying conflicts and the needs met by the maladaptive behavior interfere with actualization of goals.

Often the adolescent is sullen, angry, and withdrawn initially. Flexibility and informality are necessary to the initiation of a relationship. These young people need acceptance of *who they are* but *not* of their antisocial behavior. This distinction is difficult to communicate but necessary for the development of a trusting therapeutic relationship (see Chap. 6).

Caretakers must be sensitive to their own feelings and be aware of how they are provoked by the emotionally pained adolescent. Patience, consistency, and stability are necessary in a therapeutic relationship. These disturbed young people tend to test limits repeatedly and to manipulate staff and other clients. When their behavior interferes with acceptance by others and integration into society, they must relinquish these behaviors and learn new, more effective ways of relating to people and satisfying their needs. As they learn to do this and to cope with stressful situations, people will interact with them differently. The more socially acceptable and responsible their behavior becomes, the better the chance that they will be able to satisfy their needs and gain positive social rewards without resorting to antisocial behavior.

Some behaviors are particularly problematic in a hospital setting. Table 35-1, on the care of the adolescent, cites common problem behaviors, nursing diagnoses, goals, and suggested interventions.

Table 35-1 Care of the Adolescent

Client Behavior: Elopes from hospital unit to avoid confrontation.
Nursing Diagnosis: Impulsive avoidance of reality.
Nursing Goals: Help client develop control of impulse to flee from distressing situations.

Interventions:
- Enforce specified limits.
- Explore how feelings are managed.
- Assist clients to examine the consequences of their actions.
- Guide exploration of alternative ways of dealing with feelings and problems.
- Encourage ventilation of feelings.
- Establish contract that when pressures seem unmanageable, the nurse can be turned to for a discussion of the issues.
- Encourage client's peers to share their feelings concerning the client's elopement and its implied rejection of both treatment and their help.

Client Behavior: Aggressive, assaultive attack on another.
Nursing Diagnosis: Inadequately socialized, inability to mediate feelings.
Nursing Goals: Help client develop impulse control, manage feelings appropriately, and learn socially acceptable behavior.

Interventions:
- Use restraints to prevent assaultiveness and enforce limits.
- Facilitate verbalization of feelings.
- Suggest vigorous physical activity such as competitive sports to lessen buildup of tension.
- Help client analyze situations to identify what provokes rage.
- Explore alternative ways of managing provocative situations.
- Enforce firm limits.
- Communicate behaviorial expectations clearly.
- Assist client to establish personal goals.
- Encourage other clients to confront the adolescent on their fears and concerns and the impact on their ability to help.

Client Behavior: Violates hospital prohibition of drug and alcohol use on premises.
Nursing Diagnosis: Avoids dealing with feelings.
Nursing Goals: Help client cope with stress without resorting to drugs or alcohol.

Table 35-1 Care of the Adolescent *(continued)*

Interventions:
- Search client and belongings for drugs and alcohol.
- Confiscate drugs and alcohol.
- Supervise activities and visits.
- Explore problems and feelings.
- Confront discrepancies between what is said and actual behavior.
- Assist client to examine consequences of behavior.
- Provide opportunities for graduated assumption of responsibilities.
- Give positive feedback on effective management of frustrating situations and evidence of responsible behavior.
- Encourage other clients to verbalize the feelings of rejection and risk they experienced as a result of the behavior.

Client Behavior: Withdraws physically and emotionally from others.
Nursing Diagnosis: Low self-esteem blocks ability to relate to others.
Nursing Goals: Help client develop self-acceptance and feelings of competency.

Intervention:
- Encourage participation in unit activities by joining client.
- Select minimally demanding group activities initially.
- Provide opportunities for client to perform competently.
- Give positive feedback when tasks are handled well.
- Require client to be escorted by others for all off-unit activities until client socializes voluntarily.
- Limit time client spends in room alone.
- Limit television watching by engaging client in conversation.
- Encourage other clients to involve client in unit activities.

Client Behavior: Anxiety reaction consequent to enrollment in college in another state.
Nursing Diagnosis: Difficulty separating from family.
Nursing Goals: Help client develop independence and differentiation.

Intervention:
- Point out strengths and areas of competency.
- Give positive feedback on efforts toward independence.
- Open communication between client and parents.
- Explore with client the role she plays in the family and how it affects her.
- Help parents examine their relationship.
- Explore with client her fears and fantasies about what will happen to her and her parents if she leaves home.
- Encourage other clients to share their perceptions of the client's predicament.
- Communicate societal expectations of young people the client's age.

Client Behavior: Mutilates forearm with lighted cigarette and scratches wrist with thumbtack from unit bulletin
                     board.
Nursing Diagnosis: Poor self-concept;
                     isolated, with feelings of rage and loneliness.
Nursing Goals: Increase client's self-esteem;
                     help client establish meaningful relationships and cope less destructively with feelings.

Interventions:
- Supervise client closely.
- Remove all items which could be used for self-destructive purposes from the client's environment.
- Explore feelings and events which precipitated behavior.
- Give positive feedback when there is appropriate management of feelings.
- Confront client on use of behavior as an attention-getting device.
- Explore how client thought staff and family would respond to the mutilating behavior.
- Restrict recreational off-unit activities when mutilative behavior occurs.

Table 35-1 Care of the Adolescent *(continued)*

- Require evidence of responsible behavior before full privileges are restored.
- Set up graduated, clearly specified responsibilities.
- Encourage peers to share their perceptions and feelings about the episode with the client.

Client Behavior: Runaway consequent to learning of mother's pregnancy.
Nursing Diagnosis: Difficulty confronting parents' sexuality.
Nursing Goals: Help client cope with own and parents' sexuality as well as to confront mother's pregnancy openly and directly.

Interventions:
- Restrict to unit until pressure to elope lessens.
- Encourage client to talk about feelings related to pregnancy and peers' perception of the situation.
- Explore client's feelings about changes in body image and self-concept.
- Encourage discussion with peers about who they are and what is happening to them.
- Encourage client to confront parents with feelings.
- Help client explore changes in the family caused by pregnancy.
- Help client recognize others' acceptance of mother's pregnancy.

Client Behavior: Flaunts homosexuality; extremely effeminate behavior; makes seductive and outrageous propositions to same-sex peers and staff.
Nursing Diagnosis: Sexually seductive and provocative behavior interferes with establishment of relationships with others.
Nursing Goals: Clarify client's sexual identity and help client to abandon offensive sexual provocativeness.

Interventions:
- Confront client on use of behavior as an attention-getting device.
- Positively reinforce authentic behavior and reactions toward others that are not laden with sexual overtones.
- Ignore sexually provocative behavior when used to gain attention.
- Explore client's thoughts, feelings, and attitudes about sexual orientation.
- Explore perceptions of the consequences of choosing this sexual orientation.
- Enforce limits on socializing with other clients when seductive behavior is imposed on others.
- Encourage other clients to share their feelings about client's behavior toward them.

Evaluation

Because of adolescents' well-established, self-defeating patterns of coping, careful planning and intervention are necessary to help these youngsters follow through the treatment program. They will impulsively and often unconsciously sabotage their own progress. Setbacks are inevitable and must be accepted as part of the natural course of events. Steps forward are often small. Staff must recognize these small progressions and—more importantly—help adolescents see improvement not only in their behavior but their overall situations as well.

If nursing goals are clearly articulated and specified in terms of gradients, they can be used to measure the effectiveness of nursing interventions. For example, the assaultive client whose behavior is outlined in Table 35-1 requires interventions directed toward social conformity, the prevention of dissocial behavior, and the imposition of the consequences of acting out. The success of these interventions can be evaluated by assessing the client's progress toward impulse control and the client's ability to talk about feelings rather than acting on them.

References

1 Norman Kiell: *The Universal Experience of Adolescence,* Beacon, Boston, 1968.
2 E. Erikson: *Identity, Youth and Crisis,* Norton, New York, 1968.

3 J. Anthony: "The Juvenile and Preadolescent Periods of the Human Life Cycle," in S. Arieti (ed.), *The American Handbook of Psychiatry*, Basic Books, New York, 1974, vol. 1

4 D. Miller: *Adolescence*, Jason Aronson, New York, 1974.

5 A. Freud: *Normality and Pathology of Childhood*, International Universities Press, New York, 1966.

6 A. Freud: *The Ego and the Mechanisms of Defense*, International Universities Press, New York, 1971.

7 A. Freud: "Adolescence as a Developmental Disturbance," in G. Caplan and S. Lebovici (eds.), *Adolescence: Psychosocial Perspective*, Basic Books, New York, 1969.

8 J. Kestenberg: *Children and Parents: Psychoanalytic Studies in Development*, Jason Aronson, New York,

9 G. Blum: *Psychoanalytic Theories of Personality*, McGraw-Hill, New York, 1953.

10 W. Gadpaille: *The Cycles of Sex*, Scribner, New York, 1975.

11 H. Ginsburg and S. Herbert: *Piaget's Theory of Intellectual Development*, Prentice-Hall, Englewood Cliffs, N.J., 1969.

12 L. Wilkins: *The Diagnosis and Treatment of Endocrine Disorders in Childhood*, Charles C Thomas, Springfield, Ill., 1965,

13 H. S. Sullivan: *Interpersonal Theory of Psychiatry*, Norton, New York, 1968.

14 E. Erikson: *Childhood and Society*, Norton, New York, 1963

15 E. Hurlock: *Developmental Psychology*, 2d ed., McGraw-Hill, New York, 1959.

16 S. Feinstein: "Adjustment Reaction to Adolescence," in A. Freedman, H. Kaplan, and B. Sadock (eds.), *Comprehensive Textbook of Psychiatry*, 2d ed., Williams & Wilkins, Baltimore, 1975.

17 R. Spiegel: "Anger and Acting Out: Mask of Depression," *American Journal of Psychotherapy*,

18 P. Mullahy: *Psychoanalysis and Interpersonal Psychiatry*, Science House, New York, 1970.

19 A. Johnson: "Sanctions for Superego Lacunae of Adolescents," in *Childhood Psychopathology*, International Universities Press, New York, 1972.

20 C. Malmquist: "Depressive Phenomena in Children," in *Manual of Child Psychopathology*, McGraw-Hill, New York, 1972.

21 S. Szurek and I. Berlin (eds.): *The Antisocial Child: His Family and His Community*, The Langley Porter Child Psychiatry Series, Science and Behavior Books, Palo Alto, Calif., 1970, vol. 4.

22 H. Steirlin: *Separating Parents and Adolescence*, New York Times Book Company, New York, 1974.

23 S. Harrison and J. McDermott: *Childhood Psychopathology*, International Universities Press, New York, 1972.

24 J. Meeks: "Behavior Disorders of Childhood and Adolescence," in A. Freedman, H. Kaplan, and B. Sadock (eds.), *Comprehensive Textbook of Psychiatry*, 2d ed., Williams & Wilkins, Baltimore, 1975.

Chapter

36

The Abusive Family

Barbara Flynn Sideleau

Learning Objectives

After studying this chapter, the student should be able to:

1 Assess families and work situations for evidence of abuse

2 Discuss the dynamics of abuse, including the victims, abuser, and contributing environmental factors

3 Collaborate with other health and welfare professions in the delivery services to the abusive families

4 Plan nursing interventions to assist abusive families to cope more effectively

5 Intervene in the abusive family cycle to protect the victim and facilitate the development of more effective family coping

6 Evaluate the delivery of services to the abusive family

Violence is as old as humankind and our society is not immune to it. The prevention and control of violence presents serious and difficult problems, especially since it is the weak and the powerless who become the victims of abuse (see Chap. 15).

Violence within the family has been defined by Lystad[1] as a mode of behavior involving the direct use of physical force by some family members against others. This violence ranges from the mild spanking of a child to the commission of a homicidal act. Such behavior also varies in intent, ranging from attempts to control behavior to the venting of personal hostility. Sometimes it may be a mixture of both.

Epidemiology and Statistics

Statistics on the frequency of child abuse vary considerably and are incomplete. Estimates have suggested that child abuse may occur as often as 6 times in every 1,000 children.[1] Each year, $1/2$ to 1 million children may become the victims of abuse meted out by their caretakers.[2,3] No statistics are available on the incidence of wife battering or the fate of those in residential institutions who are abused by caretakers.

Precisely what constitutes child abuse is poorly defined. Cultural norms concerning the child's right to protection are, in practice, vague and perhaps deliberately so. Children "belong" to parents and are considered to have only limited rights. The expansion of children's legal rights is often seen by society in general and especially by parents as an infringement of parental authority.

Statistically, abuse is more common in families of low socioeconomic status and educational achievement and among those with broken homes. Such findings may be inaccurate. Abuse is known to occur in middle- and upper-class families who are financially stable and have attained high levels of education. However, cases treated in emergency rooms or clinics are more apt to be labeled and reported to child welfare authorities; in suburban communities, on the other hand, where treatment is by a family physician, reporting is less likely.[1]

In recent years the legal aspect of child protection has undergone a radical change. The Mondale bill (Child Abuse and Treatment Act of 1973) has been implemented to attack the problem. It states:

> Child abuse and neglect means the physical or mental injury, sexual abuse, negligent treatment or maltreatment of the child under the age of eighteen by a person who is responsible for the child's welfare under circumstances which indicate that the child's health or welfare is harmed or threatened thereby. . . . -

Since the passage of this bill, all states have enacted legislation to protect the child from abuse and to require health-care professionals (physicians, teachers, nurses, and social workers) to report suspected cases of abuse.

Forms of Abuse

The physical abuse which a victim may suffer includes bruising; burning; whipping; skin laceration; bone fractures, particularly of the torsion type; and trauma to the internal organs caused by punching or kicking of the abdomen or sexual molestation. However, for the victim to experience the effects of abuse it need not be as direct and overtly aggressive as a physical attack. Physical and emotional neglect can be equally destructive to the well-being of the victim. This type of abuse includes failure to meet nutritional needs. Such deprivation can result in retarded growth and development.

The infant and young child are particularly vulnerable to inadequate "mothering" and emotional and physical neglect. The consequence of maternal deprivation is *failure to thrive*. An infant or child whose nutritional, sensory, oral, and dependency needs are met satisfactorily will direct energy toward growth and development. When these basic needs are not met, the "taking in" process is disturbed. In time, the child's physical growth will be slowed or stopped, the development of motor skills will be delayed, and social and emotional withdrawal will occur. Such infants are more susceptible to infection and impaired physiological functioning, which may even result in death[4] (see Chap. 34).

Neglect can also include poor hygiene, inappropriate and inadequate clothing, failure to obtain immunization protection, and communication which is destructive of the victim's self-esteem and self-acceptance. Furthermore, runaway behavior in the latency-age child as well as teenage pregnancy have also been identified as indications of emotional neglect within the family.[5]

The problem of battered wives is only recently receiving attention. In England, refuge houses have been established where protection, counseling, and temporary shelter are provided. Although there is legal protection for the wife in our society, for a variety of reasons it is not often used and it generally fails to mitigate the husband's abusive behavior. The cultural pattern of denial operates to prevent the recognition that men beat, torture, and kill the women they live with, just as it has, in the past, operated in relation to the abuse of children. Many women live despairingly and desperately in a world of almost incredible violence. Their stories are commonplace to lawyers, doctors, psychiatrists, the clergy, and court officials. These wives delay, often for years, reporting the harrowing experiences of their married lives, even to friends and relatives, in shame, fear, and hopelessness that anyone can help.[6]

The Clients
The Victims
The victims of abuse are those individuals with the least power in society, those who, throughout the ages, have been the recipients of maltreatment. Children, adolescents, women, the institutionalized, and the aged have little capacity to defend themselves against physical assault and emotional neglect. Children from birth to 3 or 4 years of age have been identified as particularly vulnerable. Infants who cry uncontrollably because of colic pains, for instance—cannot protect themselves from the shaking and slapping inflicted by immature, frustrated parents.[7]

The victim also often possesses special characteristics which engender intense feelings in the abuser. Tom, a lively 3-year-old with curly red hair and blue eyes, clearly resembled his father. His mother also saw him as having a personality similar to that of his father, who abandoned the family shortly after his birth. Tom was frequently and severely beaten by his mother, while his two older sisters, who resembled the mother's family, were never the target of abuse. Tom's physical appearance, probably the fact he was a male, and the perceived similarity of his personality to his father's triggered the mother's anger and resentment, which she displaced onto her son.

The Abuser
The abuser is physically stronger and more powerful than the abused. In the marital dyad, the husband most often abuses the wife, while either a parent, older sibling, baby-sitter, or related adult assaults the child. In residential institutions and day-care centers, caretakers may abuse or neglect the retarded, the mentally incompetent, the aged, or children.

The Dynamics of Abuse
The dynamics of intrafamily and caretaker violence can be viewed in terms of the sociocultural, intrapersonal, and interpersonal contexts. The social-structure aspects of family and caretaker violences are (1) the power structure of the family or institution, (2) the socializing framework of beliefs and values, and (3) the power and social structure of the larger society.[1] A family and a residential institution consist of a hierarchy of

interpersonal relationships, with superordinate and subordinate roles as well as rivalries that often elicit the use of force.[1] Parents dictate family rules and regulations and mete out discipline when their children violate them, while administrators set policies for their employees and also enforce them with disciplinary measures. Parents and administrators may be punitive rather than constructive when rules are violated. Parents may abuse their children directly and physically. In the work situation, employees frustrated by insensitive and punitive administrators vent their angry feelings onto powerless clients. Employees, like children in a family, may also engage in sibling rivalry to gain the attention of authority figures. Authority relations, milieu climate, hierarchical positions in the structure, values, and beliefs influence the expression of violence in the family and work environments.

Society

Society's attitudes toward the use of force as a legitimate means of attaining ends—especially in imbalanced interpersonal relations such as male-female, caretaker-client, adult-child—and the tendency to resort to force for dealing with conflicts in our society contribute to the incidence of abuse. The abuser-abused relations are intimately linked to prevailing social attitudes and the common concept of human beings and their rights. The use of force toward women, children, the aged, and the incompetent is also related to the way in which these people are seen by society and how their rights are defined.[8] (See Chap. 15.)

In our society, the socially unacceptable and those who are unable to care for themselves are relegated to institutions out of the mainstream of life. The rights of this population are not always adequately protected. The problems of neglect and abuse these people face are often not brought to public attention except when they become a political or media issue.

Work alienation may be an influential societal factor in abuse. A work environment with a hierarchical and authoritarian structure which is compet-

itive and exploitative creates psychological stress and in some instances causes deviance in the employees. The locus most frequently perceived as safe for releasing tension generated in the workplace is the nuclear family, where the spouse or child victims become the objects of anger.[8] In residential-care settings, the caretakers may vent similar feelings on the clients.

The beliefs and values derived from the sociocultural context may foster violence. Our cultural norms of child rearing allow the use of a certain amount of physical force toward children by their adult caretakers.[1] Children in our society are not protected by the law against bodily attack in the same way as are adults. There are still some school districts in the United States where children are the recipients of physical punishment at the hands of school authorities for purposes of discipline (see Chap. 15).

The Family

Wives have historically been considered the property of their husbands. Women's child-rearing responsibilities, their own childhood experiences, their lack of financial independence, and social policies toward women have often served to maintain them in their subservient positions. Isolation in the home, a lack of awareness of alternatives, an absence of support, and shame can prevent an abused wife from seeking refuge and leaving a seemingly intolerable situation.

Many adults accept the use of physical force in the process of socializing children and dealing with their aggressive feelings and impulses. Naturally, this acceptance of violence will influence the behavior of these adults toward each other, their children, and/or their clients.[1] Parents who have been punished severely as children tend to punish their offspring in the same way. Children are more aggressive toward others as a result of observing or having been subjected to such punitive behavior, and they continue to be punitive as adults. A son raised in a home where the father assaults the mother will be apt to treat his wife similarly. A daughter from such a home will accept abuse as a part of the marital relationship. Adults provide the abusive examples that children later follow as they try to cope with frustration and anger in stressful situations (see Chap. 15 and 17).

To further complicate the family situation in our society, we have moved from the kinship structure of extended family to the nuclear family. Abusive families often live in isolation, and when alienation from the extended family exists, there is often a concomitant isolation from friends and community. When the family members are unable to share problems and solutions or to give and receive support from significant others, tension within the family builds and avenues for release tend to become focused within the family.

Maternal Dynamics

The roots of child abuse reach back to preceding familial generations. (See Chap. 11.) The behavior is learned and is brought to the fore when stresses from various socioeconomic and interpersonal sources go beyond the abusive person's capacity to cope. Asch describes a postpartum syndrome in which the mother experiences an emotional response which may range from a "blue feeling," to a deeper depression, to a massive psychotic reaction. Some hostile impulses and thoughts both toward the fetus before birth and toward the newborn infant are not unusual and well within the normal range of maternal ambivalence. They tend to evoke guilt and shame, which the woman suppresses. These reactions derive from experiences involving the person's mental representations of pregnancy, parturition, and motherhood; they are not confined to the biological mother, since this phenomenon has been observed in adoptive mothers as well[9] (see Chap. 32).

If the attachment proceeds along a healthy course, these feelings are effectively suppressed and warm, nurturing feelings emerge and predominate. Where the attachment process is weak or absent, the mother may experience obsessive infanticidal thoughts which may be manifested by the reaction formation of obsessive concern for the baby's care and health. If postpartum psychosis

occurs, the woman experiences marked negative feelings toward the baby. Disordered thought processes may impel the woman to rid herself of her "bad part," and suicide may be attempted. She may also displace these suicidal drives onto the infant; that is, the distinction between the self and the infant may be blurred. Her depression is experienced in reaction to the sense of loss after delivery, and her psychological development may be so distorted that infanticide looks to her like the only way of alleviating her pain.[9]

Although, in the majority of instances, the first act of abuse is reported when the child is about a year old, it seems reasonable to suppose that the first reported instance will have been preceded by prior incidences and that the battering may very well have begun during the postpartum period. According to Asch, this behavior derives from a reawakening of the mother's childhood conflicts. It is a renewal of an older conflict between the new mother and *her* mother, the infant's grandmother, which is acted out with the baby. She identifies with the original aggressor in the abusing relationship, only now she is not the victim but herself the aggressor.[9]

The mother may have wanted someone to love and someone to love her in return. She expects the child to gratify needs for dependency, self-esteem, love, and belonging (see Chaps. 32 and 1). These needs are intensified as the child demands nurturing. An infant does not give or return love; rather, it makes demands on the caretaker, who in this instance is emotionally impoverished and has little to give. If the infant also suffers from colic and is premature or irritable, there is even less satisfaction in mothering, and such a situation may increase the mother's feelings of inadequacy. The mother's unconscious desire for a role reversal cannot be fulfilled. As the mother reenacts with the child her own abused and rejected childhood, she feels anxiety and guilt. The loss of self-esteem threatens the mother's fragile, narcissistic equilibrium. She projects her "bad" self-image and unacceptable feelings onto the child and attacks the child, who now symbolizes her inadequacies. This identification with the aggressor in her past allows her to actively master the traumatic rejection she had passively experienced as a child.[2,7,19]

In situations where the mother is not abusive but has allowed a husband or boyfriend to batter her child, there is a variation to the psychodynamics. In this case, the interaction between mother and child is similar. However, Green points out that the bad self-image is partly retained and partly projected onto the child. The internalized bad-mother image is projected onto the abusive mate. Consequently, the mother identifies with the child victim. In most instances where the mate is abusing the child, he is also abusing the mother. These women tolerate this cruelty as a masochistic repetition of their childhood experience. Their extreme emotional dependency and linking with this mate and the extent of their feelings of worthlessness serve to bind them into this pathological relationship. However, if the mother is abandoned by the abusing mate, it is not uncommon to find such a woman assuming the aggressor role and abusing her children.[7]

Paternal Dynamics

The abusive behavior exhibited by the father at this point in the child's life may be based on envy of his wife's pregnancy, old feelings of sibling rivalry for attention which have resurfaced, and revived feelings and fears associated with the oedipal conflict. If the oedipal resolution was defective or if the ability to tolerate competition with authority has been inadequate, such a revival of feelings may precipitate neurotic or even psychotic behavior. Manifestations of this intensified conflict include transient mood changes, sudden and compulsive extramarital affairs, the breakthrough into consciousness of homosexual impulses, or severe affective or psychotic difficulties. Overwhelmed with these fears and fantasies, the father may assault his child or wife.[9]

The Parents' Dynamics

Abusive parents are immature, impulsive, and often isolated from their families of origin. Some tend to be rigid and domineering and to use violence as a way of controlling the environment. A child who fails to live up to the parents' unrealistic expectations becomes the victim of their uncontrollable rage.

Research does not support the concept of a specific "abusive" personality. Multigenerational transmission, the environmental context, the personalities of those involved, and the stresses present at the moment contribute to the abusive situation.[7]

Abusive parents are basically depressed, hostile, and aggressive. They appear to be continually angry at someone or something. Their feelings stem from their internal conflicts and are triggered by normal daily difficulties. As rigid people, they tend to lack warmth, reasonableness, and flexibility in their thinking and beliefs. Morris has identified four types of abusing parents: (1) the parent who is distressed and guilty concerning the relationship with and treatment of the child; (2) the undercontrolled, impulse-ridden parent who is angry about the relationship with the child and who blames the child for the family problems; (3) the overcontrolled parent who feels "correct" in punishing the child, even if the punishment results in injury; (4) the parent who responds to an inner psychotic world rather than to the real world and the child[2,11] (see Chaps. 15 and 17).

Parental alcohol abuse is a significant contributing factor to the abusive situation. Rage—along with impulsive, assaultive, and sexually aggressive behavior—is more easily triggered when inhibitions are diminished by excessive alcohol consumption. In some families, one parent may manipulate the other into the role of disciplinarian and establish the expectation that physical punishment must be inflicted on the child if parents are to maintain their authority in the household (see Chap. 17).

Abusive parents have many hypochondriacal complaints and frequently undergo elective surgery. They exhibit a flight from parenthood through illness and work. They seem to live in fear of their own parents' opinion of them and see their parents as threatening and destructive influences on their lives. In their marital relationships, the men are frequently sexually demanding and the women compliant but lacking in interest. There is a marked absence of satisfaction or enjoyment in their sexual acts.[12]

When speaking of their child, abusive parents reveal their ambivalent attitudes, and these are corollary to the ambiguity with which they view themselves. They describe the child as both lovable and hateful, they exhibit extreme and intense emotions as they describe incidents which illustrate the child's offensive behavior. These descriptions often sound as if the conflict had occurred between adults, reflecting their unrealistic expectations and inability to view the child as a child.[12]

Sometimes, a child in a violent family kills either the abusive parent or a sibling. The child who kills in this situation is acting as the unwitting lethal agent of an adult, usually a parent, who unconsciously prompts the child to kill so that the adult can vicariously enjoy the benefits of the act. A history of parental brutality is a significant factor in the homicidal adolescent's attack on a parent. Young children can also be provoked to and are capable of homicidal rage when there is a perceived threat to their position in the family system, but more often they are the recipients of covert messages from their adult environment to kill.[1]

The Child's Dynamics

The special characteristics of the child which generate hostility in the abusing parent are often unique to the relationship. However, the child's developmental stage and the behavioral characteristics of the phase may trigger specific conflicts in the parents. Also, control is more of an issue in certain developmental phases. The toddlers' impulsive drive to experience the environment, and their innate messiness, is disruptive to a compulsive parent who places a high value on neatness and obedience. Another critical point in the parent-child relationship is adolescence, when the child is ambivalently striving for independence.

Children who exhibit age-appropriate sexual behavior may be in conflict with their parents. Toddlers who explore or manipulate their genitals may be perceived as abnormal by their parents. This behavior evokes the parents' anxiety about their own unacceptable impulses, which lie buried in their subconscious. These impulses are ascribed to the child by denial of their ownership and projection onto the child.

Parents may administer prophylactic punishment to prevent the child from becoming delinquent or pregnant out of wedlock. The child's sex, physical appearance, or personality may have the potential for triggering a past conflict in the parent, which is then reenacted with the child (who becomes the victim). If the parent is separated, divorced, or abandoned by a mate, the child may be seen as the cause and consequently become the focus of the parent's anger.

Negative attention is better than no attention in a child's world. Although being beaten is not a healthy way of making contact with the parent, it has the elements of interaction and sensory input desired by the child. Thus, to receive attention from the adults in the environment, the child learns to be provocative and invites abuse. This dynamic becomes very evident when these children are placed in foster homes and continue to exhibit provocative behavior with the foster parents. Extinguishing such behavior requires time, patience, and understanding on the part of the surrogate parents or caretakers.

Race can be another significant variable which places the child in a special position within a family. Jamie was a 7-year-old from his mother's common-law marriage to a black laborer. His mother, who was white, was abandoned and subsequently married a white tradesman. This marriage produced two children, a boy and girl who were fair skinned and blond like their father. Jamie's skin color was café au lait and his hair dark brown and very curly. This child represented a very difficult and unhappy period in the mother's life and his mixed racial appearance was a sharp reminder of her earlier liaison. The present marriage and family life seemed stable and relatively happy except for Jamie's role in the family: he was frequently and severely beaten by the mother. On admission to the emergency room, his back—from shoulders to ankles—was severely lacerated from a beating with a belt, and his shoulder was broken. In this family, Jamie had become the scapegoat for the denied family stresses and the mother's bad self-image.

Caretaker Dynamics

Many of the interpersonal and family-type dynamics are also seen in the institutional setting. Caretakers single out the clients they abuse for reasons unique to the relationship. Identification with the client produces a negative transference. (See Chaps. 6 and 16.) Unresolved conflicts are revived, and these are reenacted in the relationship with the client. Because these caretakers are immature, impulsive, aggressive, and dissatisfied with their jobs or status in society, the demands made by the confused, incontinent, or hostile client stress their ability to provide sensitive, therapeutic care. Consequently they focus their anger and frustration on the vulnerable client, who becomes the victim of abuse.

In instances of abuse, emotional linking is an important factor. Intimate relationships involve characteristic emotional ties that can potentially generate strong feelings. The intimacy of long-term care, the dependence of the client, and the inadequacy of emotional support in both the work setting and the home situation all heighten the negative feelings of caretakers toward their clients. The proximity of family living, which tends to constrict body space and add to the normal daily irritations—compounded by environmental stress such as unemployment, poor housing, and extreme weather conditions—stresses the abuser's inadequate coping mechanisms and limited impulse control.

Primary Prevention

Primary prevention on all levels would require fundamental changes in the philosophy and values underlying our social institutions and human relationships. It requires a reconceptualization of childhood and the status of the noncontributing dependent person in society, a reconsideration of the rights of their dependence, and a recognition of their needs. It calls for a rejection of the use of force as a means for achieving social ends. Poverty must be eliminated, along with the alienating conditions in the work and housing environments. The social processes which trigger abuse must be changed, and the population needs to understand the normal growth and development of children—their needs and the importance of need fulfillment for a healthy life.[8]

Secondary Prevention

In most instances, the abused child is identified on admission to an emergency room for treatment of the injuries received in the abusive assault. Laws in every state make it mandatory that professionals in health, educational, social service, and law enforcement agencies report such incidents to the child welfare authorities. Teachers, school health and public health nurses have opportunities to recognize injuries which suggest abuse rather than an accidental cause. Health professionals in contact with families who have new babies or have recently adopted children are in a position to identify early indications of a faulty attachment process and a potential for abuse. Other family situations which have potential for abusive behavior are the addition of a new child to an already stressed environment, the death of or abandonment by a spouse, financial crisis, an alcoholic or addicted parent, or a parent whose serious illness is disruptive to family dynamics.

Parents may recognize their potential for harming their child and may ask welfare officials to have the child placed in a foster home or residential institution. These parents claim to be "at the end of their rope" and say that they "can't stand it any longer." A prompt, sensitive response to such a cry for help is vitally important if the child is to be protected from abuse. Professionals working with families in which a parent is an alcoholic or addict must find out how this person behaves when drunk or under the influence of drugs to determine the risk to spouse and children of assaultive maltreatment. In institutions, sensitive, caring, and perceptive professional supervision of those who are giving direct care is likely to uncover situations where the caretaker's ability to cope is being excessively taxed or where his or her personality structure is not appropriate to the work.

Tertiary Prevention
Assessment

At this level of prevention, the child has already been the recipient of abuse; efforts are then made to stop the battering and prevent further incidents.

When a child or adult exhibits injuries which do not fit the description of the reported accident, abuse must be considered. In the case of children, the incident that comes to professional attention may not be the first to occur. Parents who physically abuse their children frequently "shop" hospitals and agencies. The central registry for the area must be contacted to determine whether the family has been treated or is receiving services from another agency. The data obtained may help to confirm suspicions of abuse, prevent duplication of services, and/or coordinate services in the follow-up care.

If abuse is confirmed or strongly suspected, even if the injuries are not serious, hospitalization is recommended to protect the child from further injury and allow additional time for assessment of the family. The parents of these children will often refuse to permit diagnostic tests. When these tests are done, they often reveal recent and old fractures for which the parents offer either no explanation or one that fails to account for the type and extent of the injuries. These parents tend to turn the child over to the emergency room staff and withdraw to the waiting room or leave the hospital. They do not relate to the children, and if these children cry while the parents are present, there are attempts to silence them but with no offer of comfort or affection. These parents do not question treatment or prognosis and do not volunteer information regarding the child's injury or health. When confronted, they become evasive or contradict themselves regarding the circumstances of the injury. They may even appear irritated when questioned about the symptoms and become critical or angry with the child. The parents may feel guilty, frightened, and overwhelmed by personal problems and what has happened to the child. They are probably convinced that nobody would want to help them. Their defensive structure is usually denial and hostility.

The child must be carefully examined and all injuries documented on the chart. The family dynamics and the child's behavior must be observed carefully. Typical, well-nurtured children in an emergency room setting cling to their parents; they refuse or are reluctant to go to the nurse; they turn to their parents for comfort, assurance, and affection; they protest having to be in the hospital and want to go home. Abused children cry hopelessly under treatment and examination but otherwise cry very little. Sudden movements by the nurse or physician may cause them to flinch. They do not look for comfort, assurance, or affection from their parents and seem wary of any physical contact initiated by the parent. They appear apathetic but wary and alert if approached by staff or if they hear another child crying. When admitted to the children's inpatient unit, they do not protest loudly and tearfully upon their parents' departure. They settle into the unit routine quickly and usually continue to size up the situation. At some point they often state that they do not want to go home but would rather stay with the nurses.

It is not uncommon to find that these children are hyperactive or have impaired motor activity suggestive of organic brain damage. Younger children, once oriented to the unit, may exhibit a *grabbing reaction*. They will bite or grab the caretaker and shout for attention. Such behavior stems from a desire to become involved in a "belonging" relationship—a desire of such intensity as to cause the child to grab at caretakers and their property. Once the object is grabbed away, it appears to lack the attribute of property and thereby loses its value to the child, who discards it to look for more belongings. This behavior is a derivative of *lap hunger,* which is an excessive need to be held by the caretaker and suggests mobilization of desires that had been latent.[12]

The assessment process focuses on two levels, the individual interpersonal and the family dynamic. The assessment process must include the physical and physiological status of the child, the level of growth and development, and the child's behavioral response to the parents, caretakers, and treatments. The family dynamic must also be assessed: the way in which parents relate to the child and each other; the frequency and length of visits; verbalizations about parenting, the child, and the spouse; and problems the family is experiencing (strengths, weaknesses, and areas for growth). Based on the data collected by the treatment team, judgments are made as to whether the child can be returned to the family or should be placed outside the home. Community and family resources are also assessed to determine what resources and alternatives are available to the family. Clearly, knowledge of the family's past use of health and welfare services will contribute to the decisions which are made. Input from the public health nurse who makes home visits is important. The data base assembled by all who care for the child and family is used to formulate a comprehensive treatment plan.[2] Table 36-1 is an assessment guide.

Nurse's Response
When nurses and other professionals find that physical harm and emotional neglect have been inflicted, particularly on a child, they are outraged, shocked, and angry. After assessing the extent of the child's injuries, they are appalled at the depravity of the parents and are unwilling to return the child to the parents. They project their anger onto the parents and reject them, overlooking the parents' needs, and focus on the child. On the other hand, the caretakers may do all they can to treat the child and family in a humane and systematic way, making appropriate referrals and maximizing communication with the community agen-cy. Despite such involvement, however, services may not be delivered and the child may not be protected or the family helped. In these circumstances, caretakers will be apathetic and discouraged when faced with another such case. Services to children are inadequate, overloaded, and operating with limited financial resources. Consequently, the follow-up care provided to these families is often only minimal.

Self-awareness is the first step in diagnosing a human situation. This awareness contributes to a sharper and more systematic diagnostic process and more accurate analysis of the data. To understand the totality of the abusive incident, it is necessary that nurses recognize their own biases, values, conflicts, reactions, and impact on the clients. The nurses must be "tuned in" to their perceptions and how they are influencing their emotions. Self-awareness contributes to a more sensitive and effective relationship with the parents and to a more accurate data-collecting process.[2]

The vulnerability of the child and the pain caused by the abuse may lead the nurses to project their own emotional needs onto the child and to entertain rescue fantasies. If this dynamic exists, then the parents are excluded and the child is placed in an even more untenable position. The nurse cannot fulfill the rescue contract and the child is further isolated from the family.

Mike, a 3-year-old hospitalized after being abused by his mother, became the favorite of Ms. Dart, a member of the nursing staff. This nurse stayed overtime to feed him, bought him toys, and spent as much time as possible during the working day playing with him. When Mike's mother visited, Ms. Dart excluded her from her son's care and spoke to her in a curt, hostile manner. In time, the mother visited less frequently and interacted minimally with her son and the staff. When it was time for discharge, social services decided to return Mike to his home with follow-up counseling. The day Mike was discharged, he resisted being dressed by his mother and cried for Ms. Dart. The mother was visibly angry and reluctantly allowed

Table 36-1 Assessment Guide

Assessment: The Victim

---

1 Presence of injuries which do not fit the description of the accident.

2 Evidence of multiple bruises, chipped front teeth, or burns, particularly of the type inflicted by a cigarette.

3 X-ray reports which indicate old healed fractures. There is a need to determine how such fractures were incurred and whether the explanation adequately fits the extent and type of injuries present or the evidence of old healed fractures.

4 Retarded growth and/or development of the child with no history of pathology.

5 Child's clothing inappropriate in relation to weather conditions.

6 Child shows evidence of poor hygiene.

7 No immunization appropriate to the child's age.

8 Child wary of adults or caretaker from the referring facility.

9 Child adapts to hospital unit quickly.

10 Child does not seek out parents for comfort or affection.

11 Child does not cry when parents leave.

12 Grabbing behavior/lap hunger exhibited by the young child.

13 Child shows provocative behavior which generates anger in others.

14 Delinquent or runaway behavior; teen-age pregnancy.[13]

15 Adult victim reluctant to talk about injuries, particularly if spouse, parent, or caretaker from the referring facility is present.

Assessment: Abuser

---

1 Evidence of dysfunctional attachment process in new mother. Withdrawal from the child. Expresses fears that he or she will hurt the child.

2 Abused as a child.

3 Evidence of psychosis.

4 Alcohol and/or drug abuser.

5 Low self-esteem, low self-acceptance.

6 Hostile and depressed.

7 Hypochondriacal complaints; history of several minor surgical interventions.

8 Impulsivity in decision making.

9 Seductive toward child of the opposite sex.

10 Explains need for physical punishment as due to "badness" in victim.

Assessment: Family Dynamics

---

1 Behavior expected of abused child is not appropriate to child's age.

2 Abused described as "difficult" or "hateful."

3 Special negatively perceived characteristic ascribed to the abused person.

4 Lack of knowledge of normal growth and development.

5 Divorce, separation, abandonment, death of spouse.

6 Financial, housing, or personal crisis.

7 Behavior toward crying/injured child is aloof, not comforting or affectionate.

8 Expectations that child should give and be "grateful" to parents.

9 Family refuses to allow diagnostic procedures.

10 Parents withdraw from hospitalized child.

Table 36-1 Assessment Guide (continued)

Assessment: Family Dynamics

11 Parents complain of difficulty in coping with the child and/or their own lives.

12 Impaired communication: *mystification*, *pseudomutuality*, masking. (See Chap. 3.)

13 Evidence of family *fusion*. (See Chap. 11.)

14 Evidence of *family projection*, e.g., scapegoating.

15 *Emotional cutoff* from families of origin.

16 Evidence of *multigenerational transmission process*; parents give history of being physically abused as children.

17 Evidence of *societal regression*: family has been experiencing chronic sustained anxiety which has been reinforced by absent or inadequate environmental resources and support.

the nurse to dress him. Ms. Dart disagreed with the discharge plans but was unable to intervene. Mike could not remain in the hospital; no space was available in the community child-care facility; no foster home was available; and the mother agreed to counseling. Ms. Dart could not actualize her rescue fantasy and the child was returned to his mother. Because of the nurse's overinvolvement, the mother was rejected by her child. She learned nothing about her own or her child's needs and how they could be met. Since it was highly probable that she would not follow through with counseling, the risk of another abusive incident remained.

In some instances, the nurses may feel that they have betrayed the family and were punitive in making a referral. If the child's injuries are not serious and the family's socioeconomic status, educational level, and religion or ethnic background are the same as those of the nurse, there is a greater possibility of identification (see Chap. 16). The parents' sophistication and affluence also contribute to these feelings, causing nurses to feel uncomfortable about labeling them as abusive.[2]

Nurses and other professionals are generally uneasy talking with the family about the abusive incident. All concerned are often suffused with anger and anxiety. If they lack an understanding of the dynamics of abuse, they will distort the phenomena and see removal of the child and rejection of the parents as the only solution. The attitudes of the professionals have a profound influence on the parents' availability for treatment. The initial inter-

view sets the tone of the relationship between the family and the health-care delivery system. Caretakers must communicate care, concern, and a desire to understand the parents' predicament. They must define their role as supportive and assistive. Confrontation will only increase the parents' need to defend themselves. An interview technique must be employed which allows parents and child to maintain ego and family integrity. The helping process begins when the family can talk about their frustrations, anxieties, and problems. Thus, a sound, trusting relationship must be developed before the family will be able to work with the nurse and expose their fears, feelings, and problems. Once a level of trust is established, the parents will test the sincerity and commitment of the nurse. There will be times when they become closed and withdrawn, avoiding contact with the nurse. If the nurse remains available, concerned, caring, and accepting, they may venture to trust again. These depressed parents fear rejection; they possess low self-esteem and little self-acceptance. Consequently, it is difficult to get close to them and to develop a trusting relationship.[27]

The problems of an abusive family are often extensive; many community resources and much professional expertise must be used in their resolution. It is important for agencies and the multidisciplinary treatment team to work collaboratively. If communication among those involved in the treatment program is not maximized and services are not coordinated, then both the family and its care will be fragmented.

Nursing Goals

1 Protect the victim from physical abuse and emotional neglect.
2 Promote a healthy growth and development pattern in the child or adult victim.
3 Assist parents or caretakers to become aware of the importance of their own need fulfillment, feelings, and thoughts.
4 Assist the parents or caretakers as individuals to develop effective problem-solving skills.
5 Strengthen the family unit or caretakers' position by helping them deal with unresolved conflicts, feelings of inadequacy, loneliness, lack of self-esteem and self-acceptance.
6 Enhance the family's ability to help members meet their needs.
7 Develop the family's parenting skills.

Nursing Diagnosis and Intervention

In the course of these processes, data collected about the victim, the aggressor, and the family or work-setting dynamic are analyzed and nursing diagnoses are formulated. The diagnoses must encompass all those involved in the abusive incident. Table 36-2 gives examples of nursing diagnoses, interventions, and nursing orders applicable to the abusive family dynamic.

Multidisciplinary Treatment Approaches

A major effort must be made to involve the parents in the treatment program. Communication between parents and child must be maintained, if at all possible, to ameliorate the child's feelings of rejection and abandonment and to prevent weakening of the parents' ties to the child. When placement in a foster home is the only solution to an abuse case, it is not necessarily salvation for the child. In many instances, there are no homes available and the child is sent to an institution where emotional neglect cannot be remedied because of the overcrowded conditions and inadequate staffing. If the child is placed in a foster home, it may be the first in a series. When such a placement is made in the child's best interest, it should be for as brief a time as possible.[14]

The public health nurse is in a strategic position for assessing family strengths, weaknesses, and areas for growth. The nurse is often seen as a helping person. With persistence, care, concern, and rapport which is based on trust, the nurse can work effectively with the family to implement the treatment plan. When a child is removed from the home, other siblings fear for their safety and the possibility that they too will be rejected. Efforts must be made to help them cope with the separation and with their fears. They too should maintain communication with the abused child.

The abusive family needs intensive, long-term care if the treatment goals are to be met. Agencies provide family and group therapy. Home visits by the nurse provide an opportunity to assess the quality of parenting and are important to maintaining a broad data base on which to make decisions regarding the treatment plan. This information also helps to make possible the early identification of problems. Interventions focus on the resolution of old conflicts, the maintenance of a stable home environment, the development of parenting skills and feelings of adequacy as parents, effective ways of dealing with stress, ways of increasing self-esteem and self-acceptance, the reduction of social isolation, the amelioration of a faulty attachment process, the integration of the child into the family system, and the development of a healthier family dynamic which assists members to meet their needs.

Evaluation

The goals and nursing diagnosis are used by the nurse to formulate the treatment plan and guide the evaluation process. Treatment plans—stated in terms of observable, desired client behaviors—

Table 36-2 Nursing Intervention

Diagnosis	Intervention	Orders
Emotionally deprived child seeking human relationships by grabbing and exhibiting lap hunger.	Satisfy child's need for nurturance.	1 Hold, cuddle, rock child for X minutes every hour. 2 Give child what is asked for. 3 Encourage play with toys; start with child on lap and gradually make transition to play which is out of physical contact with caretaker. 4 Encourage the child to explore environment with caretaker. 5 Communicate with child while feeding and giving care. 6 Praise child for interacting and playing appropriately with toys.
Hostile parents with low self-esteem and guilt who are withdrawing from the child by remaining aloof during visiting hours.	Make therapeutic use of self; involve parents in the child's care; enhance parents' self-esteem	1 Initiate contact with family and inform them of the child's progress. 2 Involve parents in the care of the child; have them help feed and bathe child; encourage them to play with child. 3 Remain with parents; work with them, giving positive feedback for nurturing behavior. 4 Express concern about how they are managing and the turmoil in the household undoubtedly caused by the child's hospitalization. 5 Avoid seeking admission of abuse.
Immature, impulsive parents, isolated from friends and community and unable to solve daily household problems. (See Chap. 17.)	Foster maturity in the parents; teach them problem-solving process; encourage them to socialize.	1 Guide parents in solving immediate problems that they see as important, using a systematic approach; point out alternatives and explore their consequences. 2 Assist parents to find friends and become involved in the community. 3 Model discussion and analysis of problems, expression of feelings, and acceptance of differing opinions.
Rigid, dependent parents lacking knowledge of normal growth and development and with unrealistic expectations of the child. (See Chap. 33.)	Provide parent education; increase parent flexibility and reasonableness.	1 Explore their expectations of the child. 2 Describe expected behavior for a child of this age. 3 Identify the areas of parent-child conflict for this phase. 4 Explore alternatives for resolving conflicts with the child.
Grief caused by separation of child from family and placement in foster home.	Facilitate grief work (see Chap. 23.)	1 Explore feelings about the placement. 2 Encourage expression of feelings about separation. 3 Arrange for preplacement visit for parent and child to the foster home. 4 Maintain avenues of communication between parents and child during placement. 5 Assist parents to recognize and understand siblings' response to the placement. 6 Assist parents to help siblings express their fears and fantasies about the placement; provide support, reassurance, and contact with the placed child.

Table 36-3 Evaluation

Treatment plan	Behavioral criteria
Mother uses nurse as a resource when feeling stressed.	1 Mother calls nurse and requests visit because she "feels depressed and anxious and child is getting on her nerves."
Father recognizes alcohol problem and seeks help.	1 Father participates regularly in AA meetings and encourages wife to attend Al-Anon.
Mother nurtures child, parents effectively.	1 Child seek comfort from mother when finger is pinched by toy and receives cuddling, soothing, and affection.
	2 Child is clean and properly dressed.
	3 Child has gained weight and exhibits new motor-coordination skill in pedaling a tricycle.
Family participates in therapy.	1 Parents attend family and group meetings regularly (no absences or lateness).
	2 Parents share problems and frustrations with other parents.
	3 Parents engage in problem-solving activities regarding financial matters, family discipline, and housing.
	4 Each parent is supportive and comforting to others in the group.

serve as criteria for evaluation. Table 36-3 is a sample of how treatment plans may be stated in terms of observable behaviors which indicate the effectiveness of the plan and the degree of change in the client's behavior. The behavioral criteria in Table 36-3 are sample behaviors which indicate to the nurse that the treatment plan has been effective.

The abuse of the powerless in our society has roots in the past. Violence is a part of our culture and not likely to be eradicated in the near future. It is learned and passed on from generation to generation. Prevention, case finding, and treatment are challenges that nurses in all health-care settings must accept. Each member of society has the right to have his or her basic needs met and deserves the opportunity to strive to fulfill the growth-promoting needs. Nurses are in strategic positions to assist clients to optimize their potential.

References

1 Mary Lystad: "Violence at Home: A Review of the Literature," *American Journal of Orthopsychiatry*, vol. 45, no. 3, pp. 328–341, April 1973.

2 Nancy Deborah Hill Ebling: *Child Abuse: Interventions and Treatment*, Publishing Sciences Group, Acton, Mass., 1975.

3 R. J. Gelles: "The Social Construction of Child Abuse," *American Journal of Orthopsychiatry*, vol. 45, no. 3, p. 346, April 1975.

*4 Camille Legéay: "Failure to Thrive," *Nursing Forum*, vol. 4, no. 1, pp. 56–71, 1965.

5 Leila Whitling: "Defining Emotional Neglect," *Children Today*, January–February 1976, pp. 2–5.

6 Mary Van Stolk: "Beaten Women, Battered Children," *Children Today*, vol. 5, no. 2, March–April 1976.

7 A. Green: "Child Abuse: Pathological Syndrome of Family Interaction," *American Journal of Psychiatry*, vol. 131.

8 D. Gil: "Unraveling Child Abuse," *American Journal of Orthopsychiatry*, vol. 45, no. 3, pp. 363–371.

9 S. Asch et al.: "Postpartum Reactions: Some Unrecognized Variations," *American Journal of Psychiatry*, vol. 131, pp. 870–874, August 1974.

10 I. D. Melowe: "Patterns of Parental Behavior Leading to Physical Abuse of Children," presented at

*Recommended reference by a nurse author.

workshop sponsored by Children's Bureau in collaboration with the University of Chicago, Colorado Springs, Colo., March 21, 1966.

11 M. G. Morris, R. W. Gould, and P. J. Matthews: "Toward Prevention of Child Abuse," *Children*, March–April 1974.

12 Richard Gladston: "Preventing the Abuse of Little Children," *American Journal of Orthopsychiatry*, vol. 45, no. 3, April 1975.

13 Allison Friedman et al.: "Nursing Responsibility in Child Abuse," *Nursing Forum*, vol. 15, no. 1, 1976.

14 Elizabeth Davoren: "Foster Placement of Abused Children," *Children Today*, May–June 1975, p. 41.

37

The Family Coping with Hereditary Conditions

Margretta Reed Seashore   Lillie Ann Reed

Learning Objectives

After studying this chapter, the student should be able to:

1 State the frequency of genetic disease and define the four important patterns of inheritance

2 Identify five ways in which such disease has a serious impact on the family

3 Outline five stages in the response of a family to the birth of a defective child

4 State three coping mechanisms which can be utilized by families

5 State five kinds of situations where genetic diagnosis and genetic counseling might be applicable

6 Discuss the treatment for three genetic diseases

7 Discuss how the techniques of prenatal diagnosis can help families to avoid tragedy

8   Assess the needs of the family

9   Identify community resources outside the medical institution which may be helpful

10 Develop personal techniques for dealing with the anguish, fear, doubt, guilt, anger, and confusion that genetic disease may visit on a family

11 Recognize his or her own feeling and develop ways to deal with them

The decrease in infant mortality due to infectious disease has accentuated the importance of genetic disease as a cause of morbidity and mortality in infants and children.[1] Of every 100 babies born in the United States today, 3 have a serious birth defect; many of these defects have a genetic cause. About 20 percent of all pediatric hospital admissions are for disorders with a genetic component. Such infants and children may need evaluation at a major medical center. But ongoing care will take place in cities and towns, major centers, community hospitals, and doctors' offices. Nurses will need to be involved, whether on a genetic team in a major center, in a physician's office, as school nurses, or as public health nurses. They will find genetic disease everywhere, and everywhere its impact will be significant.

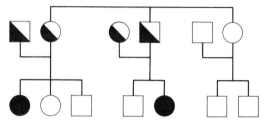

Figure 37-1 This pedigree illustrates a recessive pattern of inheritance. Circles are used to indicate females and squares to indicate males. The darkened symbols represent children affected with cystic fibrosis. The half-darkened squares and circles are heterozygous parents. Note that carrier parents can have both normal and affected children. Only parents who are both carriers can have affected children.

Mechanisms of Inheritance

Before the implications of genetic disease can be understood, some knowledge of the mechanisms of inheritance is necessary. The genetic material which controls heredity is contained in *genes:* tiny, complex molecules of DNA which are packaged into *chromosomes.* Each human has hundreds of thousands of genes, arranged on 23 pairs of chromosomes. These pairs of genes are termed *alleles.* The germ cells (ova and sperm) contain only half the genes, arranged on half the chromosomes. Thus each parent passes half his or her genes on to each child. There are endless combinations of genes which may be passed on, so no two individuals are alike. Defective genes can cause disease. Recessive disorders result when

the same abnormal gene is present in each parent and is passed by each parent to the child. In this case, parents are termed *heterozygous* and are acting as carriers (see Fig. 37-1). Such parents assume a 25 percent risk with each pregnancy of having an affected child.

Dominantly inherited disorders result when a single copy of a defective gene is sufficient to cause disease. These disorders are inherited in a vertical fashion, from parent to child (see Fig. 37-2). Statistically, the parent with a dominantly inherited condition has a 50 percent chance of passing that condition on to each child. In some cases, the defective gene resides on the *X chromosome.* In the female, such a gene is paired with a normal allele, and the woman is therefore an unaffected carrier. In the male, there is only one X chromosome (the Y chromosome forms the other one of the pair), hence no normal allele is present

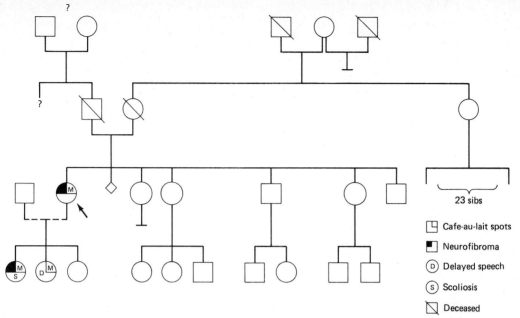

Figure 37-2 This is a pedigree of a family with neurofibromatosis (von Recklinghausen's disease). Note that the proband (*arrow*) has two affected children and one normal child. We cannot determine whether one of the proband's parents was also affected or whether she represents a new mutation.

to counteract the effects of the defective gene and disease results (see Fig. 37-3). The woman who carries a defective gene on an X chromosome has a 50 percent chance of having an affected son; the chance of having a carrier daughter is also 50 percent. Some disorders seem to "run in families" but do not demonstrate a clear pattern of Mendelian (recessive, dominant, or X-linked) inheritance. It can be shown that for some of these disorders multiple genes are involved, not just one or a pair. Such situations are termed *polygenic,* and there are many examples of them. The chromosomal disorders result not from single-gene defects but from gross deletions, duplications, or rearrangements of chromosomal structure. They are frequently severe.

Clinical Examples of Inherited Disorders

The largest group of inherited diseases is that of the recessive disorders, many of which are inborn errors of metabolism. Phenylketonuria (PKU) is an example. Affecting 1 in 10,000 infants, this disease, if untreated, leads to crippling mental retardation. Dietary treatment starting at 2 to 3 weeks of age is notably successful in reclaiming these children for useful lives. Neonatal screening for PKU, now carried out in most states, serves to detect affected infants prior to the development of brain damage. There is no practical way of screening for carriers of this recessively inherited condition.

Another example of a recessively inherited disorder is Tay-Sachs disease. By affecting lipid metabolism in brain cells, this condition leads to severe brain damage and death by age 4. No treatment is as yet available; none survive. Strategy to prevent this tragic disease utilizes screening techniques to identify carrier parents in the population at risk, which is made up largely of Ashkenazi Jews. Prenatal testing can then be offered to these people.

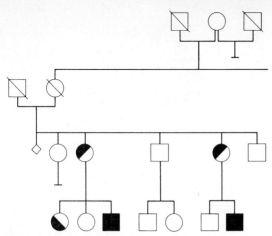

Figure 37-3 The pedigree illustrates sex-linked inheritance. The darkened squares represent boys affected with hemophilia. Note that the carrier mothers (*half-darkened circles*) have both affected and unaffected sons. Unaffected males (*clear squares*) cannot have carrier or affected children unless, of course, they themselves marry carriers.

Cystic fibrosis (CF) is the most common recessively inherited condition in those of Anglo-Saxon descent. About 1 in 20 Caucasian Americans is a carrier. This usually fatal condition, for which no molecular mechanism has as yet been defined, leads to severe pulmonary and gastrointestinal malfunction. Oral pancreatic enzyme treatment may be partially effective but does not stem the inexorable pulmonary failure. At present no carrier test is known, but much research is being devoted to the biochemical delineation necessary for the development of such a test.

In the black population, sickle cell anemia is the most common inherited illness. Characterized by defective hemoglobin A, this recessively inherited condition results in anemia, painful crises, bone infarcts, and infection. Carrier testing is available; its use can lead to a selection of reproductive options for the affected family.

Duchenne's muscular dystrophy is an example of an X-linked disorder affecting males. The individual suffering from this disease demonstrates muscle weakness, pseudoatrophy of calf muscles, and progressive intractable debilitation.

The female carrier does not usually show any clinical abnormalities but has a 50 percent chance with each pregnancy of passing the defective gene on to her sons. Not all affected males have mothers who are carriers. Some have genes that represent new *mutations* (alterations in the hereditary material). Statistical calculations based on pedigree information can help determine a woman's risk of being a carrier if she has an affected male relative. But biochemical carrier testing for this disorder remains inexact.

Another example of an X-linked disorder is hemophilia A, in which a deficiency of the clotting factor VIII leads to defective blood clotting and prolonged bleeding after injury, sometimes resulting in hemarthrosis and severe joint disability. Treatment with exogenous factor VIII is effective but costly. As in muscular dystrophy, women who are possible carriers can be tested. But the tests are difficult to interpret, so that probability calculations are necessary to estimate risk.

Huntington's chorea demonstrates a dominant pattern of inheritance. It is the prototype for the dominantly inherited neurodegenerative disorders. No biochemical mechanism is known to explain the sequence of chorea, psychosis, and relentless progressive dementia that mark the development of this condition. Even more tragic is the fact that the average age of onset is 35 to 50 years, so that affected individuals have frequently already completed childbearing before the diagnosis is made.

Neurofibromatosis (or von Recklinghausen's disease) offers another example of a dominantly inherited condition; in this disorder the degree of severity varies dramatically from one patient to another. One patient may show only café-au-lait spots, while his or her affected child may have the full range of manifestations including mental retardation, skin tumors, and tumors of the central nervous system.

Many types of multiple congenital malformations are thought to be inherited in a polygenic fashion. For example, the combination of cleft lip and palate involves a 5 percent risk of recurrence in a sibship where cleft lip and palate have already occurred. When there are two affected siblings, the recurrence risk rises to 10 percent. The same figures apply to spina bifida and anencephaly. Pyloric stenosis is another condition where multiple genes appear to be involved. Diabetes mellitus is a common disorder with a substantial genetic component. The child of two diabetic parents has a 50 percent chance of eventually developing diabetes, while a person with a diabetic sibling has a 5 to 10 percent chance of developing the disease. A strong argument can be advanced in the case of the polygenic disorders that interaction between genes and the environment is necessary to produce disease.

Down's syndrome is the prototype for the chromosomal disorders; it results from the presence of an extra number 21 chromosome (trisomy 21; see Fig. 37-4). In 5 percent of the cases, the additional chromosome may be attached (translocated) to another, apparently normal chromosome (translocation Down's syndrome). Down's syndrome occurs in 1 of every 600 babies born; half

Figure 37-4 This karyotype, stained with quinacrine and viewed using a fluorescent microscope, was performed on cells from a child with Down's syndrome caused by trisomy 21. Note that there are three number 21 chromosomes. Two have bright satellites on the short arms and are from one parent; the third is from the other parent and has no satellites.

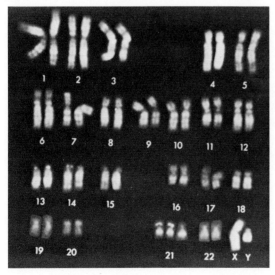

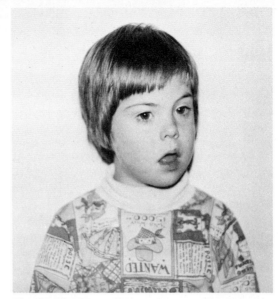

Figure 37-5 This child with Down's syndrome has the typical face, short stature, and hyperflexibility seen in this disorder.

these babies are born to women over 30 years of age. These children show the physical features depicted in Figs. 37-5 and 37-6. They often have severe cardiac disease, always demonstrate mental retardation, and run a higher-than-average risk

Figure 37-6 The transverse palmar crease shown here extends from the medial to the lateral aspect of the palm and is seen frequently on the hands of children with Down's syndrome.

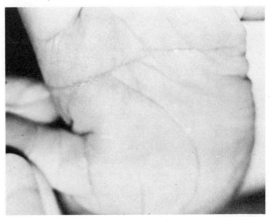

of developing leukemia. The risk of producing a second child with Down's syndrome depends on the type of chromosome abnormality present in the child. A woman who has had a child with Down's syndrome but who has a normal karyotype herself has a 1 to 2 percent chance of giving birth to another such child. The reasons for this are not known. About 2 percent of the time, a parent of a child with translocation Down's syndrome also carries the translocation chromosome but has only two number 21 chromosomes and is clinically normal. Such a parent runs a risk of 5 to 15 percent of having a child with Down's syndrome.

Of the other autosomes, numbers 13 and 18 are the only ones regularly involved in trisomies. These two trisomies are very severe and are usually not compatible with life beyond 1 year of age. Their recurrence risk is not known.

There are three common constitutions involving abnormal sex chromosomes: XO (Turner's syndrome), XXY (Klinefelter's syndrome), and XYY.

Turner's syndrome results in defective ovarian development, short stature, sexual infantilism, and, rarely, mental retardation. These patients can be treated using exogenous estrogens and progestogens, but their infertility remains unchanged.

Males with an XXY karyotype (Klinefelter's syndrome) also suffer from sexual immaturity and infertility with testicular hypoplasia. They can be treated with exogenous androgens to achieve secondary sex development, but they remain sterile.

Individuals with the XYY karyotype have reportedly been found with higher than expected frequency in maximum-security prisons. It has been suggested but by no means proved that these individuals are at greater than normal risk for developing antisocial behavior. More information is needed before the clinical significance of this karyotype is fully understood.

Social and Cultural Attitudes

Concern with the cause and implications of human birth defects has been apparent since at least Babylonian times. Old rock carvings and chalk drawings from all over the world depict malformations that we recognize today.[2,3]

In the seventh century B.C., the birth of abnormal children was used to predict the future. According to the Chaldean diviners, "When a woman gives birth to an infant that has six toes on each foot, the people of the world will be injured." The predictions extended from the city to the country and even to the king.

Theories of causations have also been important. There is much in the ancient literature to suggest that malformed children were considered evidence of divine anger with humankind. Impressions on the child by maternal thoughts were long considered to be causes of malformations. These are old ideas; Greek mothers were encouraged, during pregnancy, to look at beautiful statues to ensure the birth of beautiful children.

A particularly dangerous concept was the *hybridity theory*. When a resemblance to an animal was imagined in the defective child, the infant was thought to have been conceived by coitus with the animal. Women were punished and even killed for this supposed consorting.

Such beliefs did not die with the Babylonians. Malformed children were still considered portents in the fifteenth century, and information of this sort was widely published as late as the eighteenth century. The theory of maternal impressions was recorded in 1889 in a medical textbook, and many of these ideas have survived into the twentieth century. Even today, maternal worries and fright are thought by some anguished parents to account for their children's deformities. The mother's most frequent response to the deformed child is "What did I do to cause this?" Though often unspoken, beliefs about punishment from God for unnamed sins are common.

An explanation for the abnormality may be so important that if one cannot be provided, the parents may devise explanations of their own in which superstition and misinformation may play a large role. It is well to take these factors into account in discussions with families. A statement like this can be helpful: "Many parents fear that their child's abnormalities were caused by something they did, or that their child is afflicted for a special reason; if thoughts like these have bothered you, it might be helpful for us to discuss them." Having been told that such beliefs are common, parents may feel more free to discuss them openly.

Misconceptions about heredity confuse and confound many people. Until genetic concepts are taught more widely in the schools, this will continue to be a serious problem. Some cultures still consider failure to have a son reason for a man to divorce his wife and seek a new wife, completely ignoring the knowledge that the male determines the child's sex.

Many people believe that genetic disease is untreatable. "Well, if it's inherited, nothing can be done about it." It frequently comes as a surprise that the presence of a hereditary disorder in one child does not necessarily mean that all the children in the family will have it. The question is often asked, "You mean we could still have normal children?"

The concept of deformities or disorders being "passed through the family" brings preexisting rivalry and conflict to the fore. Defensive remarks, such as a claim that "There has never been anything on *our* side of the family," are frequently made. Questions about family history ring like accusations. Recriminations are heard, such as "If you hadn't married that girl, you wouldn't have had a child with PKU." Lynch has reported inconsistent behavior[4] in many families. One man, though stating that the appearance of cystinosis in his daughter was the will of God, nevertheless had a vasectomy to make sure that he would not have any more children.

In one study,[5] it was shown that families continue to have children, even in the presence of a chronically ill child. Where there were two affected children in a family, however, fertility greatly declined. This is in sharp contrast to Carter's results from family studies.[6] These showed that, after *genetic counseling,* families with a high risk of recurrence of genetic disease significantly curtailed reproduction. By contrast, families with a low recurrence risk did not limit their growth. Similarly, Tips and Lynch[7] reported curtailed reproduction immediately after the birth of an affected child, not only in the immediate family but throughout the kindred. This was followed by increased reproduction throughout the family after genetic counseling.

Dealing with such strong and sometimes illogical feelings is often a trying experience for everyone. The facts of inheritance must be communicated clearly and logically. The loss of self-esteem wrought by stigmatization, guilt, and feelings of fault and responsibility must be curbed by a sympathetic explanation of the facts. Patients must be reminded and convinced that they did not choose nor did they know their genetic makeup. Misconceptions about treatment, palliation, and prevention must be replaced by accurate information.

Once a family has been given a genetic diagnosis and has embarked on genetic counseling, the nurse must be able to use the knowledge of coping mechanisms to aid the family members in their attempts to meet this crisis. The experience may be so shattering that strong support by the well-informed professional is crucial. How do parents perceive their genetically defective child?

Phases of Coping

It is said that every child is a narcissistic recreation of his or her parents. In the child, they see all the things that they hoped for in themselves: beauty, personality, intelligence. The mother's hidden fears concerning the possibility of bearing a malformed child are reflected in the question "Is he [or she] all right?" heard so often in the delivery room. The mother assumes the responsibility for having a normal child; if the child is not normal, she is troubled by guilt and a feeling of inadequacy or a sense of failure. The father, too, shares her feeling of disappointment and guilt. Their initial shock and disbelief gradually give way to bewilderment and despair.[8]

Having an imperfect infant generates tension

for each of the parents and creates stress in their relationship with each other. It constitutes a crisis situation and tends to reactivate any previously unresolved emotional problems between them.

Initially, they may deny that the defect does in fact exist, perhaps claiming that the diagnosis is mistaken. Or it may be difficult for the parents to attain a realistic attitude toward either the limited life-span or altered life-style implied by the nature of the disorder. The mother may try to plan "as if" there were no disability at all. This denial, based on unreality, can result only in grief, disappointment, failure, and bitterness. Parents may develop grief and mourn for the healthy child who might have been, much as they would mourn for a dead child[9] (see Chap. 39).

Realizing that the infant is imperfect, one parent may blame the other for the disability, or they may project their feelings to someone or something else—a family member, a neighbor, or the environment. Frequently their anger is displaced to the physician, nurse, or other member of the health team.[8,9]

Parents also may withdraw from or try to avoid the situation. This is exemplified by avoiding friends and family or not visiting the infant in the nursery.[10] There are families who avoid all but their closest friends because they find it too painful to explain again their child's affliction.

How can the parents ease their disappointment? Some rationalize by saying that this particular child will give other rewards, such as "bringing the family closer together." Another oft-quoted phrase is "Everything happens for the best."

Later, when the infant or child is at home, the parents may overprotect him or her as compensation for their anger and resulting guilt. Or because of their great fear of losing the child, they may begin to view it as being more fragile or vulnerable than the facts would warrant. The nurse must take care to recognize the defense mechanisms used by the parents, realizing that inconsistencies appear in their reasoning.[11] To question their rationalizations would be to destroy their defenses, a loss they can ill afford and one that would arouse feelings of anxiety and low self-esteem. The par-

ents have the need to do something to rid themselves of their uncertainties. At this time steps may be taken to do concrete problem solving for the present and to begin planning for the future.

Klaus and his colleagues have suggested[12] that an understanding of the stages through which parents are progressing may enable the professional staff members to be more effective in their dealings with them. The length of time that parents remain in the stages of shock and denial is variable; indeed, spouses may be at different stages and thus find it difficult to understand and help each other. Sadness, anger, and anxiety may be prolonged, making it difficult for parents to get on with the tasks of adaptation and reorganization. The physical demands of caring for the defective child may push some parents apart and limit their time away from the child. The nurse, recognizing that conflict about blame is separating the spouses, may be able to intervene. The search for an explanation may lead to the development of a religious or philosophic interpretation of the experience. The nurse, recognizing this need, will try to interweave the known facts without destroying the fabric of the defense.

Nurses' Response to Client/Family Behavior

In addition to recognizing the defense mechanisms displayed by parents and family at this time, nurses must also be alert to their own feelings in response to the particular diagnosis. Such emotions as shock, disbelief, anger, and resentment can be expected. Various coping mechanisms will be used in order to deal with these frightening feelings, and the nurse's attitude may affect the behavior of the parents. If the nurse shows anxiety and discomfort in the face of the child's disorder, the parents may also display this behavior or reject the nurse. On the other hand, if the nurse shows acceptance and warmth toward the child, the parents are less likely to show rejection. McCollum[13] has warned, however, that empathy may lead to overidentification; nurses in such situations may actually mourn as if their own children had been affected. Anxiety about their own children may result. Significant past losses may be recalled and relived, and latent feelings of anxiety about the nurse's own death may be raised.

Nurses' emotions, also, may be contingent on the area in which they work as well as their developmental level or period in life. For example, the young mother with small children of her own who is working on the obstetric unit may identify with the mother who has just given birth to an infant with an obvious defect such as a cleft lip. Her natural response might be to support this mother. She might feel pity and want to protect the newborn from the gaze of curious onlookers and the mother from any unpleasant comments from others. On the other hand, the young nurse on the pediatric unit, perhaps being the father of young children himself, may experience frustration in caring for a child who, he knows, cannot get well. He may also feel depressed because he knows that long-term goals cannot be attained. Fear of the child's gradual deterioration may develop, especially in view of the fact that this decline will eventually end in death regardless of the medical treatment and nursing care given. In addition, the nurse may be distressed by the knowledge that little children do not fully understand the reasons for treatments that are frequently painful and frightening. In caring for the child with a chronic disorder such as cystic fibrosis, which requires intermittent hospitalization, the nurse may feel discouraged to realize that no total cure can be effected. The more mature nurse might easily identify with the 40-year-old mother who feels overwhelming long-term responsibility for the birth of a child with Down's syndrome.

Whatever their feelings, nurses must not deny them or turn themselves into mechanical people who are devoid of feelings or emotions. They must nevertheless keep these feelings under control so as to remain objective and able to function. By being in command of their feelings, nurses can foster meaningful communication with the client and family, encouraging parents to communicate in an open atmosphere about their feelings. With-

out this control and openness, conversation remains at a superficial level and meaningful communication is impossible. Moreover, the nurse should remain tolerant and nonjudgemental even if the client responds in a way that the nurse deems inappropriate.

Assessment

In arriving at a genetic diagnosis and treatment plan, the assessment must include information about the following: (1) the medical history of the affected client, (2) when symptoms began, (3) when signs were first seen, (4) how the disorder has progressed, (5) what abnormalities have been noted, and (6) what treatments have been tried.

A complete evaluation of the family history is also needed: (1) whether other members are similarly affected, (2) whether there are siblings, and (3) whether early or unexplained deaths have occurred.

The nurse can obtain both objective and subjective information through observation and communication, eliciting information that can be helpful to the physician in making a diagnosis or planning treatment. The nurse should review the medical records to become familiar with the diagnostic studies which have been done, the medical diagnosis, and the plan of care if this has been formulated. After greeting the patient and/or the family and becoming oriented to the situation, the nurse can obtain the nursing history including personal, socioeconomic, and social data; the patient's concept or perception of self; the patient's physiologic and emotional status, adaptation to illness, understanding of treatment and procedures, and specific fears.[14] In caring for an infant, the nurse would obtain information from the parents. It is also important to evaluate the patient's and family's reaction to the illness and/or hospitalization.[15]

It is at this time that the nurse can elicit and evaluate the interactions between family members. Perhaps there are other situations which affect the family's view of this particular disorder. What is the psychological meaning to this family of this disorder? This is of particular importance for genetic disorders because of the social and cultural implications of genetic disease. If there are siblings, what is their response? Families are usually concerned that other children may also be affected although they have not yet shown signs of disorder. There are families who do not wish their other children to be examined out of fear that they too will show signs of the dreaded illness. This behavior may deprive these families of the very reassurance they need. The siblings themselves, if past age 4 or 5, probably share these concerns, though they may be unvoiced and may be represented by behavioral problems. What is the response of the extended family? Pressures not to divulge "family secrets" may render *pedigree* information inaccurate. Hesitation to allow others to know of the patient's affliction may hinder ascertainment of important family history. The extended family may view the disorder as a social stigma and be frightened and uncooperative. Only by observation, communication, and exploration can the nurse define the problems in order to make decisions or inferences regarding deficits, potential deficits, and strengths in the patient's health status.

Planning Nursing Care

Planning the nursing care requires a clear identification of goals. It is of first importance to help the client and family accept the diagnosis as well as the imperfect child. The implementation of the therapeutic plan will require the following:

1 The nurse can support the family members in their efforts to cope with and accept the hereditary disorder by:
   a Engaging the family in the problem-solving process
   b Helping them to identify and discuss their feelings
   c Helping them to see any positive aspects of the situation that can be found

2 The nurse must communicate expectations for the future of the afflicted child.

3 The nurse must identify the community resources needed to support client and family efforts.

4 The nurse must clarify the risk of developing and means of preventing the disorder in other family members.

The patient and family will need help in coping with a hereditary disorder. Before the nurse can be of any assistance to the family, a relationship of trust with them must be established. One can begin by asking the parents to explain what they know about the disease. Then the nurse can reexplain, clarify, and interpret what the physician has told them in language that they can understand. This is especially important to the new mother of a defective infant. If the nurse can encourage the mother to talk and can determine how she perceives her infant, discussion of the infant's defect can take place in a manner that will decrease the mother's anxiety.[16] The nurse can give emotional support to the patient by displaying an attitude of what Rogers calls "unconditional positive regard" and "empathic understanding."

It is crucial at this time to help the mother accept the infant and establish a warm relationship with him or her. It is known that infants need contact in order to form a maternal attachment, and it has been shown[17] that mothers who have not touched or cared for their premature infants show different "mothering behavior" when the infants are a year old. These mothers were less responsive and used touch less for comforting than did other mothers. Parents need to get acquainted with the imperfect child at a time when they are grieving for the "perfect child" who was not born. It is extremely helpful at this time to emphasize the normal aspects of the child. One can say "You have a normal child who has an abnormality in the development of his feet." The *child* is normal; only the feet are not. All children, no matter how deformed, have positive aspects which can become a focus of attention. Family separation must be minimized and contacts between the parents and the newborn maintained.[18] Though the mother may hesitate to touch or hold the infant, the nurse can help by asking the mother if she wishes to do so and by providing the opportunity.[10] It will be easier for the mother if continuity of care is established by providing the same nurse to care for the infant each day, so that they can establish rapport. Though opportunity is provided for the mother to care for the defective infant, she should not be coerced to do so. If and when she chooses to look after her child, positive reinforcement should be given by the nurse. When the mother shows that she is ready, the nurse can teach her any special skills that will be necessary in caring for this particular infant. This will increase her self-confidence and her acceptance of the infant.[10]

Nurses frequently show their concern for mothers, but fathers, too, need help at this time. They have similar concerns and others as well; they may have financial worries and they may be called upon to make decisions concerning medical procedures.[10] If the infant has been transported to a major neonatal intensive-care center and infant and mother are miles apart in different hospitals, the strain on the father and the conflict over where he is most needed may be severe. The birth of a defective child is a drain on a family's time, energy, and financial resources. Siblings will need to be told of the birth of the imperfect child, and this may be the father's responsibility too.

Though the birth of a defective infant provides a most poignant example of the impact of genetic disease, parents are no less vulnerable to the shattering effects of such a diagnosis when the child is older. Indeed, in some respects, the fact that attachments have been strengthened by this time may make such a diagnosis even more heartrending.

Chronic disease in childhood is always a trying experience. Burnette[19] cites her own family's experience of having a child with cystic fibrosis. The burdens that she mentions include financial strain, daily treatments for the child, and the daily cleaning of equipment. She tells how parents may feel unsure about whether treatment is necessary or beneficial, how they have limited faith in themselves and resent the demands on their time. She mentions that siblings feel deprived and that this leads to conflicts. Siblings resent it if parents stay too long with the hospitalized child. She states that families need knowledge of the disease as well as emotional support. On the practical side, they need to know where they can buy equipment, how to operate it, and how to obtain funds to buy it.

Families with children with PKU need much help and support in adhering to a difficult and often unattractive diet. It may be difficult to persuade mothers that what appears to be the opposite of a balanced diet is necessary for their child's optimal development. Parents are now being trained to give their hemophiliac sons the needed factor VIII concentrate by injection at home. While this decreases hospitalization, it also places the burden of doing a painful procedure on a parent.

Some families consider it a sign of weakness to use community resources such as regional centers and counseling services. They may recoil at the idea of accepting financial assistance from foundations or state agencies. The well-informed nurse will try to understand these feelings. The nurse may express personal positive feelings about the benefits that these agencies can provide, and these views may be augmented by any personal experiences he or she may be willing to share. There are many parent organizations, such as PKU and CF parent groups, as well as organizations for retarded citizens that may be of inestimable value in helping families cope. These organizations are made up of people who have "been there"; there is little they don't know.

Families must be prepared to deal with the unhappy reality of death. This is considered in detail in Chap. 39. For other families, the prospect of prolonged disability or severe deformity may be worse than that of death itself. It may be impossible to prepare for long-term progressive deterioration such as that seen in Tay-Sachs disease. We have often heard parents say "I'll take the chance of another child if it can either be healthy or fail to survive; what I can't face is a child who will be severely deformed or handicapped."

All these problems are compounded when a

family knows that contemplated future children will also be at risk, when siblings fear that they or their future children may be threatened by the dreaded condition, or when members of the extended family fear for their own children.

Intervention

Genetic counseling is an important aspect of intervention in the management of genetic disease. Combined with *carrier testing* and *prenatal diagnosis,* it provides the opportunity for families to exercise real reproductive options in the face of inherited disorders.

The objective of genetic counseling is the communication of information to families regarding the "magnitude of, implications of, and alternatives for dealing with the risk of occurrence of a hereditary disorder within the family."[20] This entails accurate medical diagnosis, correct ascertainment of risk, and thoughtful transfer of information to the family, followed by support and assistance in implementation of their decision. Much harm can be done by optimistic reassurance that is not based on fact as well as by thoughtless admonitions against further children when the actual recurrence risk is not known.[21]

The role of the nurse on the genetic counseling team is a changing one, evolving along with the expanding development of genetic counseling facilities. There are two very different roles for the nurse on the genetic counseling team. Hsia has reviewed the early data from a counseling program in a large medical center.[21] The team is composed of a physician-geneticist, social worker, nurse coordinator, and—when indicated—other specialists. The nurse first introduces the patient to the clinic. He or she obtains a detailed history of the problem, collects relevant medical data about affected relatives, explores the family history, and constructs a pedigree. The nurse then presents these data to the physician-geneticist. Thus preliminary evaluation and literature review can be done prior to the arrival of the family. The social worker interviews the family and determines educational level, financial situation, level of anxiety,

and religious views; all these are important in the decision-making process the family is about to undertake. The family is seen by the physician-geneticist and the medical diagnosis is corroborated. Then comes the difficult task of outlining prognosis, treatment, and recurrence risk. At this time the importance of the professional, sensitive, educated nurse again surfaces.

The patient wants to know "what will happen to me (or my child)?" "What treatment is necessary or possible?" "Can others in the family develop this condition?" "Are they at greater risk?" "What about future children?"

The nurse need not be a member of the genetic team to be involved. The sensitive and informed nurse *hears* what the patient is really asking, *recognizes* the significance of questions about genetics, *understands* the need for an accurate answer. She or he may interpret the family's concerns to the physician. On the inpatient unit, the nurse may have more continuous contact with the family than does the physician and thus may gain the trust of the family, enabling members to ask questions they would otherwise not be comfortable enough to·ask. Similarly, in the outpatient department, even a student nurse who has been briefed about the family's condition may provide this opportunity for important exchange of information. In the less formal situation, either in the clinic or at the bedside, the professional nurse can act as interpreter of complex data to the family. If the nurse is informed about basic mechanisms of inheritance, he or she can clarify confusing information. If the nurse is knowledgeable about mechanisms of handling stress, she or he can help families cope more effectively (see Chap. 5).

Most genetic counseling clinics share several basic principles:

1 Medical diagnosis must be accurate.
2 Scientific knowledge must be thorough.
3 Information must be communicated.
4 A nondirective approach should be used.

At the clinic described above, the counseling team tries to be certain that families receive factual, accurate information and that they know it is up to them to make any decision about action. Families receive support regardless of whether the decisions they make seem wise to the staff. Decisions are never prescribed, and the fact that different courses of action are needed in different families is never lost sight of.

What are the options available to families coping with genetic disease? Technical advances have broadened our understanding of the biochemical and biological mechanisms of many genetic disorders. This, in turn, has increased the options available to affected families and made possible interventions that increase their chances of having healthy children.

Antenatal Diagnosis

Perhaps the most far-reaching of these techniques is that of antenatal diagnosis. Over sixty inborn errors of metabolism and virtually all the recognized chromosomal abnormalities can now be detected in the unborn fetus at risk.[22] Families who have had a child with Down's syndrome or other chromosomal abnormalities may now be assured that the next child need not be so affected. Most families who utilize the techniques for detecting inborn errors of metabolism have also had a previously affected child. Two important exceptions to this unfortunate way of ascertaining families at risk now exist: mothers over the age of 35 years are known to run a considerably greater risk than do younger women of having a child with a chromosome abnormality. They can now be offered prenatal testing of the unborn fetus and thus avoid the birth of an affected child.

Families whose ethnic background renders them more likely to carry certain defective genes and thus puts them at greater risk can also be detected. An example of this type of intervention is seen in the Tay-Sachs prevention programs that are being conducted throughout the country. Where both husband and wife are Tay-Sachs carriers, the problem can be detected and the couple offered genetic counseling. Because the disease can be detected in the affected fetus early in pregnancy, such couples need not give birth to a child who is doomed to die of Tay-Sachs disease. Other disorders also lend themselves to this type

of prevention. Sickle cell anemia in the black population and Thalassemia in those of Mediterranean background also lend themselves to carrier-detection programs. Because prenatal detection techniques for these latter two conditions are still highly experimental, mass carrier testing is proceeding more slowly. PKU and CF are still undetectable in the unborn fetus, and carriers cannot yet be consistently and reliably detected. Advances in technology may open these conditions to similar kinds of prevention. For most families who utilize prenatal detection techniques, selective abortion of affected fetuses is the preferred option. However, this is not uniformly so; the decision to abort is also affected by religious and cultural factors. Families that carry such a pregnancy to term are better prepared for the tragic outcome because of prenatal diagnostic information. Although the reassuring news of normality offers joy and relief to all involved, the waiting period between test and results can be most trying, even for the most well-adjusted, and the decision to abort an abnormal fetus is not an easy one, even for the most committed.[23] A great deal of support from the team is needed by families at this time.

For many families, prenatal diagnosis is not feasible; for some it is not acceptable. Then families must utilize other options. Traditionally, *adoption* has provided the route by which such families fulfill their desires for healthy children. This often requires much soul searching and discussion. Families must be helped through the trying period of application and the long, lonely period of waiting. Adoptable babies are becoming fewer, and this may prolong the wait.

When both parents carry a defective recessive gene or when the father has a dominantly inherited disorder, *artificial insemination* (AID) may be utilized. Though this is a biologically effective way of surmounting either situation, it may be extremely difficult for some parents to undertake. Thorough discussion of the meaning of parenthood to both spouses is extremely important in helping parents discuss this option (see Chap. 32).

Carrier detection programs have been alluded to. They present their own special problems in terms of the psychological reactions of those found to be carriers. Many people find it very threatening to be told that they are carrying a defective gene. To have an abnormal gene strikes at the very core of their selfhood. They need to know that everyone carries at least five or six abnormal genes that are, however, usually undetectable. *They* are fortunate (or unfortunate) enough to know the identity of one of theirs.

How do families respond when they receive information about their genetic risks? Several authors have commented on the concept of "burden." Families may be more likely to take a large risk of having a minor disorder than a small risk of having a very severe disorder. Burden aside, high risks tend to deter further reproduction. News of low risk tends to have a reassuring effect and to deter fewer people. But parental distortion of information may be frequent.[24] This is a possibility which needs much further study. There may be emotional resistance to the assimilation of information, and this resistance may be augmented by anxiety.

Anxiety may be a prominent response to receiving genetic information. When evidence of early maladaptation is evident, remediation may be attempted. Nonadaptive behavior may take the form of denial of a significant recurrence risk. For example, a family with a child with PKU may behave as if the recurrence risk of 25 percent for each pregnancy were unknown to them, despite frequent repetition of the facts by genetic team members. One family with a child suffering from cystic fibrosis said, upon learning of the same diagnosis in their second child, "But it was this one's turn to be normal." This is a magical way of thinking.

Rejection of the affected child is serious evidence of maladaptation. A low-phenylalanine diet may not be followed, or even more destructive behavior may be seen. Occasionally the origin of the abnormal gene is completely misunderstood. One mother insisted that she must be carrying the defective gene even though there was no rational reason to believe so. When parents are faced with a defective child, when a person learns of a serious genetic disorder in a spouse, or when a couple find out that they have a high risk of having abnormal children, a crisis in their lives is unques-

tionably reached. Sympathetic, professional, and supportive crisis-intervention techniques should be applied (see Chap 5).

It is important to regard the family as a unit. Perhaps an older sibling had wished to be rid of his younger brother. Now illness has made that old wish possible. The older child did not really want such an outcome but now fears he or she has magic power. The child's behavior may therefore become a problem, and parents need to be warned to expect this. The older sibling of a child doomed to worsen and die of Tay-Sachs disease must be told that not everyone who goes to the hospital fails to return.

Is a mother feeling guilty because she did not want the child and attempted abortion? Has a father transformed his anger at the child's disorder or at its genetic cause into insistence that the child is not his? An empathic opportunity to ventilate such frightening and disorganizing feelings is crucial. The involvement and understanding of the family is central to its protective role.[25] Open discussion and honesty about feelings will enhance the mastery of this crisis. If marital discord has resulted, this problem must be recognized. Fears of abandonment must be brought out in the open. Once the complex nature of the problem leading to the crisis is recognized, its solution may be sought.[26]

The family support sources must be identified. Can both parents be helped to support each other? Are there grandparents who can participate? Is there a family physician whose long-term trust can be utilized? Perhaps there are close neighbors. Often, parents of similarly affected children can be most supportive. The help of such parents can be sought after a new mother has been given the diagnosis of Down's syndrome in her child.

The coping ability of the family must be assessed. Are both parents synchronous in their reactions? Is their level of concern realistic or have distortions occurred? For example, a family had a child with Tay-Sachs disease. Slowly, over about 3 months, they recognized that their infant was failing but did not know the reason. Finally, when the child was 6 months old, a neurologist made the diagnosis. Both parents were overcome with anger and grief. They could not understand why this had happened to them. They told the physician of their guilt at not having the Tay-Sachs carrier testing they had known about. They talked of their increasing pain on regarding the child and knowing her fate. But they were able to discuss their feelings openly. "Are we losing our grip?" they asked. "What should we tell our older child?" They reached the stage of asking how to know when the sick child should be hospitalized. They resolved the crisis, though continuing to live with the tragedy, by ventilating their feelings, recognizing the problem, supporting each other, and seeking workable solutions. The professional nurse must be prepared to help families arrive at this kind of resolution.

Once the diagnosis of a genetic disorder has been made, the family evaluated, and a plan of action designed, this plan must be implemented. Perhaps medications are needed. Or, as in the case of PKU, a special diet may be prescribed. The nurse must help the family accept these necessary measures. As previously mentioned, the genetic aspects of the condition must be clarified to the family and the information communicated accurately. This may result in the need for other family members to be evaluated. Help may be needed in communicating this to those who need to be examined. If chronic care will eventually be needed, help toward finding this must be offered.

Evaluation of Intervention

Several measures can be used to evaluate the effectiveness of the intervention. One can ask the client if he or she thought genetic counseling was beneficial. Hsia[21] learned from questionnaires sent to clients who had received genetic counseling at a major clinic that about 80 percent found the counseling had answered most of their questions and had been helpful. The same number felt that their understanding had been improved and they had been helped to cope. Did counseling influence their reproductive attitudes? Tips and Lynch[7] found that counseling led to increased reproduction throughout the family, presumably

because risks were smaller than families had thought. Carter[6] reported dependence on size of risk and severity of disorder. Hsia[21] also reported some influence on reproductive attitudes. This effect may be estimated by the level of use of contraceptive methods and of prenatal testing. In the case of a child with a treatable disease, evaluation of the utilization of treatment can indicate the effectiveness of the intervention. Other questions can be asked: Is the marriage still intact? Have the siblings developed normally? Is the couple participating in social activities? Have community resources been utilized? If not, what kind of further help can be offered? The client should be asked. The effectiveness of intervention needs ongoing evaluation if we are to learn and improve our techniques.

References

1 M. R. Seashore: "Genetics: The State of the Art in Connecticut," *Connecticut Medicine,* in press.

2 J. V. Neel: Birth Defects Original Article Series 9:1–4, National Foundation, 1973.

3 J. Warkany: "Congenital Malformations of the Past," *Journal of Chronic Diseases,* vol. 10, pp. 84–96, 1959.

4 H. T. Lynch, T. P. Knish, A. J. Krush, and R. L. Tips: "Psychodynamics of Early Hereditary Deaths," *American Journal for the Diseases of Children,* vol. 108, pp. 605–610, 1964.

5 H. A. Sultz, E. R. Schlesinger, and J. Feldman: "An Epidemiologic Justification for Genetic Counseling in Family Planning," *American Journal of Public Health,* vol. 62, pp. 1489–1492, 1972.

6 C. O. Carter, J. A. Fraser-Roberts, K. A. Evans, and A. R. Buck: "Genetic Clinic: A Follow-up," *Lancet,* vol. 1, pp. 281–285, 1971.

*7 R. L. Tips and H. T. Lynch: "The Impact of Genetic Counseling upon the Family Milieu," *Journal of the American Medical Association,* vol. 184, pp. 183–186, 1963.

8 D. R. Marlow: *Textbook of Pediatric Nursing,* 4th ed., Saunders, Philadelphia, 1973.

9 W. S. Yancey: "Approaches to Emotional Management of the Child with a Chronic Illness," *Clinical Pediatrics,* vol. 11, no. 2, pp. 64–67, February 1972.

*10 G. C. Mills: "Supporting Parental Needs after Birth

of a Defective Child," in Brandt, Chinn, and Smith (eds.): *Current Practice in Pediatric Nursing,* Mosby, St. Louis, 1976.

11 J. C. Coleman: *Abnormal Psychology and Modern Life,* 3d ed., Scott, Foresman, Chicago, 1964, pp. 96–108.

*12 D. Drotar, A. Baskeiwicz, N. Irvin, J. Kennell, and M. Klaus: "The Adaptation of Parents to the Birth of an Infant with a Congenital Malformation," *Pediatrics,* vol. 56, pp. 710–717, 1975.

*13 A. T. McCollum: *Coping with Prolonged Health Impairment in Your Child,* Little, Brown, Boston, 1975.

14 V. K. Carrieri and J. Stigman: "Components of the Nursing Process," *Nursing Clinics of North America,* vol. 6, pp. 115–124, March 1971.

15 Sylvia Carlson: "A Practical Approach to the Nursing Process," *American Journal of Nursing,* vol. 72, no. 9, pp. 1589–1591, September 1972.

16 Gladys M. Scipien, et al.: *Comprehensive Pediatric Nursing,* McGraw-Hill, New York, 1975.

*17 M. H. Klaus and J. H. Kennell: "Mothers Separated from Their Newborn Infants," *Pediatric Clinics of North America,* vol. 17, pp. 1015–1037, November 1970.

*18 Mecca S. Cranley: "When a High-Risk Infant is Born," *American Journal of Nursing,* vol. 75, no. 11, November 1975.

*Recommended reference by a nurse author.

19 Betty Anne Burnette: "Family Adjustment to Cystic Fibrosis," *American Journal of Nursing,* vol. 75, no. 11, November 1975.

20 W. S. Sly: "What Is Genetic Counseling?" in *Contemporary Genetic Counseling,* Proceedings of a Symposium of the American Society of Human Genetics, 1972, Birth Defects Original Article Series, vol. 9, pp. 9–18, 1973.

21 Y. E. Hsia: "Choosing My Children's Genes: Genetic Counseling," in M. Lipkin and P. T. Rowley (eds.): *Genetic Responsibility,* Plenum, New York, 1973.

*22 M. R. Seashore and M. J. Mahoney: "Prenatal Diagnosis: Its Safety, Accuracy, and Indications for Use," *Connecticut Medicine,* in press.

23 J. Robinson, K. Tennes, and A. Robinson: "Amniocentesis: Its Impact on Mother and Infants: A 1-year Follow-up Study," *Clinical Genetics,* no. 8, pp. 97–106, 1975.

24 M. S. Sibinga and C. J. Friedman: "Complexities of Parental Understanding of Phenylketonuria," *Pediatrics,* vol. 48, pp. 216–224, 1971.

*25 D. M. Kaplan, A. Smith, R. Grobstein, and S. E. Fischman: "Family Mediation of Stress," *Social Work,* vol. 8, pp. 60–69, 1973.

26 G. Caplan: *Principles of Preventive Psychiatry,* Basic Books, New York, 1964.

27 J. Desforges: "Current Concepts in Genetics," *New England Journal of Medicine,* vol. 294, p. 393, 1976.

38

The Family with an Exceptional Child

Judith Meyer

Learning Objectives

After studying this chapter, the student should be able to:

1   Assess the strengths and weaknesses presented by the exceptional child and his or her family in the community
2   Recognize deviations from normal growth and development
3   Define selected terms used with the exceptional child
4   Assess selected etiological factors in relation to the exceptional child
5   Assess selected adaptations of the exceptional child
6   Assess selected family responses to the exceptional child
7   Describe selected medical regimens used with the exceptional child
8   Recognize the significance of selected factors in the environment of the exceptional child which influence adaptation
9   Use the context of the nurse-client interaction therapeutically
10   Make nursing diagnoses relating to the exceptional child
11   Work collaboratively with the client, parents, and members of the health team
12   Outline goals on a priority basis
13   Implement a plan of care for the exceptional child
14   Identify means of primary prevention in relation to the exceptional child
15   Maximize enhancement of potential in relation to the exceptional child
16   List guidelines for evaluating the care of the exceptional child

An exceptional child is a child whose growth and development deviate from the norm in some way. Traditionally the term has been applied to retarded or very bright children. In the present discussion, however, the child with minimal brain dysfunction and seizure disorders will also be included in this category. Many of the adaptational responses of the exceptional child are adopted by any child who deviates developmentally.

Regardless of the type of exceptional development the child may present, the first nursing task is to identify the strengths, weaknesses, and areas of potential growth in these children and their families, as well as the resources available in their communities.

Selected Client Behaviors
Retardation

The official definition of "mental retardation" adopted in 1958 by the American Association of Mental Deficiency states that retardation is the presence of subaverage general intellectual functioning which originates during the developmental period and is associated with impairment in adaptive behavior.[1] Retardation is not a disease entity itself but a complex of symptoms due to a variety of causes.

Mentally retarded children are as different from one another as are children of normal or superior intelligence. They are generally thought of as having an innate limitation of intellectual potential. But some children who function at a subaverage intellectual level may have potential for higher, normal, or even superior functioning. An emotional, hearing, or visual disturbance may have interfered with either their development or the expression of their development. For example, a child may be so preoccupied with conflicts within the family that concentration and absorption of learning at school is limited. If the family conflicts can be relieved, the child may be able to learn as well as an average child. A disturbance of hearing or vision may also limit a child's ability to integrate what is being taught in a regular classroom. Correction of the disturbance or special educational techniques which do not rely on the disturbed sense may reveal normal potential for learning.

Mental retardation may have the highest incidence of all childhood disorders. It is estimated that 3 percent of the population are identified as mentally retarded at some point in their lives. Some children are identified at an early age because of marked developmental lags or because their physical appearance is characteristic of *Down's syndrome* or *cri-du-chat syndrome.* However, the peak period of recognition is between 6 and 16 years of age, when the pressures of formal schooling reveal impairments. Those children recognized at this time are the higher-functioning retardates who are identified by their teachers when specific cognitive tasks are being taught and evaluated. The lack of mastery of these tasks may not interfere with social functioning and thus not be recognized by parents. The incidence of retardation may reach 10 percent or more of the school population in some deprived urban areas. Mental retardation appears to be more frequent in boys than girls, the ratio being 55 percent to 45 percent. This disparity may in part be related to biological factors (sex-linked genetic disorders) and in part to differences in social expectations for the sexes. At least 75 percent of the retarded have no obvious physical stigma. However, the group as a whole has a higher percentage of sensory defects, language disorders, neuromuscular impairment, seizures, and physical anomalies than the general population. The retarded, like other children with handicapping defects, are more vulnerable to emotional problems; conversely, children with emotional problems frequently function at a retarded level.

At present it is estimated that of the probable 6 million mentally retarded persons in the United States, 200,000 are in institutions, 300,000 are on waiting lists for such care, and an equal number in general or special hospitals or prisons. More than 85 percent live at home. Seven out of ten of these are of school age, and it is estimated that the majority receive only minimal medical care and guidance.[2] It is clear, therefore, that the thrust of the development of services, especially educational facilities, must be in the communities where the children live.

Intelligence is not the result of a single mental process but includes abstract thinking, visual and auditory memory, causal reasoning, verbal expression, manipulative capacities, and spatial comprehension. Current—but inadequate—practices quantitatively identify intelligence in terms of mental age or intelligence quotient (IQ). This is the ratio of mental age to chronologic age and supplies only averages of the composite attainments in some of these mental abilities. These tests, which reflect middle-class white culture, are biased against those whose life experience and cultural background differ from the norms used in test construction. Arrested or inadequate mental development is rarely equally distributed among the various intellectual spheres. Frequently some mental functions are within normal limits in moderately retarded children, as they are also with the very bright child. Table 38-1 illustrates the range of IQ levels and the educational, vocational, and social implications of the handicaps involved.

More than one hundred different factors have been identified as being closely or causally relat-

Table 38-1 Intelligence Quotient Classifications

IQ range	Education	Employment potential	Social implications
Borderline, 68–83	1 Regular classroom with slight program modification by a skilled teacher	1 Moderately skilled to semiskilled jobs	1 Often indistinguishable from others in a general social milieu.
	2 "Slow learner."		2 Coping skills may be limited in time of stress
Mildly retarded, 50–75 (educational) system classification).	1 "Educable"—special education classes or regular classrooms up to fourth or fifth grade with an understanding teacher.	1 Semiskilled or unskilled jobs.	1 First to be affected by economic change in society.
		2 Considered expendable by employers.	2 Normally blend in with society, function independently as adults.
		3 Marginal socioeconomically.	3 Need assistance from social agencies in times of stress—coping skills limited.
Moderately retarded, 35–50.	1 "Trainable"—rarely learn to read and write but learn self-care habits such as eating, dressing, toileting.	1 Sheltered workshop employment.	1 Adequate social adjustment in the home and neighborhood.
	2 Learn acceptable social behavior, table manners, speech, and other means of communication.	2 Economically useful at home.	2 Dependent on family.
Severely or profoundly foundly retarded.	1 Require help with most functions of daily living. They must be fed, bathed.		1 They function as infants and toddlers.
	2 They can learn to sit, stand, relate to others, and feed themselves with assistance.		2 They require continued care and protection as adults either in the home environment or in an institution.[3]
	3 Some can learn to play with toys and other children.		

ed to mental retardation, yet there is no identifiable biologic or organic problem in 65 to 75 percent of regarded children. In their case, retardation is probably caused by sociocultural or environmental deprivation and is a by-product of poverty and indadequate parenting (see Chap. 33). The majority of the mildly retarded and minimally brain-damaged children come from the more disadvantaged classes of society characterized by low income, limited educational achievement, unskilled occupations, and generally impoverished environment.

These children are, in general, poorly nourished, subject to more acute and chronic illnesses, and receive less medical and dental care than do those from the middle and upper income groups. Many of these children are born to mothers who are themselves poorly nourished and who have received little prenatal, perinatal, or postnatal care. The prematurity rate in such environments is 2 to 3 times the national average. Retardation in these underpriviliged children is largely acquired, possibly beginning in utero and becoming apparent during the second or third year of life. It is probably a consequence of lack of good interpersonal relations, the absence of psychological stimulation,

and overall sensory, emotional, environmental, and nutritional deprivation.

In contrast to the symptoms of mild retardation found in the lower sociocultural groups, the more severe degrees of retardation appear to be more evenly distributed throughout the population.[2]

Scipien outlines some of the most common etiologic factors in Table 38-2.

Minimal Brain Dysfunction

The term "minimal brain dysfunction" (MBD) is currently used to identify a syndrome in which a child has learning or behavior disabilities in spite of average, nearly average, or above-average intellectual ability. The disabilities range from mild to moderately severe and are attributable to such deviations of cerebral function as impairment in perception, conceptualization, language comprehension or expression, memory, control of attention, impulse control, or some motor functions.[2]

In the majority of cases no specific cause can be determined for the syndrome of minimal brain dysfunction, but in some instances there is an apparent link to genetic disorder, birth injury, or prenatal or postnatal illness or injury of the central

Table 38-2 Etiological Factors of Retardation[3]

1 Prenatal period
  a Chromosomal anomalies: Down's syndrome (trisomy 21), Klinefelter's syndrome
  b Errors of metabolism: Phenylketonuria (PKU), hypothyroidism (cretinism), Hurler's disease (gargoylism)
  c Malformations of the cranium: Microcephaly, hydrocephaly
  d Maternal factors: Rubella (German measles), some other viral illnesses of mother, syphilis, anoxia, blood-type incompatibility, malnutrition, toxemia

2 Neonatal or perinatal period
  a Anoxia
  b Intracranial hemorrhage
  c Birth injury
  d Kernicterus
  e Prematurity

3 Postnatal period
  a Infections: Meningitis, encephalitis
  b Poisoning: Insecticides, medications, lead
  c Degenerative diseases: Tay-Sachs disease, Huntington's disease, Niemann-Pick disease
  d Physical injury: Head injury, asphyxia, hyperpyrexia
  e Brain tumors
  f Social and cultural factors: Deprivation, emotional disturbance, nutritional deficiency

nervous system. Some dysfunction may be sex-linked, since the incidence is higher in boys than in girls. Poverty is also correlated with a high incidence of minimal brain dysfunction.

Because of continuing disagreement about how to identify the child with MBD, the frequency of the disorder is not well documented. Generally 5 to 10 percent of the population is thought to have some manifestation of the disorder. Whatever the frequency, it is thought to be increasing due to improved obstetrical and pediatric techniques which allow children to survive who previously would have died. Like mild retardation, the disorder is often not identified until the child is of school age and being taught reading and writing. What differs for the child with MBD is the "intensity, persistence, and clustering of the symptoms." A differential diagnosis is directed at determining whether the behavioral symptoms are caused by retardation, emotional disturbance, or MBD. Evidence of organic impairment must be separated from behavioral symptoms generated by the child's response to the physical disability.

Motor Signs

These most commonly include a lag in one or more of the developmental milestones. The child may be late in sitting, standing, walking, talking, or using language. The retarded child, by contrast, is consistently slow in reaching all or most developmental milestones. A second motor sign may be marked and continuous hyperactivity which may have an aimless quality. The mother may have felt the child to be very active while she was pregnant. During infancy, the child may be too restless to cuddle easily. Toddlers and school-age children may be impulsive in thoughts, feelings, and actions. This may result in tantrums that do not have the angry element of the traditional temper tantrum but rather a quality of frustration, helplessness, and deep pain. The hyperactivity of MBD is practically continuous. It may be very reassuring for a mother to know that this hyperactivity usually decreases spontaneously during puberty. In many cases hyperactivity is caused by anxiety, but it then appears primarily in association with stress.

Children with MBD may exhibit generally disruptive behavior for which there is no specific psychological term. They are called "bad" and told that they "just don't listen" by parents and teachers. Additional motor signs are difficulties in both fine and gross motor control, difficulties in sucking and swallowing, difficulties in dressing, throwing a ball, and riding a two-wheeled bike.

Cognitive Signs

These include distractability or poor attention span. The child may have difficulty differentiating important from unimportant stimuli and may respond to all equally. Or these children may consider their inner thoughts of equal importance to the teacher's word. They may then be labeled daydreamers. Or the distractibility may be visual. For example, the child may have little or no trouble reading single words presented separately but have great difficulty with a whole page of printed words. An environment where extraneous stimuli are reduced can be most helpful. Several learning sessions are better than one long one. The child with MBD may also have difficulty with the accurate perception of time, space, form, sound, and sequence. The child may have trouble separating figures from background or seeing things as a whole. Cause-and-effect relationships may be difficult to grasp. Poor retention is another common cognitive sign. Parents and teachers often complain that the child cannot remember anything for any length of time. What was taught and seemingly learned one day may have to be retaught and relearned the next. This difficulty is also characteristically erratic; that is, one day the child remembers learning from the previous day and the next day he or she does not. The child may also have difficulty forming concepts and abstractions at an age when others are doing so. Thus, age-appropriate jokes and humor or the rules of games when playing with others may not be grasped, and this may play a role in the child's lack of popularity with peers.

Diagnosis of MBD is usually made on the basis of history. Psychological and neurologic examination can confirm suspicions aroused by

the history and by assessment of school achievement and adjustment. Objective observations
made in the home and the school environment by
the nurse are significant. Direct monitoring of
behavior is helpful in diagnosing a child with MBD
only if the child is observed in a familiar environment, since both the parent and the child may act
in atypical ways in an unfamiliar one. Much to a
parent's exasperation, the hyperactive child often
sits quietly in the physician's office while the
mother tearfully describes her futile efforts to control the hyperactivity at home. Parents are then
sometimes blamed for ineffective limit setting and
discipline or intolerance of the activity level of a
normal child.

Seizure Disorders

The terms "seizure disorders," "epilepsy," and
"recurrent convulsive disorder" are used interchangeably. These terms designate a variable
symptom complex characterized by recurrent, paroxysmal attacks of unconsciousness or impaired
consciousness, usually with a succession of tonic
or clonic muscular spasms or other abnormal
behavior.[4]

The etiology and pathology of epilepsy are
unknown. The genetic inheritance of epilepsy has
been unduly emphasized. Seizures may have a
demonstrable organic pathology, suggest an emotional component, or have no identifiable cause.

Epilepsy is diagnosed primarily from a history
of seizure episodes; it is confirmed by abnormal
EEG readings, which are found in 90 percent of
children with idiopathic seizures and in almost all
children with organic seizures. The diagnostic
work-up includes an extensive neurologic assessment to determine any organic basis for the seizures. Identification of an organic cause is important prognostically because generally control of
such seizures is less satisfactory and the social
adjustment of the child who has them is less
adequate than that of children with idiopathic
seizures. Table 38-3 identifies categories of seizures and the accompanying behavioral manifestations.

Children with a history of seizures may learn to
induce them, as a way of getting attention, by
overbreathing, watching a blinking light, or some
other form of behavior. Drug therapy alone will
clearly be unsatisfactory. Complex family problems probably underlie this kind of behavior. Not
paying attention to the behavior and rewarding
more appropriate behavior has been effective in
reducing this as well as other types of seizures.[5]

Epileptic children display a wide range of
mental abilities comparable to those in the general
population, although a high incidence of seizures
does exist in retarded children. The presence of
epilepsy per se does not call for modification in
teaching methods, curriculum, or classroom
placement unless retardation is present or the
epilepsy is uncontrolled. Epileptic children without severe brain damage have the same intellectual ability as normal children and should have the
same opportunity to learn and develop within the
same school setting. The majority of epileptics are
in every other respect normal human beings. Most
authorities deny the existence of an "epileptic
personality." They maintain that any demonstrable
deviation in personality is caused by restrictions
imposed by society, mismanagement of the epileptic at home and in the community, or anxiety,
which is related to the anticipation of a seizure.

Exceptionally High Intelligence

The very bright or gifted child is defined as the
child with an IQ *above 120.* This is a practically
useful definition, but it should be remembered that
IQ alone gives a very limited picture of any child's
various strengths and abilities. Bright children are
found throughout the population, but they are more
often the children of bright parents in the middle or
upper classes of society. Brightness is correlated
with good nutrition, good health care, appropriately stimulating environments, and good schools.
Not all bright children have bright parents, and
such parents may react with feelings of inadequacy and helplessness to their child's abilities. Siblings may be jealous. They may withdraw from
competing with the brighter child or they may
tease the child for being "different."

The classic studies of Terman and Oden indi-

Table 38-3 Categories of Seizure Types

Seizure	Behavior
Grand mal	Seizure may be preceded by an aura or prodromal twitching, localized spasm, irritability, headache, digestive disturbance, or mental dullness.
	Seizure itself involves generalized convulsion with tonic and clonic phases of muscular spasms as well as involuntary urination and/or defecation from contraction of abdominal muscles.
	The convulsion is followed by sleep.
Petit mal	Seizures consist of transient loss of consciousness. Motor manifestations include upward rolling of eyes, moving of lids, dropping or rhythmic nodding of head, quivering of trunk and limb muscles.
	Clinical evidence of petit mal rarely appears before age 3 and frequently disappears by puberty.
	Intellectual development is rarely impaired.
Psychomotor seizures	This is the most difficult type to recognize and control.
	A slight aura may manifest itself in a shrill cry or an attempt to run for help.
	The seizure itself consist of purposeful but inappropriate motor acts which are repetitive and often complicated, characterized by gradual loss of postural tone.
	After 1 to 5 minutes of unconsciousness, normal activity may resume or sleep may ensue.
Status epilepticus	Seizure involves successive major convulsions without intervening recovery of consciousness.
	The most frequent cause is sudden withdrawal of anticonvulsant medication: an attack may occur 2 to 4 days after phenobarbital is withdrawn, 7 to 12 days after withdrawal of Dilantin.
	Seizure may be precipitated by an acute respiratory infection or the administration of chlorpromazine.
	An attack constitutes medical emergency requiring vigorous treatment.

cate that gifted students are physically healthier than the average, better coordinated, more attractive personally, and in general enjoying a richer, fuller life.[6] They are also slightly taller and heavier, with a wider range of both intellectual and nonintellectual interests. They have been found to be less likely to become maladjusted. The image of the isolated, tormented genius has not been validated in reality. However, gifted children may show an unevenness of achievement in different functional areas very much as children of average potential do. For example, their motor and intellectual development may be more advanced than their emotional and social development.

Early signs of giftedness in children include play which is more verbal, extensive early reading, and a greater capacity for fantasy and imaginative play. In school, gifted children may perform at levels that are two or three grades ahead of those of their peers. The bright child is likely to be the one who leads peers in fantasy play: the one who states the plot, assigns the roles, and invents the props.

Social Attitudes

Social attitudes in general and in the particular environment of the exceptional child very much influence that child's and family's adjustment. They also affect the attitudes and behavior of nurses. Our culture tends to value intellectual capacity and achievement and may view as a threat persons who are defective or who are mistakenly viewed as defective in this area. In this context, gifted children may receive special attention and advantage. However, in a culture which values equalization of opportunity, many feel it is undemocratic to provide special opportunities to the gifted.

Social attitudes toward epileptic children have been similar to those toward the retarded, but there is a greater component of fear. Epileptics have to overcome the archaic notion that they are possessed by devils. The public still retains many misconceptions about this disease; it has been confused with everything from insanity to criminality. These attitudes have led to ostracism and restrictions on the activities of people suffering from epilepsy.[7]

Blatt suggests that through the establishment of the mental health/mental-retardation dichotomy—that is, because of the nomenclature related to objectives, services, and economic support—mental retardation has been relegated to a place of secondary importance in our society.[8]

Children with minimal brain dysfunction or epilepsy are generally viewed with both greater hopefulness and greater fear than the mentally ill; perhaps fear because, often, the presenting behavior is dramatic and out of immediate control, and yet hopefulness because of the greater chance of "cure" and normal functioning.

All, including the gifted, share the effects of society's lack of emphasis on the development of each individual's maximum potential. This is particulary evident in institutions. Dybwad reports that many of our institutions strip the residents of their human dignity, identity, motivation, privacy, and basic human rights. This is not so much due to administrative incompetence or cruelty as to the belief that the residents are inferior creatures, devoid of sensitivity, to whom the usual norms of human interaction do not apply.[8]

Parental Responses

The reactions of parents to their exceptional child vary widely. The degrees and kinds of responses are influenced by such things as the attitudes of their own social group or class, marital relationships, attitudes toward deviance, past experiences, and future aspirations.

Solnit and Stark have used the mourning process as a model for understanding parental reactions to the birth or diagnosis of a defective child.[9] Psychological preparation during pregnancy includes both anticipation of a perfect child and fear of a damaged one. Thus, the birth of a defective child represents the loss of the desired child and the realization of the parents' fears. The initial phase of the mourning process is one of numbness and *denial*. Denial protects the parents from ego deflation. A child represents to parents an extension of themselves; thus, it is normal for the parents to perceive any defect in the child as a reflection of parental inadequacies and for them to utilize denial as a means of coping.

Denial is facilitated in early childhood when parents can rationalize the defect or developmental lag by saying that they have a "lazy" or a "good" baby. When parents search for the cause and a solution and they are not forthcoming, there is increasing confrontation with reality. *Anger* is generated as a defense against feelings of helplessness and frustration. A parent may blame professionals, ancestors, or spouse for the child's defect. Parents may angrily ask, "why me?" Normally, anger gives way to sadness and *depression*. Anger is abnormal when it is prolonged and replaces positive, effective action.

Preoccupied with their own sorrow and grief, many parents withdraw from others for a time. "Working through" of the loss takes time. In contrast to the parents of a dead child, these parents are, while grieving, also required to invest love in the new and handicapped child. The recognition and *acceptance* of the real child lies not so much in being told about the child's assets by professionals but in the parents' discovery of the child's positive aspects in situations which may be planned by the professional.

Parents may be able to recognize and accept their child's limitations, or they may experience what Olshansky has described as *chronic sorrow*.[10] Some believe this may occur because many of the parents' initial reactions are kept alive by guilt over their continuous, covert rejection of the defective child. Consciously they may feel they do not love the child enough. Some parents lean over backward to show love, to hide any hint of irritability or impatience, to protect the child against danger, and to minimize the slightest frustration. But behind the excessive solicitude one can see the unconscious aggression and sadness. These reactions may or may not be shared by both parents, but in either case they may lead to marital discord and an increased divorce rate. Chronic sorrow may also be kept alive by concern about what will become of the child when the parents die or are otherwise unable to provide care or protection. Even with parents who seem to have worked through the grieving process, anger, blaming, and depression may appear at various developmental milestones or life crises such as school entry, puberty, or at a time when the disability becomes more obvious.

Gardner has described parallel responses by parents of children with *minimal brain dysfunction*.[11] As part of their denial process, parents may question the diagnostician's competence and begin "shopping" for the professional who will tell them what they want to hear, which is that nothing is wrong. Parents may feel that organicity implies permanence and incurability and look for the professional who will confirm their hope that the problems are psychological and thus "curable." Some parents may insist that the child just needs stricter discipline. Fathers may blame mothers for not providing this, or parents may blame teachers. Parents need to learn that help is available for both types of problems. Another way to deny the child's MBD is by overprotection. By keeping the child an infant, the parents seek not to expose the defects he or she will show with greater maturity; thus they avoid confronting the painful reality.

Inappropriate guilt is another common reaction to MBD. Parents may feel that they did something wrong or sinful to bring this situation upon themselves. This may be related to repressed hostility toward the child, as if the parent had wished the condition on the child. Gardner believes that guilt is more often a futile attempt to control feelings of helplessness. Parents, by attributing the cause to themselves, give themselves the power to control what is otherwise uncontrollable.[11]

Siblings may share many of the reactions of their parents to the exceptional child. They will tend to imitate their parents' attitudes and behavior toward the child. Since their self-esteem is immature and fragile, they may be acutely embarrassed by the behavior or reputation of the exceptional child among their neighbors or school friends. Siblings may be either proud or resentful of any care of the child that is delegated to them, depending on the way the parents assign the task and whether they provide the siblings with adequate nurturing. Neighbors also, more often than not, tend to be more tolerant and understanding if they receive a clear, matter-of-fact explanation rather than being led to believe that the child is "strange" or "bad."

Parents of very bright children will not share the mourning response of parents of other exceptional children unless they view the child's intelligence and behavior as deviant, strange, or defiant. Some parents may simply not see their child's special qualities and needs. Others may tend to exploit their child's cleverness or be pushy and overstimulating. Still others may be possessive and overprotective, while those who feel threatened by their child's intelligence may be repressive.

Chronic parental adaptive reactions are deep and complex. If adaptive responses interfere with appropriate nurturing, referral for psychiatric counseling may be indicated.

Children's Responses

Exceptional children themselves may also have adaptive reactions that become problematical. Because of the mutuality of the parent-child relationship, both sides experience difficulties and each feels that some of these problems stem from the other.

These children may have fear reactions when exposed to many frustrations and humiliations that the normal child does not face. They may dread each new undertaking because of the disappointment to which it may lead, foreseeing failure even in areas of capability. Therefore the child must be helped to become aware of his or her capabilities, so that activities which will reveal limitations can be minimized. There will be improvement through training, treatment, and growth. Early educational experiences can give these children the head start in a preschool setting or at home they so sorely need.

The child with MBD or retardation needs much more supervision and regulation than the average child. Without these controls, the child not only fears but may suffer guilt for what he or she does when uncontrolled. An orderly, predictable environment with appropriate limits can be beneficial. The child may withdraw to avoid fear, humiliation, and rejection. It can help to adapt the environment in ways that will make it less threatening and more inviting. Placing the child in a special class with others who have similar difficulties can help the child to feel more acceptable and reduce his or her sense of exclusion and embarrassment. Social and recreational groups for children with MBD or retardation can serve a similar purpose.

Regression to more immature behavior than expected is common. The behaviors most often seen are enuresis, rocking, baby talk, whining, silliness, clinging, temper tantrums, thumbsucking, and balking at assuming age-appropriate responsibilities such as dressing, making one's bed, and doing chores. Through regression, the child is protected from the embarrassment and rejection that he or she might encounter when trying to function at a higher level. Overcoercive parenting also leads to resistiveness in the child and regressive behavior. The overprotective mother may encourage this regression. Pointing out the negative consequences of these behaviors may help the child assume more control. Similarly, some children will engage in clowning behavior to gain a sense that they are initiating and controlling the ridicule and laughter that they fear. If this behavior or any other is not rewarded by attention, it will decrease. Children who overreact to the laughter or bullying taunts of other children or to

disappointments can be rewarded for greater self-control. It may also help them to rehearse anticipated situations through role playing. Very bright children may also have difficulty making friends and need to have acquaintances of similar ability. However, these children also need to understand and accept less gifted children.

Impaired children may develop feelings that their disability is total rather than partial. They must repeatedly be told that their deficits are in certain areas only and that everyone has areas of strength and weakness. Gardner reports that low self-esteem is almost universal in children with brain dysfunction. Neurotic symptoms that are formed to support feelings of adequacy only result in a further lowering of self-esteem. For example, the unpopular boy who lies to his peers and describes interesting and unusual exploits may enjoy more ego-enhancing attention at first; but as soon as his peers learn of his lies (and they inevitably do), he suffers more rejection than when he was unpopular but truthful.

Children base their self-appraisal primarily on the views of the people around them, and children need the good opinion of others. They develop their own criteria for self-appraisal gradually. They need to be helped to accept opinions that are accurate and to reject those that are not. Feelings of competence must ultimately be based on some realistic attribute or skill. Compliments that the children know are inaccurate will further lower their self-esteem. Marginal self-esteem is often reflected by an absence of assertiveness. Adults must encourage children to be assertive and speak up when they are taken advantage of.

Children with limitations may become especially aware of how different they are from their peers as they become adolescents. The handicapped child has even more difficulty dealing with the normal problems of adolescence. Normal adolescents struggle for independence from parents and the achievement of a sense of identity—including a sexual identity. But adolescents with brain dysfunction or retardation may be much slower to achieve autonomy or incapable of being totally independent of their parents. They, therefore, may not risk rebellion and be much more passive and dependent in their relationships with their parents or other adults. They may rely more on adults than on peers, who tend to reject them. Independent functioning however, remains the goal. Skills that others seem to learn automatically, such as riding the train or simple social amenities, may need to be broken down into their component parts and patiently taught.

Decisions may have to be made as to whether the exceptional adolescent should pursue relationships with others who are normal—relationships that are often frustrating—or whether he or she would find it more satisfying to cultivate children who have similar problems. This decision calls for the evaluation of many factors, including the adolescents' adaptive capacity, the general attitudes of the others involved, and the environment.

A job experience may be much more rewarding than school if it is chosen in an area which capitalizes on the adolescent's strengths and requires minimal functioning in areas of weakness. Aptitude testing may be helpful in making an appropriate choice of training and employment.

Nurses' Responses to the Exceptional Child

Nurses' responses to the exceptional child and family will be colored by their own social and familial backgrounds. They may share some of the responses of parents to their children. In responding to the parents of a defective child, their own mourning experiences may help them to empathize with parents. Nurses have the same potential as anyone else for getting "stuck" in one phase of the mourning process. Unlike most parents, however, they have the option of avoiding the children and their problems altogether. Children whose physical appearance is distorted or who have unappealing habits may elicit insurmountable revulsion. Slow or hyperactive children may create intolerable frustration and impatience in some nurses. Unconscious guilt over feelings of revulsion, anger, or depression may lead the nurse to criticize these reactions in parents or other professionals. Nurses, of course, may also share social attitudes of hopelessness or insensitivity. Scipien states that before nurses deny having prejudices and negative feelings about the deviant child, they should ask such questions as:

1 What is my first reaction when I am told that a child is mentally retarded?
2 Do I tend to agree with the professional or family member who advises the mother to institutionalize her newborn mongoloid child before she becomes too emotionally involved?
3 What are my feelings about caring for a 6-year-old who is not toilet trained?
4 Can I warmly touch or embrace a child with grotesque physical features?
5 Do I believe that retarded people can really be helped?[3]

This personal assessment must be followed by experiences in working with retarded children—experiences that develop the ability to react to each child in terms of individual needs and potential rather than in terms of physical features or level of functioning.

A similar process is required of the nurse who is to work with children with MBD or epilepsy. In response to the disorderly, unmanageable behavior of a child with MBD, the nurse may experience frustration, anger, or helplessness when efforts to intervene fail or proceed at an extremely slow rate. Nurses may also experience similar feelings about the parents if they feel the parents are responsible for the child's behavior or that they should be able to effect better control. A nurse's own initial efforts to intervene may be met with screaming or retreating and crying. Nurses should use their responses as a valuable part of the assessment process. This will help them to empathize with parents or teachers. Otherwise, the nurse may enter a degenerating spiral of mutual rejection and hostility.

Nurses may also have a variety of responses to very bright children. They may favor them in a way that creates jealousy in the children's peers or may overestimate their capacity for independence or performance. Nurses may be jealous or resentful of their potential. Of course, the nurse may respond with delight or a sense of challenge to aspects of any exceptional child.

Assessment

The nursing assessment involves collection of the data base. The development of assessment criteria assists the nurse in identifying areas of strength and weakness for the exceptional child and the family. The nurse's assessment is based on a thorough knowledge of the normal milestones and sequences of growth and development (see Chap. 5). The following criteria will facilitate the assessment process as the nurse serially observes the child and family:

1 Identify parental concerns and the child's problems.
2 Determine whether the parents can care for the child at home or should plan for placement in an institution
3 Determine parental feelings about interpreting their child's problems to others
4 Evaluate parents' perceptions about the child's potential for independent living and appropriate social and sexual relationships
5 Determine parents' attitudes and beliefs about the medication regimen
6 Assess family patterns of interaction
7 Assess parent decision-making process
8 Identify how responsibility for care is determined and how delegation of responsibility is received
9 Assess the family's emphasis on educational and vocational achievement for their exceptional child
10 Identify the family's strengths, weaknesses, and potential areas for growth
11 Assess the child's self-esteem
12 Identify the child's response to environment settings: home, school, play

13 Identify problem behaviors

Nursing Diagnosis

Most often the care of an exceptional child involves a team of professionals in health and educational settings. The nurse, especially in a clinic setting, may be the most appropriate person to work directly with the family to coordinate and interperet the treatment plan, acting as a liaison between the many services utilized by the family. The nurse may become a person with whom the family feels able to share fears, feelings, and fantasies. Consequently, the nurse will be able to amass a considerable data base regarding the child's and family's functioning. In many instances, the nurse may become the family's advocate in the health-care system.

Nursing diagnosis involves identifying the client's and family's total problems as well as assets. These problems and assets are most effectively defined by describing them behaviorally. Goals can then be formulated and an effective plan of intervention can follow. Some of the nursing diagnoses for exceptional children are:

1 Decreased self-esteem and self-confidence reflecting parental shame and guilt
2 Developmental lag relating to organic/perceptual impairment
3 Denial of seizure potential
4 Family isolation from social and community supports
5 Chronic grieving process impairing parental participation in effective intellectual and sensory nurturance of the child
6 Parental ambivalence regarding the need to institutionalize the adult offspring who needs more care than the parents are physically able to provide
7 Unrealistic parental expectations of the exceptional child: a Motor, b Cognitive, c Social

8 Family experience of stress that may affect the accuracy of their perceptions of the child

Planning and Intervention
Primary and Secondary Prevention

Nursing intervention begins with prevention and case finding. The quality of the genetic pool determines the health of offspring. Parents need to be aware of the expected outcomes of their particular inheritance patterns. Programs promoting physical well-being contribute to health among children. Effective parenting will promote maximum attainment of a child's potential. The nurse is involved as resource person and educator for families in all three areas (see Chaps. 33 and 37) while working in antepartum and postpartum centers, well-child clinics, pediatricians' offices, schools, home settings, and hospitals. Additionally, the nurse in these settings can contribute to the early identification of deviation so that remediation can be instituted and maladaptive coping patterns can be minimized.

Tertiary Prevention

A key goal for nursing intervention is the *enhancement of parental effectiveness.*[12] This may be accomplished by helping parents learn how to assess the child's ability and plan for promoting optimal development. For example, parents need to understand that although their child does not have a specific major skill such as speaking words, small, preliminary skills such as babbling and cooing or turning of the head toward others who are speaking may be present. These preliminary skills are components of the major one. Parents who understand this may respond and reward the preliminary behavior and physically guide and model the next behavior in the hierarchy, thus promoting its development.

Nurses may also teach the need for early environmental stimulation (see Chap. 33). This may involve offering the child safe, appropriate objects of varying color, size, texture, and noise-making potential. It may involve offering different tastes and opportunities for cuddling, rocking, and swinging. It may involve modifying the environment to reenforce the child's strengths and skills; for example, providing the child who is beginning to walk with a space where it is safe to fall. This approach attempts to capitalize on a child's readiness to learn new tasks and skills.

Providing for the needs of an exceptional child is a demanding task for most parents and often beyond what can be expected of one parent alone. Communicating observations and recommendations to both parents can show them how both can be involved in the child's care in a cooperative way.

Parents need information that they will find both useful and interesting. For example, books have been written specifically to give parents and lay people the facts about retardation and MBD and to outline techniques of intervention and behavior modification. There are also general books about parenting that are written in a lively, easily understood style.

Parents also need to talk about the future and to be encouraged in reasonable hopes. Nurses can arrange for opportunitites to listen and validate plans and hopes that seem reasonable. Many exceptional children will achieve full independence and lead satisfying, productive lives. In almost all situations, problem behaviors can be reduced and desired new behaviors developed.

Parents in similar situations have much to offer one another in terms of sympathetic support and information or even the sharing of child supervision and care. Group discussions can be part of a clinic's or school's services. Clinic-sponsored social functions can enable parents to establish supportive relationships which they may pursue independently thereafter. Nurses act as resource people, referring parents to those agencies that exist within the family's geographic area. Parent groups have often been the initiators of new schools or services for their children. Parents can sometimes appropriately channel the anger they feel about their child's disability onto a negligent political or social group and effect political change to enhance some aspect of their situation.

Parents may also be less paralyzed and depressed by new episodes of stress if they have anticipatory guidance regarding when to expect problems and how to deal with them. For example, a young girl may begin to have more seizures when she begins to menstruate. Parents can be warned of this and assured that an adjustment of medication may again alleviate the seizures.

An additional acute problem for parents is what to tell people, especially the affected child. Gardner advocates telling the MBD child the truth in simple, age-appropriate terms, so that the child will not imagine his or her disability to be worse than it really is. The child who fears the worst may develop anxiety-alleviating symptoms such as severe withdrawal or preoccupation with activities which seem to offer magical control of fears. Vagueness also leads children to distrust their parents, and this may have serious consequences. These observations apply to the epileptic child as well. Openness with siblings is advocated for the same reasons.

It is important for the nurse to work within the family strategy, strengthening it and not imposing recommendations foreign to their orientation or methods of problem solving. For example, a poor family may not be able to buy special toys but may be helped to adapt household objects that they already have.

A second key goal of nursing intervention is *enhancement of the child's self-esteem.*[12] The exceptional child's growth and development, like that of the normal child, will be influenced by an adequate self-concept. A child with low self-esteem may be fearful of trying new tasks or may overcompensate and attempt tasks beyond his or her present abilities; thus the child fails to learn the intermediate steps that would lead to success. Children's self-esteem will be enhanced by consistent expectations in accord with their capacities—expectations by which they are appropriately challenged. It is also helpful to such children to facilitate positive experiences with peers, school, and community. Like any child,

exceptional children need the praise and positive reeinforcement of parents and teachers in order to accept themselves as important, understood, and loved human beings. Social experiences need to be guided to ensure reasonable acceptance and to protect these children against unmanageable rejection and misunderstanding.

As the child reaches functional latency level, appropriate friends are needed as well as participation in the household division of labor, achievement in school, and beginning psychological separation from the family. During the functional adolescent stage, children and parents may need assistance in acknowledging and appropriately expressing their sexuality. Adolescent independence and extrafamilial social relationships become important issues relating to self-esteem. Opportunities for such experiences should be sought within the ability level of each child. Community clubs, halfway houses, and group homes may provide the gradual experience needed by these children.

A third key goal is to provide *opportunities for learning.*[12] The learning of new skills tends to enhance self-esteem, and developmental age-appropriate play is an important preliminary to learning. Every child needs objects, experiences, and playmates. Barnard has identified major points to be considered in planning opportunities for learning by the retarded child, but it is equally important to consider the parents' motivation and readiness to carry out such a teaching plan. An unsophisticated woman who is already overwhelmed by the demands of her children will not be able to carry out a complex behavior-modification program at home. But she may be able to imitate a professional person who demonstrates age-appropriate play with her child.

If, for example, a 7-year-old child is severely retarded, activity of the sort that is ordinarily appropriate for an infant—such as cuddling and visual and tactile stimulation—may be needed. On the other hand, a precocious 2-year-old may thrive in a preschool class with the 3- and 4-year-olds. Or a bright 10-year-old who requires medical hospitalization might be more comfortable with the youngsters on an adolescent unit than those on a children's unit.

The physical, physiological, and neurological factors that indicate the child's readiness to learn a task must be considered. For example, a child is not ready for toilet training until the physical strength to stand and walk alone and the ability to control sphincters have been developed.

When the nurse and parents decide it is appropriate and desirable to teach the child a specific skill, the first step is to analyze the small-component aspects of the total skill. For example, toilet training involves taking pants down, sitting quietly on the toilet, releasing the urine and feces into the toilet, wiping with toilet paper, pulling pants up, and washing hands. A child may have some of these component skills but not others. The first components are prerequisites for later ones and must be taught first.

On the basis of the initial assessment, realistic goals should be set. A very involved, intelligent mother who has already toilet-trained her child and guided the child to age-appropriate play may be taught to systematically reward her child in an increasingly complex hierarchy of dressing skills. It must be remembered that gross motor skills, such as throwing a ball, physically and neurologically precede fine motor skills such as buttoning.

The nurse may identify the component steps of a learning task and work to achieve small goals that lead to larger goals. In the language of behavior modification, this is called *shaping*. For example, in teaching a child to eat with a spoon unassisted, the nurse would first reward attending to the spoon and food, later grasping the spoon, and then scooping and filling the spoon, and so on. The nurse must be careful, when teaching a higher-level skill, to avoid inadvertently rewarding less developed, inconsistent behavior such as finger feeding. This mistake would only confuse the child and slow progress.

Another method of teaching is *fading*. In this method the teacher physically guides the child through the motions of the new skill and gradually reduces the strength of guidance as the child performs the task independently. In feeding, for example, the teacher would hold the child's hand around the spoon and guide the hand to scoop the food and deliver it to the mouth. As the teacher feels the child proceeding in the right direction, the pressure of the guidance is reduced. Learning must always progress from simple to complex tasks. A system of recording progress is useful to provide accurate assessment and to demonstrate to the mother that slow but steady progress is being made. Such a record may also serve to show when a method is not working and must be reevaluated or modified.

Attention must be secured and maintained in order to teach a child. When teaching self-feeding, this may be done by making a noise such as tapping the spoon, calling the child's name and giving a simple direction, or demonstrating that a desired reward is available when the task is complete. A child is not learning to dress independently if a teacher pulls on the clothes while the child gazes at toys across the room. Distractions may have to be removed, or the child's head may have to be guided to look in the desired direction. Expectations should be demonstrated to the child as clearly as possible, and verbal cues should be as simple and short as possible. A flow of chatter, even if it is intended to be encouraging, may be distracting and confusing. Verbal cues may be accompanied by others that are visual, auditory, or physical. Rewards must be tailored to each individual child, since an effective reward is something that the child likes and will work to get. Not all children will work for candy and most tire of only one reward, so it is most effective to have several available. Children need repeated practice of the skills they are in the process of learning. Also, parents need to be supported as they adapt to changes that are occurring in their child.

As with other exceptional children, early identification of giftedness is advocated in order to nurture special talents and avoid wastage and later difficulty. A child who is bored in the classroom may withdraw into fantasy or engage in disruptive behavior with other students. School may become a hated requirement rather than a stimulating channel for abilities. All children need stimulation, challenge, and education at their level of ability. Educators still debate whether this is better achieved by advancing these children early or providing "enriched" programs for them. A decision must be made for each child depending on individual needs and the resources available in the school and community. Whatever a child's exceptional characteristics may be, the developmental needs of the average child (see Chap. 5) must be used as a baseline.

The special physical needs of the child must also be considered. Retarded infants and young children often have a greater susceptibility to infection, and extra precautions may therefore be necessary to protect them. Retarded, MBD, and epileptic children are more prone to have accidents and therefore require greater supervision and more safety precautions. Seizures require the usual care and precautions, and these must be taught to all those who care for the child throughout the child's day. The nurse may have a specific task related to the need for medication in some children with MBD and most with epilepsy. Where medication is prescribed, all concerned—the child, parents, and in some cases teacher—need to know the drug's action, dosage, schedule, and possible side effects as well as the long-range plan of usage. Some children—especially adolescents—and their parents discontinue a regimen of medication as part of their denial of their problem.

The stimulant drugs have been demonstrated to be highly effective with MBD children. The most effective agents are the amphetamines and methylphenidate (Ritalin). Hyperactivity may actually increase when attempts are made to reduce it with sedatives such as the barbiturates. When stimulants do not successfully reduce hyperactivity, one of the tranquilizers usually will. Reducing the child's hyperactivity enhances receptivity to learning. These stimulants also have an alerting effect which helps concentration.

Parents have many concerns about using stimulant drugs on their MBD children. They need specific teaching to understand how the medication works. Some parents are reluctant to undertake a trial of medication because they fear addiction or that the child will suffer side effects. Current evidence indicates that the chances of addiction are minimal. The side effects of the stimulant drugs, especially anorexia and insomnia, usually do not persist if the medication dosage and schedule of administration are adjusted correctly.

Successful medical management of the epileptic child requires determination of the most appropriate drug or combination of drugs as well as the most appropriate dosages. To achieve this result, a systematic program for a trial of the various anticonvulsant drugs is necessary. Phenobarbital or Dilantin are the most common drugs of choice. Gas-liquid chromatography has become a valuable adjunct for determining the optimal dosage of the anticonvulsant drug. Seizures can be controlled or significantly reduced with anticonvulsant drugs in more than 80 percent of epileptics.

Another significant nursing role in regard to medication is that of coordinator in determining optimal dosage and schedule of administration. In this capacity, the nurse can provide the physician with specific data obtained from parents and teachers and from observing the child at home or in other familiar settings. As the child grows, medication needs may change; the nurse can help the family anticipate behavioral differences and plan with the physician for dosage changes.

Institutional Care

Such care of children involves special advantages and obstacles. Institutionalized children may have insufficient opportunities to develop self-esteem and independence. On the other hand, they may receive specialized services that no family or day school could possibly provide. Families facing the prospect of institutionalizing their child need special support and guidance in handling the extreme guilt and shame they often feel. The decision should not be rushed. The family needs time to consider whether this is really the best solution for the child and the family. They need to talk to people who can describe what the institution offers, and they ought to see it if possible. They may also be reassured by talking with other parents who have already mastered their ambivalence regarding institutionalization and who are satisfied with the decision they have made. In general, institutional care is recommended less frequently than care within the family and community. For example, a group home located in the family's own community may enable a child to have more frequent contact with his or her family than an institution would, provide access to more community facilities, and yet also afford the close supervision and 24-hour care that the family cannot provide at home. The more complete the facilities within the community are, the less likely it is that institutional care will be required.

Evaluation

Evaluation of the care of an exceptional child involves renewed comparisons of growth, development, and behavior against the original assessment and nursing diagnosis. It may involve a reassessment and change in the diagnosis or the problem list. The evaluation, like the plan, should be made in collaboration with the child, the parents, and other involved adults. Evaluation with most exceptional children will be a lifelong process; this should be a specific expectation and plans for it should be made.

References

1 R. Heber (ed.); "A Manual on Terminology and Classification in Mental Retardation," *American Journal of Mental Deficiency,* vol. 64, no, 2, p. 3, 1958, monograph supplement.

2 Waldo Nelson (ed.): *Textbook of Pediatrics,* Saunders, Philadelphia, 1969.

*3 Gladys Scipien et al.: *Comprehensive Pediatric Nursing,* McGraw-Hill, New York, 1975.

4 W. G. Lennox and M. A. Lennox: *Epilepsy and Related Disorders,* Little, Brown, Boston, 1960, 2 vols.

5 Steven Zlutnick et al.: "Modification of Seizure Disorders: The Interruption of Behavioral Chains," *Journal of Applied Behavioral Analysis,* Spring 1975, pp. 1–12.

6 James Magary and John Eichorn (eds.): *The Exceptional Child,* Holt, New York, 1960.

7 L. D. Lippman: *Attitudes toward the Handicapped,* Charles C Thomas, Springfield, Ill., 1972.

8 Frank Menolascino: *Psychiatric Approaches to Mental Retardation,* Basic Books, New York, 1970.

9 A. S. Solnit and Mary H. Stark: "Mourning and Birth of a Defective Child," *Psychoanalytic Study of the Child,* vol. 16, International Universities Press, New York, 1961.

10 S. Olshansky: "Chronic Sorrow: A Response to Having a Mentally Defective Child," *Social Casework,* vol. 43, pp. 191–194, 1962.

11 Richard A. Gardner: *MBD—The Family Book about Minimal Brain Dysfunction,* Jason Aronson, New York, 1973.

*12 Kathryn Barnard and Marcene Powell: *Teaching the Mentally Retarded Child,* Mosby, St. Louis, 1972.

*Recommended reference by a nurse author.

Chapter

39

The Nurse's Response to the Family System with a Dying Child

Karen Davis Frank

Learning Objectives

After studying this chapter, the student should be able to:

1 Identify sociocultural factors related to death and dying inherent in contemporary Western culture

2 Differentiate the normal phases of coping with the dying process

3 Identify how children and adults handle death in terms of their levels of growth and development and their concepts of body image

4 Construct relationships between concepts mentioned above and the responses of the dying child and his or her family

5 Identify his or her own feelings and behavior concerning death and dying

6 Construct a nursing-care plan for the dying child and his or her family which promotes the normal resolution of grief

Death always brings one suddenly face to face with life. Nothing, not even the birth of one's child, brings one so close to life as his death. . . . The impending death of one's child raises many questions in one's mind and heart and soul. It raises all the infinite questions, each answer ending in another question. What is the meaning of life? What are the relations between things: life and death? the individual and the family? the family and society? marriage and divorce? the individual and the state? medicine and research? science and politics and religion? man, men and God? All these questions came up in one way or another, and Johnny and I talked about them, in one way or another, as he was dying for fifteen months. He wasn't just dying, of course. He was living and dying and being reborn all at the same time each day. How we loved each day. "It's been another wonderful day, Mother!" he'd say, as I knelt to kiss him good night.[1]

Frances Gunther poignantly tells the reader in the above excerpt how she felt when her 17-year-old son was dying. Her response is in marked contrast to that of many grieving parents today, who have great difficulty working through their feelings. Her son's behavior is inspiring; he reveals how he found meaning in his life, in spite of the tragic limitations of his future. Their example illustrates an ideal response of a dying child and his family. The professional nurse can help each family, in their own way, strive toward this ideal as they struggle painfully through one of life's most difficult experiences, a child's dying and death.

People will speak easily one day of death and dying with their loved ones and with members of the helping professions. They will no longer consider public discussion of dying obscene as they begin to understand that like birth, death is a part of life. This discussion aims to provide nurses with a conceptual framework for understanding the needs of dying children and their families.

Sociocultural Context of Dying
Western Culture and Death

As the West became industrialized, the urban nuclear family replaced the rural extended family as the basic unit of society. The decline of religion and religious rituals converged with this development, leaving the modern family increasingly isolated at the time of bereavement. The relationships between members of such a small family have become necessarily more intense. The pain of losing a family member becomes correspondingly severe.

While the structure of the contemporary Western family changed, attitudes toward death also changed. Contemporary culture finally acknowledges that people of all ages are concerned with dying and death. The Victorian taboo against expressing one's feelings about so-called delicate subjects had been firmly established until recently. A survey of the lay and professional literature reveals an awakening interest in the feelings of dying patients and their families.

Western culture still tries very hard to keep the reality of death from children and adults alike. Families, especially highly educated ones, often do not allow their children to attend the funeral of a family member. Most hospitals refuse to extend visiting privileges to children. Many children are told by a well-meaning parent that their dead sister or brother has gone on a long journey or has gone to sleep, or some other fantastic explanation may be offered. Such explanations, while they are culturally acceptable, do not promote mental health. It can be quite costly and damaging to children's personalities to shut them out of their experience of sorrow. To deprive children of their sense of belonging at this very emotional moment is to shake their security.[2]

This exclusion of children from death and dying is a relatively recent phenomenon. Until the eighteenth century, children were always a part of the deathbed scene. Perhaps modern adults deny the significance of death to their children as a reflection of their own denial of death. Aries feels that the American preference for embalming is a clear indication of our refusal to accept the finality of death:

> During the wakes or farewell "visitations" which have been preserved, the visitors come without shame or repugnance. This is because in reality they are not visiting a dead person, as they traditionally have, but an almost living one who, thanks to embalming, is still present as if he were awaiting to greet you or to take you off on a walk.[3]

The Conflict between Curing and Caring

Influence of Technology on Caretaking

In recent years, with the introduction of life-support systems, dying has become more complex. "Death with dignity" is an idea whose time has come. Yet, it is a goal which often appears hopelessly out of reach. The helping professions, including nursing, are oriented to maintaining life, not terminating it. Bergman writes that for physicians the "ethos is to cure rather than care, and death, after all, represents failure."[4]

A dramatic ethical dilemma arises when a critically ill child is kept alive by an array of machines. An electroencephalogram taken at this time may indicate little or no brain activity. Painful experimental medications and treatments often precede this state of affairs. For parents to witness, passively, their child's terrible suffering and subsequent deterioration has to be the worst kind of torture. Death usually takes place at the hospital, among strangers.

To help their clients, nurses need to explore new alternatives and to examine their own feelings about life and death carefully. Perhaps children and their parents need to be offered more choices, such as whether or not to accept painful medications, treatments, and heroic measures. Remaining at home should be a legitimate alternative to recurrent hospitalization.

A Child's Death Is a High Social Loss

The death of a child is always tragic, representing a high social loss to the family, the community, and the nurse. Glaser and Strauss state that social loss is indicated by the "total of the valued social characteristics which the dying client embodies," such as "age, skin color, ethnicity, education, occupation, family status, social class, beauty, 'personality,' talent, and accomplishments."[5]

Age seems to be the most significant factor in determining social loss in Western culture, as a long, full life is highly valued. Children who are dying have their future stolen from them. They can no longer dream of whom they will marry, how many children they will have, or what careers they will pursue.[5]

A low-social-loss factor, such as brain damage, can obliterate the impact of a high-social-loss factor, such as youth. The death of a severely retarded 6-year-old child may be perceived as a low social loss, in spite of the child's age.

The quality of nursing care the client receives may be directly dependent upon how highly the client is valued by the community. An adolescent who is comatose because he or she was shot while robbing a gas station would perhaps be viewed as a low-social loss client. The quality of care received by such a client may be below par, as the nurses unconsciously devote more of their time to more highly valued clients.

High-social-loss clients are generally the recipients of extraordinary attentions, but not always. These same clients may be avoided when the staff needs to avoid the intense feelings aroused by the high-social loss situation. An 18-year-old student nurse with leukemia who has just been admitted to the hospital could certainly provoke such an avoidance pattern.

The concept of social loss can help nurses identify and resolve their feelings concerning their dying clients. The process of categorizing clients according to their social value—certainly not a constructive, professional way to evaluate the needs of clients—is not usually a conscious process. For nurses to consistently deliver high-quality care to dying children and their families, it is essential that they analyze how they perceive their clients in terms of social loss. Careful self-evaluation and validation of his or her own behavior with colleagues can help each nurse to provide the finest care for all clients, based on an objective assessment of client needs.

The Meaning of Death to Children

The literature concerning the way children perceive death and dying is controversial. Some authorities do not believe that children can comprehend the finality and irreversibility of death until they are at least 8 or 9 years old.[6]

Other writers have published dialogues with young children that demonstrate a concrete grasp of the finality of death. An 8-year-old girl tells us: "The thing that worries me most about being dead is that I wouldn't be here anymore. I would miss my mother and family. When someone dies, they aren't around anymore. . . . They get buried and they rot."[7]

Waechter asked sixty-four sick children to tell stories about selected pictures, and she discovered that children who were seriously ill discussed loneliness, separation, and death more often. The following story was told by a 7-year-old boy with cystic fibrosis:

> The little boy had to stay in the hospital because the doctor wanted it. He got a shot in the back; a big needle. He was scared of shots, and didn't want it. And the doctor did it hard. His lungs are gone—he can't breathe. His lungs got worse and he didn't get well. He died and he was buried with a big shovel."[8]

Nagy studied 378 children between the ages of 3 and 10 and identified three distinct phases. To the child between 3 and 5 years of age, death was clearly reversible, not final. Between 5 and 9 years, the children comprehended the finality of death but had difficulty accepting that everyone would eventually die, including themselves. Children 9 years of age and older understood that they would die one day, like everyone else.[9]

Another view is offered by Anthony, who perceives children's reactions to death in terms of an age-specific crisis:

> . . . crises regarding death may occur during childhood in sensitive children living in a family in which free emotional expression is accepted and even encouraged. The first . . . based on a separation anxiety and fear of abandonment, occurs between four and six years of age . . . The second crisis, an existential crisis is at an age between nine and eleven years, is brought about by the realization of the irreversibility of death, in relation to both the self and loved ones.[10]

The nurse can observe the following behaviors in children, reflecting these crises. Children under 9 years personify death in an attempt to make an abstract concept concrete. Nagy, for example, discovered that to children death is perhaps a skeleton, a woodcutter, or a man in a white coat. These children understand that a dead person can neither move nor speak. They feel, however, that the deceased can hear people talking. Children of 10 and above begin to verbalize and fantasize about rebirth, reunion, and reincarnation.[9]

What does death and dying mean to children? It may be impossible to give a clear-cut answer to this question. The degree to and way in which a child is exposed to death determines the child's perception of death. Young children who experience death and starvation as constant companions perceive quite easily that everyone's life is indeed finite. In highly industralized societies, the contemplation of death is removed from the everyday life of children; consequently, their perception of death is not as clear. Nurses must each draw their own conclusions in context and constantly reevaluate their findings.

How Do Children Respond to Death?

When the adults in a family are torn with grief, they are often too upset to observe and respond helpfully to the children participating in the painful drama. Children have feelings too and respond in their own way to their loss.

Following are some examples contributed by Grollman which illustrate some typical responses:

Denial "It is just a dream. Daddy will come back. He will! He will! . . ."

Bodily Distress "I have a tightness in my throat! . . ."

Hostile Reactions to the Deceased "How could Daddy do this to me? . . ."

Guilt "He got sick because I was naughty. I killed him."

Hostile Reactions to Others "It's the doctor's fault. He didn't treat him right. . . . It's God's fault. . . ."

Replacement "Uncle Ben, do you love me, really love me?"

Assumption of Mannerisms of the Deceased "Do I look like Daddy? . . ."

Idealization "How dare you say anything against Daddy? He was perfect. . . ."

Anxiety "I feel like Daddy when he died. I have a pain in my chest. . . ."

Panic "Who will take care of me now? Suppose something happens to Mommy? . . ."[2]

The child's actual behavior may not always appear to reflect the above conflicts. The child's open expression of feeling may elicit negative parental responses. For example, when a child asks to play with the toys that formerly belonged to the deceased brother or sister, for example, the parents may become distraught. They interpret their child's behavior as the worst kind of disloyalty.

A similar difficulty arises when the child laughs freely at a favorite television cartoon program. The parent wonders how the child can be so callous as to laugh easily while the adults negotiate their painful grief experience. Or the parents may misinterpret the laughing behavior in another way. They may feel the child has successfully worked through his feelings of grief: "Well, I'm so glad to see Tom laughing. It means he's taking things well."

Children, of course, are capable of feeling the great loss of a loved one one moment and yet becoming fully absorbed in something funny the next. Children do not expect, like adults, to stop loving, living, and enjoying for a prescribed mourning period. They do not feel that their behavior demonstrates disloyalty at all.

An adult usually has difficulty understanding how a child can truly mourn the loss of someone dear and yet still eat with a hearty appetite, sleep soundly each night, and attend school as usual. Superficially the parent may seem pleased with such a "fine" adjustment. But on a deeper level the parent may rage that a child can continue to function so adequately while the adult cannot.

Normal Phases in Coping with the Dying Process
Acute Death: No Opportunity for Anticipatory Grief Work

Learning to live with the loss of a child is hard enough. The task can be overwhelming when death comes with no warning. There are always regrets, things the parents wish they could have said or done, feelings they wish they could have shared had they the opportunity. Even when the parent-child relationship has been consistently rich and warm, the feeling remains that the relationship is somehow incomplete. When the parent-child relationship has been uneven, threaded with subliminal hostility and rejection, the guilt experienced by the newly bereaved parent can be terrifying, and professional help may be indicated.

When the cause of death is accidental and the parent feels there is a remote chance it could have been prevented, the self-imposed guilt can be crushing. The author worked with one mother who could not forgive herself for telling her 4-year-old daughter to play in the basement that morning. The little girl was fatally injured falling down the stairs to the play area.

Because the loss is unexpected, the parents'

normal grieving responses may telescope into a shorter time interval than usual. The intensity and sudden onset of strange physical and mental symptoms may frighten the bereaved parents. Patterson and Pomeroy describe how parents of babies who succumb to the sudden infant death syndrome (SIDS) fear they are losing their minds:

> Parents often experience strange bodily sensations, such as dizziness, pressure in the head, heartache, and stomach pain. These sensations are accompanied by a sad expression, sighing, insomnia, and restlessness. They may engage in excessive ritualistic activity such as repetitive sweeping, washing or folding clothes.
>
> The parents' mood may also fluctuate widely. They may have difficulty concentrating and frequently express hostile feeling towards their closest friends and relatives. In some instances mothers deny their infant's death. For example, they may continue to draw the baby's bath or prepare food for the child. The parents may dream about the dead child or be afraid to stay in the house alone. One mother sat in the yard for many days when no one else was at home. Parents with neither business nor family ties usually move soon after the child's death.[11]

This grieving process is also experienced by parents who have time in advance to deal with the fact that their child is dying. But then the process is spread out over a longer period of time.

Long-Term Death: Anticipatory Mourning

Parents who have just learned that their child has a fatal illness, unlike the parents of a child who has suddenly died, can learn to cope with and adapt to the loss over a period of time. Lindemann calls this *anticipatory grief*. Time gives the stricken parents a chance to accept the diagnosis intellectually first and then, later, emotionally. It is believed that grieving behavior following an expected death is a continuation of the coping behaviors demonstrated while the child was ill rather than an entirely new cluster of behaviors.[12]

Futterman and Hoffman describe this process as *anticipatory mourning*. They have defined anticipatory mourning as "a set of processes that are directly related to the awareness of the impending loss, to its emotional impact, and to the adaptive mechanisms whereby emotional attachment to the dying child is relinquished over time."

They develop five concepts to help the student better understand the process of anticipatory mourning: *acknowledgement, grieving, reconciliation, detachment,* and *memorialization*.[13] Parents may be involved in several of these processes simultaneously, or they may experience them serially, with overlapping.

> *Acknowledgment* is the process of gradually accepting the reality that the child will die soon.
>
> *Grieving* is the expression of feelings concerning the anticipated death.
>
> *Reconciliation* implies the ability to find meaning and worth in the child's and parents' lives, in spite of the guarded future
>
> *Detachment* indicates that the parents are learning to redirect their emotional energies away from the dying child and toward other relationships.
>
> *Memorialization* means that the parents have identified a well-defined concept of their child which will remain in their memory after his or her death. This concept is usually idealized.

Anticipatory grieving is usually a constructive process. In certain cases, however, this process rapidly becomes destructive if there is no appropriate nursing intervention. When a child suffers from an illness such as leukemia, for example, he or she may have many useful years during a series of remissions. If the parents begin their grieving too early, they may stop their child and themselves from living full lives. They may actually begin to withdraw from the parent-child relationship too early. A nurse's informed intervention can help the family live with meaning in spite of an uncertain future.

Phases of Coping with Death

Although each family deals with its tragic situation in its own characteristic way, there are enough similarities between family responses to permit their classification into distinct phases of adaptation. Kübler-Ross has identified these phases as *denial, anger, bargaining, depression,* and *acceptance.*[14]

Most children and their families do not follow a neat progression from one phase to the next. Elements of several phases may occur concurrently, or some phases may be skipped altogether. The following discussion develops a conceptual framework to help the nurse understand on a deeper level the dying experience as seen from the view of the child and the child's family. Each of these phases is illustrated with the help of case histories of children who were admitted to a concentrated care unit. Many examples come from the N family, whose 13-year-old son Keith was admitted in a deep coma due to Reye's syndrome.*

Denial

During their initial interview with the physician and the nurse, the N's learned that their son had only a fifty-fifty chance of recovering. Mrs. N needed the defense of denial several times to help her cope with her sorrow. She responded, "He's not going to die, is he? He can't! He's so intelligent!" Later in the evening both parents needed to use denial when faced with the knowledge of the possible deterioration of their son's condition. The physician explained that there was some clinical evidence of mild cerebral edema. Although a cousin present at the discussion recalled the reference to cerebral edema, the parents did not. Similarly, after Keith had received an exchange transfusion,

---

*Reyes syndrome is a severe viral illness which produces liver dysfunction and subsequent cerebral edema. This illness often follows a mild infection such as pharyngitis.

the term "critical" was used to describe his condition. With surprise in her voice, Mrs. N responded, "Critical? I didn't know he was critical!"

After the first exchange transfusion was completed and Keith's condition seemed stable, Mrs. N made plans to return home for the evening, "to get the children to bed and get them ready for school tomorrow." Mrs. N did need to get home, but not for the reason she claimed, since a cousin was already with the other children to care for them that night. Mrs. N needed to get home so she could focus on something besides Keith's illness, escape the intolerable situation, and thus, in effect, deny it temporarily. Mr. N actually avoided visiting the client's room, although he was extremely concerned about his son. Like Mrs. N, he seemed relieved to be told that it would be a good idea for him to return home for a while, as he had a severe upper respiratory infection which Keith could contract.

Kübler-Ross feels that denial is usually a temporary defense that enables the individual to mobilize his or her emotional resources.[14] This seemed true of the N's, since they returned early the next morning and kept their vigil until late that night.

The dying child may also use denial. Kübler-Ross states that "maintained denial does not always bring increased distress if it holds out until the end."[14] Sharon, a mildly retarded 9-year-old who came to the unit each time she had an exacerbation in the course of her illness, never used the word "leukemia." Although she had frequent bone-marrow aspirations and alopecia due to radiotherapy, she insisted to the end that she was hospitalized for a virus. Her mother encouraged this use of denial, for she had told Sharon, over the preceding years, that "most children get leukemia sometimes, just like they get colds." Sharon had no mirror, and so she was unaware that she had lost her hair. She never requested a mirror. Her mother further stated, "I'm an actress, and I've been active in many community and professional theater productions so pretending is not difficult for me. The public health nurse brought me a book to read about another family in our situation, but I told her I'm not interested in reading anything so depressing as that. It's too morbid."

Sharon was happiest playing board games with her interested mother and staff members and never indicated to anybody a desire to deal with her situation on a deeper level. Denial was an effective defense mechanism for this family.

Anger

When denial no longer works for the family, anger and rage usually follow close behind. When Mrs. N could finally accept the fact that it was indeed her son who was in a coma, perhaps an irreversible one, she slammed her fist into her hand as her face tightened with pain, exclaiming "Damn it!" Later she added, "Keith was always such a good son, always helping everyone, so kind." The implicit message is anger that this illness has struck her son instead of someone less worthy. Mr. N never demonstrated anger externally but seemed to internalize it instead. He had colitis long before Keith became ill. During this crisis he had many attacks of acute abdominal pain and diarrhea, all the while thanking everyone for everything they had done so far.

Richard, a 12-year-old hospitalized for systemic lupus erythematosus, and his mother manifested another form of angry behavior. They constantly used the call bell to request nursing assistance and complain. Richard had been transferred to the concentrated care unit after being treated in another hospital. He felt the nurses in the other hospital let him participate in his care, but that at this hospital he was excluded. He became enraged, for example, when a nurse refused to inform him of his temperature.

Mrs. T was beginning to feel helpless in the face of her child's poor prognosis and his constant demands. The anger began to spill over to the rest of the family too. Mr. T, displacing his own anger, claimed that his son's problems were his wife's fault. He began to demand that his wife maintain a 24-hour vigil each day. He "forbade" her to run the bingo games at their community church, as she had done once a week for 10 years. This was Mrs. T's only activity outside her family. The inability of Richard's family to control the course of his illness made them angry; they expressed this anger by trying to control others in their environment more closely.

Bargaining

Kübler-Ross has defined bargaining as one of the less well known stages of dealing with death. Clients at this stage feel that they may escape death if only they demonstrate good behavior.[14] One mother promised God that if her son recovered from his life-threatening crisis, she would dress him in white always, as proof of his purity and faith. Mr. N remarked, almost to himself, "If Keith makes it out of this, I'll never ask for anything again, ever. We asked for help before when there was sickness, but that was nothing. We'll never expect anything more after this."

Depression

Kübler-Ross speaks about two types of depression. The first is *reactive depression,* which develops in response to changes in body image, loss of sexual identity, financial loss, or inability to function as breadwinner or caretaker. The second type is *preparatory depression,* which develops as a way of dealing with the expected loss of all love objects.[14]

To help a person experiencing reactive depression, the nurse can provide opportunities to reinforce the client's self-esteem and help the client to maintain his or her dignity and identity. Concrete steps to resolve real social and financial problems will also help lift the depression.

When a client is experiencing preparatory depression, however, the needs are quite different. People need to be able to share the sorrow they are feeling. If the nurse is comfortable with silence, nonverbal sharing may be the best kind to offer. It is difficult for the living to accept this phase of sorrow and beginning detachment. Very often staff and family members unwittingly obstruct the client at this point by trying to create an optimistic atmosphere.[14]

Robert was a cachectic 9-year-old boy admitted to the pediatric service for a jejunal biopsy to confirm clinical evidence of a malignancy. Although the parents describe his premorbid personality as outgoing and interested, Robert at this point was detaching himself from his environment. He lay in bed in the fetal position with his eyes open, yet not responding to anyone verbally. His only activity was to visit the lavatory. His parents were able to accept this behavior, explaining to the staff that "He's exhausted, he's been through a lot and just wants to rest." The maternal grandparents, however, had great difficulty accepting the terror of the situation and at one point rushed in desperately to tell Robert, "When you come home next week, we're getting you that 10-speed bike you've always wanted." Robert did not answer.

Mr. N was overtly depressed as he maintained the vigil for his son Keith. He stayed in the same chair in the waiting room for most of the evening, hardly lifting his head when he finally spoke in a barely audible voice. He felt he was unable to eat and did not wish to lie down. He continued to utilize denial concurrently, as he would visit his comatose son's room only when strongly encouraged to do so by the physician.

Acceptance

Kübler-Ross feels strongly that most patients can reach this phase if they have had an opportunity to work through the earlier phases of denial, anger, and depression successfully. It is at this stage that interest in the outside world is severely diminished. The number of visits is reduced, less verbal communication takes place, television becomes irrelevant, and so forth.[14]

The quiet presence of the nurse at this time can indicate to the client that he or she is not alone. Noise and activity are unnecessary to communicate that the nurse indeed cares. It is crucial for the nurse to help the child's family to understand that the patient's withdrawal from worldly concerns at this time does not indicate rejection of them but rather an acceptance which reflects maturity.

Factors Which Influence Family Dynamics
Premature Grieving

The painful process of gradual emotional detachment from the dying child is necessary for the future mental health of the survivors.[13] If it is completed too soon, however, the effects can be disastrous. This process needs to be distinguished from anticipatory mourning, which is a healthy way of preparing for a future loss.

Carried to its extreme, premature grieving may be manifested as a growing reluctance to visit the sick child, culminating perhaps in abandonment altogether. Susan, a 2-year-old girl admitted to the pediatric service because she bruised easily, was visited almost daily by her mother while her diagnosis was being determined. Once the illness was diagnosed as thrombocytopenia and Susan's mother was told that the child might hemorrhage to death at any time because her platelet count was so low, the mother's visits slowed to a trickle. A splenectomy was done in a final attempt to keep the platelet count up to levels compatible with life. Susan had no visits prior to her surgery and few afterwards.

Premature grieving can also be manifested as total absorption in the child's physical condition, to the exclusion of all other concerns. The astute nurse can try to help such a family regain its perspective. Many illnesses permit the client years of enjoyable and useful life before he or she ultimately succumbs. The timetable is often a variable one, for no professional can accurately predict how a particular child will respond to medications and treatments.

It is the nurse's task to help each family find their own way to continued meaning and joy in their own lives and the life of their child. As the family is assisted by the nurse to learn to ventilate and accept their positive and negative feelings concerning the traumatic situation, they will begin to find some peace. They should then be able to give up their premature grieving and learn to live again.

Marital Discord

The couple struggling to adapt to the news that their child has a fatal illness often discover that their marital relationship is under severe strain.

The very young couple is surprised to find little comfort from others their age. Their close friends, couples they socialize with regularly, probably feel threatened by the thought that tragedy can strike their children too. The parents of the dying child may find their peers withdrawing from them in an attempt to deny the vulnerability of their own children. It is helpful when the anguished parents can meet with others whose children are seriously ill. They can usually discover the support they need through identification with this new group.

The author's observations seem to support the principle that stress intensifies relationships in their already established directions: good marriages improve while poor ones crumble. Each family member seeks to meet his or her own needs while trying to meet the needs of other family members in a complementary way.

Some individuals, overwhelmed by the magnitude of their own needs, have little ego strength remaining to meet the needs of their spouses or their other children. The denial, anger, and depression identified as phases of coping with the dying process may not be expressed directly but projected or displaced instead. This situation creates further strain.

One grief-stricken mother was so fully engrossed in the nursing needs of her child at the hospital that she was totally unresponsive to her husband's needs. He felt that he had failed in what he thought was his role, to protect his family from harm. He retaliated, compensating for his feelings of helplessness by barking orders to everyone whenever he came to visit his child.

The wife may displace anger. Instead of raging at the gods she feels have deserted her, she may rage at her husband because the bills are accumulating mercilessly. The husband, in turn, may feel helpless and therefore depressed that his child is dying. He may manifest this depression by being unable to function at home and assume his rightful share of the household tasks.

These are the internal strains which begin to weaken the marital relationship. If there is no nursing intervention to promote direct expression of feelings and resolution of conflicts, the family members may no longer be able to provide each other with love and support when they need them most.

The external strains upon the couple stem from Western culture's unwritten expectations of behavior when a family member is dying. According to Gourevitch, the parents are "forbidden to lose hope, to amuse themselves, or to leave the child at all."[15] These standards are unrealistic and not compatible with mental health. It comes as no surprise in light of both the internal and external strains upon each marriage that, for many couples, separation or divorce may follow their child's death.[16]

The thoughtful nurse tries to minimize the marital stress which can arise by trying to keep the channels of communication open. When parents are given an opportunity to share their feelings with other couples in the same predicament, they often discover that their problems are not so unusual and that they can be solved.

Sibling Responses

The other children in the family sense the tension in the home. The parents may get angry at them more often, may ignore their needs more than usual, and may leave them in the care of others for long periods while they visit the sick child at the hospital. This negative change in parental behavior may be difficult for the other children to accept, as it makes them feel abandoned.

The child between 1 and 3 years of age, for example, may fear that each separation may be a permanent one. For children this age, the concept of time is poorly understood. Each moment they are separated from their parents can seem like an eternity, since terms like "tonight" or "tomorrow" have little meaning for them yet. Only a visual experience, such as actually seeing mother or father, is real to the toddler. When children this age cannot see a parent, they may fear they have lost that parent forever. Only repeated separations and reunions gradually alter the young child's perception of relationships.

Each child reacts to the altered family dynamics in a manner reflecting the child's own personality strengths and weaknesses. Children who have successfully mastered the developmental tasks for their age may continue to function adequately in spite of the family stress. Children with preexisting emotional difficulties, however, may find their problems to be increasingly insoluble. For the child whose thinking is in the prelogical phase, such as the preschooler, comprehending the impending death of a beloved sibling becomes a most difficult task. After repeated explanations, the puzzled preschooler may still ask, "Will Johnny be able to play with me when he leaves the hospital?" If the parent and nurse continue to offer simple, concrete, repeated explanations, the youngster will eventually be able to incorporate the reality of the expected loss and begin to deal with feelings about the loss.

Regardless of his or her age and maturity, each sibling at home will probably experience the following uncomfortable feelings, as described by Gourevitch: (1) *guilt* stemming from death wishes toward the sick brother or sister, (2) *fear* of also becoming ill, (3) *jealousy* at the exclusive attention paid to the patient, and (4) *rage* at the leniency with which he or she (the sick child) is treated at home during remissions.[15]

The following passage illustrates the dialogue which took place between Mr. and Mrs. N and a nurse when the parents began to learn how they could help their other children resolve their conflicts about Keith's condition. Keith's parents were initially concerned only with who would put the other children to bed and get them ready for school the next day.

At the nurse's suggestion, they began to consider what they would tell the children about Keith's illness. "What should I do? Should I tell him he's going to die?" The nurse suggested that they share their distress and fears with the children. The parents needed to be certain that the children knew their brother was very sick, and that although people at the hospital were doing everything possible to help him, no one knew yet whether he would recover. The parents planned to be able to communicate this in a realistic yet hopeful way.

"But Susan is too young to understand dying. She's only 5 years old," said Mrs. N. Then her husband reminded her, "Five seems young, but Susan has been asking a lot of questions lately. She's been obsessed with death." Then Mrs. N supported her husband, "That's right! Only yesterday, before Keith was even sick, she asked how long our dog would live."

The N's soon identified another problem. Susan had been glad when her brother had left for the hospital "because he always picks on me," she said. They were soon aware that Susan could easily blame herself for Keith's illness and possible death, since she was at the age when children indulge in magical thinking. Susan would probably conclude that her negative wishes had had a direct magical effect upon Keith's health. The distinction between fantasy and reality is still blurred for the 5-year-old.

The physically healthy siblings may express their feelings indirectly in terms of psychosomatic problems, difficulties in school, or interpersonal problems with chums. The sensitive nurse tries to intervene to help the parents listen more perceptively to their children, so that they can better understand the experience from the child's point of view.

A special problem arises for the sole surviving child in a family. In such a situation, the parents may be more reluctant than usual to expose the child to the ordinary risks of childhood. They may be afraid that this beloved child could also be taken from them, as the first one was. The nurse can help the parents become aware of their feelings and of the ways in which these feelings have affected their behavior. As their insight into themselves grows, the parents will become progressively more ready to change their attitudes toward their child in a positive direction.

Jane, an 8-year-old girl admitted to the pediatric service for vague stomach pains, was on the verge of hysteria despite the absence of painful treatments. The reason for the hysteria became clear as Jane's mother explained that she had lost a child 4 years before Jane was born. The child had a congenital heart defect and died in the hospital. The family talked openly about the dead child and still had her photographs prominently displayed. Relatives and friends constantly remarked on the strong resemblance between the two girls. "Jane could have been her twin," they would say.

Nursing intervention in this case was directed toward helping the parents see that Jane feared she would die in the hospital, as her deceased sister had done. After Jane's mother helped Jane to clarify her feelings about hospitalization and explained the differences between her own health situation and that of her deceased sister, Jane improved markedly.

The affected siblings need above all to know that their feelings are quite normal. The children need reassurance that they are still worthy people, even though they have thoughts and feelings they fear are quite unacceptable to others.

The Right to Know

The question is not, "Should we tell . . .?" but rather, "How do I share this with my client?"[14] Ideally the child's primary nurse should be present when the physician shares for the first time the nature of the child's diagnosis with the child and the family. In this way the nurse can more accurately assess the family's strengths and weaknesses under stress and help validate reality for the family later. Parents often have a selective memory under stress, and the nurse can later clarify misunderstandings.

It is most important to maintain hope for the family. Everyone needs to feel that all available treatments and medications will be tried and that the client will be carefully followed. In most cases it is destructive to tell children how long they will live. In any event, this is really an unknown quantity. Diseases affect each person differently, as do medications and treatments.[14]

Two excerpts from dialogues with children suffering from leukemia illustrate clearly that children need to participate in learning about their illness as well as understanding and planning their care:

> All of a sudden I got my room redecorated and all new clothes for school. . . . When we came back from the doctor's office, things were all different at home. I started getting lots of things I never could have before. I never could have a big machine gun that shoots BB's, but the next day my father comes home and he has this gun for me. . . . Relatives who never used to visit started coming around and bringing me all kinds of things. . . . Sometimes when I walked into the room, my mother and father would stop talking and look at me.

> I knew that something was up after the first few visits to the doctor. My parents talked it over and decided not to say anything to me until they were sure, and when they found out for sure, my mother told me. I know that there is no cure for leukemia, but I feel better knowing what I have.

This child later explained, "I still have a lot to worry about, but I was even more worried before because I was thinking a mile a minute about what I had."[17]

The nurse and physician who have worked through their own feelings about death and dying will be the most helpful to the families in crisis. They would be most objective while assessing each family's needs at this sensitive time and be able to respond to them therapeutically.

Role Relationships

Roles within the family may become more fixed as the child's illness increasingly limits the possibilities for change. Older children may have to assume parent surrogate roles temporarily and to defer their own developmental needs. The parents may feel themselves to be failures in their roles of caretaker and provider. At the same time, as the child's illness continues to demand more time and money, the family's circle of interests may narrow to include fewer roles outside the family constellation.

If everyone in the family assumes mutual nurturing roles, then every family member can have his or her needs met. It often happens instead that one person, usually the wife and mother in our culture, must assume the nurturing role for the entire family. This can be a heavy burden. The nurse can provide some relief by teaching family members to help each other and helping the mother to learn that it is OK to accept help from others and delegate responsibility.

Within the hospital, the family has to adapt to a cluster of new role relationships. The sick child is now told by the nurse instead of a parent when to eat and when to sleep. The parent, in turn, discovers that the power relationships have changed. The nurse tells the mother and father when they may visit, what procedure they may assist with, and what information they may have. Some families have great difficulties adapting to any change. These families may chafe under the role upheavals caused by the child's hospitalization.

Nurses' Response to Client and Family Behavior

Nurses' responses to dying children and their families are colored by their unique socioeconomic and cultural backgrounds. As nurses become progressively more capable of understanding their own feelings and consequent behavior, they become increasingly professional in their relationships with clients. As Vernick discovered in his extensive work with leukemic children, youngsters wish to deal with their feelings. Nurses need to be certain that they are as receptive to the children as they think they are.

Chronically ill and seriously ill children readily and realistically can and wish to speak about their fears, concerns, and ideas about death and dying. . . . It was rare to find a young patient who fled from the opportunity and chose to remain silent. . . . Even with their youngest patients, straightforward, simple communication techniques were used. They found no need to become involved in complicated symbolic and interpretive techniques. This latter approach . . . is used (often) because of the interviewer's anxiety about dealing directly with the grim subject matter. . . .[7]

Below are sample questions nurses need to ask themselves:

1 In which situations do I feel most comfortable? Least comfortable? Why?
2 What are my feelings about childhood? What do I feel are the capabilities of children at different ages?
3 What kinds of experiences have I had with death and dying as a child or young adult? Was I included in funeral ceremonies? At what age? How did my family deal with the death of my pets? Has someone close to me died? How do I feel about it?
4 How do I feel about pain and suffering? Euthanasia? Autopsies? Organ transplants?

After identifying problem areas, nurses need to resolve the conflicts which the painful feelings may provoke. It is important to remember that feelings can never be right or wrong; they just exist. Many nurses now feel that sharing one's own feelings with the clients and their families can be therapeutic when it is purposeful.

Nurses need to use all available resources to discover new ideas to use when resolving problems. It helps to talk feely with coworkers in purposeful conferences to obtain support. Role playing and role reversal with coworkers and clients help nurses discover how they feel and how others feel. Another helpful technique is recording dialogue and nonverbal communications between the nurse and the family. When the nurse studies these records away from the situation, he or she may discover discrepancies between the verbal and nonverbal messages which have been sent.

In addition to gaining insight into how nurses respond as individuals to the dying child and his or her family, it is helpful if we understand how nurses react as a group. Quint tells us that "it is common practice for the nursing staff to protect themselves from awkward situations by minimizing contact with patients who are not to be told their diagnosis." Such avoidance also enables nurses to avoid identifying and resolving their own feelings.[18]

Nurses as a group tend to value certain traits in people. These traits include being independent, lovable, active in ward activities, and making few emotional demands on the staff. Nurses tend to stay longer with such clients during each client-nurse interaction because people who have these favored traits build the nurse's self-esteem. They make the nurses feel they have indeed done a good job.[17]

Other traits in clients tend to provoke negative responses from nurses. Clients who whine or are angry, demanding, or tearful are first on the list to be rejected by the professionals. Nurses who are profoundly religious may feel threatened by clients and families who find no solace in their faith. Persistent denial of serious illness and its necessary treatment makes nurses feel constrained. Finally, nurses conclude that some clients exhibit exacerbations of their illness, such as a choking spell, only when there is an audience.[17]

Nurses must eventually learn that the patient's anger, directly or indirectly expressed toward her, is usually displaced anger. An immature nurse will feel that the dying client is directly criticizing him or her in complaining that the bath water is too cold. The more secure nurse will try to look beyond the facade of constant complaints and try to empathize with the client.

Tension and conflict will probably always be with us in the life-and-death situation of the hospital unit. Nurses must, therefore, constantly work at gaining insight into their underlying feelings. If nurses are aware of their own behavior—and how it is influenced by their underlying feelings and preconceived notions of valued client behavior—they can relate to clients in an open, meaningful way.

Nursing Diagnosis

Careful observation helps each nurse to assess the needs of children and families accurately. It is important to note which *behavior constellation* seems to dominate their responses. *Sociocultural factors* pertinent to the particular family need to be identified. The nurse needs to assess how children and their families perceive *body image* at this time. Finally, the nurse needs to evaluate the child's developmental level and the family's responses to growth and development (see Chap. 5).

Behavior Constellation
Aggression
Although children and parents will demonstrate a wide range of behaviors, some of these will emerge as the dominant ones. An angry child who feels aggressive and resistant may refuse painful treatments and tests when consulted. The angry parent may demand frequent room changes, new meal trays, and so forth.

Regression
Children who are regressing to a safe level may appear excessively dependent. They may withdraw and avoid eye contact or verbalizing. The parent who regresses or withdraws may try to have the nursing staff make parental decisions: "Please tell Johnny to be still for the biopsy. He'll listen to you better than he will to me." Or, "Should I consent to the laparotomy tomorrow? I'll do whatever you suggest."

Denial
Children who use denial may seem passive and unconcerned, as though the entire experience were happening to someone else and hence of no consequence. Parents may avoid discussing the

nature of their child's illness directly or may fail to note negative changes in his or her condition.

Acceptance

Children whose behavior is characterized by acceptance will be unhappy when faced with painful but necessary procedures; however, they will also be able to share positive experiences. Similarly, parents who have begun to accept the illness situation will deal with their feelings openly and be able to accept assistance from others. There is a realistic balance between independence and dependence which is appropriate for both children and family members when they approach true acceptance.

Sociocultural Factors

It is important for the nurse to assess and evaluate the child's sociocultural background and its influence upon the course of the illness. Following are some questions nurses need to ask themselves about each child:

1 Does the child feel at home at the hospital? Is the child's background substantially different from that of the primary nurse? Is there a language barrier? Is there a racial barrier? Is there an economic barrier? For example, if the child has grown up in the "culture of poverty," it may be difficult for him or her to share feelings with the nurse, a professional. The child may be distrustful of all official agencies, including the police and fire departments, courts, schools, and hospitals. The child's superstitious beliefs may lead to feelings that the illness is a punishment.

2 Is the child's typical day at home radically different from one at the hospital? At home, were there three structured meals each day or many snacks? Has there been a pattern of naps and a regular bedtime?

3 What is the child's personal experience with authority figures? Have authority figures been loving, trustworthy, reliable? Have parents leaned toward overprotectiveness? Are they

reluctant to encourage the child to take risks he or she is capable of taking? Has peer-group experience been fostered constructively? What self-care is within the child's capability. Is it appropriate to the child's age?

4 What have the child's personal experiences with health professionals been? Has the child had annual physical checkups? Has health care been mostly of an emergency nature? Has the child been hospitalized before? Has the child needed painful treatments before?

Body Image

The nurse needs to assess how children perceive their body image in relation to their illness. Are they concerned with function and mobility, attractiveness, sexuality, the need to look similar to others, or a combination of these?

Parental figures are most significant during the toddler period. Their approval or disapproval of the toddler's behavior and physical appearance is conveyed verbally and nonverbally. "Children who are accepted by their parents usually do not overvalue or undervalue their bodies." On the other hand, if mastery of the environment is not achieved, the child may experience such negative feelings about himself as helplessness, pain, inadequacy, and guilt.[18]

Adolescents are especially vulnerable to conflicts concerning their altered body image. They are worried about looking like their peers of the same sex and being sexually attractive to the opposite sex.

While toddlers need the acceptance of their parents for a healthy body image, adolescents yearn for the full acceptance of their peers. Adolescents, indeed, feel threatened by the changes in their appearance that serious illness and its treatment can bring. They feel abandoned as they sense their friends withdrawing from them. Friends do not wish to identify with someone whose altered body image reminds them that they too are vulnerable to death.

Nurses who accurately assess their clients'

needs in terms of behavior constellations, socio-cultural factors, developmental levels, and body image concepts will be well prepared to develop an informed plan of nursing care.

Goals

Four objectives summarized by Cain and Cain capture in a nutshell the goals for nurses who work with dying children and their families. The following behaviors can be expected from a family which has come to terms with its grief: "(1) full realization and acceptance of the loss, (2) resolution of anger and irrational guilt related to the loss, (3) significant withdrawal of emotional investment from the lost person, and (4) a redirection of interest and involvement with the bereaved's environment."[19]

The time needed to achieve these objectives can vary widely, but at least 2 to 4 months following the child's death are necessary as a rule. Important days in family life may remind the family of the child they lost, and grieving may begin again. This renewed grieving is still exquisitely painful but should not be as disruptive as the original grieving period.[19]

Nursing Interventions

Nursing interventions that may prove to be particularly helpful are outlined below:

1 *Be sure the child has a primary nurse during each shift,* to develop a close relationship. Being involved in such an intense relationship is stressful, so be sure to take time off from the case occasionally. Communicate your feelings openly to other staff members.

2 *Observe changes in child's and parents' behavior, and interpret these in relation to the child's age level and perception of body image.* Body-image distortion can be magnified by fantasy. Projective play techniques such as drawing, storytelling, or play with puppets can elicit the child's current feelings. "Repeated personal inspection can reduce body image distortion. . . . Explanations offered to children should be simple and brief, since children cannot tolerate prolonged concentration upon threatening events."[18]

3 *Help the patient and family to make use of all available resources,* such as extended family members (grandparents, aunts and uncles, cousins), the clergy, and family service agencies. Try to provide a group experience for the child or parents when available and appropriate.

4 *Express your continued availability.* "I know this must be a horrible experience for you. No one likes to endure so much pain and uncertainty. If you'd like to talk about it with me, perhaps you won't feel so alone."

5 *Try to anticipate the child's responses: a* "Perhaps you feel it is your fault you became so sick." *b* "It must be hard for you to understand how you can be sick when your body looks fine outside. Maybe I can help explain it to you. Shall I draw a picture?" *c* "You seemed to have so much pain and be so frightened during your liver biopsy this morning. Let's talk about it." or, "Why don't you draw us a picture of what it felt like?"

d "Have you ever seen a television program about a person with the same illness you have? How did you feel about it?" *e* "Do you ever feel your parents have been treating you differently since you were hospitalized? How do you feel about this?" *f* "Since it is your body that is sick, we would like to help you understand what is wrong and why certain diagnostic tests and treatments are necessary. We will always tell you in advance what test you will have, when you will have it, what it is for, and how you can help us. Whenever possible, we will try to consult you to find out when you would prefer to have the tests done and to determine whether you have any preference in premedications."

6 *Try to anticipate the parents' responses: a* "It seems your child became sick so suddenly. Perhaps you've been wondering if he was sick earlier and you and your physician hadn't noticed it." *b* "How much do you think your child understands about her illness? How do you think we can best help her through this?" *c* "You must be exhausted. Life has changed so much for you in such a short time. Has it changed for the whole family?" *d* "Mrs. G is sitting in the next room with her son, who has also been very sick. Would you like to speak with her? She has been very interested in meeting you." *e* "Your child seems to be suffering so these past few weeks. Perhaps sometimes you think it would be kinder if her suffering were all over." *f* "With Johnny so sick between remissions, it must be hard to treat him as normally as possible. Do you find this difficult?" *g* "Johnny has a younger brother and sister. Have they been asking a lot of questions about Johnny's hospitalization? Has their behavior changed? Perhaps they are more reluctant than usual to let you leave, or perhaps they have been 'too good'?"

7 *Give other children on the unit a chance to work through their feelings about the death and dying of their fellow patients.* This can be done verbally or via projective play techniques. "I'm sure you noticed that Johnny's bed is empty this morning. Let's talk about it. You were such good friends, weren't you?"

When the nursing interventions identified in the above discussion are applied consistently, most clients are able to cope with their loss adequately. When the clients' behavior seems resistant to change in spite of the most creative nursing approaches, and the behaviors are threatening to be destructive to themselves or others, then long-term counseling with a mental health professional is indicated.

Evaluation

When nursing diagnosis has been accurate and nursing intervention has been appropriate, the nurse should be able to evaluate to what extent nursing care has been helpful to the family in crisis. When families are functioning at an optimal level, they are able to meet most of the following criteria. The family members can:

1 Be all they can be
2 Successfully negotiate each stage of growth and development
3 Get in touch with their feelings; identify and handle them
4 Develop and maintain a healthy self-esteem
5 Handle stress constructively
6 Develop and maintain healthy interpersonal

relationships with each other and people outside the family

7 Resume adequate functioning—as much as possible—at home, at work, or in school

These criteria apply to all families and provide a useful benchmark to help the nurse measure how the family is growing and changing.

References

1 John Gunther: *Death Be Not Proud*, Harper, New York, 1949, pp. 250–252.

2 Earl A. Grollman (ed.): *Explaining Death to Children*, Beacon, Boston, 1967.

3 Philippe Aires: "A Moment That Has Lost Its Meaning," *Prism*, vol. 3, pp. 27–37, June 1975.

4 Abraham Bergman: "Psychological Aspects of Sudden Unexpected Deaths in Infants and Children," *Pediatric Clinics of North America*, vol. 21, pp. 115–121, February 1974.

5 Barney G. Glaser and Anselm L. Strauss: "The Social Loss of Dying Patients," *American Journal of Nursing*, vol. 64, pp. 119–121, June 1964.

6 Stanford B. Friedman: "Psychological Aspects of Sudden Unexpected Death in Infants and Children," *Pediatric Clinics of North America*, vol. 21, pp. 103–111, February 1974.

7 J. Vernick: "Meaningful Communication with the Fatally Ill Child," in E. James Anthony and Cyrille Koupernick (eds.): *The Child in His Family: The Impact of Disease and Death*, Wiley, New York, 1973.

*8 Eugenia Waechter: "Children's Awareness of Fatal Illness," *American Journal of Nursing*, vol. 71, pp. 1168–1172, June 1971.

9 Maria Nagy: "The Child's Theories Concerning Death," *Journal of Genetics and Psychology*, vol. 73, pp. 3–27, 1948.

10 E. James Anthony: "A Working Model for Family Studies," in E. James Anthony and Cyrille Koupernik (eds.): *The Child in His Family: The Impact of Disease and Death*, Wiley, New York, 1973.

*11 Kathy Patterson and Margaret Pomeroy: "SIDS," *Nursing '74*, vol. 74, pp. 85–88, May 1974.

12 Erich Lindemann: "Symptomatology and Management of Acute Grief," *American Journal of Psychiatry*, vol. 101, pp. 141–148, 1944.

13 Edward H. Futterman and Irwin Hoffman: "Crisis and Adaptation in the Families of Fatally Ill Children," in E. James Anthony and Cyrille Koupernik (eds.): *The Child in His Family: The Impact of Disease and Death*, Wiley, New York, 1973.

14 Elisabeth Kübler-Ross: *On Death and Dying*, Macmillan, New York, 1969.

15 Michael Gourevitch: "A Survey of Family Reactions to Disease and Death in a Family Member," in E. James Anthony and Cyrille Koupernik (eds.): *The Child in His Family: The Impact of Diseases and Death*, Wiley, New York, 1973.

16 N. Alby, G. Raimbault, and H. L. Friedman: "Les parents devant la mort de l'enfant," *Concours Medical*, vol. 11, pp. 1874–1883, 1971.

*17 Jeanne C. Quint: "Obstacles to Helping the Dying," *American Journal of Nursing*, vol. 66, pp. 1568–1571, July 1966.

*18 Irene Riddle: "Nursing Intervention to Promote Body Image Integrity in Children," *Nursing Clinics of North America*, vol. 7, pp. 651–657, December 1972.

19 Albert C. Cain and Barbara S. Cain: "On Replacing a Child," *Journal of the American Academy of Child Psychiatry*, vol. 3, pp. 443–456, 1964.

*recommended reference by a nurse author.

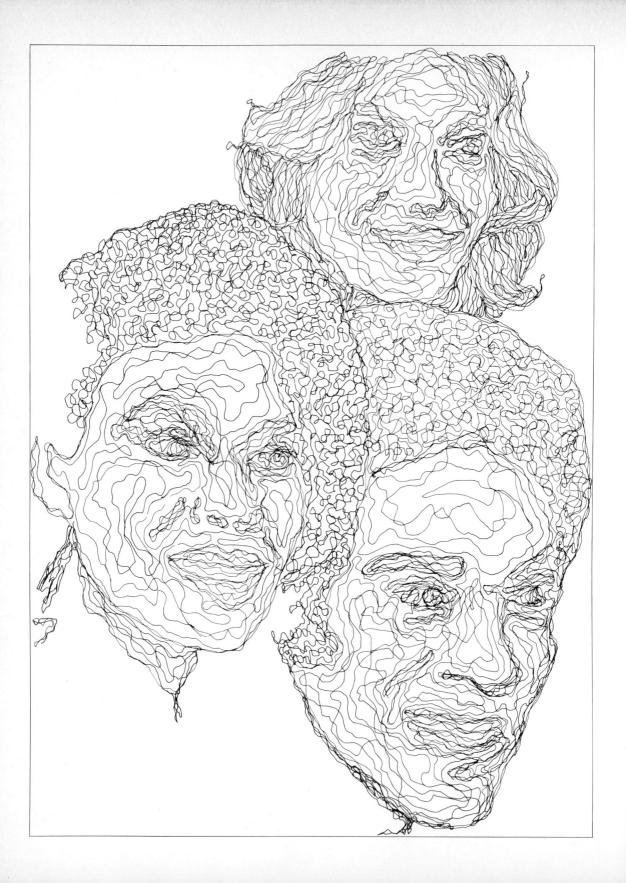

Six

Future Directions

40

Nursing Research

Judith Belliveau Krauss

Learning Objectives

After studying this chapter, the student should be able to:

1 Articulate the purpose of research in nursing

2 Define nursing research

3 Differentiate nursing research from other types of research

4 Name the steps involved in analyzing clinical nursing problems

5 Identify at least one major problem in psychiatric–mental health nursing practice

6 Differentiate between exploratory, hypothesis-testing, and measurement studies

7 Classify areas of nursing practice into their component parts or factors to be studied

8 List the rights of human subjects participating in research studies

9 Name at least two major issues which influence the conduct of nursing research in psychiatric–mental health nursing

Recent psychiatric nursing literature documents that this is a time of role expansion in psychiatric nursing. As members of a professional subspecialty, psychiatric nurses are taking on increasing responsibility for the assessment, evaluation, treatment, and follow-up of psychiatric clients in institutional and community settings. Carnegie, editor of *Nursing Research,* has pointed out that as a profession takes on increased authority for its practice, so too does it take increased responsibility to improve that practice. That responsibility in professional nursing is believed best fulfilled through the conduct of empirical research by nurses themselves.[1]

Research is no longer a new concept in nursing, although the concept of the nurse-researcher has gone through some significant changes over the last decade. It was not until recently (1973–1974) that the studies addressing the practice of nursing as it influences clients outnumbered the studies of teaching, curriculum, career orientation, and administration in nursing. Most studies reported in *Nursing Research* in its early years were conducted by sociologists, physicians, and psychologists and were concerned with the workers. In contrast, by January–February 1973, only 13 of 108 authors in *Nursing Research* were not nurses, and the focus of the study began to shift from the workers to the work of nursing.[1]

Necessity of Research

The rapid role expansion in nursing, coupled with the shift in emphasis of nursing research from educational and administrative studies to clinical studies, suggests that the reasons nurses and nursing research exist may be the same: for the improvement of client care and the discovery of nursing strategies which will assist clients in the attainment and maintenance of health. It remains true, however, that the majority of nurses and

*The author gratefully acknowledges the influence of Donna Diers, MSN, under whose tutelage the field of nursing research was clarified and the formulation of the ideas expressed in this chapter became possible.

nurse-educators are consumers rather than producers of research.[2] Schlotfeldt[3] has suggested that:

> Systematic inquiry is a responsibility of both practitioners and of investigators. Both types of inquirers need the wisdom to select from among the many hypothetical notions and practical problems that present themselves, those about which inquiry is likely to yield knowledge most important to [humanity]. Both need to understand the nature of objective, systematic, inquiry.

One could extend Schlotfeldt's reasoning to suggest that the degree to which the investigator and practitioner are the same people is the degree to which nursing, as a practice discipline, will promote research which holds promise of improving the services of the practitioners. If it is the delivery of quality health-care services to clients through the practice of nursing that the professionals must continually examine and change, then it follows that clinical research could draw nurses closer to their practice through a systematic approach to problem solving and conscious movement toward planned rather than random change.

Nursing Research

Research is a process, a way of thinking about the problems of one's practice, as well as an outcome, an assimilation of findings which, when connected by the appropriate theory, sheds new light on relationships and associations between and among facts and predicts the occurrence of yet unobserved events and relationships. Many nurses, particularly those educated at baccalaureate and higher levels, intuitively if not knowingly involve themselves in the process. Their purpose for study is to make the process and the outcome of nursing research explicit, to examine the nature of researchable nursing problems, and to highlight some potential areas in need of systematic investigation in psychiatric–mental health nursing practice.

There are at least two kinds of researchers in nursing today: one is the nurse who does research and tries to fit the practice of nursing into the study designs created for the pure scientists and the laboratory setting; the other is the practitioner who is struggling with live nursing problems and attempting to create systematic methods of studying those problems almost at the same moment they are being experienced. The former is a nurse who does research; the latter is doing nursing research.

Jacox has emphasized that much of what is taught in nursing is in the realm of untested theory.[4] Research is one way to test and create theory. It stands to reason that nursing places itself on more solid ground each time it tests and then implements theory designed to affect practice—that is, to improve client care.

The researching of nursing practice presents many problems in methodological design, procuring samples, and measuring clinical phenomena in accurate and sensitive ways. This makes the generating of empirical theory a more complex (although not insurmountable) problem. In a practice profession such as nursing, research falls short of the well-controlled laboratory setting with its isolated variables and precise measurements. It becomes incumbent on the researcher not only to study the nursing-practice problems but also to continually search for and develop the most appropriate methods for the conduct of nursing studies. Any definition of nursing research must include both processes. The following definition of nursing research has been formulated by borrowing from a number of nursing research authorities:

> Nursing research is the systematic study of the practice of nursing, using scientific methods to ensure that the findings represent reality and that facts are collected with as much objectivity as possible; with the express purpose of describing and effecting nurse-client phenomena, developing appropriate and sensitive methodologies which fit the nurs-

ing problems, and testing and developing theory whose implementation improves practice.[25-7]

Research as Process

The word "research" often raises visions of complicated tables and lists of statistical findings, to say nothing of the image of the researcher as a dusty intellectual tucked away in the library stacks. In actuality, "research" when modified by "nursing" means something quite beyond the *findings;* it places the researchers in the practice settings. As a tool or way of approaching problems, nursing research offers a new way, and some would argue the best way, of thinking about and dealing with one's practice.

An integral part of the research process is the identification and analysis of clinical-practice problems, followed by posing the research questions and/or hypotheses, designing ways to collect the necessary information, designing or discovering the most appropriate measures, collecting data, processing and analyzing it, interpreting the findings, and generalizing them to like situations. Diers points out that this process goes beyond the mere practical solution of an individual difficulty; it places the particular clinical problem in a broader framework and relates it to other phenomena that are thought to be in the same class of problems in the larger universe of nursing practice.[6]

The research process enables a clinician to relate one clinical situation or phenomenon to another and to apply like solutions or interventions to like situations on the basis of a broad theoretical understanding of the facts or factors involved. Diers further suggests that by placing particular client-care problems on a more abstract plane, we deemphasize the idiosyncratic nature of the client's problem and make available other knowledge such as literature, previous studies, and relevant theories which enable the nurse to transfer learning from one situation to another and to treat the client in the broadest context of client-centered nursing.[6] Through this process, client-centeredness comes to mean a growing base of knowledge concerning how clients and nurse-client interactions are alike or different. Given a set of circumstances which guides practice and enables nurses to make complex clinical judgments is of overall benefit to the client.

By way of illustration, take the situation of a nurse in a chronic psychiatric outpatient setting carrying a large caseload of clients. Over the past year, the nurse has noted that a seemingly large number of clients have had to be rehospitalized or have required an increase or significant change in their medication regimen.* This observation is shared with the nursing supervisor. One typical response to such a "problem" would be to institute a series of policy changes such as reducing the clinician's caseload, instituting the practice of seeing all clients more often, changing the treatment program, or accepting into treatment only those clients whose prognosis was good. Any of these "solutions" would be based on untested assumptions about what causes clients to relapse. The cause may be overworked nurses, infrequent contact, the wrong intervention, or the wrong client. All these solutions, while potentially useful, are examples of immediate random responses to a particularized client-care problem without benefit of a systematic examination of the problem in its broadest context and an application of other sources of knowledge.

In applying the research process to this situation, such questions may be raised as: "Won't valuable time be wasted searching for solutions while clients continue to experience difficulties? Would it net different results in the long run?" Another look at the original problem employing the research process would attempt to analyze it and answer these questions. Having noticed that a large number of clients have relapsed, the clinician feels that there is a discrepancy between the goals of the treatment program and *what is*. The goals of the program are to keep clients out of inpatient settings and to maintain them on low

doses of psychotropic medication that will enable them to adjust to community living. In fact, however, clients are being hospitalized in large numbers and are requiring higher than maintenance levels of psychotropic medication, thus hampering their ability to live in the community.

Up to this point, the clinician has only a hunch or a feeling that something is wrong. How can one be sure? In this situation, it might be a good idea to check records over the last 12 months to validate the impression that large numbers of clients have been rehospitalized or experienced major medication changes. Suppose that such a survey led to the conclusion that 49 percent of all clients in a particular caseload did have some form of relapse in the last year. How does one know that this is a discrepancy that matters? Maybe this situation is peculiar to the particular caseload or just a chance occurrence. One way to further validate that there is a problem that matters is to ask *all* clinicians on the service to systematically check their records over the last year to determine a relapse rate. Having determined everyone's relapse rate and observing that all were similar, the clinician can now take an average of all the relapse rates to determine the average rate for the service over a full year's time. Assume that the overall unit relapse rate turns out to be 48 percent. Since the problem has moved from a caseload-specific situation to the unit level, the clinician might turn to the literature to discover that recidivism or relapse statistics for chronic clients on a local, regional, and national basis suggest that the problem is a large one and one that matters on a variety of levels. Through the literature, it is discovered that relapse in a chronic population has been found to be associated with age, sex, living situation, the occurrence of certain kinds of life events, medication noncompliance, problem-solving ability or social competence, and certain types of symptom exacerbation. It is also discovered that most of the literature addresses only an *untreated* chronic population, those clients who are discharged from inpatient settings with no follow-up or outpatient treatment. Clinicians wonder whether the factors identified in the literature as related to relapse

*This case example is taken directly from the grant "Nursing with Chronically Ill Psychiatric Outpatients," NU 00370-04, USPHS, Slavinsky and Krauss, co-investigators.

would apply to *their* clients, a *treated* chronic population. Further questions then occur: "Which factors, in which combinations, are most likely to predispose clients to relapse? And are there adequate tools to gather the necessary information which could be adapted to these clients' capabilities and used by nurses without disrupting their practice?"

A number of other questions might be raised, and a number of statements known as *hypotheses* might be formulated which would predict certain relationships between facts, based on the clinician's understanding of the literature and on previous studies. It is likely that clinicians have raised so many questions and hypotheses that they will have to select those few which need to be answered first and for which they have the time, experience, money, and resources to gather, process, and analyze the necessary data.

The case example could be continued to further illustrate the process of designing and implementing the appropriate nursing study to address the problem, but first it is necessary to return to the original questions which prompted the analysis. It is hoped that the case example itself has answered the question, "How might the research process be applied in this situation?"

The research process introduces a way of systematically analyzing clinical problems; it enables the nurse to become something more than a "reactor" in the nurse-client interaction. On one level, using the process illustrated in the example is nothing more than good practice. Sound clinical judgments require the use of observation and of consistent criteria by which to describe and interpret those observations. Feinstein points out that in caring for clients, clinicians constantly perform experiments. Although they do not usually regard ordinary client care as a type of experiment, every aspect of clinical management can be designed, executed, and appraised with intellectual procedures identical to those used in any experimental situation.[8] The research process illustrated in the example offers one way for nurses not only to observe the same phenomena but also to process them in similar fashion using the same criteria for

making clinical decisions. Beyond the issue of making isolated clinical decisions, this process enables nurses to convert their clinical problems into research problems, examining them at a level of abstraction removed from the particular situation and generalizing the learning to similar situations. Table 40-1 summarizes the process employed in the case example and is designed as a guide for thinking about a clinical problem and converting it into a research problem, research questions, and/or hypotheses.

On the face of things, it would seem that the quickest and easiest solution for the nurse in the case example might have been to institute an immediate change in the situation which would seem logically (and intuitively) to address the problem of relapse. For example, the nurse might have decided that all clients who had relapsed during the previous year would be seen three times per month instead of the usual two, assuming that increased contact would offer the necessary support to decrease clients' anxiety and thus lower their relapse rate. The nurse would be "experimenting" with an intervention that might or might not produce the wished-for results. In short, hunch, intuition, or something nebulously referred to as "previous clinical experience" would guide the clinical judgment and result in the experimental intervention. Feinstein aptly suggests that this form of experimentation under the guise of the conventions of accepted clinical practice may mask flagrant imprecisions, vagueness, and inconsistency in the practice of the most reputable clinicians.[8]

Time would have to elapse in order to evaluate the effect of the selected intervention; in this instance, just about a year would have to pass before the nurse could assess whether or not the intervention had any influence on relapse rates (assuming the nurse would recall that there was a problem and a solution to be evaluated). However solutions to nursing problems are arrived at, and whatever form they take, time must elapse before evaluation can take place. If the evaluation is not a formal part of the process (as it is in the research process), there is a good chance that it will not

Table 40-1 Guide for Analysis of Clinical Problems[7]

1 Identify and state the discrepancy.
   - Why or how do you know there is a discrepancy? How did you come to feel it as a discrepancy?
   - How do you know it is a difference *that matters?*
   - If the discrepancy were removed, what would the result look like? What are the implications of removing the discrepancy? Of not removing it?
2 Describe the significance of the discrepancy to practice and theory.
   - How big is it? How big a gap is there between what is and what should be, or what is known and what needs to be known?
   - What is this problem an instance of?
3 Analyze the nature of the discrepancy.
   - What are the two conditions?
   - What factors are involved in each?
   - How are the factors related? How do you know?
4 What questions need to be answered to remove the discrepancy?
   - What are the most important questions? Why?
   - How practical will obtaining the answers be? Consider your own resources — energy, time, money, interest, experience.
   - Select the questions to be answered.
5 Specify the type of study that is appropriate.
   - Have you identified factors? Relationships?
   - Do you have hypotheses or predictions or are you looking for them?
   - If you have hypotheses, what form do they take?

take place and nothing at all will be learned from the particular situation that could be applied to other situations. The next time a similar problem arises, the nurse will be in the same position, picking a solution and hoping it works. This hit-or-miss process takes time and often nets inconsistent and ineffective results over the long haul, doing little for the overall improvement of client care.

The research process clearly takes time as well. It is easy to see from the case example that one can generate enough questions about aspects of practice to spend a lifetime searching for answers. Nevertheless, each step of the research process nets usable, transferable knowledge and enables the nurse to establish a network of related theories and knowledge which can explain the occurrence of certain events and predict the occurrence of other events.

Given that all approaches to practice take time, the real question becomes: "Which approach to practice holds out the most promise for improving client care?" Diers states that in a service profession like nursing, research without practice

is sterile and irrelevant; practice without research is ritualistic and intellectually empty.[6] There can be only one conclusion: good practice is good research, and vice versa. The criteria for each process are the same.

Research as Outcome

The final question which prompted an analysis of the problem was: "Would the research process net different results in the long run?" It can best be answered by examining the outcomes of that process.

The outcomes of the research process depend to a large extent on the way in which the original problem was analyzed and the methods that were employed to study it. Various methodological designs are useful in addressing clinical problems. For the student who wishes to pursue research methodology, it has been the subject of many texts.[2,5,9–11] In general, the methodology selected is governed by how much is already known or understood about the clinical problem. There are essentially three major types of methodological design: exploratory, hypothesis-testing, and measurement designs.

Exploratory Designs

Exploratory design is most often employed when little is known about the problem or when the nurse-researcher wishes to take a fresh look at a long-standing situation. This type of design is prompted by questions concerning what facts or factors exist in the situation which would best describe it or what relationships might exist between and among certain factors. For instance, if an inpatient adolescent service was having increasing difficulty with clients who were eloping (running away) but had little idea as to the causes of this behavior, an exploratory design might be employed which would enable the clinicians to take a systematic, broad look at all possible factors (age, sex, time of hospitalization, diagnosis, etc.) which might be related to a client's eloping from the hospital. Many questions would be raised about the similarities and differences between elopers and nonelopers and about such issues as the frequency and time of elopement as these might relate to other factors. The outcomes of such exploratory studies are descriptions of clinical phenomena (like elopement), comparisons of one group to another (elopers to nonelopers), discovery of potential relationships (i. e., diagnosis to elopement), theory development, and more questions and hypotheses to be tested about relationships between and among factors.

Hypothesis Testing

Hypotheses are predictions that certain events will occur given the right conditions or that certain relationships exist among the phenomena being studied; they are tentative explanations of the occurrence of events based on the prediction of relationships among a complex set of data. Hypothesis-testing designs are utilized to test pre-dictions (1) of cause-effect relationships and (2) of the relationships between variables. An example of a cause-effect relationship that might be tested is this: "Medication maintenance plus group psychotherapy will cause increased community socialization in chronic psychiatric outpatients as compared to medication maintenance alone with a similar group of clients." A relationship between variables is exemplified by the hypothesis that chronically ill psychiatric outpatients who, in a previous 12-month period, have had stressful life events will be more likely to relapse in the subsequent year than similar clients without such events. This hypothesis tests the relationship between life events and relapse. The outcomes of these designs are explanations, tested interventions, evaluation and demonstration of procedures, the articulation of cause-effect relationships leading to the design of new programs and interventions, tested clinical theory, and more questions and hypotheses.

Measurement Designs

Measurement designs are, of course, used to develop and test nursing measures useful for the gathering of research and clinical data. The outcomes of such studies enable a clinician to evaluate the *reliability* (the extent to which the measure gives the same results with repeated use and the extent to which two measurers get like results), *validity* (the extent to which the measure measures what it claims to measure), *meaningfulness* (the extent to which the measure fits the practice situation), and the *sensitivity and precision* (the extent to which the measure picks up the full range of occurrences on a continuum and the extent to which it distinguishes between cases) of a measure. Ultimately, such studies contribute to the improved data-collection methods for other studies and lead to the development of useful clinical measures which enable clinicians to predict the occurrence of certain events in their clients' treatment.

Each methodological approach offers a multiplicity of outcomes or results, and each can be utilized to gain a different perspective on parts of the same problem. Some methodological approaches are more rigorous than others and allow the transfer of knowledge from one situation to another to occur with more certainty of its applicability, while other approaches produce tentative answers and more questions which must be tested at higher levels before knowledge would be transferred to other situations. Regardless of the methodology used, the results of the research process enable the nurse to test assumptions about practice and about nurse-client interactions. Very often the results of a research study are not in the predicted or expected direction, thus challenging certain long-standing assumptions of the profession.

Research in effect transforms nursing from a practice based on assumption and tradition to a profession based on theory. One of the overriding results of the research process is to link practice and theory, where theory is a mental invention to the purpose of guiding practice.[12] The relationship of research, practice, and theory is not a linear but a circular one. Practice stimulates research and theory development, while research mines the data from practice which test or further build on theory; theory, in turn, contributes to different practices and provides the foundation for more advanced research; and practice, once again, provides the validation of research results and the backdrop for the further generation of theory.[7]

Clearly the research process offers results quite different from and more far-reaching than the mere practical solutions to individual, isolated problems. Systematic inquiry, or research, is essential not only to the survival of the nursing profession but also to the survival and optimal health of the people nurses serve.

Research Problems in Psychiatric–Mental Health Nursing
Researchable Questions

Since most research problems are discovered by asking questions about practice, it is important to examine the nature of those questions which lend themselves to research. Research deals with statements of what is or could be, of what relationships exist among facts, and of comparisons between and among phenomena. Research is a way of examining and evaluating work, gathering information, anticipating change, and modifying practice. However, none of these goals will be achieved unless the nurse-researcher asks the right questions. Research seeks answers to questions related to fact, to tangible, observable phenomena whose meaning can be validated by others. Not all questions can be addressed by research. Specifically, research cannot address questions of value, that is, questions about what one *should* do or about what is *best* for clients or what may be *better* than something else.[5] Research will never tell nursing what it should do; nurses will still have to make those important value judgments. But research will provide nurses with some of the data necessary to make them. For example, nurses working with chronic psychiatric outpatients often wonder whether medication maintenance, group psychotherapy, individual psychotherapy, social rehabilitation, or some combination of treatment modalities would be best for their clients. It is not unusual to find psychiatric nurses interested in the question, "What is the *best* treatment mode for my clients?" You may be surprised to learn that no amount of research will provide the answer to that question.

A question of value can often be reworded and reformulated into several questions of fact which can then be addressed through the research process. For instance, one could ask, "What are the differential effects of medication maintenance alone versus medication plus biweekly supportive therapy with a consistent nurse therapist?" Or, "What is the incidence of relapse for chronic psychiatric outpatients treated with medication alone as compared to similar clients treated with medication and weekly individual supportive psychotherapy?" Or, "What factors are related to relapse and symptomatic exacerbation in a treated chronic psychiatric outpatient population?" Answers to these and many more questions of fact would begin to assimilate the data needed to make policy decisions related to the original question, "What treatment is best for clients?" The answers to the research questions would tell the nurse what effects certain treatment modalities had on certain types of clients. These answers would further elucidate the complex set of factors which contribute to clients remaining asymptomatic or experiencing exacerbation, staying out of the hospital or being rehospitalized, taking their medications or not taking their medications, holding a job or losing it, adjusting to community life or withdrawing, and so forth. Obviously, there is no *one* answer, right for all clients and all nurses, to the question, "What is best . . . ?" It is through the research process—the accumulation of answers to questions of fact—that nurses begin to assimilate the necessary data vital to the everyday professional value judgments that must be made toward promoting optimal health in their clients.

Research Needs

The marriage between psychiatric–mental health nursing and research is young enough that all facets of practice are open to study. There are as many researchable questions about practice as there are practitioners to raise them. With that in mind, the table of Contents of this book can be used as a guide to considering some potential areas in need of research. The text contains material on six major areas of psychiatric-mental health nursing: (1) the client, (2) the family, (3) the nurse, (4) theoretical models, (5) therapeutic modalities, and (6) treatment environments, not necessarily in that order. Each of these six areas could be characterized in a variety of ways depending on the research interest or questions, and each individually or in any combination with the others would open avenues of nursing research. The following schema illustrates possible, though not exhaustive, ways that these areas might be characterized, classified, or categorized for the conduct of a research study.

The clients might be looked at in terms of their (1) demographic characteristics: age, sex, race, socioeconomic status, diagnosis, occupation, education, living situation, marital status, etc.; (2) behavior: silent, aggressive, abusive, withdrawn, isolated, abusers of alcohol or drugs, confused, hyperactive, anxious, etc.; (3) illness: severity, duration, prognosis, symptom constellation, etc.

The family might be looked at in terms of its (1) role as client; (2) role in client's social adjustment; (3) composition: sexual distribution, head of household, size, number of children, number of children living at home, etc.; or (4) dynamics: interaction patterns, inclusiveness, emotional investment in the client, decision-making patterns, information sharing, etc.

The nurses might be looked at in terms of their (1) role: group therapist, individual therapist, milieu manager, team leader, medication giver, administrator, etc.: (2) therapeutic style or manner: authoritarian, laissez-faire, egalitarian, democratic, open, closed, distant, personal, interested, uninterested, etc.: (3) experience: number of years, number of previous cases, faculty rank or institutional status, etc.; (4) personal characteristics: age, sex, race, etc.; or (5) training: psychiatric aide, resident, graduate prepared nurse, etc.

The theoretical models might be looked at in terms of their (1) authors: Erickson, Freud, Peplau, Sullivan, etc.; (2) framework or subject matter: interpersonal theory, intrapsychic theory, behavioral modification, gestalt, transactional analysis, etc.

The treatment modalities might be looked at in terms of their (1) boundaries: inpatient, outpatient, open, closed, structured, unstructured, etc.; (2) function: assessment and evaluation, crisis intervention, day treatment, resocialization, etc.; (3) geographic location: catchmented or noncatchmented; or (4) institutional affiliation: general hospital, community mental health center, home-visit agency, satellite clinic, state facility, university facility, etc.

As one begins to examine any area of practice from a research perspective, one must conceptualize it in terms of its various parts or factors which can then be described, compared, and contrasted with other factors. The research process actually begins at this level for every study, where the investigator must search out those factors which best characterize the phenomena or problem under study. For some, this process in itself constitutes an exploratory study whose sole goal is to describe a little-understood phenomenon in detail; for others, this process has already been achieved by investigators or theorists who have published their findings. These findings become the foundation for research at higher levels with goals beyond description, including the testing of predicted relationships and experimental interventions.

Utilizing the six-part schema of psychiatric–mental health nursing, let us trace the development of a number of research inquiries which could emerge from aspects of the same clinical problem: *"relapse in a chronic psychiatric outpatient population."* Very little is known about *the clients* in this population beyond their diagnosed chronicity. The *treatment environments* often vary according to state or local preference for serving this usually large group and may be located in community mental health centers, state institutions, home-visit services, satellite clinics, supportive living/work settings, or general hospital psychiatric clinics. The *therapeutic modalities* most often employed for this population include medication maintenance, supportive group therapy, social rehabilitation therapy, supportive individual therapy, or some combination of these.

The nurse is very often the professional who has a good deal of contact with this population and who is responsible for many aspects of their care including medication supervision, supportive therapies, crisis intervention, and social therapies (where social workers or occupational therapists are unavailable). *The families* of these clients often exhibit multiple psychiatric difficulties which may also require therapeutic intervention, and they experience a variety of problems around integration of the client into the family unit. The *theoretical models* which have been employed in examining the problems of chronicity and relapse include stress theory, life-change theory, social-adjustment theory, and problem-solving theory, to name a few.

To begin, much is still needed by way of description of phenomena related to the problems of chronicity and relapse. For example, an explor-atory study could be designed which would follow large numbers of chronic psychiatric outpatients who relapsed in the previous year and compare them to equally large numbers of similar clients who did not relapse in the previous year. Several factors in each client's life might be looked at and described simultaneously. These factors could include certain demographic characteristics (age, sex, race, socioeconomic status, marital status, living situation, diagnosis); the illness in terms of its duration, severity, and symptom patterns; the family setting in terms of size, responsibilities of the client and its emotional investment in the client; and certain theoretical phenomena thought to be important, such as problem-solving ability, social competence, and the occurrence of life events. Interviews with the clients, their families, and their therapists and the use of chart information might be employed to gather the data. The data could be compiled in a way that would characterize the relapsed and nonrelapsed clients as groups according to the above-mentioned dimensions. The two groups could then be compared as to similarities and differences, thus leading to some hypotheses about what factors in a chronic psychiatric outpatient population might be related to relapse.

Still further descriptive studies could be conducted comparing groups of similar clients in a variety of therapeutic modalities, using symptom exacerbation, life events, relapse, and a measure of problem-solving ability as a means of comparison. The outcomes of such a study might include hypotheses about which modalities are related to improved problem-solving ability, lower relapse rates, the occurrence of fewer symptomatic exacerbations, or the occurrence of fewer life events.

Using the knowledge gained from the descriptive studies, an hypothesis-testing study could be designed predicting the occurrence of relapse in clients who had low problem-solving ability, high numbers of life changes, and a previous relapse history as compared to similar clients who had high problem-solving ability, few life changes, and no previous relapse history. In such a study, the data might be collected through interviews of clients and therapists as well as chart review, and the prediction of relapse or no relapse might be made for the year following data collection. Should predictions prove accurate (assuming they were tested in a variety of settings under similar conditions by several researchers), then another line of study might begin.

The investigator might decide to design a data-collection instrument which could be used by nurse-clinicians in their treatment of chronic psychiatric outpatients that would enable them to determine whether their clients represented high risks for relapse. Knowing that each client has a different "risk status" for relapse might lead to experimental intervention studies to discover therapeutic modalities or nursing roles useful in reducing risk of relapse.

Clearly, the possibilities for research in this one small area of psychiatric–mental health nursing could continue ad infinitum. No one study addresses all facets of a clinical problem. While one group of investigators is conducting research which describes a particular client behavior, another group is developing an instrument to measure that behavior and still another group is testing experimental interventions to alter the behavior. Each set of studies might produce results which would influence the other studies. Those studies which are developing instruments or testing hypotheses need to be repeated several times in different settings by different researchers under similar circumstances in order to ensure their repeatability and accuracy.

This kind of effort requires an increase in the numbers of psychiatric–mental health nurses engaged in the research process and involved in clinical practice. An attempt must be made on local, state, regional, and national levels to identify the major psychiatric–mental health nursing-care problems which impinge on clients' health. Priorities must then be set which will guide the conduct of nursing research into those areas that are most important to the optimal health of patients.

Psychiatric–mental health nursing is in need of systematic research conducted at all levels of design, ranging from descriptions of phenomena to the experimental testing of interventions based on what is already known about the problem. In 1975, six of thirty *Nursing Research* clinical research studies were classified as psychiatric–mental health research.[13] *Nursing Research* is only one forum for reporting findings, and those figures represented an overall increase from the previous year in the conduct of clinical and psychiatric nursing studies. The figures are a long way from representing a concerted effort on the part of psychiatric nurse-clinicians to systematically question and examine their practice and report their findings. If nursing in general and psychiatric–mental health nursing in particular is to keep pace with the rapid changes in health-care delivery, practitioners must make a more systematic effort to address client-care problems and communicate the results of their inquiries in a way that influences further study of the same problems.

Issues Influencing the Conduct of Nursing Research in Psychiatric Settings

Whole texts and chapters can and have been written about a variety of issues which directly influence a person's ability to conduct research. Three major issues which directly shape the conduct of nursing research in psychiatric mental health settings are: (1) the issue of access and control; (2) the need for appropriate nursing measures; and (3) the rights of human subjects.

Access and Control

In order for any profession to conduct research, the problems selected for study must be within the realm of that professional practice, within its access and its control. "Access" refers to the training, educational background, and clinical experience unique to a profession which makes it privy to the understanding of certain phenomena. "Control" refers to the ability of a profession to observe and manipulate certain phenomena which affect practice. There is a temptation on the part of beginning researchers and professionals new to research to attempt to study someone else's clinical problems while ignoring their own.[7] For instance, the nurse (with no special background in biochemistry or psychopharmacology) who is interested in examining the biochemical effects of psychopharmacologic agents is choosing a field of study beyond the access and control of nursing. In most states, nurses cannot legally prescribe medications, and nursing education does not provide the necessary theoretical background to conduct such studies. A nurse interested in psychopharmacologic intervention might appropriately choose to study the role of the nurse in administering such agents or the nurse-client interaction around their administration. Experimentation with psychosurgical intervention is beyond the access and control of nursing, while experimentation with the postsurgical management of such clients is within the access and control of the profession.

In many psychiatric–mental health settings, the issue of access and control is made explicit through the use of institutional review committees whose purpose is to review research proposals and make decisions as to their appropriateness and usefulness to the setting. Very often such committees make judgments as to whether the researchers possess the capabilities (theoretical and clinical) to conduct the study as well as whether the study fits in with the other research needs of the institution.

Need for Appropriate Nursing Measures

In psychiatric–mental health settings, nursing research most often and most appropriately studies some aspect of nurse-client interaction. Before assessing, evaluating, or describing such phenomena, one must obtain satisfactory measures and develop impartial, unbiased ways of using them. As demonstrated in the six-part schema of psychiatric–mental health nursing, there are many sources of data and many ways to measure them. Nursing, as a profession new to research, has been in the position of simultaneously studying clinical problems and finding ways to measure

them; and nurses have had to borrow or adapt measures developed by other professions toward different ends. Borrowed measures, like borrowed methodologies, often shape the problem to the study instead of the study to the problem. A nurse interested in the effects of a nurse-run treatment program on the community adjustment of chronic psychiatric outpatients cannot rely on the usual psychiatric outcome measures of symptom exacerbation, days out of the hospital, medication compliance, etc., to measure the quality of the life a client leads in the community. Psychiatric nurses familiar with community intervention, who understand the problems of everyday living with which clients must cope and who see the conditions and standards under which these people function, must develop measures sensitive to change in these areas. Only those types of measures will ultimately record the effects of *nursing* interventions as opposed to *medical* interventions. An issue central to the future of research in psychiatric–mental health nursing is the conduct of measurement studies and the development of instruments which can sensitively and accurately measure phenomena unique to nursing practice.

Rights of Human Subjects

Human beings—the clients being treated—have the right to privacy, confidentiality, anonymity, safety, and informed consent. These rights are protected by law and they must be safeguarded during the conduct of research studies in which clients participate. In psychiatric–mental health settings perhaps more than other settings, the nurse must be particularly vigilant in ensuring not only the protection of these rights but also the clients' understanding of them. The nurse is further obliged to make sure that these clients are capable of making informed choices about participation in research projects.

The issue of privacy in psychiatric settings is a particularly knotty one for researchers. Meltzoff and Kornriech point out that therapeutic relationships are thought to be so unique as to make experiments nonreproducible and so private as to make them inaccessible to outside scrutiny. This, they feel, tends to discourage research and to prevent acceptance of research findings.[14] The therapist-client relationship in psychiatric settings has traditionally been a confidential, private, and in some cases anonymous one. Many therapists argue that the introduction of anyone or anything (one-way screen, tape recorders, video equipment) into the treatment relationship so drastically alters conditions as to make progress difficult (if not impossible). Ironically, research studies of this problem are inconclusive as to the detrimental effects of external recording devices. They lean toward suggesting that such devices have some effects, not necessarily detrimental, on the therapeutic process which could influence research results, but not treatment results (see Meltzoff and Kornreich for a thorough review of this literature). It is possible to conduct research studies and gather data while maintaining confidentiality and anonymity and respecting the privacy requirements of clients and therapists alike. Data can be grouped and coded in such a way as to mask any identification of individuals. Data can be collected in ways that minimize disruption of treatment and maximize the amount of information gathered in a given period of time. It is clear, though, that psychiatric nurses as well as other professionals must clear avenues for scrutiny of their most important work if they are to benefit from their mistakes and successes and develop a body of clinical practice theory.

Informed consent is another issue which requires more vigilance in psychiatric–mental health settings. The DHEW Policy on Protection of Human Subjects, June 16, 1971, defines informed consent as "the agreement obtained from a subject, or from a subject's authorized representative, to the subject's participation in an activity."

The basic elements of informed consent are as follows:

1 A fair explanation of the purpose of the study and adequate introduction of the researcher
2 A fair explanation of the procedures to be followed, including an identification of those which are experimental

3 A description of the attendant discomforts and risks
4 A description of the benefits to be expected
5 A disclosure of appropriate alternative procedures that would be advantageous for the subject
6 An offer to answer any inquiries concerning the procedures and purpose
7 An instruction that the subject is free to withdraw consent and to discontinue participation in the project or activity at any time and instruction that refusal and/or withdrawal to participate in or to continue with the study will produce no negative consequences at that time or in the future

Most psychiatric and educational institutions now have human-subject review committees whose sole purpose is to see that all conditions of informed consent are met and that the research study is within reasonable limits of safety and risk to the human participants. The question arises, "Can a committee, however thorough in its review, monitor on paper a process which must take place between a researcher and a subject?" It would seem ultimately incumbent on the nurse-researcher to make sure that what goes on the paper is dynamically translated to the client and/or subject who must make an informed choice to participate in a project. Nurse-investigators must also be skilled nurse-clinicians in order to make judgments about clients' ability to make decisions and their capacity to understand information being offered. The investigator must offer information in such a way that it can be processed by the client or that the client can seek the assistance of a guardian who could act in the client's best interest in deciding about participation. A client who has been fully informed and chooses to participate in a research project may be more likely to complete the project. The subject who is not fully informed but agrees to participate out of fear, ignorance, or intimidation may drop out or be unavailable for interview later. Ultimately, informed consent is of benefit not only to the research subject but also to the investigator who can ill afford to lose subjects and valuable data necessary to the completion of a project.

It should be clear that the nurse-researcher must be just as strongly motivated toward human welfare as the nurse-clinician. The researcher may more often be concerned with the welfare of groups of people, while the clinician is concerned with the welfare of particular individuals. When the researcher and the clinician are one and the same, as in nursing research, these distinctions become artificial. Nursing research, if it is to address the pressing and ever-changing client-care problems of our profession, must be the embodiment of sound inquiry, competent practice, and relevant theory.

References

*1 M. Elizabeth Carnegie: "The Shifting of Research Emphasis and Investigators," *Nursing Research,* vol. 23, p. 195, May–June 1974.

*2 David J. Fox: *Fundamentals of Research in Nursing,* 2d ed., Appleton-Century-Crofts, New York, 1970.

*Recommended reference by a nurse author.

*3 Rozella M. Schlotfeldt: "Cooperative Nursing Investigations: A Role for Everyone," *Nursing Research,* vol. 23, pp. 452–456, November–December 1974.

*4 Ada Jacox: "Nursing Research and the Clinician," *Nursing Outlook,* vol. 22, pp. 382–385, June 1974.

*5 Faye Abdellah and Eugene Levine: *Better Patient Care Through Nursing Research,* Macmillan, New York, 1965, part 2.

*6 Donna Diers: "This I Believe about Nursing Research," *Nursing Outlook,* vol. 18, November 1970.

7 Donna Diers: Unpublished teaching materials, by permission

8 Alvan R. Feinstein: *Clinical Judgment,* Williams & Wilkins, Baltimore, pp. 21–24.

9 Claire Selltiz: *Research Methods in Social Relations,* Holt, New York, 1959.

10 Mabel Wandelt: *Guide for the Beginning Researcher,* Appleton-Century-Crofts, New York, 1970.

*11 Eleanor Treece and William Treece, Jr.: *Elements of Research in Nursing,* Mosby, St. Louis, 1973.

*12 James Dickoff and Patricia James: "A Theory of Theories: A Position Paper," *Nursing Research,* vol. 17, pp. 197–203, May–June 1968.

*13 M. Elizabeth Carnegie: "The Editors Report—1976," *Nursing Research,* vol. 25, January–February 1976.

14 Julian Metzoff and Melvin Kornreich: *Research in Psychotherapy,* Atherton, New York, 1970, p. 11.

41

Collected Papers

Learning Objectives

After studying this chapter, the student should be able to:

1 Outline the mandates of the National Institute of Mental Health
2 Describe the influence of federal legislation and funding on psychiatric–mental health education and service
3 Understand the consequences of present legislation for psychiatric–mental health practice
4 Define graduate education and the preparation of clinical specialists
5 Understand the influence of graduate education on psychiatric–mental health nursing, both historically and in current practice
6 List the motivations and reasons of nurses who enter private practice
7 List the qualifications of the private nurse practitioner
8 Identify the practical considerations to be kept in mind when undertaking private practice
9 Describe the future impact of nurses practicing in the private sector

FEDERAL FUNDING AND LEGISLATION*

M. Leah Gorman

The impact of three decades of federal funding legislation on professional development in psychiatric–mental health nursing is most dramatically seen in a projected increase of master's-prepared psychiatric nurses from no more than a dozen in 1948 to approximately 10,000 by 1978. It is indeed doubtful that, without federal funding under the National Institute of Mental Health, this significant increase of advanced psychiatric–mental health nurses would exist. (*Advanced psychiatric–mental* health nurses are those holding master's or higher degrees with specialization in psychiatric–mental health nursing.)

The National Institute of Mental Health

Major factors leading to the passage of the National Mental Health Act—which was signed into law by President Harry S Truman in 1946—included the public impact of World War II's psychiatric casualties; the staggering number of people rejected by the draft because of psychiatric problems; and the awareness of deplorable, dehumanizing conditions in the nation's public mental hospitals. This act authorized the establishment of the National Institute of Mental Health, which was mandated to carry out the following objectives:

1 To foster and aid research relating to the cause, diagnosis, and treatment of neuropsychiatric disorders

2 To provide for training of personnel through the award of fellowships to individuals and of grants to public and nonprofit institutions

3 To provide aid to states through grants and other assistance to establish new treatment facilities

4 To make provision for demonstration projects

*The views presented by the author do not necessarily reflect the opinions or official position of NIMH or DHEW. References 1–6 for this section appear on p. 694.

and pilot studies dealing with the prevention, diagnosis, and treatment of mental illness

Federal Legislation and Funding

The Congress enacted the first appropriation to launch a national mental health program in 1947. The Psychiatric Nursing Training Branch (now called Psychiatric Nursing Education Branch) was established under the leadership of Esther Garrison in 1947, and in 1948 nine psychiatric nurse-training grants were awarded, totaling close to $212,000. From that beginning, the program has made significant progress in fulfilling its stated goals: (1) to increase the number of educationally prepared psychiatric–mental health nurses; (2) to improve the quality of training of psychiatric nurses, including the expansion of psychiatric nursing content in baccalaureate schools of nursing; and (3) to provide psychiatric–mental health education in all areas of nursing confronted with mental health problems.

From the time of the first nine grants to the last count in fiscal year 1976, the Psychiatric Nursing Education Branch has awarded close to $143 million. From this amount, a total of 22,675 traineeships were awarded. (Traineeships do not represent individuals. Programs vary in the number of years required for completion; therefore a student may receive from 1 to 5 actual traineeships.) Of the total, 3,779 of these traineeships went to undergraduate programs; 16,325 were given to graduate nursing programs (including both master's and doctoral levels); and 2,571 were awarded to pilot projects, special projects, and continuing education projects.[1]

In 1956 approximately one-fifth[2] and in 1974 close to one-third of all nurses enrolled in graduate education were in psychiatric–mental health nursing.[3] Excluding medical-surgical nursing, there tend to be more students specializing in psychiatric–mental health nursing than in any other area of concentration.

Influence on Nursing Education

On recommendation of the January 1953 Committee on Review and Training policies, a long-range, intensive study of the integration of social science and psychiatric nursing concepts in prebaccalaureate curricula was undertaken at the University of North Carolina in 1955. This study culminated in publication of *Unity and Nursing Care,* a widely used classic in nursing for many years. In 1956 an award of $10,000 was given to two collegiate nursing schools to integrate psychiatric–mental health nursing content throughout the curriculum and to strengthen the basic psychiatric nursing course. From this beginning, support in basic undergraduate education expanded rapidly. By 1973, 70 percent of existing baccalaureate programs in this country were receiving NIMH support for the integration of psychiatric–mental health concepts. A total of 3,779 traineeships were awarded to baccalaureate students between 1963 and 1976.

It is clear that the early emphasis on training for leadership in psychiatric nursing was instrumental in developing sound curricula in psychiatric nursing at the baccalaureate level. The endeavors made in this field have had a major impact on all nursing education at this level.

The National Mental Health Act of 1946 has been the most significant piece of legislation affecting the development of psychiatric–mental health nursing as an area for specialization in professional nursing. While the need for special preparation in the field of mental health was evident long before legislation was passed, education in psychiatric–mental health nursing as a clinical specialty grew from nonexistence to a current total of 65 master's programs for clinical specialization in psychiatric–mental health nursing. The expansion of psychiatric nursing content in baccalaureate schools of nursing and the provision of mental health training in the various other areas of nursing practice is directly related to program activities of the Psychiatric Nursing Education Branch of NIMH.[4]

Influence on Nursing Service
To date, surveys of health personnel have failed to differentiate psychiatric nursing distribution according to academic preparation. This fact has led to an incomplete count of actual graduates who have completed master's requirements in psychiatric nursing. A 1974 survey reports that there are 28,000 active registered nurses with master's and/or doctoral degrees, or 3.3 percent of the total active pool of registered nurses. From these 28,000 nurses, about 6000 to 8000 are advanced psychiatric–mental health nurses.[5]

Registered nurses, numbering 39,228, represent the largest category of professional staff employed in mental health facilities. A hidden pool of clinical specialists in psychiatric–mental health nursing—estimated at over 2,000 in number—are those working in such nonpsychiatric settings as schools, public health agencies, comprehensive health centers, HMOs, medical-surgical or pediatric units of general hospitals, drug and alcohol services, and gerontology centers.

A 1974 national survey reports a total of 39,228 registered nurses employed in a variety of mental health facilities.[6] This represents an increase of over 21,000 registered nurses working in mental health facilities in the 11 years between 1963 and 1974. This increase was due to a variety of factors:

1 Increased emphasis on and expansion of psychiatric nursing content in undergraduate nursing programs

2 Availability of traineeships for advanced study in psychiatric nursing

3 Influence of the community mental health movement beginning in 1963

4 Changes in treatment approaches

5 Changes in types of treatment settings—away from long-term institutionalization and toward short-term, community-based treatment facilities

New Directions and New Priorities
With increasing public awareness of inadequate, ineffective, and inequitable health services, of severe maldistribution of health providers, of narrowly defined medical specialties, and of skyrocketing escalation of medical costs, the essential directions for reform in the health-care industry

emerge with startling clarity. New models of health personnel development and utilization, measures to ensure quality of health care, provision of comprehensive health services for underserved areas, and authentic consumer participation in the design of health service systems are all reflected in Public Law 93-641, the National Health Planning and Resource Development Act of 1974. This legislation has far-reaching ramifications in the health-care arena and raises many issues for the continued development of psychiatric–mental health nursing. The principal issues for those concerned with mental health care include the following:

- The need to link and transmit national mental health concerns to the new statewide health systems agencies
- Mental health care consumers and psychiatric nurses will need to cultivate skill in the development of health personnel, in mental health policy making, and in representing mental health issues and concerns on all levels of governance
- Training grants in psychiatric–mental health nursing will need to emphasize development of expertise for mental health planning and resource development

High among national priorities is the improvement of primary health care, particularly for underserved populations. Current and proposed legislation, supported by many analyses from experts inside and outside the government, stresses the need to train large numbers of primary-care physicians, physician extenders, and primary nurse practitioners; to expand their utilization; and to train and expand the utilization of other paraprofessional and allied health personnel. A basic level of mental health training is necessary for all generic health providers. Two of the major primary health-care providers in the United States are the nurse and the physician. Nursing has the largest potential pool of personnel who are able to provide primary care.

The Psychiatric Nursing Education Branch currently expends close to 20 percent of its efforts

increasing knowledge and skills in the mental health aspects of primary nursing care. It is anticipated that this level of effort will be increased in the next 5 years, with particular program emphasis in the following areas:

- Continuing education programs to upgrade the mental health aspects of primary nursing care for practicing registered nurses in a variety of health-care settings
- Liaison and consultation role training to ensure the appropriate and continuous application of psychiatric–mental health principles in direct generic health-care delivery
- Development of programs to prepare psychiatric–mental health nursing trainers for primary nurse-practitioner programs

While the need to ensure a continuing supply of highly qualified psychiatric–mental health nursing specialists will continue, an appropriate balance must be obtained in the Psychiatric Nursing Education Branch's mission to increase and expand the mental health training of primary nurses, to encourage the development of special and experimental projects which will address the mental health problems of minorities and other such underserved populations as the aging and children, and to encourage the development of training programs to prepare psychiatric nurses for strategic roles in state mental health personnel development and planning activities.

GRADUATE EDUCATION*

Donna Kaye Diers

Graduate education means formal study for a degree in nursing beyond the bachelor's degree. The bulk of higher degree programs in nursing are at the master's level.

Generally, graduate education in any field of

*References 7–14 for this section appear on pp. 694–695.

nursing practice aims to produce a specialist. A *clinical nurse-specialist* is primarily a clinician with a high degree of knowledge, skill, and competence in a specialized area of nursing. These skills are made directly available to the public through the provision of nursing care to clients and indirectly through the guidance and planning of care with other nursing personnel. Clinical nurse-specialists hold a master's degree in nursing, preferably with an emphasis in clinical nursing.[7]

Graduate education prepares specialists and also equips nurses for more independence in practice, enabling them to exercise more decision-making ability and authority. The baccalaureate graduate might be said to practice nursing in a psychiatric setting; the master's graduate practices psychiatric nursing, a fine but important distinction.

History and Education

Psychiatric nursing was one of the first specialties in nursing to develop a unique body of nursing knowledge.

Peplau's book *Interpersonal Relations in Nursing* made it clear that intensive, in-depth, psychoanalytically oriented work with clients could be done effectively by nurses as well as physicians.[8] Other forces for the development of specialized content at the graduate level in psychiatric nursing came from the more general movement in nursing education away from hospital schools of nursing and into baccalaureate degree programs. People in the university settings took more responsibility for providing abstract, theoretical content based on the analysis of student-client encounters.[9]

When, with the use of psychotropic medications, therapeutic treatment for the mentally ill became more possible and the public demand for more than merely custodial care became focused, nursing education had to move in the direction of educating nurses for more responsibility in the direct care of clients.

Psychiatric nursing, as a very young specialty, followed other movements in psychiatry closely, at first borrowing the well-developed psychothera-peutic-medical model for teaching young graduate students. Outside the hospital-unit situation, however, it was hard to distinguish differences between medical and nursing intervention in what happened privately with clients in a closed room.

The facts that nurses had the 24-hour responsibility for clients and that there was considerable need for improving the quality of care for hospitalized clients did not have much impact on graduate education in nursing until quite recently. In group psychotherapy and to a lesser extent in family and couples therapy, nursing moved ahead somewhat faster, and graduate students in nursing were offered experience as well as theory courses in group work.[10]

The community mental health movement offered nursing a chance to return to its roots of caring for the whole client, and it capitalized on nurses' comfort in going out of the institutional walls to give service. Various programs developed creative ways to involve students in community mental health. In rural areas, the role of the psychiatric nurse was broader than in urban medical centers, where there were more professionals with territorial prerogatives.

Current Practice

Graduate education in psychiatric nursing currently prepares graduates for insight-oriented psychotherapeutic work with individual clients. Beyond this basic core, some programs have developed highly sophisticated community psychiatry orientations, some have concentrated on group and family therapy, and some have developed subspecialties in child psychiatry or psychiatric liaison consultation.[11,12] Some programs prepare nurses not only to do therapy but also to make initial assessments of clients, to prepare diagnostic formulations, and to prescribe treatment and disposition.

Graduate students in psychiatric nursing now have formal courses in psychopharmacology as well as in the major theories in the field—those of Freud, Erikson, Horney, Sullivan, Glaser, etc. Many programs include considerable material on human development as courses have moved away from a

Freudian emphasis on intrapsychic explanations for psychiatric illness to a more eclectic inclusion of social-psychological theories of crisis, adult development, racial and sex-based attitudes, and the like (see Chap. 4). Study of mental health delivery systems—how people find and receive the services they need—is becoming more common as psychiatric nursing begins to take more seriously an obligation to prepare graduate students for leadership roles.

Unlike other specialties in nursing, psychiatric–mental health nursing employs the preceptorship or tutorial (called *supervision* more often in psychiatry) as a major method of teaching. There continues to be a focus on student-teacher examination of the nature and effect of the student's own personal beliefs, skills, experience, attitudes, and behavior. Some programs require the student to enter individual or group psychotherapy for personal growth and learning, and many students elect to do so out of personal motivation.

Certification

Clinical specialties in nursing have been concerned with guaranteeing to the public a high quality *product*. In New Jersey and New York, psychiatric nurses first organized a procedure for *certifying* the excellence of the practice of psychiatric nurses; their system preceded the American Nurses' Association certifying mechanism. Determining the criteria for certification has caused internal strife within the ranks of the ANA. There are some who believe certification should be for the general practice of psychiatric nursing, with an additional level of recognition for specialization within the field, as in group psychotherapy. Others believe that certification should imply highly specialized competence, with the entry credential of a master's degree. There are also disagreements within the professional organization about whether certification should signify *excellence* or *competence.*

Credentialing will become more necessary in the future, to provide a guideline for reimbursement for costs of service by third parties. Although nurses are able to demonstrate that they deliver the kinds of service clients need, they cannot be paid for them under insurance coverage, including Medicare. The only fees for service they obtain if they wish to practice outside an institution are from a client's own resources.

Doctoral Preparation

Doctoral programs in nursing are growing at a very rapid rate.[13] Since most doctoral programs are designed to begin after the bachelor's degree, many include the opportunity for clinical specialization as part of the course and clinical work. Few go beyond the master's level for depth in the clinical area of psychiatry unless the student pursues it individually.

There is very little research in psychiatric nursing to date. It may be anticipated that as doctoral programs develop in nursing, new knowledge will be developed through research. This new knowledge may then become the content of study beyond the master's degree.

The National League for Nursing's master list is the place to start looking for graduate education opportunities.[14] College catalogues can also help nurses select programs suited to their unique needs. Graduate education can provide the psychiatric nurse with the knowledge and skills to turn America's health system in the direction of client-centered care.

INDEPENDENT PRACTICE*

Margaret A. Colliton

Lucille Kinlein hung out her shingle in 1971 as one of the nation's first independent medical nurse-practitioners. Since then, growing numbers of nurses representing other clinical areas are becoming independent practitioners. This phenomenon results from several interrelated factors:

1 Twenty years of graduate education preparing clinical specialists in nursing

*References 15–26 for this section appear on p. 695.

2 Changes in nurse practice acts which foster autonomy equal to accountability in nursing practice

3 Consumer and women's liberation movements

4 Concentrated efforts to ensure quality control in health care

5 Emphasis on prevention in health care[15]

Psychiatric nurses have implemented their private practice in a variety of ways. Some have formed teams with other clinical specialists, others have joined an interdisciplinary group practice, and others have ventured out entirely on their own.[16] Most independent practitioners report having to rely on at least a part-time position either in a mental health facility or on a faculty in order to survive financially. However, at least one practitioner has been exceedingly successful in the coestablishment of a mental health facility which offers a diversity of services including family therapy; individual therapy; group therapy for children, adolescents, adults, and persons over 60 years of age; school and community consultation; counseling on sex, divorce, death and dying; and dance-bioenergetics movement therapy.[17]

Diversity in the operating structures and in the scope of practice characterizes many of the private practices described by psychiatric nurses. They work with other professionals; they do family therapy by themselves or they work with hospitalized clients or make home visits; they practice individual, family, and group therapy.

Nurses in private practice with doctoral or postdoctoral preparations offer services that are more focused, continuing to draw on the holistic view fostered by their nursing backgrounds.[18–20]

Motivation for Private Practice

Some clinical specialists enter private practice as an antidote to their dissatisfaction with the standard of health care in certain bureaucratic systems. Underutilization of skills and and frustration resulting from outdated stereotyping of *the nurse's role*—prompts many nurses to enter private practice. Others seek greater independence as a result of satisfying experiences within a facility.

Clinical specialists may have difficulty finding an institution willing to hire a master's-prepared nurse to work directly with clients, so they turn to private practice. Clinical specialists teaching on university faculties undertake part-time private practice in order to keep in touch with clinical work. Others, finding their clinical time eroded by administrative tasks, the demands of "publish or perish," and teaching responsibilities completely sever formal ties with institutions in favor of private practice.[21,22]

Qualifications for Private Practice

Not everyone who is motivated to begin private practice in psychotherapy may be qualified to do so. Present certification procedures are too general to guarantee the level of competence necessary for an independent private practice by psychiatric nurses.

A prototype for national or state certification includes the following qualifications:

- RN licensure
- Membership in ANA
- A master's degree in psychiatric nursing
- Academic and postacademic theoretical and clinically supervised preparation in psychotherapy
- Successful completion of a board examination
- Evidence of continuing practice in psychotherapy
- Ongoing supervision of practice
- Personal psychotherapy
- Proof of continuing education[23–25]

Only a small percentage of graduates at either the master's or doctoral level of any advanced psychiatric nursing program will enter private practice.

Practical Considerations

Considerations beyond adequacy of professional qualifications and legality are numerous. For example, is there need and are there resources in the community to support an additional private psychotherapist? Must a part-time or full-time position be maintained for economic security? Which services will benefit the well-being of the practitioner and the community? For example, a nurse-psychotherapist within the protection of a mental health facility might work quite successfully with psychotic clients yet be unwilling to shoulder such therapeutic responsiblilty working in private practice.

Fee setting is an issue related to personal and community needs. Traditionally nurses have treated persons regardless of ability to pay, but in private practice fee-for-service considerations are in relation to the nurses' need to earn an adequate wage. Nurse-psychotherapists, when eligible for third-party payment, will be able to increase the range of clients they treat and continue to have secure incomes.

Nurses frequently work well with the poor and those overlooked by others. The nurse in private practice must not lose touch with the needs of these individuals but must consider the time and effort spent from an economic vantage point.[25] A sliding scale which can meet the caseload and vary with it is most appropriate. Work to hasten the possibility of third-party payment for nurses includes investigation and making visible the similarities and differences in care rendered by nurse-psychotherapists in private practice and that given by other reimbursed individuals.

Once a nurse decides on private practice, it is advisable to consult a lawyer and an accountant. Provision should be made for other legal and economic ramifications such as adequate insurance coverage, tax changes, pension plans, etc. The advantages and disadvantages of solo practice, joining with a partner or partners, full-time or part-time practice, renting an office or using a space where one lives should be considered. An answering service of some kind is essential. Whether one is to adopt a low-profile approach to letting people know one is available for referrals and whether to establish a sliding-scale or fixed fee are other decisions one makes before setting up practice.[26]

Future Directions

As private nurse-practitioners grow in number, one hopes that the best of nursing tradition will infiltrate the private sector, bringing with it a humanistic, holistic, interpersonal emphasis in the prevention and treatment of emotional disorders. The greater freedom and depth that the nurse in private practice is privileged to experience in the intimate relationship with the client builds on the fundamental idealism that motivates the best in nursing. Future creative innovations may include institutes with nursing clinicians, educators, and researchers working together in a complete nursing–health-care center. Freedom from institutional constraints and full accountability for professional actions undoubtedly will uncover leaders capable of making a profound impact on the delivery of psychiatric–mental health care services.

References

1 Unpublished data from the Psychiatric Nursing Education Branch, Division of Manpower and Training Programs, National Institute of Mental Health, Alcohol, Drug Abuse, and Mental Health Administration (ADAMHA), DHEW, 1976.

2 *Facts About Nursing,* 1956–58, American Nurses' Association, Kansas City, Mo., 1958.

3 *Facts About Nursing,* 1974–75, American Nurses' Association, Kansas City, Mo., 1976, p. 87.

4 *Master's Education in Nursing: Route to Opportunity in Contemporary Nursing,* 1974–75, National League for Nursing, Department of Baccalaureate and Higher Degree Programs, New York, 1975.

5 *Source Book—Nursing Personnel,* U.S. Department of Health, Education, and Welfare Publication HRA 75-43, Bureau Health Resources Development, Division of Nursing, Bethesda, Md., 1974, p. 69.

6 Carl A. Taube: *Staffing of Mental Health Facilities—United States, 1974,* Division of Biometry and Epidemiology Survey and Reports Branch, National Institute of Mental Health, Series B, No. 8, ADAMHA, DHEW, 1974.

7 *Definition: Nurse Practitioner, Nurse Clinician, and Clinical Nurse Specialist,* American Nurses' Association, Congress for Nursing Practice, Kansas City, Mo., May 8, 1976.

8   Hildegard Peplau: *Interpersonal Relations in Nursing,* Putnam, New York, 1952.

9   Mabel Wadelt: *Outcomes of Basic Education in Psychiatric Nursing,* Wayne State University College of Nursing, Detroit, 1966.

10 Shirley Armstrong and Shiela Rouslin: *Group Psychotherapy in Nursing Practice,* Macmillan, New York, 1963.

11 Jill K. N. Nelson and Dianne A. Schilke: "The Evolution of Psychiatric Liaison Nursing," *Perspectives in Psychiatric Care,* vol. 14, no. 2, pp. 60–65, 1976.

12 Lisa Robinson: *Liaison Nursing—Psychological Approaches to Patient Care,* Davis, New York, 1974.

13 Madeleine Leiniger: "Doctoral Programs for Nurses—Trends, Questions, and Projected Plans," *Nursing Research,* vol. 25, pp. 201–210, May–June 1976.

14 *Master's Degrees in Nursing: Routes to Opportunities in Contemporary Nursing,* National League for Nursing, New York, 1976 (pamphlet).

15 Faye G. Abdellah: "Nurse Practitioners and Nursing Practice," *American Journal of Public Health,* vol. 16, pp. 245–246, March 1976.

16 Carolyn R. Aradine: "The Challenge of Clinical Nursing Practice in an Interdisciplinary Office Setting," *Nursing Forum,* vol. 12, pp. 290–302, Summer 1973.

17 Maddy Gerish: Co-Clinical Director of Expansion, Inc., personal conversation.

18 Margaret A. Colliton: *A Case Study in Nursing Therapy,* unpublished doctoral dissertation, Boston University, Boston, 1964.

19 Margaret A. Colliton: "The Nurse as Psychotherapist," paper presented at Yale University School of Medicine, Department of Psychiatry Research Conference, New Haven, Conn., April 1968.

20 Margaret A. Colliton: "The Use of Self in Clinical Practice," *The Nursing Clinics of North America,* vol. 6, pp. 691–694, December 1971.

21 Harriet Goodspeed: Private practice in family therapy, personal conversation.

22 Suzanne Lego: "Nurse Psychotherapists: How Are We Different?" *Perspectives in Psychiatric Care,* vol. 11, pp. 144–147, Winter 1973.

23 Sheila Rouslin: "On Certification of the Clinical Specialist in Psychiatric Nursing," *Perspectives in Psychiatric Care,* vol. 10, p. 201, December 1972.

24 Marcia Stachyra: "Self-Regualtion Through Certification," *Perspectives in Psychiatric Care,* vol. 11, pp. 148–150, Winter 1973.

25 Gertrude B. Ujhely: "The Nurse as Psychotherapist: What Are the Issues?" *Perspectives in Psychiatric Care,* vol. 11, pp. 155–160, Winter 1973.

26 Mary F. Kohnke et al.: *Independent Nurse Practitioner,* Trainex Press, Garden Grove, California, 1974.

Appendix I

Draft of Axes I and II of DSM-III Classification* as of March 30, 1977 American Psychiatric Association

*The traditional neurotic subtypes are included in the Affective, Anxiety, Somatoform, and Dissociative Disorders. (From Task Force on Nomenclature and Statistics, American Psychiatric Association, *Diagnostic and Statistical Manual of Mental Disorders*, 3d ed., APA, New York, April 15, 1977.)

Note: For multiaxial diagnosis, each patient is coded on each of the five axes.

ORGANIC MENTAL DISORDERS

1. This section includes those organic mental disorders in which the etiology or pathogenesis is listed below (taken from the mental disorders section of ICD-9-CM).

Senile and pre-senile dementias

Code organic mental disorder in fifth digit as 1 = (uncomplicated), 2 = with delirium, 3 = with delusional features, 4 = with depressive features, 9 = unspecified.

290.0x	Senile dementia
290.1x	Pre-senile dementia
290.4x	Repeated infarct dementia

Drug induced

Alcohol

291.60	intoxication
291.40	idiosyncratic intoxication (Pathological intoxication)
291.80	withdrawal
291.00	withdrawal delirium (Delirium tremens)
291.30	withdrawal hallucinosis
291.10	amnestic syndrome (Wernicke-Korsakoff syndrome) Barbiturate or related acting sedative or hypnotic
292.01	intoxication
292.81	withdrawal syndromes
292.31	amnestic syndrome

Opioid

292.02	intoxication
292.82	withdrawal

Cocaine

292.03	intoxication

Amphetamine or related acting sympathomimetic

292.04	intoxication
292.14	delirium
292.44	organic delusional syndrome
292.84	withdrawal

Hallucinogen

292.05	intoxication
292.45	organic delusional syndrome
292.65	organic affective syndrome

Cannabis

292.06	intoxication
292.46	organic delusional syndrome
292.76	organic personality syndrome

Tobacco

292.87	withdrawal

Caffeine

292.08	intoxication (caffeinism)

Other, mixed, or unspecified drug

292.09	intoxication
292.19	delirium
292.29	dementia
292.39	amnestic syndrome
292.49	organic delusional syndrome
292.59	hallucinosis
292.69	organic affective syndrome
292.79	organic personality syndrome
292.89	withdrawal
292.99	unspecified organic brain syndrome

2. This section includes those organic mental disorders in which the etiology or pathogenesis is either noted as an additional diagnosis from outside of the mental disorders section of ICD-9-CM (Axis III) or is unknown.

293.00	Delirium
294.10	Dementia

294.00	Amnestic syndrome
293.20	Organic delusional syndrome
293.30	Hallucinosis
293.40	Organic affective syndrome
310.10	Organic personality syndrome
294.80	Other or mixed organic brain syndrome
294.90	Unspecified organic brain syndrome

DRUG USE DISORDERS
(including alcohol)

Code course of illness in fourth (Alcoholism) or fifth digit as 1 = continuous, 2 = episodic, 3 = in remission, 9 = unspecified.

303.x0	Alcohol dependence (Alcoholism)
305.0x	Alcohol abuse
304.1x	Barbiturate or related acting sedative or hypnotic dependence
305.4x	Barbiturate or related acting sedative or hypnotic abuse
304.0x	Opioid dependence
305.5x	Opioid abuse
304.2x	Cocaine dependence
305.6x	Cocaine abuse
304.4x	Amphetamine or related acting sympathomimetic dependence
305.7x	Amphetamine or related acting sympathomimetic abuse
305.3x	Hallucinogen abuse
304.3x	Cannabis dependence
305.2x	Cannabis abuse
305.1x	Tobacco use disorder
304.7x	Combination of opioid type drug with any other dependence
304.8x	Combinations of drug dependence excluding opioid type drug
304.6x	Other specified drug dependence
304.9x	Unspecified drug dependence
305.9x	Other, mixed, or unspecified drug abuse

SCHIZOPHRENIC DISORDERS

Course of illness may be coded in fifth digit as 1 = acute, 2 = subacute, 3 = subchronic, 4 = chronic, 5 = in remission, 9 = unspecified.

295.1x	Disorganized (Hebephrenic)
295.2x	Catatonic
295.3x	Paranoid
295.7x	Schizo-affective, depressed
295.8x	Schizo-affective, manic
295.9x	Undifferentiated
295.6x	Residual

PARANOID DISORDERS

297.10	Paranoia
297.30	Shared paranoid disorder (Folie à deux)
297.00	Paranoid state
297.90	Unspecified paranoid disorder

AFFECTIVE DISORDERS
Episodic affective disorders

Code severity of episode in fifth digit as 1 = mild, 2 = moderate, 3 = severe but not psychotic, 4 = severe and psychotic, 5 = in partial remission, 6 = in full remission, 9 = unspecified.

Manic disorder

| 296.0x | single episode |
| 296.1x | recurrent |

Depressive disorder

| 296.2x | single episode |
| 296.3x | recurrent |

Bipolar affective disorder

296.4x	manic
296.5x	depressed
296.6x	mixed

Intermittent affective disorders

301.11	Intermittent depressive disorder (Depressive character)
301.12	Intermittent hypomanic disorder (Hypomanic personality)
301.13	Intermittent bipolar disorder (Cyclothymic personality)

Atypical affective disorders

296.80 Atypical depressive disorder
296.90 Atypical manic disorder
296.70 Atypical bipolar disorder

PSYCHOSES NOT ELSEWHERE CLASSIFIED

298.80 Brief reactive psychosis
298.90 Atypical psychosis

ANXIETY DISORDERS
Phobic Disorders

300.21 Agoraphobia with panic attacks
300.22 Agoraphobia without panic attacks
300.23 Social phobia
300.24 Simple phobia
300.29 Unspecified phobia
300.01 Panic disorder
300.30 Obsessive compulsive disorder
300.02 Generalized anxiety disorder
300.09 Atypical anxiety disorder

FACTITIOUS DISORDERS

300.15 Factitious illness with psychological symptoms
300.16 Chronic factitious illness with physical symptoms (Munchausen syndrome)
300.17 Other factitious illness with physical symptoms
300.18 Unspecified factitious illness

SOMATOFORM DISORDERS

300.81 Somatization disorder (Briquet's disorder)
300.11 Conversion disorder
307.80 Psychalgia
300.70 Atypical somatoform disorder

DISSOCIATIVE DISORDERS

300.12 Amnesia
300.13 Fugue

300.14 Multiple personality
300.60 Depersonalization
300.19 Other or unspecified

PERSONALITY DISORDERS

Note: These are coded on Axis II.

301.00 Paranoid
301.20 Asocial (Schizoid)
295.50 Schizotypal (Latent, Borderline schizophrenia)
301.50 Histrionic
301.81 Narcissistic
301.70 Antisocial
301.83 Unstable (Borderline personality organization)
301.82 Avoidant
301.60 Dependent
301.40 Compulsive
301.88 Other, mixed, or unspecified

PSYCHOSEXUAL DISORDERS
Gender identity or role disorders

Indicate sexual history in the fifth digit of Transsexualism code as 1 = asexual, 2 = homosexual, 3 = heterosexual, 4 = mixed, 9 = unspecified

302.5x Transsexualism
302.30 Transvestism
302.61 Gender identity or role disorder of childhood
302.62 Other gender identity or role disorders of adult life

Paraphilias

302.81 Fetishism
302.10 Zoophilia
302.20 Pedophilia
302.00 Dyshomophilia
302.40 Exhibitionism
302.82 Voyeurism
302.83 Sexual masochism
302.84 Sexual sadism
302.85 Other

Psychosexual dysfunctions

302.71	with inhibited sexual desire
302.72	with inhibited sexual excitement (frigidity, impotence)
302.73	with inhibited female orgasm
302.74	with inhibited male orgasm
302.75	with premature ejaculation
302.76	with functional dyspareunia
302.77	with functional vaginismus
302.78	other
302.79	unspecified

Other psychosexual disorders

302.90	Psychosexual disorder not elsewhere classified

DISORDERS USUALLY ARISING IN CHILDHOOD OR ADOLESCENCE

This section lists conditions that usually manifest themselves in childhood or adolescence. However, any appropriate adult diagnosis can be used for diagnosing a child.

Mental retardation

Code a 1 in the fifth digit to indicate association with a known biological factor which must be coded on Axis III. Otherwise code 0.

317.0x	Mild mental retardation
318.0x	Moderate mental retardation
318.1x	Severe mental retardation
318.2x	Profound mental retardation
319.0x	Unspecified mental retardation

Pervasive developmental disorders

299.00	Infantile autism
299.80	Early childhood psychosis
299.20	Pervasive developmental disorder of childhood, residual state
299.90	Unspecified

Attention deficit orders

314.00	with hyperactivity
314.10	without hyperactivity

Specific developmental disorders

Note: These are coded on Axis II.

315.00	Specific reading disorder
315.10	Specific arithmetical disorder
315.30	Developmental language disorder
315.40	Developmental articulation disorder
315.50	Coordination disorder

Indicate course in the fifth digit as 1 = primary, 2 = secondary, 9 = unspecified.

307.6x	Enuresis
307.7x	Encopresis
315.60	Mixed
315.80	Other
315.90	Unspecified

Stereotyped movement disorders

307.21	Motor tic disorder
307.22	Motor-verbal tic disorder (Gilles de la Tourette)
307.29	Unspecified tic disorder
307.30	Other

Speech disorders not elsewhere classified

307.00	Stuttering
307.91	Elective mutism

Conduct disorders

Code severity in fifth digit as 1 = mild, 2 = moderate, 3 = severe, 9 = unspecified.

312.0x	Undersocialized conduct disorder, aggressive type
312.1x	Undersocialized conduct disorder, unaggressive type
312.2x	Socialized conduct disorder

Eating Disorders

307.10	Anorexia nervosa
307.51	Bulimia
307.52	Pica
307.53	Rumination
307.58	Other or unspecified

Anxiety disorders of childhood or adolescence

309.21	Separation anxiety disorder
313.20	Shyness disorder
313.00	Overanxious disorder

Disorders characteristic of late adolescence

309.22	Emancipation disorder of adolescence or early adult life
313.60	Identity disorder
309.23	Specific academic or work inhibition

Other disorders of childhood or adolescence

313.50	Oppositional disorder
313.70	Academic underachievement disorder

REACTIVE DISORDERS NOT ELSEWHERE CLASSIFIED

309.81	Post traumatic disorder

Adjustment disorders

300.40	with depressed mood
309.28	with anxious mood
309.24	with mixed emotional features
309.82	with physical symptoms
309.30	with distrubance of conduct
309.40	with mixed disturbance of emotions and conduct
309.83	with withdrawal
309.90	other or unspecified

DISORDERS OF IMPULSE CONTROL NOT ELSEWHERE CLASSIFIED

312.31	Pathological gambling
312.32	Kleptomania
312.33	Pyromania
312.34	Intermittent explosive disorder
312.35	Isolated explosive disorder
312.38	Other or unspecified impulse control disorder

SLEEP DISORDERS

Non-organic

307.41	Temporary insomnia
307.42	Persistent insomnia
307.43	Temporary hypersomnia
307.44	Persistent hypersomnia
307.45	Non-organic sleep-wake cycle disturbance
307.46	Somnambulism
307.47	Night terrors
307.48	Other non-organic dyssomnias
307.49	Unspecified non-organic sleep disorder

Organic

780.51	Insomnia associated with diseases elsewhere classified
780.52	Insomnia with central sleep-apnea
780.53	Other organic insomnia
780.54	Hypersomnia associated with diseases elsewhere classified
780.55	Hypersomnia associated with obstructive or mixed sleep-apnea
780.56	Other organic hypersomnia
780.57	Organic sleep-wake cycle disturbance
780.58	Organic dyssomnias
780.59	Unspecified organic sleep disorder

OTHER DISORDERS AND CONDITIONS

Unspecified mental disorder (non-psychotic)

307.99	Unspecified mental disorder (non-psychotic)

Psychic factors in physical condition

Specify physical condition on Axis III and degree of psychological component in the fourth digit as 1 = probable, 2 = prominent, 9 = unknown or unspecified degree.

316.x0	Psychic factors in physical condition

No mental disorder

V71.00	No mental disorder

Conditions not attributable to a known mental disorder

V65.20	Malingering
V71.01	Adult antisocial behavior
V71.02	Childhood or adolescent antisocial behavior
V61.10	Marital problem
V61.20	Parent-child problem
V62.81	Other interpersonal problem

V62.20	Occupational problem
V62.82	Simple bereavement
V15.81	Noncompliance with medical treatment
V62.88	Other life circumstance problem

Administrative categories

799.90	Diagnosis deferred
V70.70	Research subject
V63.20	Boarder
V68.30	Referral without need for evaluation

American Nurses' Association Standards of Psychiatric and Mental Health Nursing Practice

Psychiatric Nursing is a specialized area of nursing practice employing theories of human behavior as its scientific aspect and purposeful use of self as its art. It is directed toward both preventive and corrective impacts upon mental illness and is concerned with the promotion of optimal mental health for society, the community, and those individuals and families who live within it. The dependent area of Psychiatric Nursing Practice is implementation of physicians' orders. The independent areas are assessment of nursing needs and development and implementation of nursing-care plans, including initiation, development and termination of therapeutic relationships between nurses and patients. Psychiatric Nursing is practiced largely in collaboration and coordination with those in a variety of other disciplines who are working concomantly with the patient. Thus, a high degree of interdependence with colleagues from other professions is inherent.

The Practice of Psychiatric Nursing is characterized by those aspects of clinical nursing care that involve interpersonal relationships with individuals and groups as well as a variety of other activities. These activities include: providing a therapeutic milieu, concerned largely with the sociopsychologic aspects of patients' environments; working with patients concerning the here-and-now living problems they confront; accepting and using the surrogate parent role; teaching with specific reference to emotional health as evidenced by various behavioral patterns; assuming the role of social agent concerned with improvement and promotion of recreational, occupational and social competence; providing leadership and clinical assistance to other nursing personnel. Joint planning or cooperative and collaborative efforts with other professionals are an essential part of providing nursing service. Most psychiatric settings employ an interdisciplinary team approach which requires highly coordinated and frequently interdependent planning.

Direct nursing-care functions may involve individual psychotherapy, group psychotherapy, family therapy and sociotherapy. Psychiatric Nurs-

es engaged in these therapies may employ a variety of approaches, particularly in the rapidly emerging area of sociotherapy and community mental health. With the national trend toward community mental health Psychiatric Nurses are more and more involved in providing services aimed toward prevention of mental illness and reinforcement of health adaptations in addition to corrective and rehabilitative services.

The indirect nursing-care roles of the Psychiatric Nurse are those of administrator with emphasis on leadership functions; clinical supervisor with emphasis on leadership functions as well as clinical teaching; director of staff development and training in a clinical facility; consultant or resource person, and researcher. In some of these indirect care roles, nurses will also be involved in providing some direct nursing care services to improve their own clinical skills and to serve as role models. All of these roles require coordinative and collaborative efforts with other disciplines.

The purpose of Standards of Psychiatric Nursing Practice is to fulfill the profession's obligation to provide and improve this practice. The Standards focus on practice. They provide a means for determining the quality of nursing which a client receives regardless of whether such services are provided solely by a professional nurse or by professional nurse and nonprofessional assistants.

The Standards are stated according to a systematic approach to nursing practice: the assessment of the client's status, the plan of nursing actions, the implementation of the plan, and the evaluation. These specific divisions are not intended to imply that practice consists of a series of discrete steps, taken in strict sequence, beginning with assessment and ending with evaluation. The processes described are used concurrently and recurrently. Assessment, for example, frequently continues during implementation; similarly, evaluation dictates reassessment and replanning.

These Standards of Psychiatric Nursing Practice apply to nursing practice in any setting. Nursing practice in all settings must possess the characteristics identified by these Standards if patients are to receive a high quality of nursing care. Each Standard is followed by a rationale and assessment factors. Assessment factors are to be used in determining achievement of the Standard.

Standard I

Data Are Collected Through Pertinent Clinical Observations Based On Knowledge Of The Arts and Sciences, With Particular Emphasis Upon Psychosocial And Biophysical Sciences.

Rationale: Clinical observation is a prerequisite to realistic assessment of a client's needs and for the formulation of appropriate intervention. Observations can be facilitated through knowledge derived from a broad general education. In addition, scholarship acquired in the study of psychosocial and biophysical sciences fosters acuity of perception and alerts the nurse to psychologic, cultural, social, and other relevant clinical data.

Assessment Factors:

1. Data collecting activities involve observation, analysis and interpretation of behavior patterns of clients which indicate a need for growth promoting relationships.
2. Data collecting activities involve identification of significant areas in which clinical data are needed.
3. Data collecting activities involve utilization of knowledge derived from appropriate sources to gain a comprehensive grasp of the client's experience.
4. Data collecting activities involve inferences drawn from observations, which contribute to a formulation of therapeutic intervention.
5. Data collecting activities involve inferences and treatment observations which are shared and validated with appropriate others.

Standard II

Clients Are Involved In The Assessment, Planning, Implementation, And Evaluation Of Their Nursing-Care Program To The Fullest Extent Of Their Capabilities.

Rationale: To a very large degree, the therapeutic process is a learning process. The same principle that applies to learning also applies to therapy; that is, the learner or client must be an active participant in the process. The ability to participate in such a process will vary from person to person and, at times, even within the same person. The word "therapy" is used here in its broadest sense; that is, any behavior or planned activity that promotes growth and well-being. Thus, "nursing-care program" and "nursing therapy" are interchangeably used, although it is recognized that many other forms of therapy exist.

Assessment Factors:

1. Clients' capabilities to participate at any given time are assessed, always keeping in mind the ultimate goals mutually determined by the client and nurse.
2. Plans for achieving and re-examining the goals are developed with the client, making whatever readjustments are necessary to progress toward them.
3. Problems are identified in collaboration with the client to determine needs and to set goals.
4. Progress of clients toward mutual goal achievement is assessed.

Standard III

The Problem-Solving Approach Is Utilized In Developing Nursing Care Plans.

Rationale: A nursing diagnosis is based on pertinent theories of human behavior. It is used to plan therapeutic intervention taking into consideration the characteristics and capacities of the individual and his environment in order to maximize the treatment program for the client.

Assessment Factors:

1. The individual's reaction to the environment is observed and assessed.
2. Themes and patterns of the behavior are observed and assessed.
3. Nursing care plans are used as a guide to nursing intervention.
4. Nursing-care plans are interpreted to professional and nonprofessional persons giving care.
5. Observations and reports of others are incorporated in the nursing care plans.
6. Nursing care plans are designed, implemented, and reviewed systematically by the nursing staff.

Standard IV

Individuals, Families, And Community Groups Are Assisted To Achieve Satisfying And Productive Patterns Of Living Through Health Teaching.

Rationale: Health teaching is an essential part of a nurse's role in work with those who have mental health problems. Every interaction can be utilized as a teaching-learning situation. Formal or informal teaching methods can be used in working with individuals, families, the community and other personnel. Emphasis is on understanding mental health problems as well as on developing ways of coping with them.

Assessment Factors:

1. The needs of individual, family and community groups for health teaching are identified and appropriate techniques are used in meeting these needs.
2. The principles of learning and teaching are employed.
3. The basic principles of physical and mental health and interpersonal and social skills are taught.

4. Experiential learning opportunities are made available.
5. Opportunities with community groups to further their knowledge and understanding of mental health problems are identified.

Standard V

The Activities Of Daily Living Are Utilized In A Goal Directed Way In Work With Clients.

Rationale: A major portion of one's daily life is spent in some form of activity related to health and well-being. An individual's developmental and intellectual level, emotional state and physical limitations may be reflected in these activities. Therefore, nursing has a unique opportunity to assess and intervene in these processes in order to encourage constructive changes in the client's behavior, so that each person may realize his full potential for growth.

Assessment Factors:

1. An appraisal is made of the client's capacities to participate in activities of daily living based on needs, strengths, and levels of functioning.
2. Clients are encouraged toward independence and self-direction by various skills such as motivating, limit setting, persuading, guiding and comforting.
3. Each person's rights are appreciated and respected.
4. Methods of communicating are devised which assure consistency in approach.

Standard VI

Knowledge Of Somatic Therapies And Related Clinical Skills Are Utilized In Working With Clients.

Rationale: Various treatment modalities may be needed by clients during the course of illness. Pertinent clinical observations and judgments are made concerning the effect of drugs and other treatments used in the therapeutic program.

Assessment Factors:

1. Pertinent reactions to somatic therapies are observed and interpreted in terms of the underlying principles of each therapy.
2. A patient's responses are observed and reported.
3. The effectiveness of somatic therapies is judged and subsequent recommendations for changes in the treatment plan are made.
4. The safety and emotional support of clients receiving therapies is provided.
5. Opportunities are provided for clients and families to discuss, question and explore their feelings and concerns about past, current or projected use of somatic therapies.

Standard VII

The Environment Is Structured To Establish And Maintain A Therapeutic Milieu.

Rationale: Any environment is composed of both human and nonhuman resources which may work for or against the person's well-being. The nurse works with people in a variety of environmental settings, e.g. hospital, home, etc. The milieu is structured and/or altered so that it serves the client's best interests as an inherent part of the overall therapeutic plan.

Assessment Factors:

1. The effects of environmental forces on individuals are observed, analyzed and interpreted.
2. Psychological, physiological, social, economical and cultural concepts are understood and utilized in developing and maintaining a therapeutic milieu.
3. Communications within the environment are congruent with therapeutic goals.
4. All available resources in the environment are utilized when appropriate in the therapeutic efforts.

5. Nursing participation and its effectiveness in establishing and maintaining a therapeutic milieu are evaluated.

Standard VIII

Nursing Participates With Interdisciplinary Teams In Assessing, Planning, Implementing And Evaluating Programs And Other Mental Health Activities.

Rationale: In addition to the nurse, the number and variety of people working with clients in the mental health field today make it imperative that efforts be coordinated to provide the best total program. Communication, planning, problem solving and evaluation are required of all those who work with a particular client or program.

Assessment Factors:

1. Specific knowledge, skills and activities are identified and articulated so these may be coordinated with the contributions of others working with a client or a program.
2. The value of nursing and team-member contributions are recognized and respected.
3. Consultation with other team members is utilized as needed.
4. Nursing participates in the formulating of overall goals, plans and decisions.
5. Skills are developed in small group process for maximum team effectiveness.

Standard IX

Psychotherapeutic Interventions Are Used To Assist Clients To Achieve Their Maximum Development.

Rationale: People with mental health problems fashion many of their patterns of living and relating to others on a psychopathologic basis. In order to help clients achieve better adaptation and improved health, a nurse assists them to identify that which is useful and that which is not useful in their modes of living and relating. Alternatives available to them are identified.

Assessment Factors:

1. Useful patterns and themes in the client's interactions with others are re-enforced.

2. Clients are assisted to identify, test out and evaluate more constructive alternatives to unsatisfactory patterns of living.

3. Principles of communication, problem solving, interviewing and crisis intervention are employed in carrying through psychotherapeutic intervention.

4. Knowledge of psychopathology and its healthy, adaptive counterparts are used in planning and implementing programs of care.

5. Limits are set on behavior that is destructive to self or others with the ultimate goal of assisting clients to develop their own internal controls and more constructive ways of dealing with feelings.

6. Crisis intervention is used to reduce panic of disturbed patients.

7. Long-term psychotherapeutic relationships with clients are undertaken.

8. Colleagues are utilized in evaluating the progress of the psychotherapeutic relationships and in formulating modification of intervention techniques.

9. Nursing participation in the therapeutic relationship is evaluated and modified as necessary.

Standard X

The Practice Of Individual, Group Or Family Psychotherapy Requires Appropriate Preparation And Recognition Of Accountability For The Practice.

Rationale: Acceptance of the role of therapist entails primary responsibility for the treatment of clients and entrance into a contractual agreement. This contract includes a commitment to see a client through the problem he presents or, if this becomes impossible, to assist him in finding other appropriate assistance. It also includes an explicit definition of the relationship, the respective roles of each person in the relationship, and what can realistically be expected of each person.

Assessment Factors:

1. The potential of the nurse to function as a primary therapist is evaluated.

2. The accountability for practicing psychotherapy is recognized and accepted.

3. Knowledge of growth and development, psychopathology, psychosocial systems and small group and family dynamics is utilized in the therapeutic process.

4. The terms of the contract between the nurse and the client, including the structure of time, place, fees, etc., that may be involved, are made explicitly clear.

5. Supervision or consultation is sought whenever indicated and other learning opportunities are used to further develop knowledge and skills.

6. The effectiveness of the work with an individual, family or group is routinely assessed.

Standard XI

Nursing Participates With Other Members Of The Community In Planning And Implementing Mental Health Services That Include The Broad Continuum Of Promotion Of Mental Health, Prevention Of Mental Illness, Treatment And Rehabilitation.

Rationale: In our contemporary society, the high incidence of mental illness and mental retardation requires increased effort to devise more effective treatment and prevention programs. There is a need for nursing to participate in programs that strengthen the existing health potential of all members of society. In this effort cooperation and collaboration by all community agencies becomes imperative.

Such concepts as early intervention and continuity of care are essential in planning to meet the mental health needs of the community. The nurse uses organizational, advisory or consultative skills to facilitate the development and implementation of mental health services.

Assessment Factors:

1. Knowledge of community and group dynamics is used to understand the structure and function of the community system.

2. Current social issues that influence the nature of mental health problems in the community are recognized.

3. High-risk population groups in the community are delineated and gaps in community services are identified.

4. Community members are encouraged to become active in assessing community mental health needs and planning programs to meet these needs.

5. The strength and capacities of individuals, families and the community are assessed in order to promote and increase the health potential of all.

6. Consultative skills are used to facilitate the development and implementation of mental health services.

7. The needs of the community are brought to the attention of appropriate individuals and groups, including legislative bodies and regional and state planning groups.

8. The mental health services of the agency are interpreted to others in the community. There is collaboration with the staff of other agencies to insure continuity of service for patients and families.

9. Community resources are used appropriately.

10. Nursing participates with other professional and nonprofessional members of the community in the planning, implementation and evaluation of mental health services.

Standard XII

Learning Experiences Are Provided For Other Nursing-Care Personnel Through Leadership, Supervision, And Teaching.

Rationale: As leader of the nursing team, the nurse is responsible for the team's activities, and must be able to teach, supervise and evaluate the performance of nursing care personnel. The focus is on the continuing development of each member of the team.

Assessment Factors:

1. Leadership roles and responsibilities are accepted.

2. Team members are encouraged to identify strengths and abilities. A climate is provided for the continuing self-development of each member.

3. A role model in giving direct nursing care is provided for the team.

4. The supervisory role is used as a tool for improving nursing care.

5. The client's needs, as well as the abilities of each member of the nursing team, are evaluated and assignments are based on these evaluations.

Standard XIII

Responsibility Is Assumed For Continuing Educational And Professional Development And Contributions Are Made To The Professional Growth Of Others.

Rationale: The scientific, cultural and social changes characterizing our contemporary society require the nurse to be committed to the ongoing pursuit of knowledge which will enhance professional growth.

Assessment Factors:

1. There is evidence of study of one's nursing practice to increase both understanding and skill.

2. There is evidence of participation in inservice meetings and educational pro-

grams either as an attendee or as a teacher.

3. There is evidence of attendance at conventions, institutes, workshops, symposia and other professionally oriented meetings and/or other ways to increase formal education.

4. There is evidence of systematic efforts to increase understanding of psychodynamics, psychopathology, and avenues of psychotherapeutic intervention.

5. There is evidence of cognizance of developments in relevant fields and utilization of this knowledge.

6. There is evidence of assisting others to identify areas of educational needs.

7. There is evidence of sharing appropriate clinical observations and interpretations with professionals and other groups.

Standard XIV

Contributions To Nursing And The Mental Health Field Are Made Through Innovations In Theory And Practice And Participation In Research.

Rationale: Each professional has responsibility for the continuing development and refinement of knowledge in the mental health field through research and experimentation with new and creative approaches to practice.

Assessment Factors:

1. Studies are developed, implemented and evaluated.

2. Responsible standards of research are used in investigative endeavors.

3. Nursing practice is approached with an inquiring and open mind.

4. The pertinent and responsible research of others is supported.

5. Expert consultation and/or supervision is sought as required. Judgment is used in assessing abilities as well as limitations to engage in research.

6. The ability to discriminate those findings which are pertinent to the advancement of nursing practice is demonstrated.

7. Innovations in theory, practice and research findings are made available through presentations and/or publications.

Glossary

A

Abreaction The expression of emotions connected with distressing, anxiety-provoking, repressed ideas. This often occurs when such ideas are brought up during therapy.

ACTH (adrenocorticotrophic hormone) Substance produced by the pituitary which stimulates the adrenal cortex.

Acting out The active expression (through *actions,* not words) of emotion that occurs when the client relives or reproduces the feelings, wishes, or conflicts which are operating unconsciously.

Adaptational energy The body's capacity to cope with stressors.

Addiction Compulsive use of chemical substances, involving physical and psychological dependence.

Adjustment A person's relation to society and to his or her inner self.

Adolescence Period of growth and development from puberty to maturity.

Adultery Voluntary coitus on the part of a married person with someone other than his or her spouse.

Adulthood stage Stage of growth and development that follows adolescence.

Affect Emotional feeling tone attached to an object, idea, or thought; includes inner feelings and their external manifestations.

Affective psychosis A psychotic reaction in which the predominant feature is a disturbance in emotional feeling tone, usually depression or elation.

Aggression A feeling or action that is self-assertive, forceful, or hostile.

Agitation State of anxiety associated with severe motor restlessness.

Agnosia Disturbance of perception characterized by inability to recognize a stimulus (e.g., a familiar object) or to interpret the significance of its memory impressions.

Agoraphobia Fear of the outdoors or going out; especially alone. It is the most common phobia.

Akathisia Continuous uncontrolled muscular movements and restlessness.

Alienation The feeling of being detached from oneself or society, the avoidance of emotional experiences, or generalized estrangement.

Ambivalence The simultaneous presence of strong, often overwhelming, but contradictory attitudes, ideas, feelings, and drives toward an object, person, goal, or situation.

Amenorrhea Absence of menstruation.

Amnesia A dissociative experience in which a person's recollection is lost or split off from conscious recall. The cause of amnesia may be organic or functional.

Amniocentesis Procedure whereby a sample of amniotic fluid is obtained from the uterus during pregnancy.

Anabolism Constructive metabolism in which body substances are repaired and/or built up.

Anal stage In Freud's framework, the stage of growth and development lasting from 18 months to 3 years.

Analogic communication Nonverbal communication.

Anger A feeling of displeasure which results from a challenge to one's perceived rights of authority and influence in interpersonal situations and which enables one to defend against the powerlessness of anxiety.

Anilingus Oral stimulation of the anal area.

Anovulation Absence of ovulation.

Anxiety Continuum of discomfort ranging from mild to panic level; unpleasurable affect consisting of psychophysiological changes in response to an intrapsychic conflict.

Apathy Lack of feeling or affect; lack of interest or emotional involvement in one's surroundings.

Aphasia Disturbance or loss of ability to comprehend, elaborate, or express speech concepts; inability to speak, comprehend, name an object, and/or arrange words in proper sequence.

Artificial insemination Process of medically instilling sperm, from a donor who may or may not be her husband, into a woman's cervix.

"As if" behavior Superficially acceptable behavior that is adopted in a defensive effort to conceal unacceptable feelings and aims and to ignore one's underlying feelings of powerlessness in interpersonal situations.

Assaultiveness Violent behavior involving a physical or verbal attack on another.

Assertive behavior An expression of emotion that is appropriate to the existing situation, as opposed to the expression of subjective anxiety (anxiety unrelated to the facts of the matter).

Ataxia Incoordination or involuntary movement.

Attachment phase Bonding of mother and infant.

Atypical developmental psychosis Psychotic process in early childhood characterized by autistic and/or symbiotic behaviors.

Aura A sensation—such as fear or olfactory, auditory, or visual hallucinations—experienced by a person just before a grand mal seizure; a peculiar epigastric sensation or a welling up in the throat.

Autistic thinking A form of thinking that attempts to gratify unfulfilled needs and desires in a way that is not reality-oriented. Objective facts are distorted, obscured, or excluded to varying degrees and personal and private meanings are applied to situations and words.

Autoaggression Aggression directed against the self.

Autoeroticism Sexual self-arousal without the participation of another person. The term "autoeroticism" is sometimes used interchangeably with "masturbation."

Autonomy A condition characterized by independence or self-governance.

Autosome Any chromosome other than X or Y, the sex chromosome.

Aversion therapy Therapy that involves the giving of unpleasant or obnoxious feedback to inhibit an undesired response.

B

Behavior modification A method of re-education based on the principles of Pavlovian conditioning. Some of the methods are response prevention, modeling, desensitization, shaping, flooding, and implosion.

Birth defect Structural abnormality appearing in an infant at birth; may or may not be genetic in origin.

Bisexual A person who enjoys sexual contacts with members of both sexes.

Bizarre behavior Eccentric behavior, or actions which do not conform to social expectations in a particular situation.

Blocking Involuntary cessation of thought processes or speech because of unconscious emotional factors; also known as thought deprivation.

Blunting of affect A disturbance of affect manifested by dullness of externalized feeling tone.

Body image One's perception, conscious and unconscious, of one's own body.

C

Castration Surgical removal of testes in male and ovaries in female.

Catatonic state (catatonia) A state characterized by immobility, with muscular rigidity or inflexibility. The catatonic state may also be manifested by excitability.

Cathexis A conscious or unconscious investment of psychic energy in an idea, concept, or object.

Change agent An outside force or person acting for another in a deliberate effort to improve a situation.

Childhood psychosis A basic disorder of personality manifested by disturbances in thinking, affect, perception, motility, speech, reality testing, and object relations.

Circumstantiality Disturbance in associative thought processes in which the person digresses into unnecessary details and inappropriate thoughts before communicating the central idea.

Cognition Mental process of knowing or becoming aware.

Cohesiveness Group phenomenon; the resultant of all forces acting on members to remain in the group; a sense of group belongingness.

Coitus The sex act; copulation; intercourse; penetration of penis into vagina.

Commitment The act of hospitalizing persons for psychiatric treatment through legal means.

Community meeting Large group meeting held at regularly scheduled intervals; prime characteristic of a therapeutic community.

Complementarity Term referring to the two-sidedness of relationships, where both parties provide both stimuli and responses. All interaction involves complementarity.

Compulsion An irrational urge to act which cannot be resisted without extreme difficulty.

Concreteness The clear, direct expression of personally relevant perceptions, values, and feelings as they exist in the present relationship.

Conditioning A process which involves associating a certain stimulus (or stimuli) with a predictable behavioral response or response pattern.

Confabulation Compensating for memory loss by filling in the memory gaps with imaginary stories which the teller believes to be true.

Confirmation True positive or negative information relevant to the current situation; validation.

Conflict Clash between two opposing emotional forces.

Confrontation Communications that call attention to significant discrepancies in another's experience; verbal messages which are intended to help another to recognize information which is not consistent with the other's self-image.

Confusion A state of mental perplexity or bewilderment resulting from disorientation.

Conscious A term describing all the elements of thought that come to mind readily.

Consensual validation The verification of reality with someone else.

Consumer Client or person accepting health services; the public.

Conversion A process whereby repressed instinctual tendencies are expressed through (or "converted" into) sensory or motor manifestations, such as paralysis of a limb or blindness, which has no organic basis.

Counterphobia Denoting a state of actual preference on the part of the phobic person for the very situation of which he or she is afraid.

Countertransference Conscious or unconscious emotional response of the therapist to the client; through countertransference, the therapist transfers onto the client feelings, wishes, and conflicts which originated in the therapist's own relationships with significant others.

Crime Conduct that is in violation of the law.

Crisis A turning point in a person's life; a conflict or problem of basic importance perceived as hazardous which cannot readily be solved by using the usual coping mechanisms; a state of psychological disequilibrium.

Crisis intervention Intervention process aimed at reestablishing a level of functioning equal to or better than that of the precrisis level.

Culture The organized set of customs, habits, ideas, and beliefs shared by a group of people.

Cunnilingus Oral stimulation of female genitalia.

D

Defense mechanisms Operations outside of awareness which the ego calls into play to protect against anxiety; coping mechanisms.

Delirium A disturbance in the state of consciousness that stems from an acute organic reaction.

Delirium tremens (alcohol withdrawal syndrome) Delirium induced by prolonged and excessive use of alcohol.

Delusion A false, fixed idea that arises within the individual without appropriate external stimulation; an idea that is inconsistent with the person's knowledge and experience. The following are examples of delusions:

Delusion of control/influence False belief that one is being controlled by others

Delusion of grandeur/importance A false belief in which one's own importance is greatly exaggerated

Delusion of infidelity A false belief that one's lover or spouse is unfaithful

Delusion of persecution A false belief that one is being harassed by others

Delusion, somatic A false belief about one's body or organ systems wherein the focus is on one's physical condition

Dementia Organic loss of mental functioning.

Denial An unconscious mental mechanism whereby one refuses to acknowledge or attempts to deny some anxiety-provoking aspect of self or external reality.

Dependency An individual's reliance on others to meet basic needs for love, affection, mothering, shelter, protection, security, food, and warmth.

Depersonalization An affective disturbance in which the individual experiences feelings of unreality or strangeness concerning either the environment, the self, or both.

Depression A pathological state precipitated by feelings of loss and/or guilt, characterized by sadness and a lowering of self-esteem.

Detachment The condition of being separated or apart.

Detumescence The penis's return to its flaccid state following erection and ejaculation.

Developmental lag Physical or emotional development which is less than that expected for a child's chronological age.

Deviance A marked difference (e.g., in behavior or endowment) from what is considered acceptable or normal in a given society.

Differentiation A process characterized by increasing complexity, integration of functions, and sense of uniqueness in an individual. Under optimal conditions, an individual moves from a relative lack of differentiation to a more highly differentiated state.

Digital communication Verbal communication.

Disconfirmation A transpersonal defense mechanism whereby a person denies the truth and confirms false images held by another.

Discrimination The ability to notice the similarities and differences in like situations.

Disjunction The process of refusing to fall in with the views of a group, or insisting on an image that is different from the group's collective image.

Disordered thinking Cognitive ideational or informational experience characterized by lapses from logical thinking, use of neologisms, circumstantiality, primary-process thought, and blocking.

Disorientation A loss of one's bearings or position with respect to time, place, and/or identity.

Displacement Unconscious defense mechanism; refers to the discharge of emotions, feelings, or ideas upon a subject other than the one that elicited the feelings.

Dissociality Sociopathic behavior patterns evident in criminals, prostitutes, and others who ignore societal restrictions; lack of awareness of right and wrong.

Dissociation The unwitting splitting off from conscious awareness of those aspects of experience that are intensely anxiety-provoking; such experience comprises the "not-me" component of the self-system.

Double-bind communication A message in which a person is commanded both to do and not to do something, so that no adequate response is possible.

Dream analysis A technique used in helping unconscious material to become conscious; the interpretation of the symbolism contained in the reported dream.

Drive Motivation; can be either biological or learned.

Dysattention A failure to focus attention on those elements of the environment that are most relevant to the tasks at hand, ranging from distractibility to complete inattention to, or loss of contact with, the environment.

Dysmenesia Impairment in the ability to retain and recall information.

E

Echolalia Automatic repetition by one person of what is said by another.

Echopraxia Meaningless imitation of motions made by others.

ECT (electroconvulsive therapy) Therapeutic use of an electric current to produce a convulsive seizure and unconsciousness.

EEG (electroencephalogram) A tracing to record electrical discharges in the brain.

Ego The aspect of personality that appraises the environment, assesses reality, stays in touch with bodily and environmental changes, and directs the motor activity of the body.

Ego ideal Part of the developing ego that eventually fuses with the superego.

Ego strength The relative ability of the ego to maintain a sense of reality, to keep unconscious material buried, and to deal effectively with the forces of id and superego.

Ejaculation In the male, the transport of semen out of the body.

Electra complex Erotic attachment of female child to father.

Elope To leave a treatment setting without the awareness of the caretakers or permission from them.

Empathic understanding The temporary experiencing of another's feelings; expressions which convey recognition of the feelings, motives, and meanings underlying another individual's communications.

Empathy An objective and insightful awareness of the feelings, emotions, and behavior of another person, their meaning and significance; to be distinguished from sympathy, which is usually more subjective.

Environment The patterned wholeness of all that is external to an individual (i.e., persons, places, or things). A change in any part of the environment affects the total system and the behavior of persons, places, or things.

Environmental supports Those material objects in the environment that the client depends on in time of stress. Examples include financial supports, adequate housing, and employment.

Euphoria Exaggerated feeling of physical and emotional well-being that is not congruent with objective stimuli or events. It may have a psychogenic origin or be due to organic brain syndrome.

Extended family The nuclear family and others related by descent, marriage, or adoption.

Extinction Lack of reinforcement of behavior patterns, designed to decrease the rate of response.

F

Family ego mass The undifferentiated aspect of the family system which retards the individual's growth as a separate, unique person.

Family therapy Treatment which involves the total family or specific family members who meet to explore relationships and process; focus is more on the resolution of current reactions to one another than on individual members.

Fantasy Daydream; fabricated mental picture.

Fear An experience having both psychological and physiological components, stimulated by an awareness of impending danger in the environment; an activating emotion.

Fellatio Oral stimulation of male genitalia.

Fetishism The association of sexual pleasure with inanimate objects.

Fixation The concentration of psychic energy at the stage(s) of psychosexual development where one's needs have been over- or undergratified.

Flat affect A form of mood change in which there is a loss of feeling tone, so that the individual often feels "blah," inert, and incapable of any emotional display.

Flight of ideas Sudden, rapid shift from one idea to another before the preceding one has been concluded.

Flooding The use of real or imaginary situations to evoke strong anxiety responses.

Fornication Voluntary coitus between a man and a woman who are not married.

Free association A technique used in encouraging unconscious material to become conscious; unselected verbalization by the client of whatever comes to mind.

Freezing A technique in family therapy; a family member pantomines a situation that is problematic, then freezes at that point.

Frigidity Inability of the female to achieve orgasm.

Frustration A feeling which results when barriers interfere with one's attainment of goals.

Fugue state A dissociative state characterized by amnesia and actual physical flight from an intolerable situation.

Fusion An emotional oneness with the family ego mass; enmeshment of family members.

G

Generalization The tendency to transfer the things learned in one situation to other, similar situations.

Genetic endowment Inherited traits, potentials, and capacities.

Genital stage In Freud's framework, the stage of growth and development lasting from 12 years to early adulthood.

Genuineness Spontaneous expressions which convey an individual's inner experience.

Gestalt therapy The treatment of persons as wholes. It focuses on the person's sensory awareness in the here and now rather than on past recollections or future expectations.

Grandiosity An exaggerated and unrealistic sense of one's worth, powers, or influence.

Grief A normal emotional response to recognized loss; it is self-limiting and gradually subsides within a reasonable time as new object investments occur.

Grieving Process of separating from a highly valued person, place, object, or ideal.

Group norm An idea in the minds of group members that can be put in the form of a statement specifying what the members ought or are expected to do under given circumstances.

Group therapy Type of treatment involving two or more clients participating together in the presence of one or more psychotherapists.

Guilt A global feeling of incompetence and self-blame generated by the acceptance of responsibility for wrongdoing or losses which have occurred. The person usually judges self by unrealistic criteria.

H

Habituation Repeated use of substances such as drugs or alcohol, accompanied by psychological dependence.

Hallucination A false sensory perception involving any of the senses, without corresponding stimuli.

Hebephrenic state A state characterized by disorganized thinking, superficial and inappropriate affect, unpredictable laughter, silly and regressive behavior and mannerisms, and frequently hypochondriacal complaints. Delusions and hallucinations, if present, are transient and not well organized.

Helicy Homeodynamic principle which states that the life process evolves unidirectionally in sequential stages; encompasses the concepts of rhythm and evolution and the unitary nature of the individual-environment relationship.

Helplessness Global feeling of inability to act on one's own behalf and inefficiency in making an impact on one's environment to create change.

Homeostasis A tendency to uniformity or stability in the individual's normal body states.

Hopelessness A companion feeling to helplessness; consists of feelings of being doomed to live in the eternal present with no opportunities for change.

Hostility A feeling of animosity or enmity toward another which is subjectively similar to anger but is of longer duration and characterized by wishes to harm the other.

Hyperemia Excess of blood in a body part.

Hyperphagia Overeating.

Hypomania A mild form of mania in which the person appears to be highly energetic, happy, friendly, outgoing, lively, witty, and productive.

Hypochondriasis A morbid preoccupation with one's state of health, either physical or emotional, accompanied by various bodily complaints without demonstrable organic pathology.

Hysteria A category of psychoneurosis characterized by sensory, motor, or psychic disturbances.

I

Id In psychoanalytic theory, a term used to denote the unconscious part of the personality that contains primitive urges and desires. It is ruled by the pleasure principle.

Ideas of reference Ideas stemming from the incorrect interpretation of incidents as having direct reference to the self.

Identification Unconscious defense mechanism in which a person becomes like something or someone else in one or several aspects of thought or behavior. This adds to ego development but does not replace the person's own ego. The personality consists of multiple identifications that have been tested for their ability to reduce anxiety.

Identity Gestalt of self-awareness made up of experiences, memories, perceptions, emotions, and a mass of sensory input.

Illusion The misinterpretation of a real, external sensory experience.

Immediacy A dimension of communication which deals with the relationship-building element of the helping process; expressions emphasizing immediacy point to relationships between clients' overt communications and their underlying impressions of what is going on between the nurse and client in the here and now.

Impotence The inability of the male to achieve or maintain erection; erectile dysfunction.

Impulsiveness A tendency to act suddenly, without conscious thought.

Inappropriate affect A display of emotion that is out of harmony with reality. The mood shown and experienced is incongruous with the situation or the accompanying thought content.

Inauthentic emotions Affective reactions which are acted out in an exaggerated fashion and serve as a reaction formation to actual feelings, which are experienced only superficially.

Incest Sexual relations between parents and offspring or between close relatives.

Individuation The developmental process of emerging as a person who recognizes his or her distinctness from other persons.

Infantile autism A neurological, perceptual, and physiological dysfunction characterized by a psychotic state in the young child.

Insight A perception of the connection between conscious behavior and previously unrecognized feelings, wishes, and conflicts.

Intimacy Loosening, to some degree, the firmness of the distinction between one's own boundaries and those of another.

Intrapsychic Within the mind.

Introjection An unconscious defense mechanism; a symbolic taking in or incorporation of a loved or hated object or person into the individual's own ego structure.

Intuition The act or faculty of knowing without the use of rational processes.

Isolation Unconscious defense mechanism; the exclusion from awareness of the feelings connected with a thought, memory, or experience. The person remembers the experience or thought but does not reexperience the emotion that originally accompanied it.

K

Kinesthesia The sense by which one is aware of the position and movement of the various body parts.

Kin network Groups of nuclear families living close enough to exchange goods and services.

L

Labeling A sociological concept for the description or designation of behavior on the basis of culturally determined norms.

Lability Emotionally unstable; rapidly changing emotions.

Latency In the Freudian and Eriksonian framework, the stage of growth and development lasting from age 6 to age 12.

Lesbian Female homosexual.

Libido Psychic energy; sexual motivation; urge or desire for sexual activity.

Looseness of association A type of disordered thought process in which the individual expresses successive ideas which appear to be unrelated to each other or perhaps only slightly related to each other. The person does not indicate an intention to change the subject or explain transitions as they are communicated.

Lust dynamism Term used by Sullivan to describe clearly stated sexual desires and abilities.

M

Magical thinking A type of primitive thought process in which an individual attaches personal meaning or power of unrealistic proportions to objective events or neutral situations. To the person involved, the thought may be the same as the act.

Malevolence A combination of spite, hate, and malice.

Mania A mood state of extreme euphoria and excitement with loss of reality testing. Can be one of the phases of manic-depressive psychosis.

Manic-depressive psychosis A major emotional illness marked by severe mood swings alternating from elation to depression.

Manipulation The process of influencing another to meet or comply with one's own needs and wishes, regardless of the needs and wishes of the other.

Masochism Sexual pleasure or gratification obtained by experiencing physical or mental pain and humiliation.

Masturbation The sexual arousal of oneself or another through manual, oral, or mechanical stimulation of sexual organs.

Maternal deprivation Inadequate or absent physical and emotional care of the infant or young child by a consistent caretaker.

Maturational crises Developmental crises; predictable life events or turning points which occur for most individuals.

Melancholia Severe depression.

Mental health The ability to cope effectively with the life process.

Mental illness Maladaptation to the life process.

Metacommunication Communication about communication.

Metarules Rules about rules.

Migraine Intensely painful episodic headache.

Milieu therapy Treatment that emphasizes appropriate socioenvironmental manipulation for the benefit of the client. The term "milieu" refers to those (social and cultural) aspects of a treatment setting which can be influential in reducing the behavioral disturbances of clients.

Minimal brain dysfunction (MBD) A syndrome characterized by deviations in cerebral function such as impairment of perception, conceptualization, language comprehension, control of attention, impulse control, and motor function.

Mother measures Those actions taken by the "mothering" figure which nurture the child and fulfill the child's needs.

Mystification A transpersonal process which consists of misdefining issues.

N

Narcissism A psychoanalytic term meaning self-love or self-interest, which is normal in childhood but pathological when seen in a similar degree in adulthood.

Negativism Strong resistance to suggestions or advice.

Neologism A made-up word or condensation of several words that has special meaning for the person using it and which lacks consensual validation.

Neurosis A mental disorder characterized by anxiety which may be experienced and expressed directly or through an unconscious psychic process; the anxiety may be converted, displaced, or somatized.

Nuclear family The husband-wife dyad plus any children they may have.

O

Object relation An emotional attachment between one person and another.

Obsession A repetitive thought which the individual is unable to control.

Occupational therapy Form of therapy in which clients are encouraged to perform useful tasks and develop interests which may either reestablish old skills and knowledge or initiate new ones.

Oedipus complex In psychoanalytic theory, that issue in a child's psychosexual development characterized by erotic attachment to the parent of the opposite sex and jealousy toward the parent of the same sex.

Oligospermia Deficiency of sperm in the semen.

Operational mourning A technique in family therapy which highlights loss of significant members and points out how insufficient mourning for them has caused current problems.

Oral phase In psychoanalytic theory, that phase of an infant's psychosexual development characterized by a concentration of psychic energies in the oral zone and strong dependent needs for oral gratification.

Organic brain syndrome Disorder caused by impairment of brain tissue. May be either psychotic or nonpsychotic.

Orgasm Highly pleasurable sexual peak response; feeling of physiological and psychological release from maximum levels of sexual excitement.

Orientation Phase of a therapeutic relationship in which the nature and purpose of the relationship is explained.

P

Panic An attack of acute, intense, and overwhelming anxiety accompanied by a considerable degree of personality disorganization.

Paradoxical injunction A technique in family therapy prescribing the symptom or reversal; therapist instructs family members to do consciously what they had been doing unconsciously.

Paranoid behavior Behavior characterized by grandiose delusions, suspicion, and mistrust of others. Paranoia also involves persecutory delusions, hostility, and hallucinations.

Parataxic mode The mode of perception in which the undifferentiated whole is broken into parts that are momentary, illogical, and disconnected.

Parental coalition Union of parents for the common purpose of rearing the children so as to best meet the latter's needs.

Perception Mental processes by which data—intellectual, sensory, and emotional—are organized meaningfully.

Phallic stage In Freud's framework, the stage of growth and development lasting from ages 3 to 6.

Phantom pain Perception of pain in a body part which has been surgically or accidentally separated from the body.

Phobia An irrational fear of an object or an environmental situation.

Plasticity Quality of being capable of being molded or changed.

Play therapy Type of therapy used with children which employs toys and games to reveal the problems, fears, and underlying conflicts.

Preconscious Elements that are difficult to remember but can be recalled with help.

Precocity Unusually early development of mental or physical traits.

Premature grieving Early withdrawal of emotional investment from the relationship with the dying person.

Premorbid Occurring before development of disease.

Prescription of the symptom A therapeutic technique in which the therapist suggests that the client increase or in some way manipulate the manifestation of symptomatic behavior; therapeutic technique used by Watzlawick.

Prevalence The number of established or diagnosed cases of an illness in a given population at a particular time.

Primary gain The reduction of tension or conflict through neurotic illness.

Primary prevention Actions taken to reduce the incidence of disease in populations at risk. Primary prevention emphasizes promotion of healthy personality development, healthy families, and healthy communities through the reduction of factors considered harmful to these systems.

Primary-process thinking Illogical thinking with a tendency toward concreteness, condensation of separate psychological items into one item, and displacement of feelings from one item to another.

Projection An unconscious defense mechanism in which a person attributes his or her feelings, impulses, thoughts, and wishes to others or the environment in an effort to deny their existence in the self; used in a wide variety of normal situations; used excessively by clients with paranoid thought patterns.

Prophylactic activities Activities designed to prevent disease or harmful events.

Prototaxic mode The mode of perception in which the self and the universe form an undifferentiated whole.

Psychoanalysis The treatment modality based on Freudian constructs; the analysis of the relationship that the client develops with the psychoanalyst.

Psychodrama A structured, directed, and dramatized acting out of a client's personal, emotional, and interactional problems.

Psychodynamics Theoretical assumption that present behavior is influenced by past experiences; science of the mind, mental processes, and affective components that influence human behavior.

Psychogenic Originating in the mind.

Psychopathology Morbidity of the mind; mental illness.

Psychosexual development The maturation and development of the psychic phase of sexuality from birth to adult life.

Psychosis State in which a person's mental capacity to recognize reality, communicate, and relate to others are impaired, thus interfering with the person's capacity to deal with the demands of life.

Psychotic depression A state of depression of great intensity, in which reality testing is impaired and physiological disturbances are pronounced.

R

Rage A feeling of overpowering, uncontrolled fury which is subjectively similar to anger and has its roots in early infantile responses to restraint of freedom of movement.

Rallying around Supportive family behavior manifested by frequent visiting, supplying of resources, and a show of concern.

Rape The act of intercourse or penile-vaginal contact forced upon an unwilling victim.

Rationalization An unconscious defense mechanism that is universally employed; an attempt to make one's behavior appear to be the result of logical thinking rather than of unconscious impulses or desires; utilized when a person has a sense of guilt or uncertainty about something that has been done; a face-saving device that may or may not deal with the truth. Rationalization relieves anxiety temporarily.

Reaction formation Unconscious defense mechanism; occurs when an individual expresses an attitude that is directly opposite to unconscious feelings and wishes.

Reactive depression A state of depression for which the precipitating stress or loss can be identified and seen to be of some magnitude.

Reality testing Fundamental ego function that consists of the objective evaluation and judgment of the external environment.

Reciprocy Homeodynamic principle that postulates the inseparability of the person and the environment and holds that sequential changes in the life process are continuous, probabilistic revisions occurring out of the interactions between the individual and the environment.

Regression Defense mechanism in which the ego returns to an earlier stage of development in thought, feeling, or behavior. Regression is a normal component of the developmental sequence and appears transiently during times of stress, when it is utilized as a retreat from anxiety and conflict.

Reinforcement Reward for a response.

Rejection Refusal to acknowledge, accept, or consider a person or idea.

Repression A widely used unconscious defense mechanism. Through repression, painful experiences, disagreeable memories, and unacceptable thoughts and impulses are barred from consciousness. Selfish, hostile, and sexual impulses are also usually repressed. A constant expenditure of energy is required to keep repressed material out of awareness; consequently, less energy is available for constructive activity.

Rescue fantasy Unrealistic belief in one's ability to help or save a client from his or her problem or resolve the client's conflict.

Resentment A feeling of indignation which is an outgrowth of unexpressed or unresolved anger at having been, in one's own perception, injured or unfairly treated.

Resistance Active opposition to the uncovering of unconscious material.

Resolution A phase in the development of a relationship during which the events that have occurred in the relationship are summarized.

Resonancy Homeodynamic principle that postulates that change in the environmental and human fields is propagated in waves. Predicts that the life process is an unending flow of wave patterns.

Resonancy phenomena Mechanisms that perpetuate characteristic behavior in a family.

Respect Communication of acceptance of another's ideas, feelings, and experiences. Recognition of another individual's potential for self-actualization.

Ritual Automatic activity of psychogenic or cultural origin.

Role Socially assigned or personally adopted patterns of behavior and responsibility.

Role modeling An exhibition of behavior which can be adopted by those observing.

Role playing A technique in family or group therapy in which members act out the parts of other members.

Role reversal Exchange of assigned patterns of behavior and responsibility between two related individuals.

Rumination Persistent thinking about and discussion of a particular subject.

S

Sadism Sexual pleasure and erotic gratification derived from the infliction of pain.

Scapegoat A family or group member who acts out unconscious family issues and is perceived as bad or sick by the others.

School phobia Young child's sudden fear of attending school and refusal to go to school.

Sculpting A technique in family therapy; family members arrange others as they perceive them relationally.

Secondary gains The "fringe benefits" individuals derive from the environment as a result of their physical or emotional illness.

Secondary prevention Aims to reduce the prevalence of disease through early case finding and effective treatment; secondary prevention places emphasis on referrals and appropriate health services, accessibility of services for clients, and rapid initiation of active treatment.

Security operation A term used in interpersonal theory to denote those behaviors which are used to avoid or lessen anxiety; analogous to the terms "coping mechanism" and "defense mechanism."

Selective inattention A phenomenon in which, due to heightened anxiety, the individual is not aware of what is going on in situations peripheral to the immediate focus of attention.

Self-actualization Process of becoming everything one is capable of becoming.

Self-esteem The degree to which one feels valued, worthwhile, or competent.

Self-image What and who one thinks one is.

Self-mutilation Destructive, disfiguring actions toward one's own body.

Self-system An organization of experiences that exists to defend against anxiety and to secure necessary satisfaction. The total organization and integration of the self, comprising the interrelationships of organic, emotional, and social components.

Sensorium   Consciousness; awareness of environment.

Sensory deprivation   Lack of adequate external stimuli and opportunity for the usual perceptions.

Sensory overload   Sensory input beyond the person's capacity to integrate and cope with the stimuli.

Sex therapy   The active treatment of sexual dysfunctions by a qualified therapist.

Sexual dysfunction   A psychosomatic disorder which makes it impossible for the individual to have and/or enjoy coitus; impotence and ejaculatory problems in the male; vaginismus, frigidity, or orgasmic dysfunction in the female.

Sibling position   The placement of one child in a family in relation to brothers and sisters in terms of birth order (i.e., oldest, youngest, etc.).

Sick role   The adoption of an identity by an individual which classifies the person as a client and requires a specific set of expected behaviors, usually of a dependent and compliant nature.

Signal anxiety   The ability to anticipate wrongdoing by connecting a wish with its consequence.

Situational crisis   Unanticipated or sudden external event in a person's life which threatens that person's biological, social, or psychosocial integrity.

Social loss   Loss of all the valued social characteristics embodied in the dying patient.

Sodomy   Any sex act other than face-to-face coitus between a man and a woman; the legal meaning varies from state to state.

Somatic therapy   Treatment of the emotionally ill or incapacitated client by physiological means.

Status   Collection of rights and privileges attributed to a group member by other members of the group.

Stereotyped behavior   (also referred to as stereotypy) Persistent mechanical repetition of speech or motor activity, commonly seen in schizophrenia. Examples include echolalia and echopraxia.

Stressor   Factor capable of eliciting a stress reaction in the body.

Structuring   A term used to describe activities aimed at establishing a working partnership with a client.

Sublimation   Transformation of psychic energy associated with unwanted sexual or aggressive drives into socially acceptable pursuits. The activity or its object is changed, but the energy is nevertheless discharged.

Substitution   Unconscious defense mechanism involving the replacement of a highly valued, unacceptable object with a less valued object that is acceptable.

Suicide   Self-inflicted harm or endangerment which results in death.

Superego   The aspect of the personality that contains the rigid, absolute rules directing the person's thoughts, feelings, and actions. The superego is that part of the personality which is associated with internalized parental and societal controls (that is, standards, morals, and self-criticism).

Symbiosis   The close interdependence of two individuals to the point where the psychic differentiation between them is blurred. Symbiosis is normal between infant and mother.

Symptom substitution   The replacement of one (extinguished) maladaptive behavior with another.

Synchrony   Homeodynamic principle that states that change in the human field depends upon the state of the human field and the simultaneous state of the environment field at any given point in space-time.

Syntaxic mode   The mode of perception that forms whole, logical, coherent pictures of reality that can be validated by others.

System   A complex of components in interaction; a group of people, issues, and feelings in interaction with one another. This interaction as a whole is greater than the sum of its parts.

T

Territoriality A form of behavior in which the individual lays claim to a defined space.

Tertiary prevention This form of prevention aims to reduce, through rehabilitation, the disability associated with disease. Emphasis is placed on preparing clients and families for the client's discharge from an institution and return to the community.

Therapeutic community A complex system which provides an effective environment for behavioral changes in clients through emphasis on their interpersonal functioning. The therapeutic community views illness as an interpersonal and social phenomenon.

Tolerance The phenomenon occurring in drug or alcohol addiction where increasing amounts of the substance must be used in order to achieve the desired effects.

Transaction A communication sequence between two people consisting of a stimulus and a response.

Transactional analysis A treatment modality developed by Eric Berne; it involves the analysis of communications between two people.

Transference Unconscious phenomena in which the feelings, attitudes, and wishes originally linked with significant figures in one's early life are projected onto others who have come to represent these people in current life.

Triangle A predictable pattern of interaction among three persons, two of whom are enmeshed and the third of whom is in a distant position. Rigid triangles are the building blocks of emotional illness.

Tumescence The erectile process in the male.

U

Unconscious Thoughts, feelings, actions, dreams, and unremembered experiences. It is very difficult to become conscious of this material, which is not recognized if one is told of it.

Undoing Unconscious defense mechanism closely related to reaction formation. A person negates an act by behavior which is the opposite of what was done before.

V

Vaginismus Irregular and involuntary contraction of the muscles of the vagina whenever there is an attempt at coitus.

Values Measure of worth; individualized rules by which people live their lives. Values govern and influence the way people behave.

Value system A set of priorities.

Vigilance A state of watchfulness.

Violence Physical force used to injure or damage others.

W

Waxy flexibility (cerea flexibilitas) A condition (found in catatonic schizophrenia) in which the extremities have a waxlike rigidity and will remain for long periods of time in any placed position, no matter how uncomfortable.

Withdrawal A person's pattern of facilitating escape from relatedness through physical and emotional distancing maneuvers.

Word salad A form of speech in which words and phrases have no apparent meaning or logical connection.

Index

AID (artificial insemination by donor),
537–538
AIH (artificial insemination with
homologous sperm), 537, 538
Akathisia as extrapyramidal reaction to
major tranquilizers, 123
Akinesia as extrapyramidal reaction to
major tranquilizers, 123
Alanon, 285, 303
Alarm reaction to stress, table, 408
Alateen, 285, 303
Alcohol:
contraindicated:
with MAO inhibitors, 128
with minor tranquilizers, 125
with phenothiazines, 123
effects of circadian cycle on intake of,
392
Alcoholics Anonymous (AA), 285
Alcoholism:
adolescent, 282
anger and, 282–287
assessment factors, 292
behavioral manifestations of, 282
child abuse and, 608
detoxification process, 285
family problems, 302–303
nurses' response to, 291
nursing diagnosis and goals, 293
nursing intervention, 298–302
psychodynamics of, 283
rape and, 196
rehabilitation for, 444
suicide and, 341, 350
violence and, 254–255
table, 255
Aldomet, effects of, on ejaculation, 363
Aldosterone, 408
Alertness, effects of mild anxiety on,
212–213
table, 213
Alleles, 620
Allergies:
alcoholism and, 283
cyclicity and, 392
psychosomatic, 423
as reactions to major tranquilizers,
124–125
table, 125
stress and, 420
Altruistic suicide, defined, 342
Alzheimer's disease (senile dementia),
table, 481
Ambivalence:
defined, 228–229
depression and, 315
intervention in, 320–321
schizophrenia and, 228
suicidal behavior and, 342
Amenorrhea:
and drug abuse, table, 291
as side effect of major tranquilizers,
124–125
table, 125
stress and, 424, 425
American Association of Mental
Deficiency, 636

American Civil Liberties Union (ACLU), 398
American Nurses' Association (ANA), 153,
692
American Psychiatric Association (APA),
12, 199, 480
diagnostic classification of, 24
Americans View Their Mental Health (Joint
Commission on Mental Health), 22
Amine theory:
of manic states, 326
of schizophrenia, 222
Amitriptyline hydrochloride:
for depression, 323
table, 127
Amnesia (fugue states), 264–266
Amobarbital for violent behavior, 257
Amphetamine psychoses, 222
Amphetamines:
for MBD children, 650
table, 288
Amplitude of rhythm, defined, 390
Amputees, rehabilitation of, 445
Amyl nitrate, table, 288
ANA (American Nurses' Association), 153,
692
Anaclitic depression, 311, 312
Anal stage of development:
development of depression in, table, 311
Freud's theory of, table, 35
origin of obsessive-compulsive neuroses
in, 269
Analgesics:
contraindicated: with MAO inhibitors,
128
with phenothiazines, 123
nonnarcotic, as drugs of abuse, table,
288
Analogic communication, defined, 50
Analysis as intervention technique with
anxious clients, 219
Analytic therapy (see Intensive group
therapy)
Anancephaly, 623
Anatomy of Melancholy, The (Burton), 310
Androgens:
anti-androgen effect of steroids, 358
prepubertal increase in, 580
in treatment of Klinefelter's syndrome,
624
Anesthetics:
contraindicated: with major tranquilizers,
121
with phenothiazines, 123
effect of circadian cycle on, 392
Anger, Dianne, 457
Anger:
allergies and, 423
of chronically disabled clients, 447
assessment of, 458
clients generating (see Alcoholism; Drug
addicts; Psychopaths; Substance
abusers)
nurses' response to, 291–292
nursing diagnosis, 293–298
defined, 281–282
depression and, 308, 315
intervention in, 321

Anger:
in dying process, 502
of dying child and the family, 665
as means of coping with death, 659
of terminal clients, 512, 513
of hospitalized clients, 400, 401
in parents of high-risk infants, 537
problematic cycle of, illustrated, 283
(See also Irritability)
Anniversary reactions, defined, 217
Anomic suicide, defined, 342
Anomie, defined, 342
Anorexia nervosa, 424–425
anxiety and, 211, 214
Antabuse (disulfiram), 285
Antenatal diagnosis (prenatal diagnosis) of
genetic diseases, 630–633
Anthony, E. James, 655
Anticipatory grief, 501, 656–657
Anticipatory guidance, 16, 551, 554
Anticipatory mourning, 657–658
Antidepressants, 126–128
for depression, 323
for OBS, 494–495
table, 127
Antiemetic properties of phenothiazines,
121, 123
Antihistamines, table, 288
Antihypertensive drugs:
effects of, on mental function, 453
impotence and, 363
Antisocial behavior:
defined, 289–291
phenothiazines for, 121–123
(See also specific forms of antisocial
behavior, e.g.: Psychopaths)
Anxiety, 33, 211–220
adolescent, 185
as adjustment reaction, 588–590
alcoholism and, 284
DTs and, table, 287
allergies and, 423
anger and, 271, 281–282
assessment of, 215–217
in atypical childhood psychoses,
564–565
as basic response to conflict and
change, illustrated, 415
behavioral manifestations of, 211
(See also Schizophrenia)
body image, self-image and, 387
as child's response to death, 656
of chronically ill clients, 447, 453
assessment of, 458
deconditioning of, 41–43
methods used in, 42–43
table, 43
defined, 211
depressive (see Depressive anxiety)
diagnosing, 217–220
drug abuse and, 289
effects of major tranquilizers on, 121, 123
effects of minor tranquilizers on, 124
ego strength and, 35
following hysterectomies, 361
grief and, 395
headaches and, 426